Head and Neck Radiology

A Teaching File

Head and Neck Radiology
A Teaching File

Anthony A. Mancuso, M.D.
Professor and Chairman
Department of Radiology
Professor of Otolaryngology
University of Florida College of Medicine
Gainesville, Florida

Hiroya Ojiri, M.D.
Department of Radiology
Jikei University School of Medicine
Tokyo, Japan

Ronald G. Quisling, M.D.
Professor of Radiology
Chief of Neuroradiology
University of Florida College of Medicine
Gainesville, Florida

LIPPINCOTT WILLIAMS & WILKINS
A **Wolters Kluwer** Company
Philadelphia • Baltimore • New York • London
Buenos Aires • Hong Kong • Sydney • Tokyo

Acquisitions Editor: Joyce-Rachel John
Developmental Editor: Michael Standen
Production Editor: Deirdre Marino
Manufacturing Manager: Tim Reynolds
Cover Designer: Christine Jenny
Compositor: Maryland Composition
Printer: Maple Press

530 Walnut Street
Philadelphia, PA 19106 USA
LWW.com

Printed in the USA

Library of Congress Cataloging-in-Publication Data

Mancuso, Anthony A.
Head and neck radiology : a teaching file / Anthony A. Mancuso, Hiroya Ojiri, Ronald G. Quisling.
p. ; cm.
Includes index.
ISBN 0-683-30144-6
1. Head—Radiography—Case studies. 2. Neck—Radiography—Case studies. I. Ojiri, Hiroya. II. Quisling, Ronald G. III. Title.
[DNLM: 1. Head—radiograpy. 2. Neck—radiography. WE 705 M269h 2001]
RC936 .M34 2001
617.5′107572—dc21

2001050231

---

10 9 8 7 6 5 4 3 2 1

CONTENTS

INTRODUCTION

The 100 cases in this volume, *Head and Neck Imaging: A Teaching File*, comprise a comprehensive core curriculum in head and neck radiology. The crossover areas between traditional neuroradiology and ENT imaging (e.g., skull base and cranial nerve assessment) are covered thoroughly. This book is intended to be used as a guide in the daily practice of head and neck radiology.

Any overlap in the case material is intentional and meant to reinforce key principals of interpretation. The questions accompanying each set of images are meant to provoke thought about the clinical situations and the diagnostic process. "Making the diagnosis" is an important, but secondary, concern.

The goal of this book is to help you, the radiologist, become an even more effective consultant to your clinical colleagues who treat head and neck diseases. Excellent quality images are the substrate for meaningful interpretation and consultation. The beneficiaries of our best possible work are the patients, who trust us to perform at the highest levels of competence. The stakes are high in head and neck pathology because of potential functional and cosmetic losses due to disease and/or treatment.

Each case contains a summary of the original imaging findings, pertinent anatomic material, and specific questions and answers. In addition, they outline and encourage a highly ordered and disciplined approach to evaluating disorders commonly encountered in an active head and neck radiology practice. The sections in each case present a portion of the diagnostic/consultation process that, when taken together, will help ensure accurate diagnosis and the best possible outcome. The rationale behind each section is as follows:

1. Problem: It is essential to put summary imaging findings in a clinical context. This practice will help focus the remainder of the process.
2. Anatomy: Head and neck anatomy is complex. It must be understood in detail before one can even begin to interpret images. This section breaks the anatomy into small "bites" that can be linked to specific clinical-diagnostic problems. This helps reduce the need for isolated, rote study of the anatomy and creates a clinical framework for understanding and retaining anatomical details necessary for accurate diagnosis and treatment planning.
3. Diagnostic Approach: There is an intended redundancy in this section from case to case. The repetition will reinforce the need for logic and discipline in the interpretative method that is chosen for evaluating head and neck imaging studies.

The diagnostic process as presented in this section is, in most cases, anatomically driven at the outset. The disease extent and morphology are then factored together with relevant clinical issues. A differential diagnosis is described when appropriate. However, the differential diagnosis is not normally the endpoint. One must also consider the impact of the information on patient care, and comment appropriately on these issues in responding to the case material (or, in a true clinical situation, to the report). A search for expected complications of the diagnosed disease, or a suggestion for further study, is just as relevant as producing an accurate diagnosis or differential diagnosis. This section will encourage such thought.

4. Diagnosis: A summary statement of the basic disease process and pertinent associated findings will help focus the clinician on the radiologist's understanding of the problem, the implications for treatment, and a need for further diagnostic evaluation.
5. Clinical Points of Importance: Some of these are clinical-radiologic bites of information essential for appreciating the clinical context of the problem. Others are just "pearls" that may help the clinician or a patient some day.
6. Additional Case Material: Accompanying cases appear in the last section of each case. These may illustrate conditions in the differential diagnosis and/or show variations in the pathology of the original case. This section will help remind the reader of the importance of logic and discipline in the diagnostic process and of the clinical considerations that have a significant impact on each clinical setting.

Head and Neck Radiology

A Teaching File

CHAPTER 1

ORBIT / EYE AND VISUAL PATHWAYS

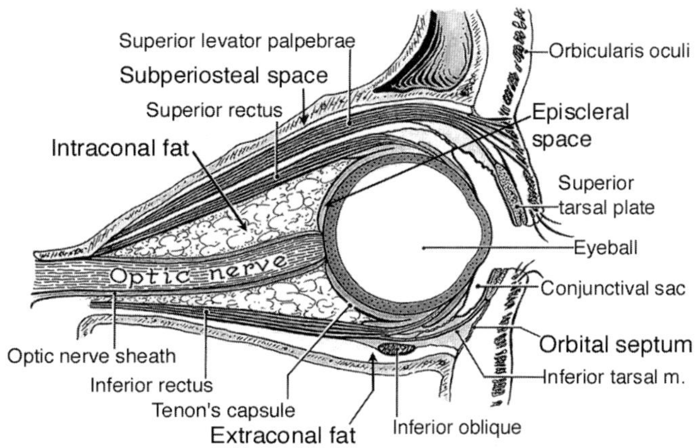

CASE 1

Clinical History: A 3-year-old presents with leukokoria.

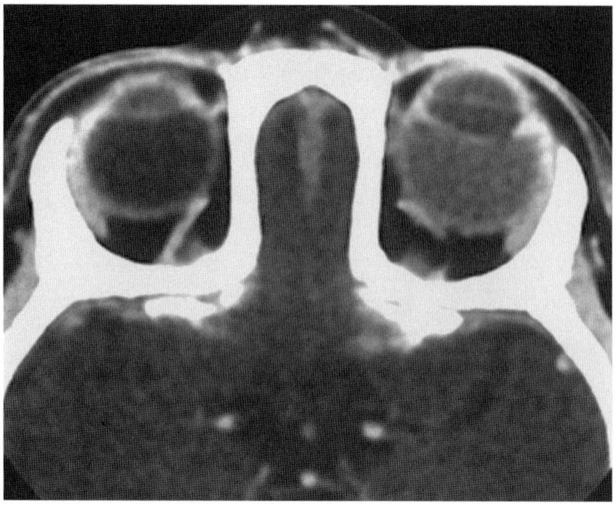

Figure 1A

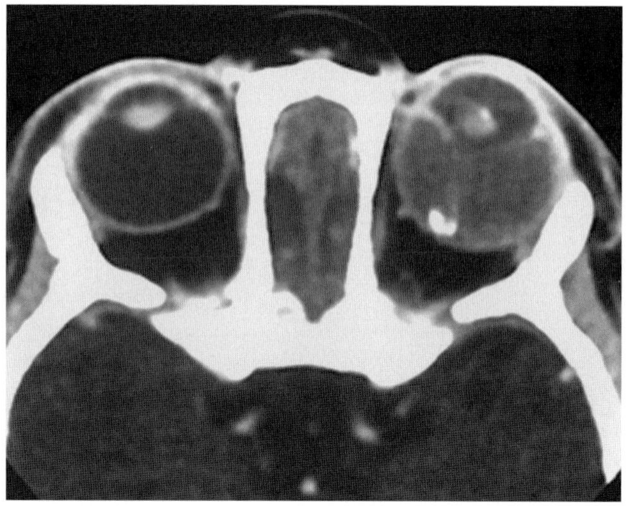

Figure 1B

1. What is leukokoria?
2. Name three major causes of leukokoria in a child under 5 years of age.
3. Name the retinal layers and potential spaces for the accumulation of effusion and hemorrhage.

Findings

Complete retinal detachment involving the left eye, which is related to a small, calcified mass along the posterior aspect of the retina. The lens is dislocated and the anterior and posterior chambers are enlarged.

Problem

Child with leukokoria (a white reflex caused by ocular pathology seen during funduscopy) secondary to retinal detachment associated with an apparently causative calcified retinal lesion

Anatomy

Three potential spaces of the eye

1. Posterior hyaloid space (between the posterior hyaloid membrane and the inner or sensory retina)
2. Subretinal space (between the inner and outer or pigmented retinal layers)
3. Suprachoroidal space (between the choroid and the sclera)

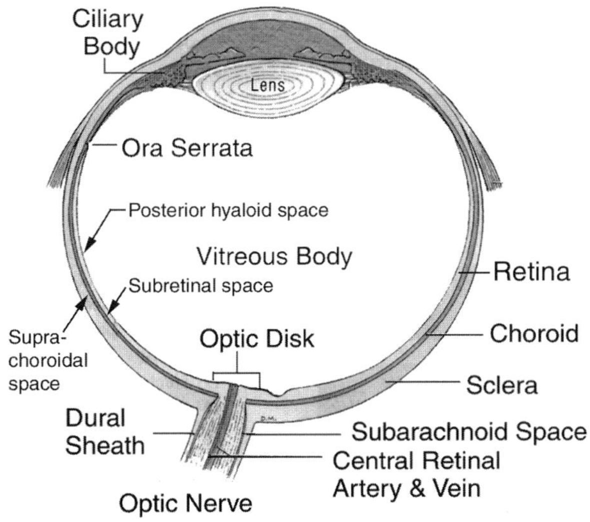

Figure 1C

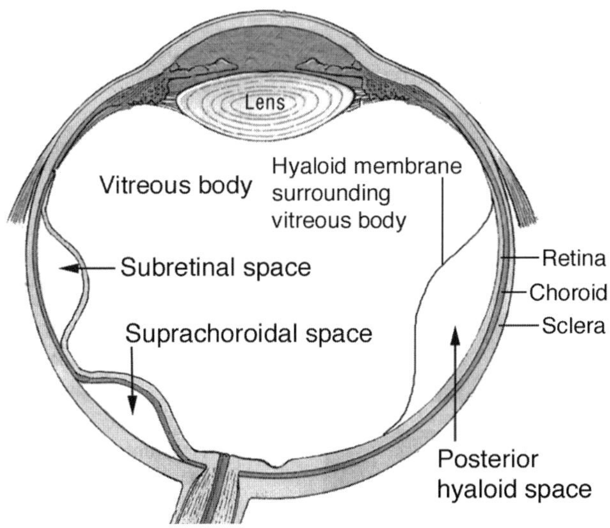

Figure 1D

Differential Diagnosis

Retinoblastoma, persistent hyperplastic primary vitreous (PHPV), Coat's disease, ocular toxocariasis, retinopathy of prematurity (ROP),

Diagnosis

Retinoblastoma with complete retinal detachment

Diagnostic Imaging Approach

A. With respect to retinal detachment
   1. Determine type of retinal detachment
   2. Identify causative pathology
B. With respect to leukokoria, the most important aids to accurate diagnosis are:
   1. Age
   2. History
   3. Uni- vs. bilaterality

Clinical Points Of Importance And Supplemental Information

A. Accurate differential diagnosis of leukokoria is essential because treatment and prognosis vary widely according to the causative pathology.
B. It is important to establish whether retinoblastoma is confined to the eye. The disease may include the following:
   1. Bilateral or trilateral (pineal region)
   2. Spread out of the eye directly through the sclera (see companion case)
   3. Seed within the subarachnoid space via the optic sheath
C. Retinoblastoma is now considered one of several primitive neuroectodermal tumors (PNET); medulloblastoma, ependymoblastoma, and olfactory neuroblastoma are some others.
D. Retinal astrocytoma (associated with tuberous sclerosis) has been confused with retinoblastoma, with unfavorable consequences.

Answers To Questions

1. White reflex at funduscopy
2. Retinoblastoma, PHPV, Coat's disease
3. Layers: hyaloid membrane, retina, choroid. Spaces: posterior hyaloid, subretinal, suprachoroidal

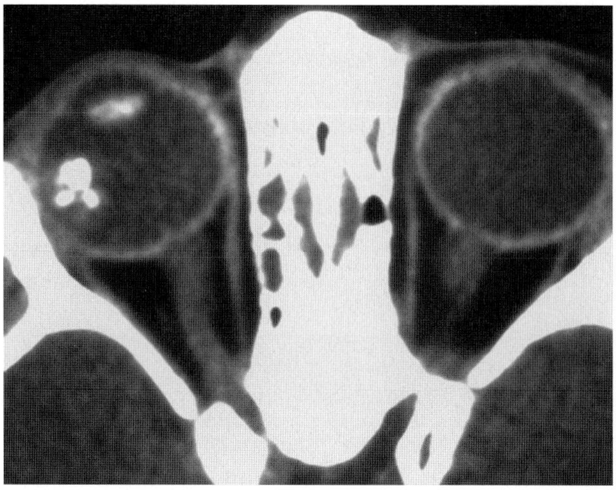

Figure 1E. Patient 1 with retinoblastoma penetrating sclera, showing a calcified mass in the vitreous body. Computed tomography (CT) image without contrast.

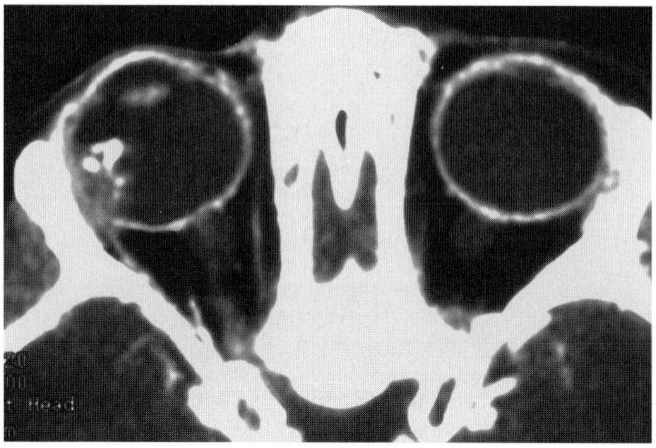

Figure 1F. Patient 1 with retinoblastoma. Contrast-enhanced CT image showing enhancing mass with calcification in the vitreous body, extending into the extraocular soft tissue and penetrating the sclera.

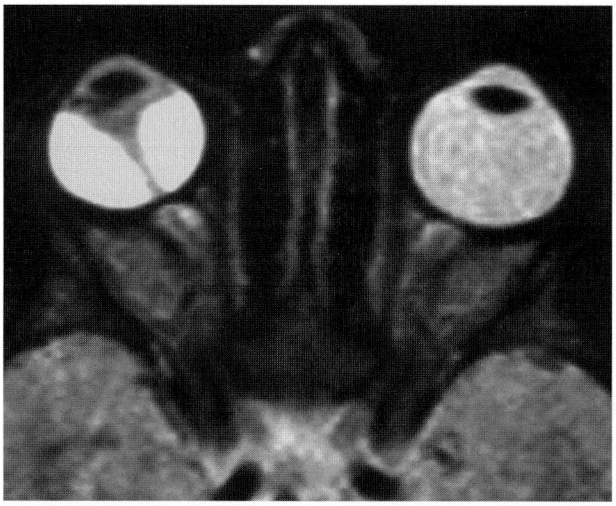

Figure 1G. Patient 2 with persistent hyperplastic primary vitreous, showing a retinal detachment with fluid collection in the subretinal space. Fat-suppressed T2-weighted axial image.

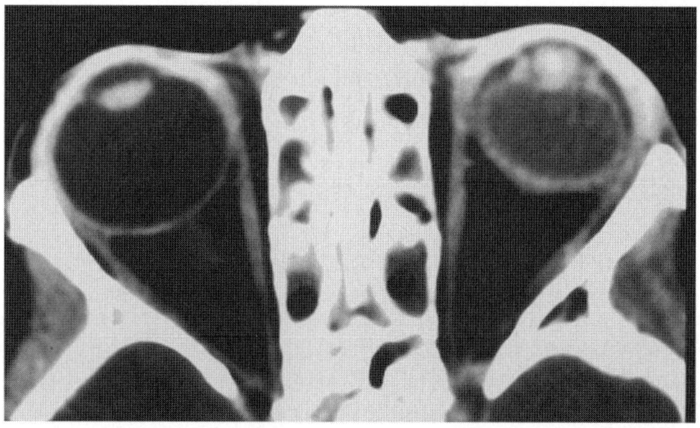

Figure 1H. Patient 3 with *Toxocara canis,* showing microphthalmia with increase in attenuation of the vitreous body on the left. Contrast-enhanced CT image.

CASE 2

Clinical History: A patient who was struck in the eye during a domestic argument presents at 2 a.m. with deteriorating visual acuity.

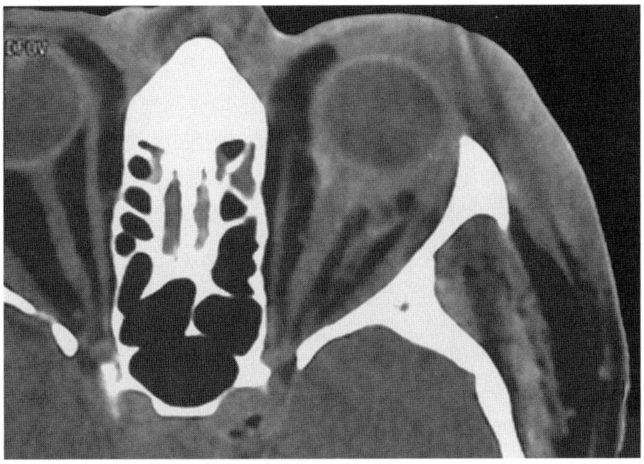

Figure 2A

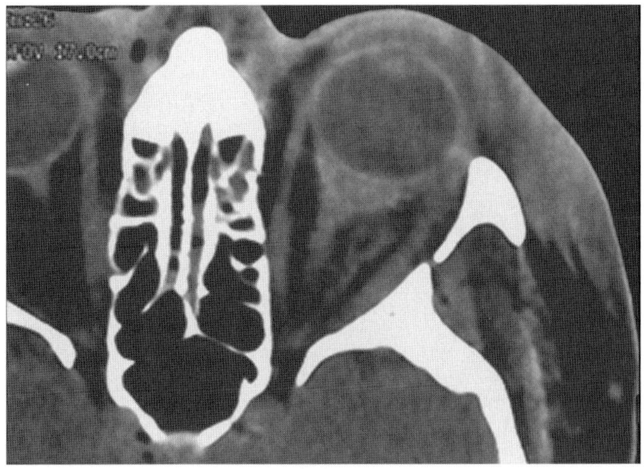

Figure 2B

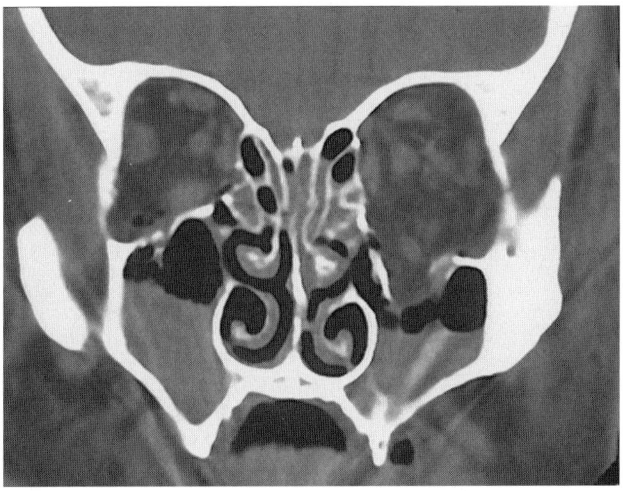

Figure 2C

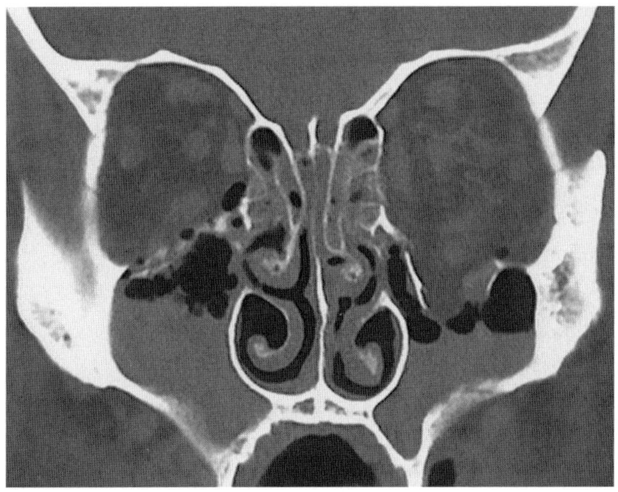

Figure 2D

1. Do the films explain the visual loss? If so, why?
2. Should you call the ophthalmologist immediately or wait until the morning?
3. What is Tenon's space?

Findings

Bilateral orbital floor blowout fractures are seen. The one on the patient's left is associated with extensive herniation of orbital fat and the inferior rectus muscle into the maxillary antrum. The axial views show a thickening within Tenon's space, which is centered at the junction of the eye and optic nerve or sheath, with the abnormal thickening spreading proximally for about 1 cm along the sheath. A small subperiosteal hematoma is associated with the minimally displaced right orbital floor fracture.

Problem

Diminished visual acuity secondary to significant orbital trauma with pathologic thickening at the optic sheath–eye junction, within Tenon's space and without obvious bony compression of the optic nerve

Anatomy

Tenon's space and the optic nerve–globe junction

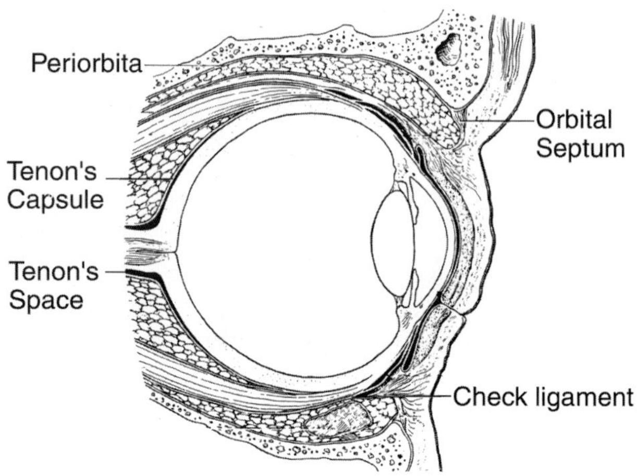

Figure 2E

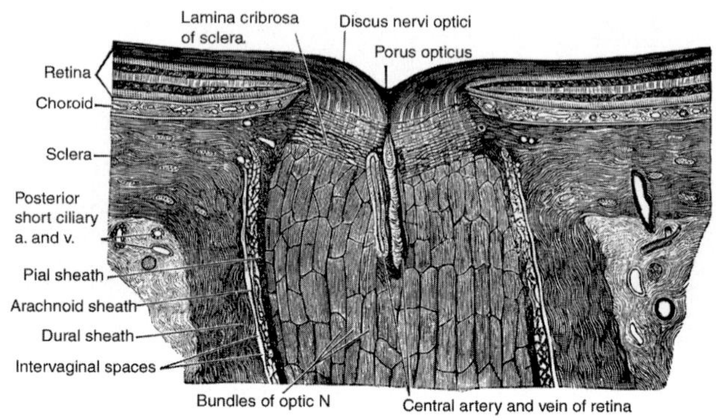

Figure 2F

Differential Diagnosis

Not applicable, but other diseases can be manifest as changes seen primarily in Tenon's space.

Diagnosis

Tenon's space and optic sheath hematoma with visual loss (vision returned following surgical decompression)

Diagnostic Imaging Approach

A. Systematically evaluate visual pathways for cause of visual loss.
   1. Eye: tension, compression, rupture, foreign body, hemorrhage, subchoroidal hemorrhage or effusion
   2. Optic nerve–sheath complex: compression, hematoma
   3. Optic canal–orbital apex: unstable fractures, bony compromise

B. Ocular dysmotility
   1. Muscle or fat entrapment
   2. Intraorbital, intramuscular hematoma

Clinical Points Of Importance And Supplemental Information

A. Optic sheath hematoma can be decompressed emergently by surgically opening a "window" in the sheath (call the ophthalmologist at 2 a.m.). Fluid or blood in Tenon's space has no significant clinical consequence.

B. A traumatic arachnoid cyst of the optic sheath can cause progressive visual loss; it requires urgent surgical decompression as well.

C. Choroidal effusion can be a sign of eye rupture and will often be treated surgically.

D. A subperiosteal orbital hematoma may go on to form a cholesterol cyst (granuloma).

E. Tension orbit is manifest on diagnostic imaging studies as a cone-shaped deformity of the eye. It is often an indication for emergency surgical decompression of the orbit if the patient's vision is salvageable.

Answers To Questions

1. Yes. Optic sheath hematoma.
2. Immediately
3. Space between fascia bulbi and eye

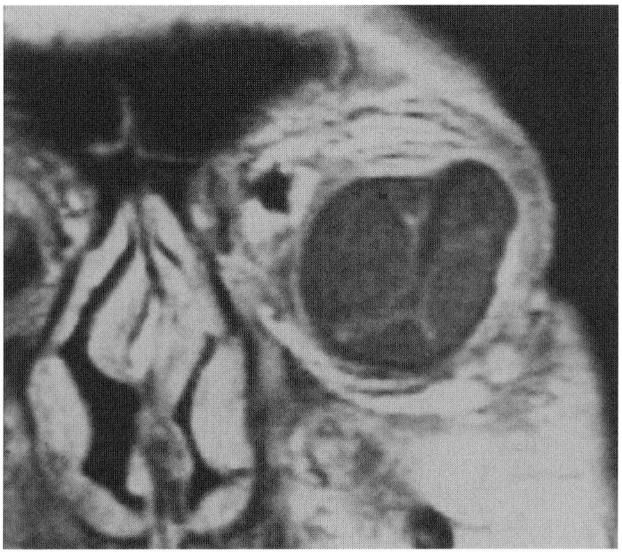

Figure 2G. Patient 1 with choroidal detachment with a staphyloma showing choroidal detachment and fluid collection in the suprachoroidal space with enhancement of the detached choroid. T1-weighted coronal image with contrast.

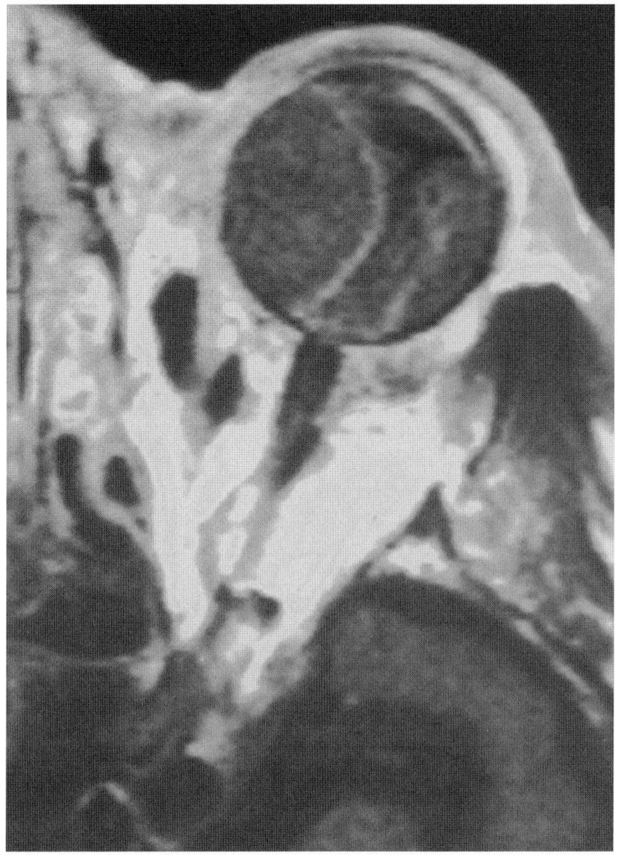

Figure 2H. Patient 2 with choroidal detachment, shown before surgical decompression. T1-weighted axial image with contrast.

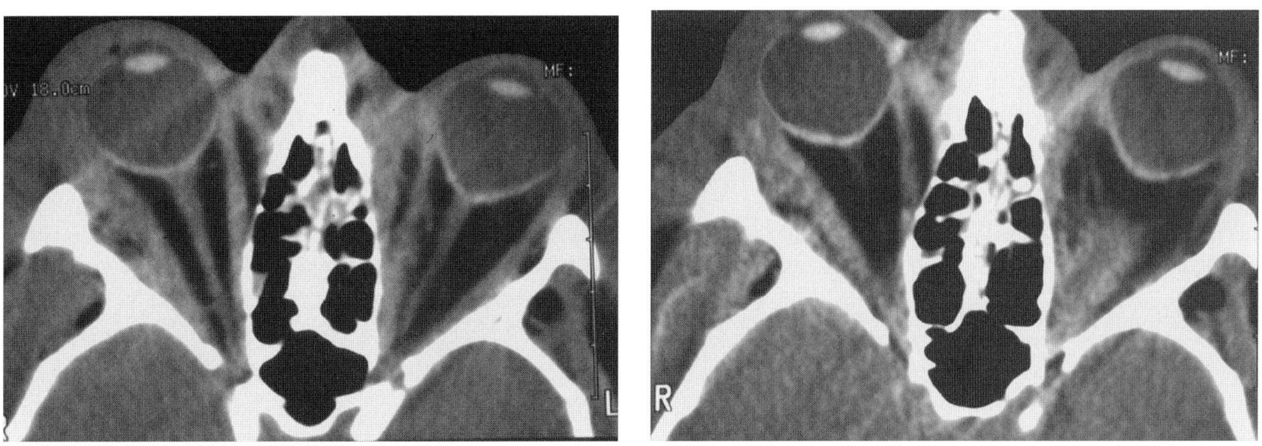

Figure 2I and **2J.** Patient 3 with bilateral tension orbit with an orbital apex hematoma on the left and an orbital sidewall hematoma on the right. Computed tomography image without contrast.

CASE 3

Clinical History: A 4-year-old girl with no history of eye problems presents with an orbital mass.

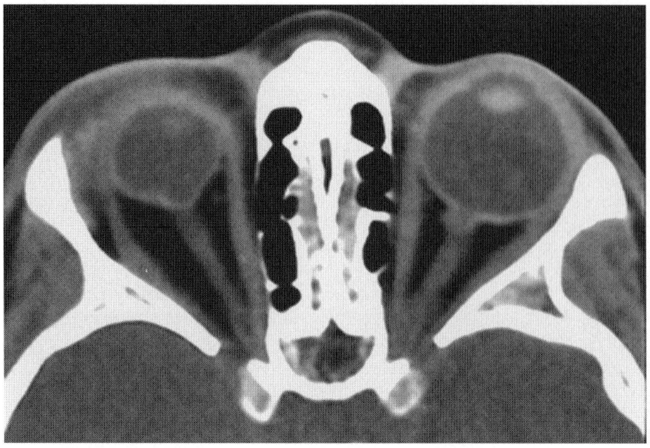

Figure 3A

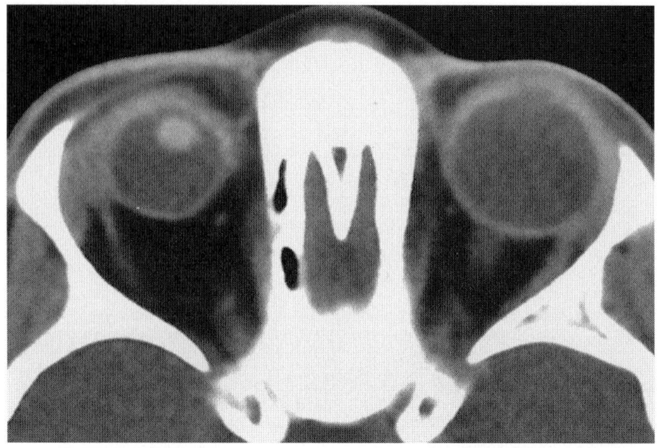

Figure 3B

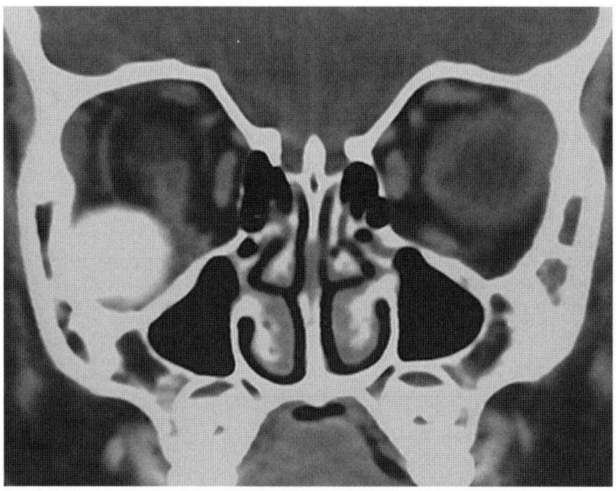

Figure 3C

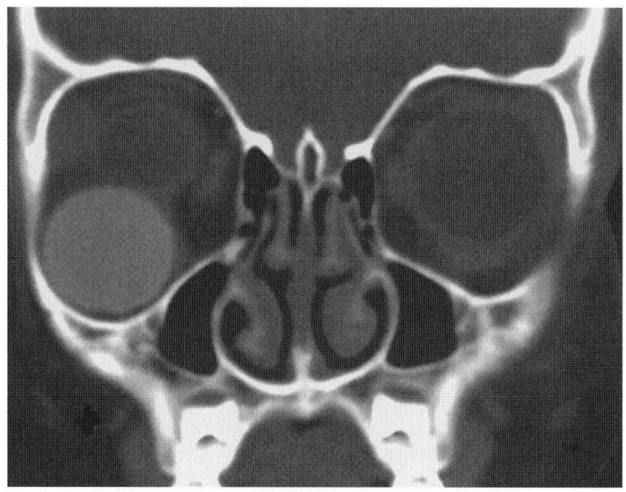

Figure 3D

1. Give a complete diagnosis.
2. What is a staphyloma? Does it differ from a coloboma?

Findings

On the right is seen a small eye and a deformity of the globe at its junction with the optic nerve/sheath. The right orbit is enlarged and a well-circumscribed high attenuation mass separate from the eye is seen within the “expanded” lower outer quadrant.

On the left is a deformity at the junction of the optic nerve-sheath complex and the eye.

Problem

Unilateral enlargement of the right orbit, an asymmetric appearance of the eyes, a high-density cyst, and bilateral colobomas in a child

Anatomy

A. Bony limits of the orbit
B. Optic nerve–eye junction

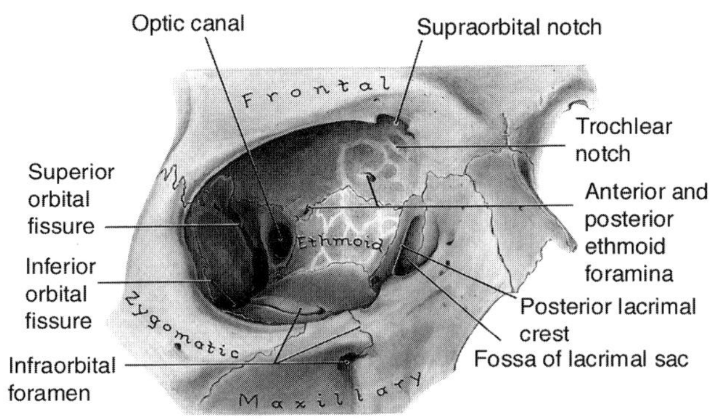

Figure 3E

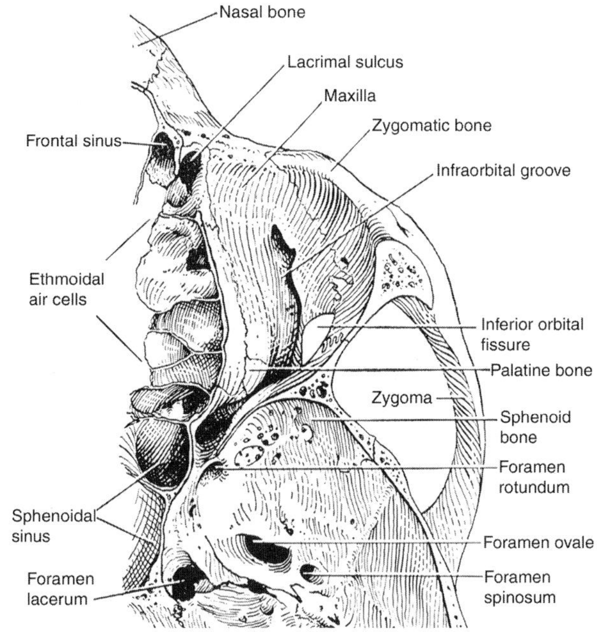

Figure 3F

Differential Diagnosis

Not applicable

Diagnosis

Developmental abnormalities of the orbit, including a dermoid (causing orbit enlargement), bilateral colobomas, and microphthalmia

Diagnostic Imaging Approach

A. Orbit
   1. Is the orbit enlarged?
   2. Are there specific areas of bony remodeling (e.g., superior orbital fissure, optic canal)?
B. Mass
   1. Intraconal, extraconal, transcompartmental
   2. Morphology (margins, vascularity, attenuation or signal intensity)
C. Nerve–sheath eye junction
   1. Eye (size, contour, internal anatomy)
   2. Nerve / sheath (size, contours, signal changes)

Clinical Points Of Importance And Supplemental Information

A. The surgeon always needs to know which compartment is involved and what needs to be done to restore the integrity of the orbit.
B. Any information related to the prognosis of vision is key.
C. Optic disc malformations are associated with forebrain anomalies, including basal encephalocele and midface anomalies. Bilateral coloboma is associated with retrobulbar cysts and Dandy-Walker cysts. Vascular abnormalities (e.g., carotid) may also be present. Brain imaging is indicated when these ocular abnormalities are discovered.
D. Patients with a highly myopic eye or congenital glaucoma can appear proptotic; such a "pseudoproptosis" should be considered in the differential diagnosis when no mass is found at imaging.
E. Dermoid lesions of the orbit are common and present in a variety of orbital locations. They are almost always relatively smoothly marginated, but their internal morphology varies greatly with their tissue content.

Answers To Questions

1. Later
2. Outpouching of sclera. Yes, a coloboma is developmental and near the sheath–eye junction.

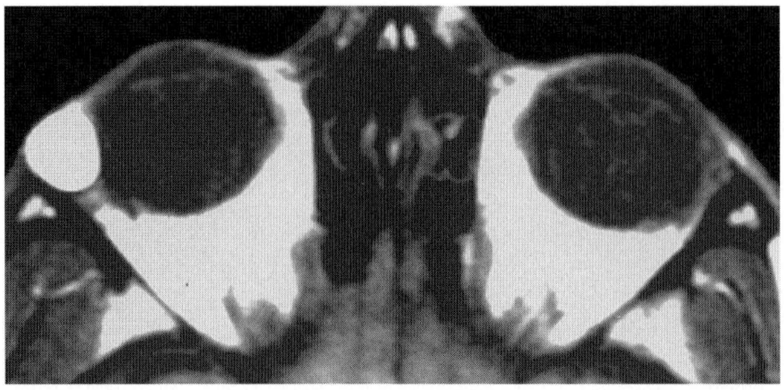

Figure 3G. Patient 1 with dermoid cyst showing a fat equivalent, high-intensity mass in the lateral aspect of orbit on the right. T1-weighted image.

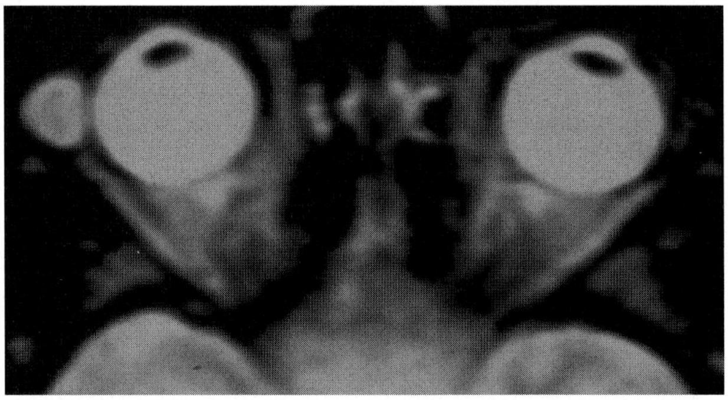

Figure 3H. Patient 1 with dermoid cyst. Fat-suppressed T2-weighted image.

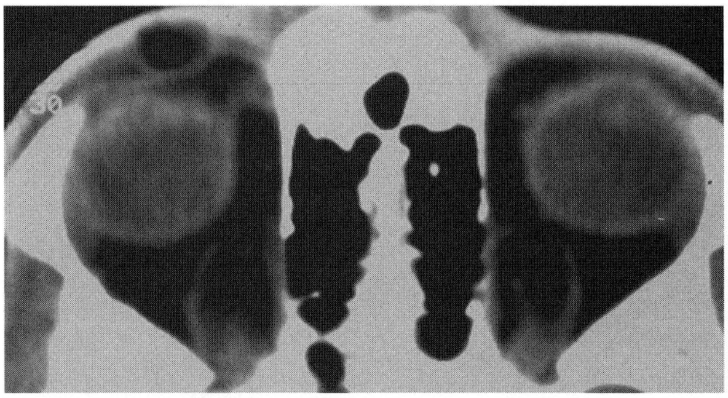

Figure 3I. Patient 2 with dermoid cyst, showing a mass of fat equivalent attenuation projecting into the conjunctival sac.

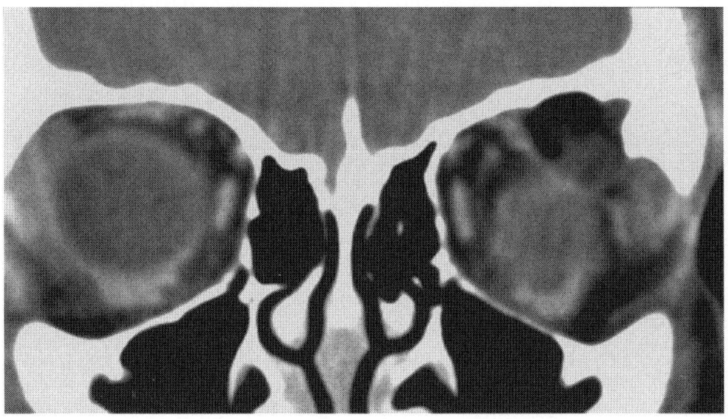

Figure 3J. Patient 3 with complex dermoid cyst, showing a mass partially containing a fat attenuation component in the superolateral aspect of the orbit on the left. Coronal computed tomography (CT) image at soft tissue window setting.

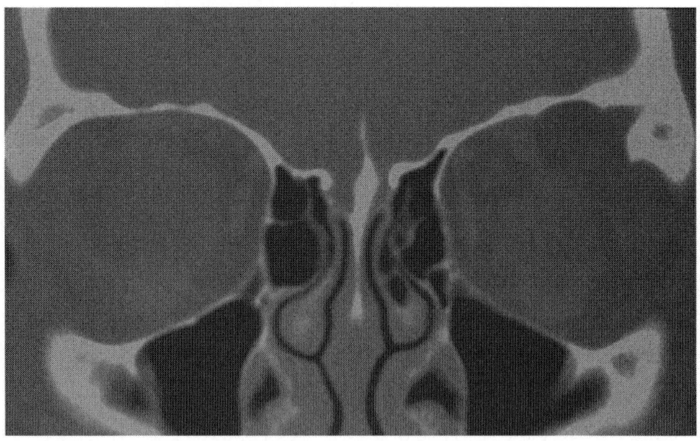

Figure 3K. Patient 3 with a complex dermoid cyst. Coronal CT image at bone window setting.

CASE 4

Clinical History: A 2 1/2-year-old girl presents with proptosis.

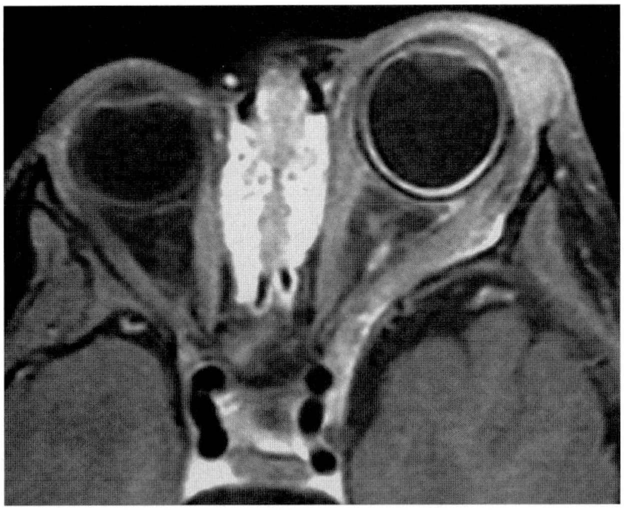

Figure 4A

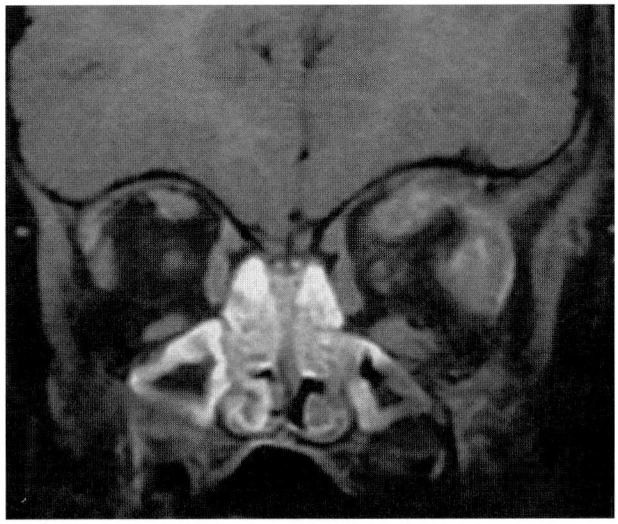

Figure 4B

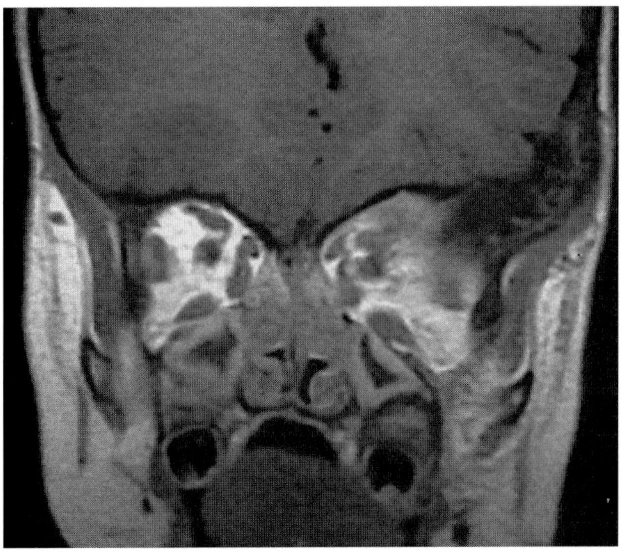

Figure 4C

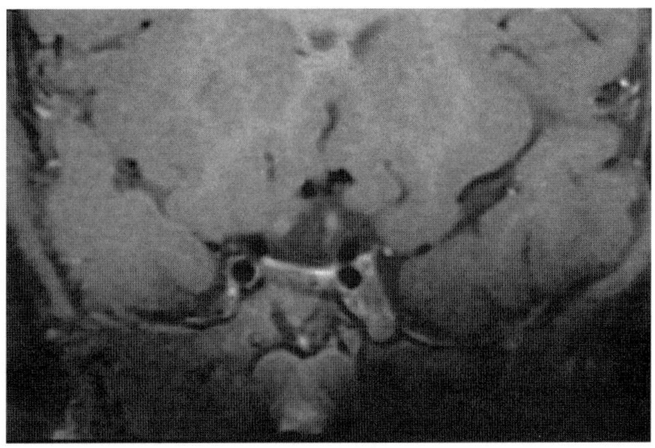

Figure 4D

1. What is the specific cause of the proptosis and what is the full extent of the lesion?
2. How do you explain the appearance of the left eye (besides the proptosis)?
3. This child has what disease? Name four manifestations of this disease.

Findings

A solid, moderately enhancing mass involving both the preseptal soft tissues and the periphery of the orbit. The mass extends to the orbital apex and eventually involves the anterior cavernous sinus, producing three distinct defects in the cavernous sinus as seen on the most posterior section.

Additional findings include dysplasia of the greater wing of the sphenoid bone, diffuse enhancement and thickening along the uveal tract of the left eye, and incidental inflammatory changes in the sinuses.

Problem

Unilateral, chronic proptosis in a young child, caused by a combination of a mass, bony dysplasia, and abnormalities of the eye

Anatomy

A. Greater wing of sphenoid
B. Superior orbital fissure
C. Trigeminal nerve (all three divisions)–anatomy within the cavernous sinus region and peripheral course of each division, including exit foramina of divisions and major branches of divisions

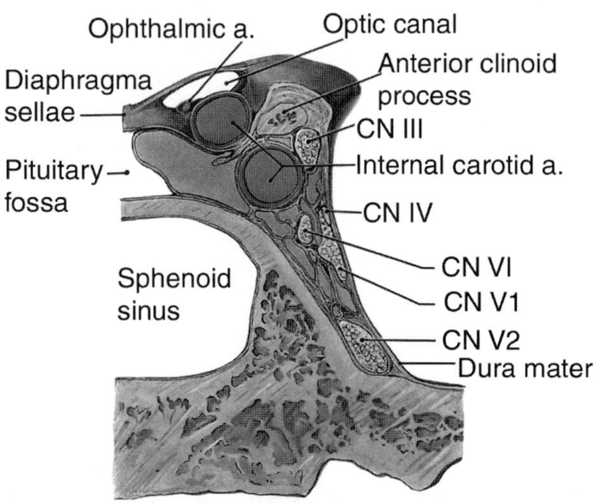

Figure 4E

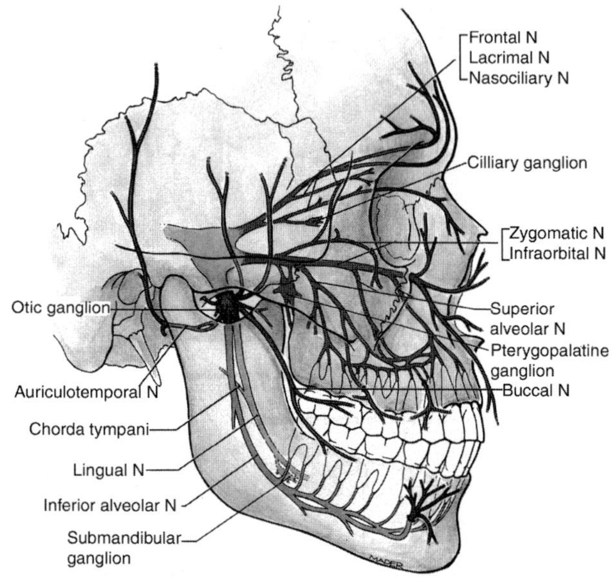

Figure 4F

Differential Diagnosis

Not applicable

Diagnosis

Neurofibromatosis type 1 (NF1 [von Recklinghausen disease]) with:

1. Neurofibroma of the trigeminal nerve: ophthalmic and maxillary divisions extending to the trigeminal ganglion
2. Bony dysplasia: greater wing of the sphenoid
3. Enlarged eye (caused by glaucoma) with membranous cyclitis

Diagnostic Imaging Approach

A. Confirm proptosis
B. Account for the vector of displacement
C. If a mass is present:
   1. Intraconal, extraconal, or transcompartmental
   2. Internal morphology
   3. Full extent

Clinical Points Of Importance And Supplemental Information

A. Chronic proptosis in a child is usually caused by a developmental lesion; rapidly developing proptosis may be caused by a complication (e.g., hemorrhage) arising in a developmental mass; however, aggressive imaging evaluation and confirmation of diagnosis are necessary because malignant disease is also a likely cause of rapidly progressive proptosis.
B. Patients with neurofibromatosis require initial evaluation of the neural axis and periodic follow-up, depending on the type of neurofibromatosis, lesions discovered, symptoms, and age.
C. Neurofibromas have a variable range of enhancement, internal morphology, and growth pattern compared with the usually homogenously enhancing, round to oval schwannomas.
D. Many of the intraaxial abnormalities visible in patients with NF1 are transient.
E. Manifestations of NF1 include:
   1. Optic glioma, gliomas at other sites, bony dysplasia, dural ectasia, nerve sheath tumors, altered signal intensity areas in the brain, the cause of which is not fully understood and which may be transient.
   2. The abnormalities in NF1 arise from primary constituents of the central nervous system (i.e., astrocytes and neurons).

Answers To Questions

1. The full extent of the plexiform neurofibroma is from the trigeminal ganglion region (cavernous sinus region) to the distal branches of V1 as they innervate the orbital region.
2. Membranous cyclitis, glaucoma
3. NF1. Optic and other gliomas, NF, dysplasia

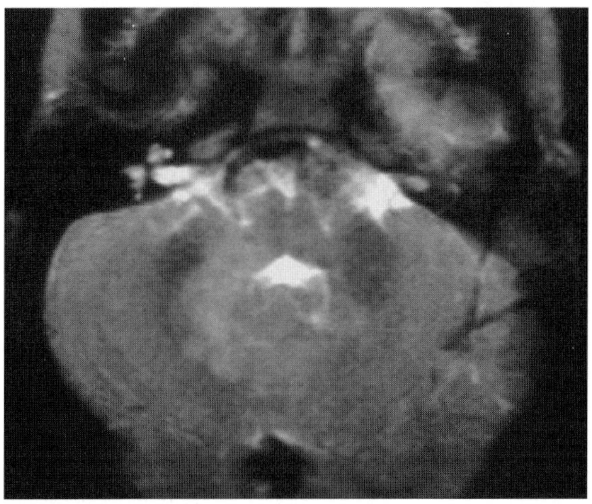

Figure 4G. Patient 1 with neurofibromatosis type 1, showing abnormally increased signal intensity in the cerebellum. T2-weighted axial image.

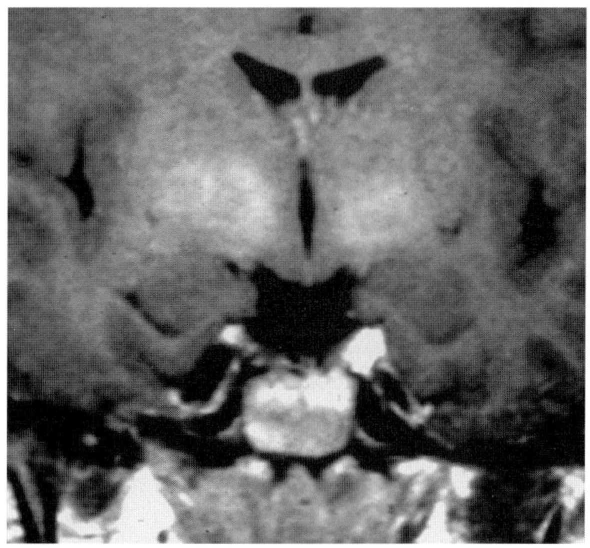

Figure 4H. Patient 1 with neurofibromatosis type 1 (NF1). T1-weighted coronal image without contrast, showing areas of increased sinal intensity in the basal ganglia caused by NF1; these subsequently disappeared.

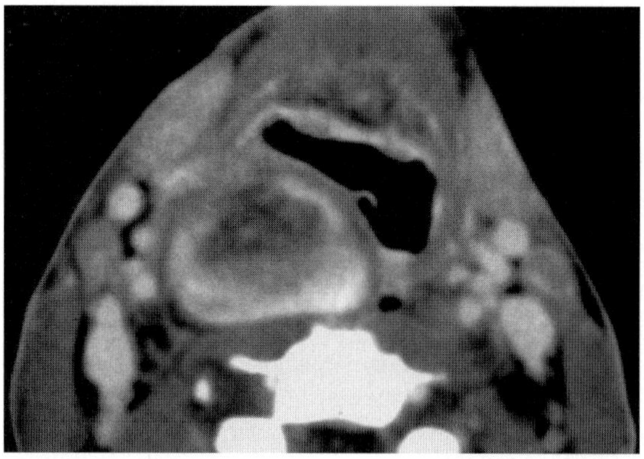

Figure 4I. Patient 2 with neurofibromatosis type 1, showing a mainly peripherally enhancing mass in the retropharyngeal space at the level of the oropharynx. Contrast-enhanced computed tomography image.

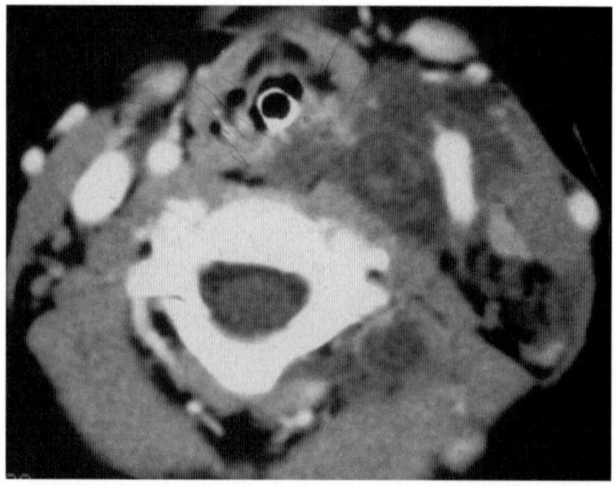

Figure 4J. Patient 3 with neurofibromatosis type 1, showing plexiform neurofibromas involving the retropharyngeal space, posterior triangle, anterior triangle, and paraspinous muscle on the left. Contrast-enhanced computed tomography image.

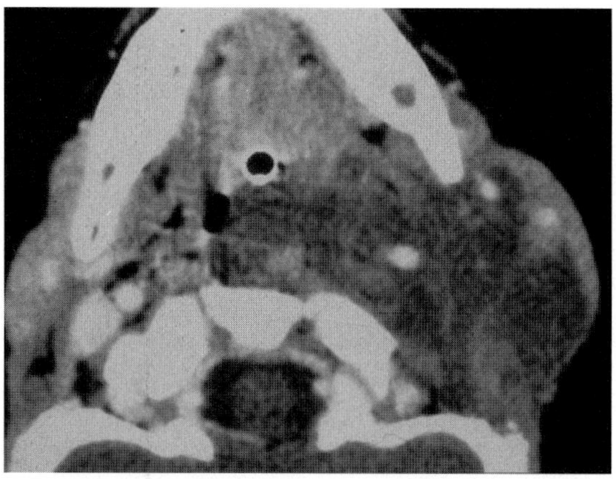

Figure 4K. Patient 3 with neurofibromatosis type 1. Contrast-enhanced computed tomography image superior to 4J.

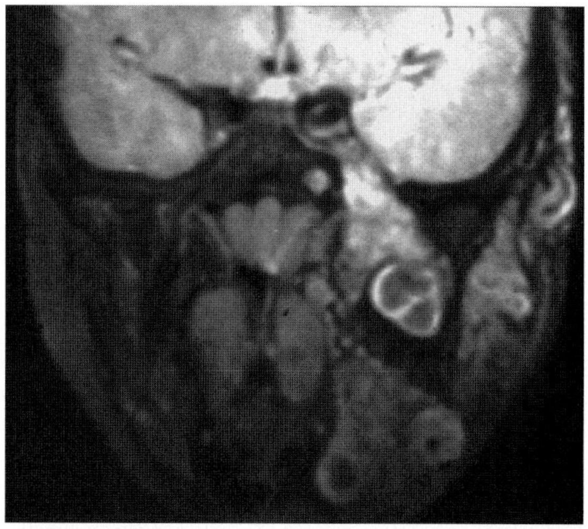

Figure 4L. Patient 4 with neurofibromatosis type 1: neurofibroma of the mandibular division of the trigeminal nerve, showing a mixed internal morphology and enhancement pattern. Fat-suppressed T2-weighted coronal image.

CASE 5

Clinical History: A middle-aged woman presents with intermittent proptosis. The images, which are at the same level, were made differently.

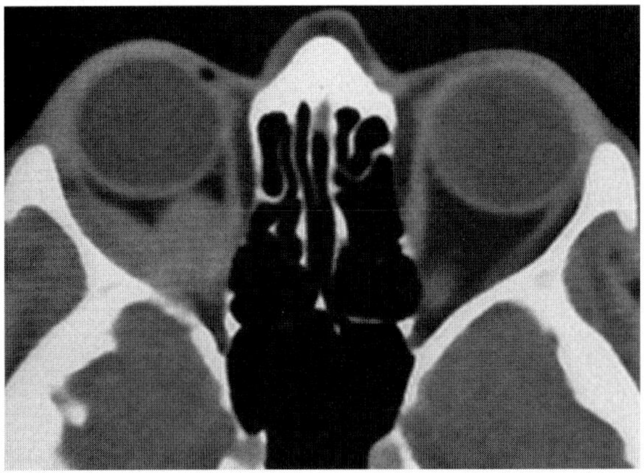

Figure 5A

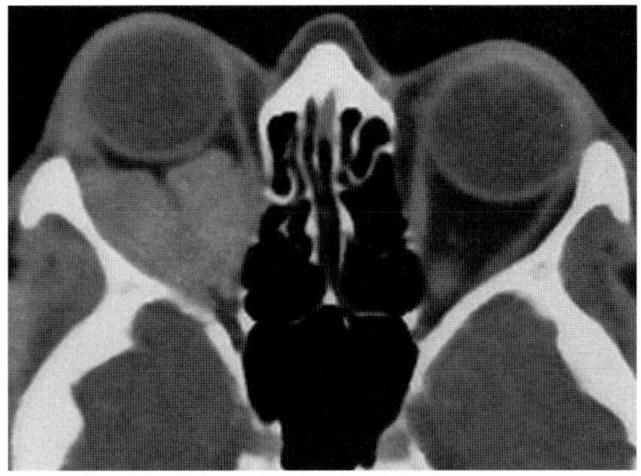

Figure 5B

1. What is the difference between the images?
2. What is your complete diagnosis? (Two related entities are present.)

Findings

A smoothly marginated, well-circumscribed intraconal mass and a second elongated mass that parallels the course of the lateral rectus muscle and may be both intra- and extraconal. The right eye may be slightly proptotic.

A second image showing definite proptosis. Both components of the mass have increased in size and are altered in shape. The second image was acquired with the patient in the prone rather than the supine position.

Problem

Intermittent (gravity, flow-related) proptosis in an adult with a transcompartmental mass, which changes with Valsalva maneuver, and possibly a separate intraconal orbital mass(es).

Anatomy

A. Veins of the orbit
B. Muscle cone and extraconal compartment of the orbit

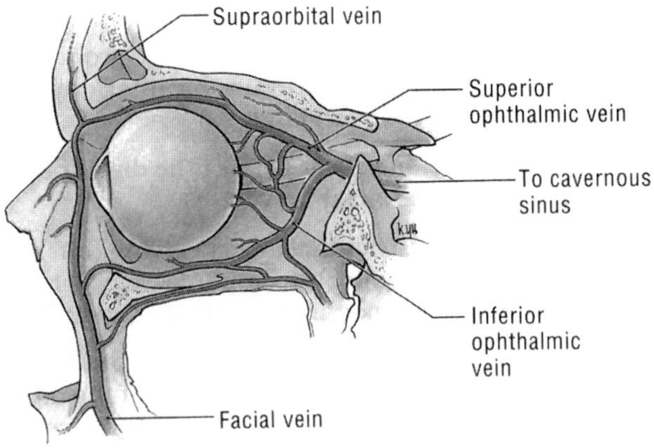

Figure 5C

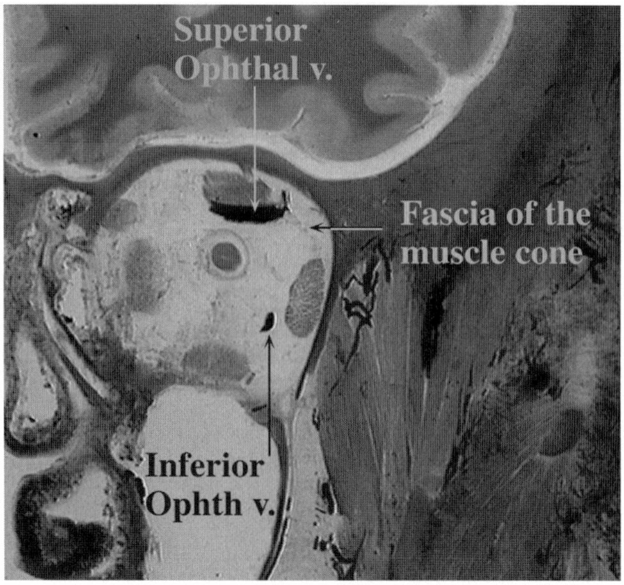

Figure 5D

Differential Diagnosis

Orbital varix, orbital varix combined with a vascular malformation

Diagnosis

Orbital varix and cavernous vascular malformation "hemangioma"

Diagnostic Imaging Approach

A. Recognize this unusual but usually clinically obvious situation and confirm the diagnosis, which can be done with baseline supine scan followed by scanning with the patient prone or during head hanging, Valsalva maneuver, or restriction of orbital venous outflow.
B. Establish whether the varix is isolated or associated with a vascular malformation.

Clinical Points Of Importance And Supplemental Information

A. Treatment is often conservative.
B. Establishing the diagnosis and determining whether the lesion is isolated (orbital varix simplex) or associated with another vascular lesion (e.g., hemangioma or lymphangioma) is useful to the ophthalmologist.
C. A simple varix or encapsulated hemangioma is resectable.
    1. The surgeon usually tries to avoid resecting a lymphangioma or hemangioma because of its normally poorly encapsulated, microscopically infiltrative growth pattern.
D. A large superior ophthalmic vein may be a normal variation and does not usually approach the size of a varix. A large vein may also be a clue to the presence of cavernous sinus thrombosis, a vascular mass in the cavernous sinus or a cavernous carotid fistula.

Answers To Questions

1. One is with and one is without the Valsalva maneuver.
2. Cavernous vascular malformation with an orbital varix

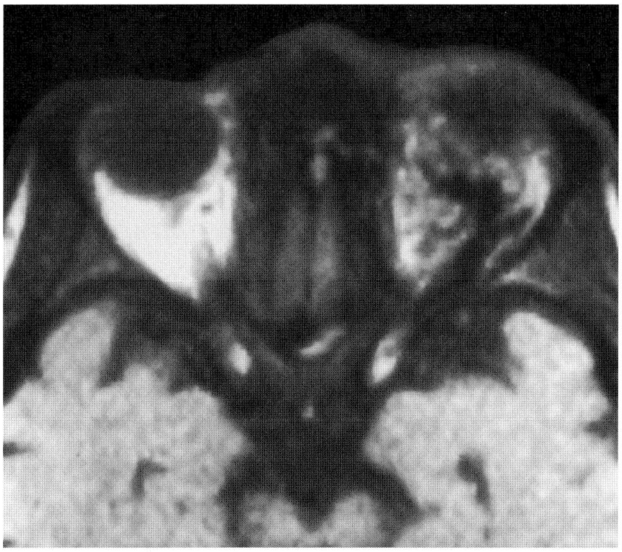

Figure 5E. Patient 1 with orbital arteriovenous malformation with varix showing enlarged tortuous vessels in the orbit on the left. T1-weighted axial image without contrast.

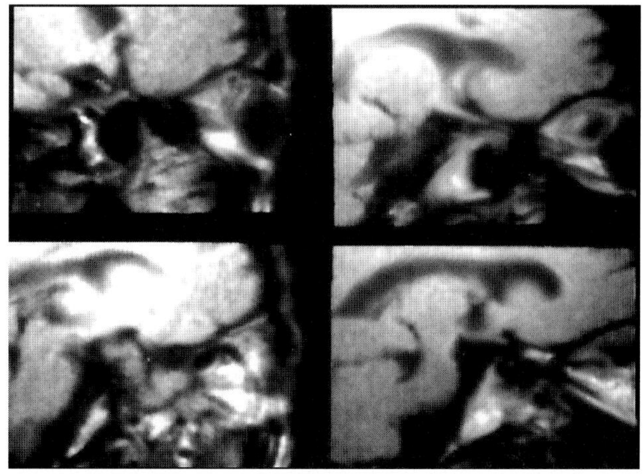

Figure 5F. Patient 1 with orbital arteriovenous malformation with varix. T1-weighted sagittal images without contrast.

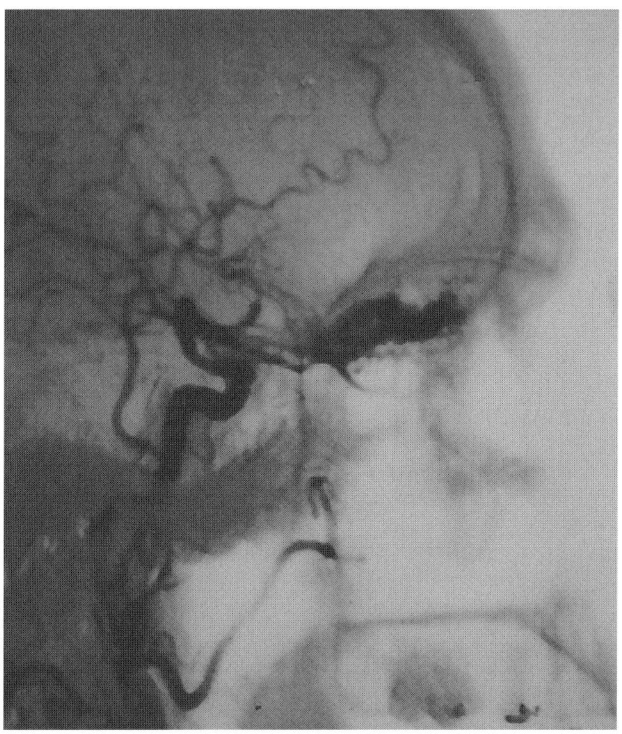

Figure 5G. Patient 1 with orbital arteriovenous malformation with varix. Arterial phase of the left internal carotid angiogram showing the nidus and enlarged draining veins in the superior aspect of orbit.

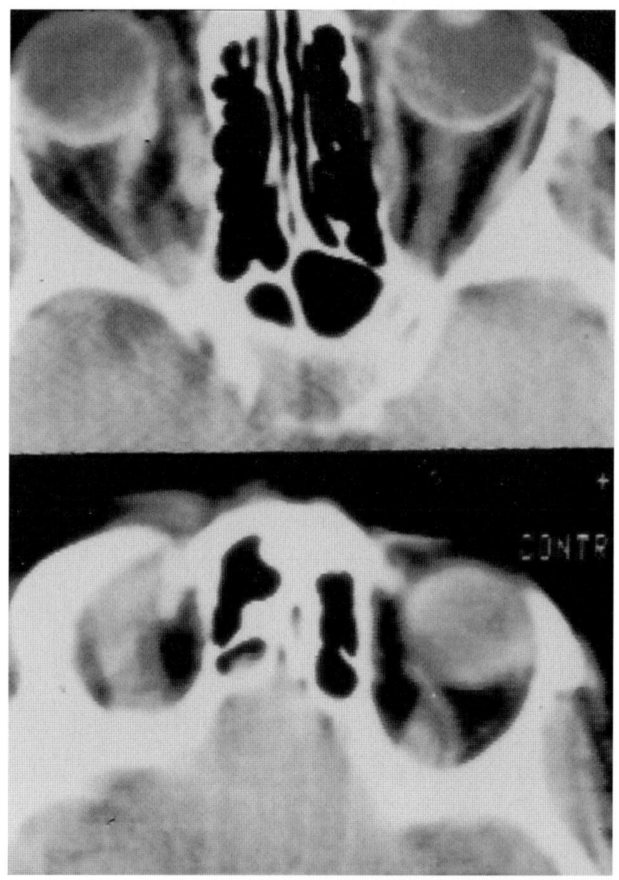

Figure 5H. Patient 2 with a cavernous carotid fistula, showing the enlarged superior ophthalmic vein on the right. Axial computed tomography image with contrast.

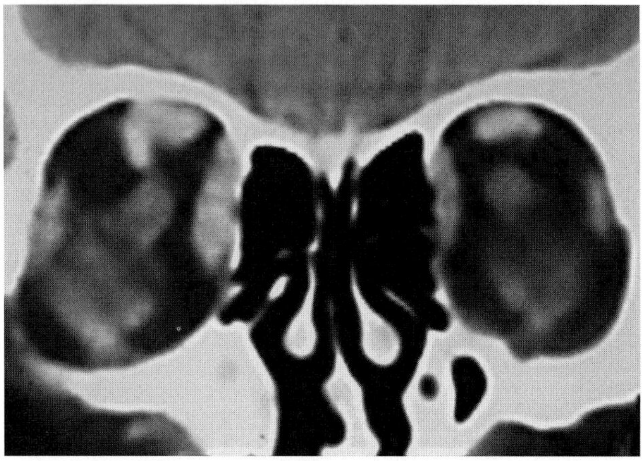

Figure 5I. Patient 2 with cavernous-carotid fistula with an enlarged superior ophthalmic vein. Contrast enhanced, coronal CT image.

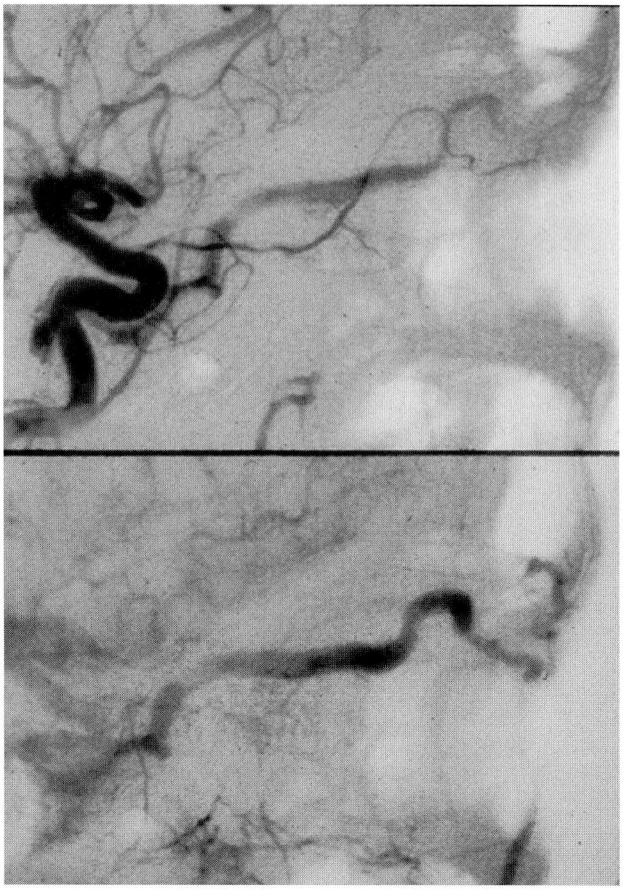

Figure 5J. Patient 2 with a cavernous carotid fistula with an enlarged superior ophthalmic vein. Right internal carotid angiogram shows early filling of the enlarged superior ophthalmic vein.

CASE 6

Clinical History: A middle-aged woman presents with diminishing visual acuity in the right eye.

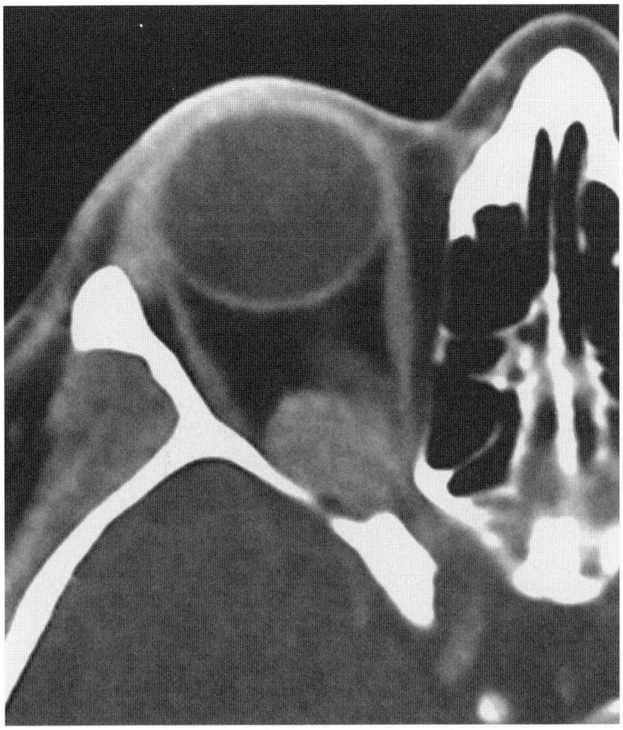

Figure 6A

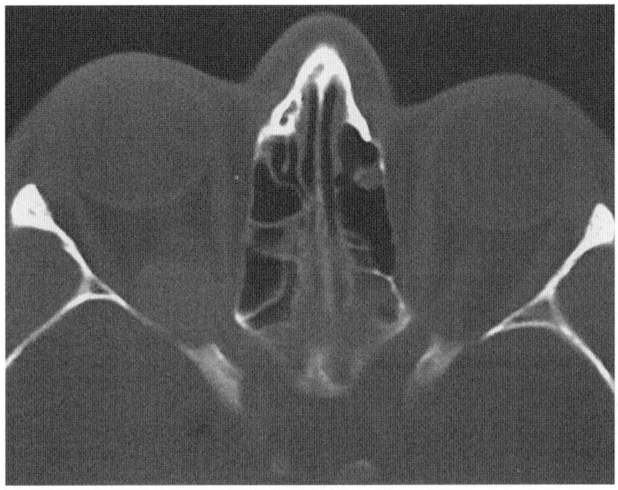

Figure 6B

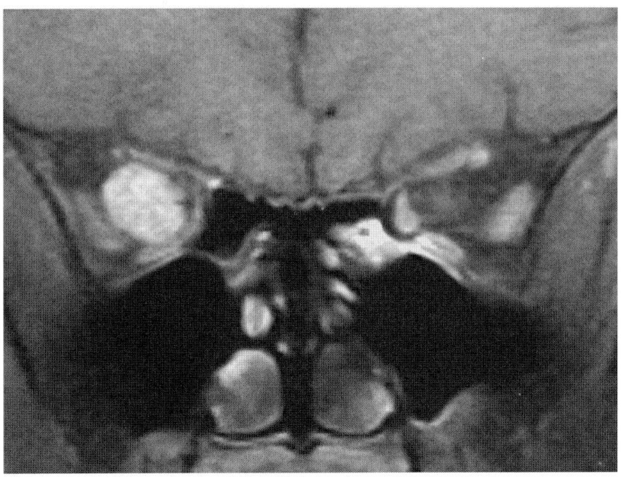

Figure 6C

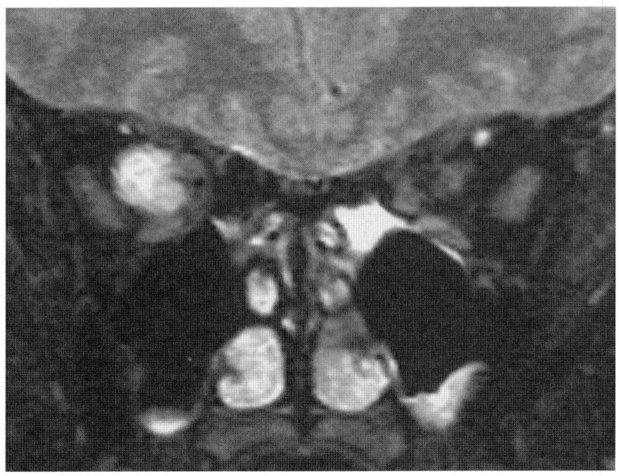

Figure 6D

1. Outline your approach to evaluating orbital masses.
2. Is this mass intraconal or extraconal?
3. Why is the lesion bright on T2-weighted images?
4. List the two most likely diagnostic possibilities.

Findings

A well-circumscribed intraconal mass with sharp margins at the orbital apex. There appears to be some remodeling of the adjacent greater wing of the sphenoid. The mass seems to be in contact with, but mainly displaces the optic nerve–sheath complex. The mass enhances homogeneously and is bright on the T2-weighted coronal image.

Problem

Unilateral diminished visual acuity in an adult caused by an intraconal mass that is in contact with and displacing the optic nerve–sheath complex

Anatomy

A. Details of intraconal (central surgical space) compartment of the orbit including:
   1. Optic nerve–sheath complex
   2. Ophthalmic artery and veins at the orbital apex
   3. Relationship of the superior orbital fissure and optic canal at the orbital apex

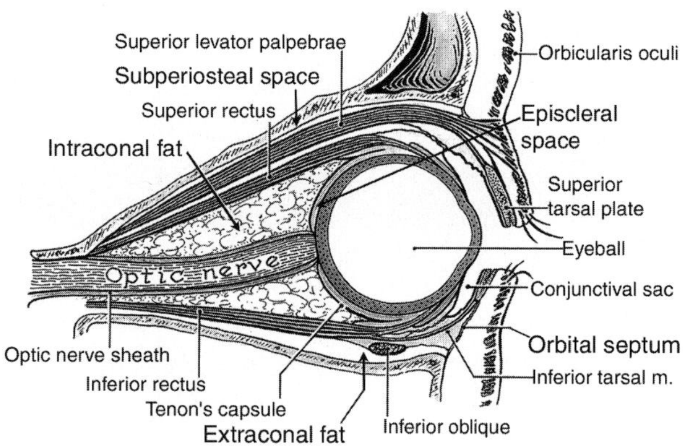

Figure 6E

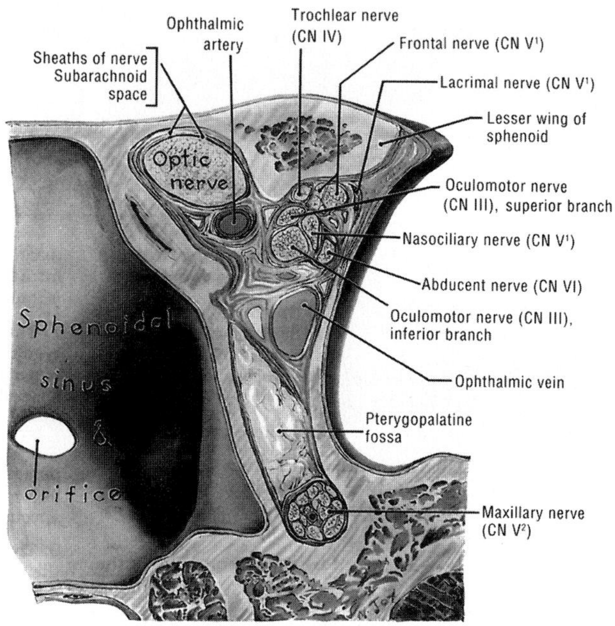

Figure 6F

Differential Diagnosis

1. Cavernous vascular malformation "hemangioma"
2. Meningioma
3. Hemangiopericytoma
4. Schwannoma or neurofibroma
5. Metastasis (rare with this morphology)

Diagnosis

Optic sheath meningioma

Diagnostic Imaging Approach

A. Evaluate the entire optic pathway in two planes to identify the cause of diminished visual acuity.
B. If a compressive mass or disease process outside the optic nerve or brain is identified:
   1. Mass vs. infiltrative process
   2. If a mass, then consider its:
      a. Location
      b. Morphology
      c. Extent
   3. If infiltrative, then consider if the lesion is:
      a. Localized or multifocal
      b. Unilateral or bilateral
      c. Dural, meningeal, bone, soft tissue origin

Clinical Points Of Importance And Supplemental Information

A. Cavernous vascular malformation "hemangioma" is much less likely to produce visual loss than other, less common intraconal masses.
B. Establish the relationship of the mass to the optic nerve–sheath complex as clearly as possible to help with surgical planning, in particular, extension to the optic canal and prechiasmatic segment of the nerve must be identified to assess risk to the other eye.
C. Avoid biopsy of an optic sheath meningoma because it can lead to orbital spread and eventual exenteration for control.

Answers To Questions

1. Intraconal, extraconal, nerve, or sheath
2. Intraconal
3. Because mass lesions can have a wide range of signal intensity, depending on their composition, especially with regard to relative water content.
4. Cavernous vascular malformation, meningioma (nerve sheath possible but rare)

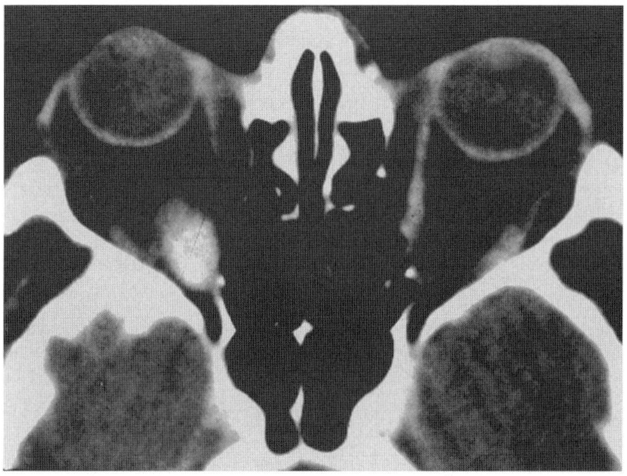

Figure 6G. Patient 1 with cavernous vascular malformation, showing an enhancing intraconal mass in the orbit on the right. Contrast-enhanced computed tomography image.

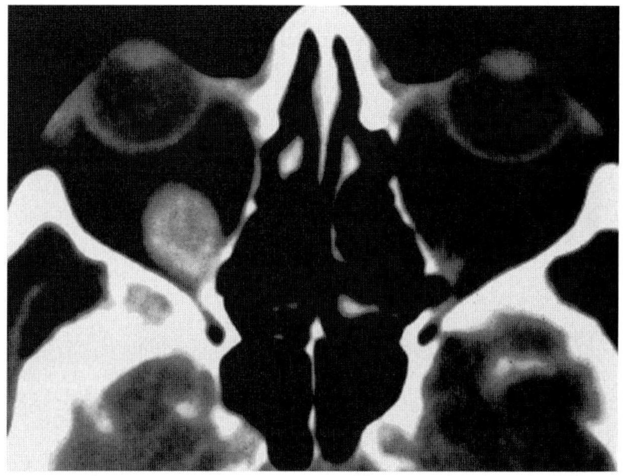

Figure 6H. Patient 1 with cavernous vascular malformation. Contrast-enhanced computed tomography image inferior to 6G.

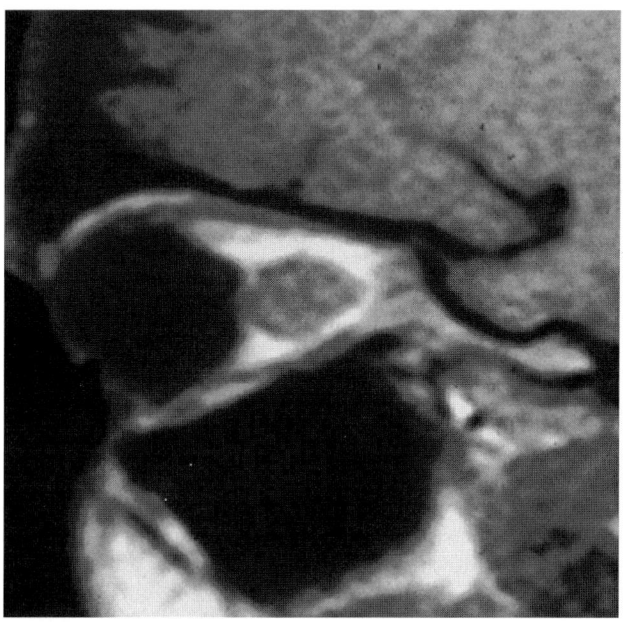

Figure 6I. Patient 2 with cavernous vascular malformation. T1-weighted sagittal image without contrast showing an intraconal mass.

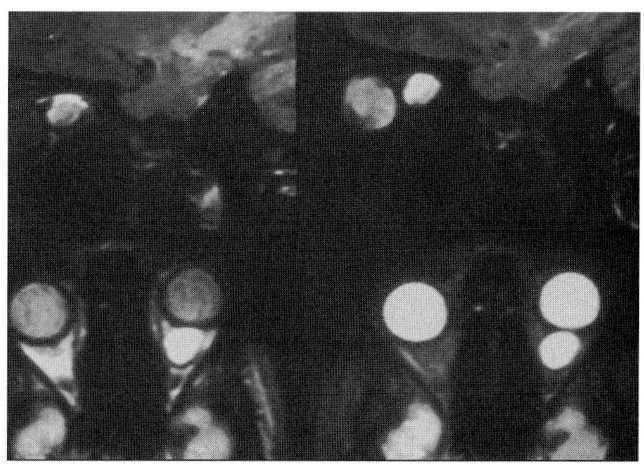

Figure 6J. Patient 2 with cavernous vascular malformation. T2-weighted images showing a high intensity, intraconal mass.

CASE 7

Clinical History: A 6-year-old boy presents with a low-grade fever and acute, slightly painful proptosis. The axial T1-weighted, contrast-enhanced image was made about 3 weeks after the other three images.

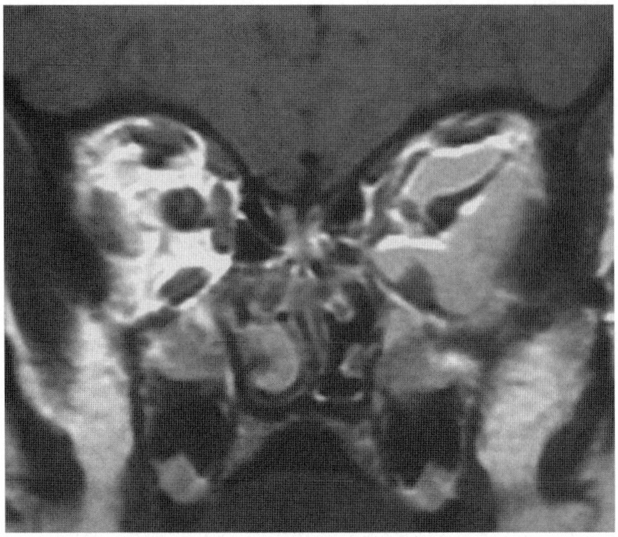

Figure 7A

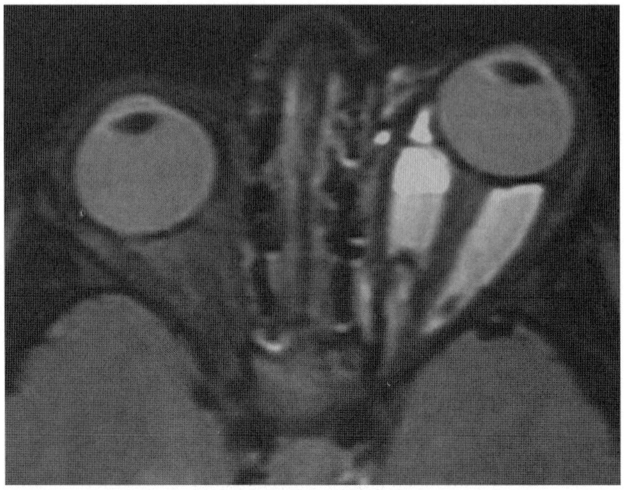

Figure 7B

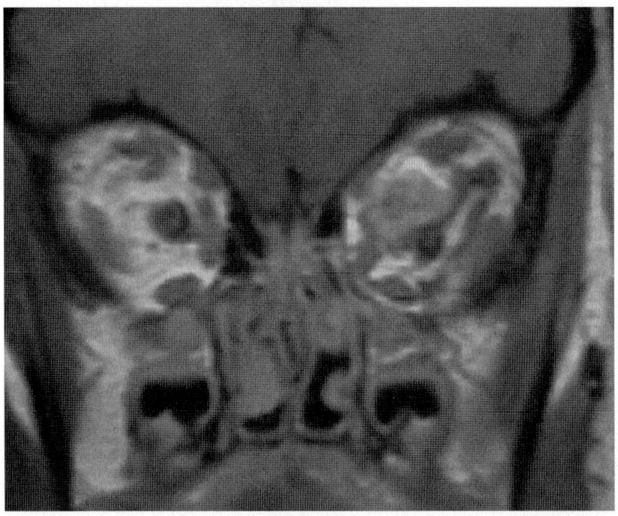

Figure 7C

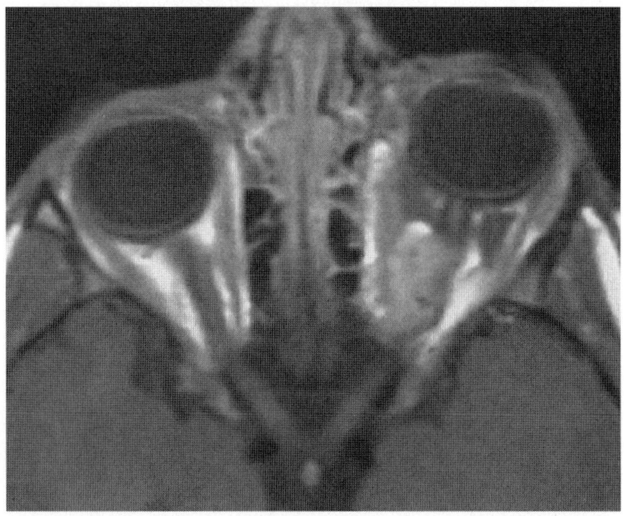

Figure 7D

1. Is this lesion intraconal, extraconal, or transcompartmental?
2. Give two possible reasons for the acute enlargement of the lesion that caused the proptosis.
3. What is your diagnosis? From the clinical factors alone, what would be the other major diagnostic concern?

Findings

A multiloculated, transcompartmental orbital mass containing a fluid/fluid level. Some enhancement is present, but the mass is predominantly composed of nonenhancing cystic spaces. Some proptosis is less obvious on the axial, contrast-enhanced T1-weighted image that was made weeks after the acute episode during which the other three images were obtained.

Problem

A young child with potentially rapidly progressive proptosis caused by a multiloculated, cystic, and partially enhancing transcompartmental mass

Anatomy

A. Compartments of the orbit
   1. Extraconal
      a. Bone
      b. Subperiosteal
      c. Extraconal fat
   2. Intraconal

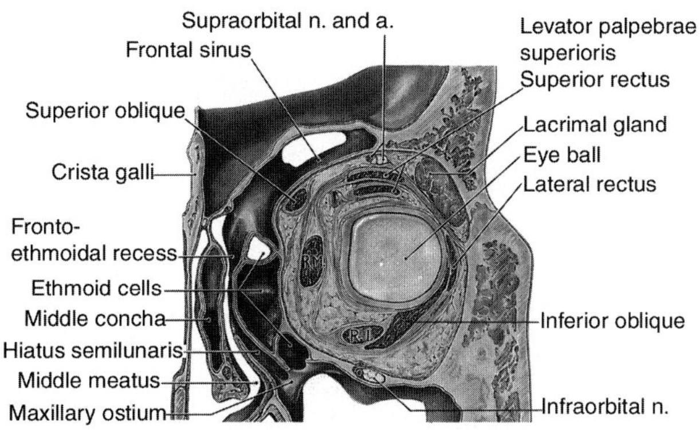

Figure 7E

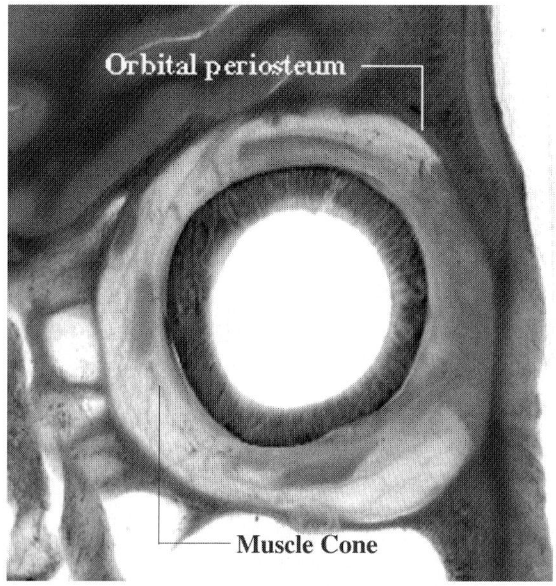

Figure 7F

Differential Diagnosis

Virtually none (rarely, parasitic cyst)

Diagnosis

Orbital venolymphatic malformation with hemorrhage

Diagnostic Imaging Approach

A. Confirm presence and establish probable cause of proptosis.
B. If a mass, consider whether the mass is:
   1. Intraconal, extraconal, or transcompartmental (origin and extent)
   2. Internal morphology (e.g., fluid levels, blood products, septa)

Clinical Points Of Importance And Supplemental Information

A. Acute enlargement of a venolymphatic malformation can occur during an upper respiratory infection (reactive lymphoid tissue present) or be caused by hemorrhage.
B. Presentation, especially in a child, can mimic that of a rapidly growing orbital neoplasm (i.e., rhabdomyosarcoma, lymphoma, granulocytic sarcoma), orbital cellulitis, or a more unusual disease such as Langerhans' cell histiocytosis.
C. Complete surgical removal of these masses is usually not possible. Treatment is aimed at preserving vision while maintaining acceptable cosmesis.

Answers To Questions

1. Transcompartmental
2. Bleed, inflammatory reaction
3. Venolymphatic malformation. Cancer or inflammation.

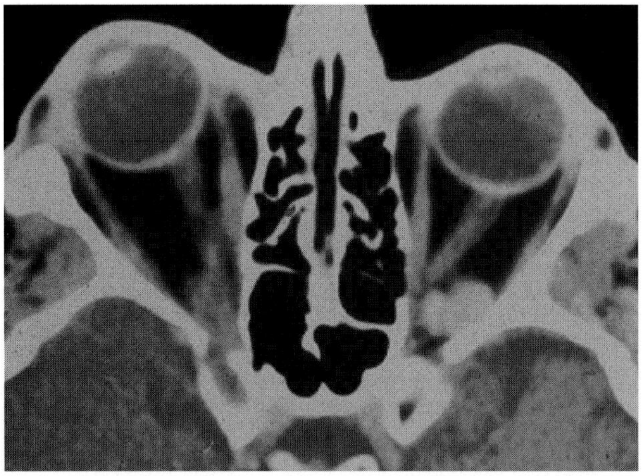

Figure 7G. Patient 1 with bilateral cavernous vascular malformation at the orbital apex, showing lobulated, enhancing masses bilaterally. Contrast-enhanced CT image.

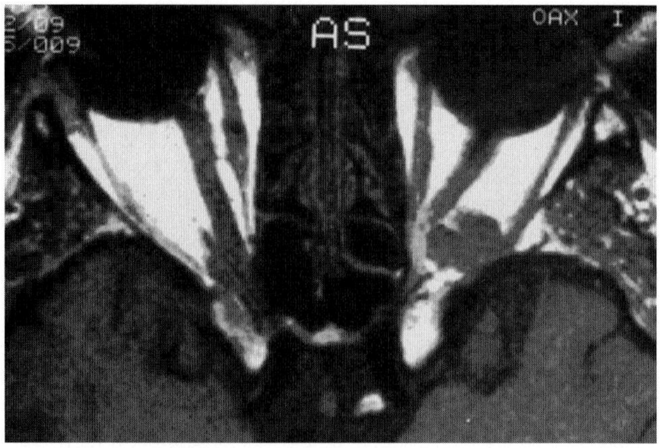

Figure 7H. Patient 1 with bilateral cavernous vascular malformation at the orbital apex. T1-weighted image without contrast.

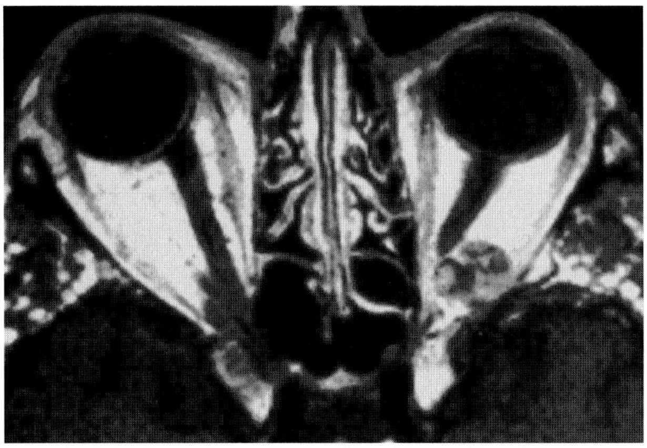

Figure 7I. Patient 1 with bilateral cavernous vascular malformation at the orbital apex. T1-weighted image with contrast.

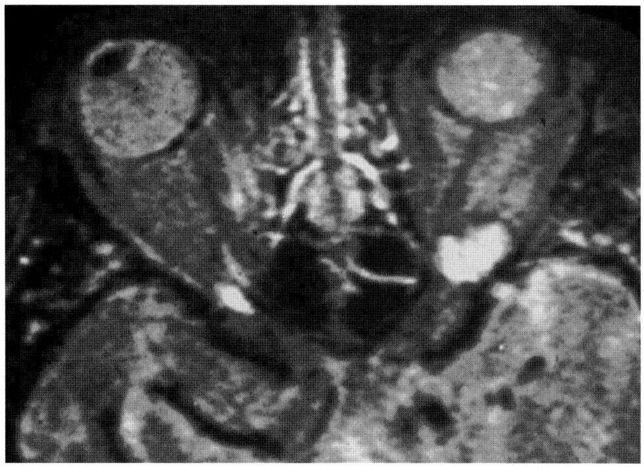

Figure 7J. Patient 1 with bilateral cavernous vascular malformation at the orbital apex. Fat-suppressed T2-weighted magnetic resonance image.

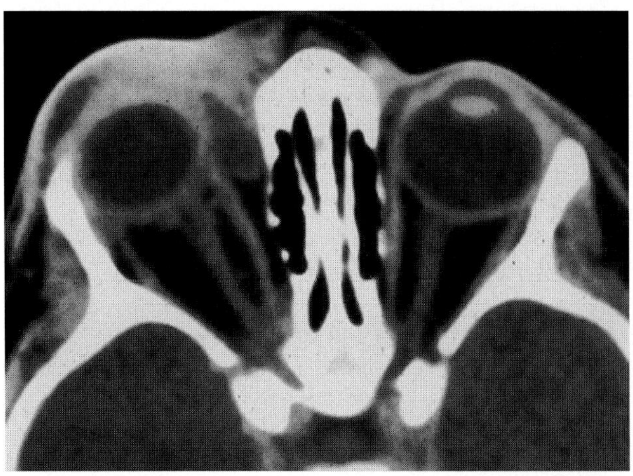

Figure 7K. Patient 2 with mixed venolymphatic malformation presenting as an acute enlarging orbital mass, showing a partially enhancing mass in the preseptal and postseptal portions of the orbit on the right. Contrast-enhanced computed tomography image.

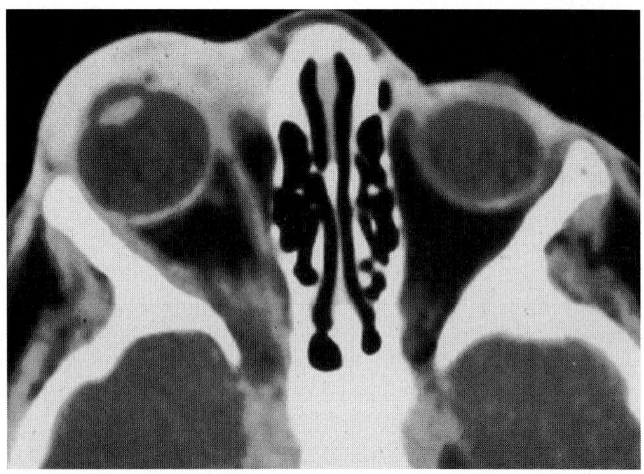

Figure 7L. Patient 2 with mixed venolymphatic malformation presenting as an acute enlarging orbital mass. Contrast-enhanced computed tomography image inferior to 7K.

CASE 8

Clinical History: A 40-year-old woman with bilateral proptosis.

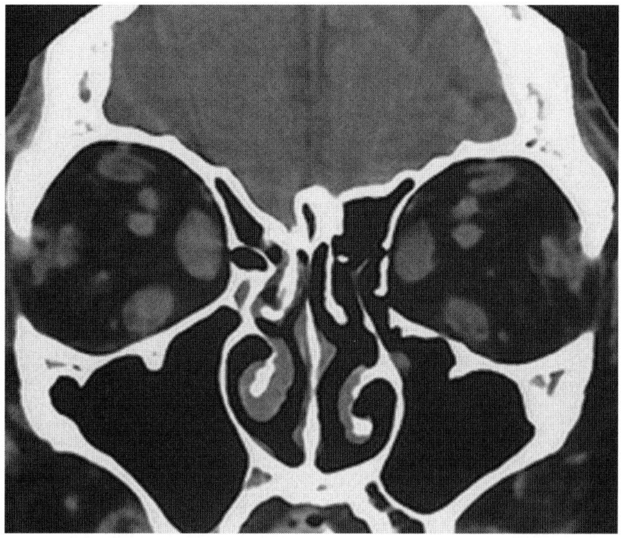

Figure 8A

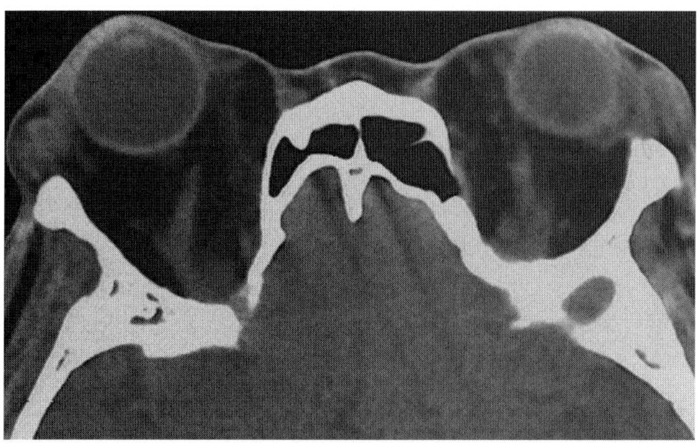

Figure 8B

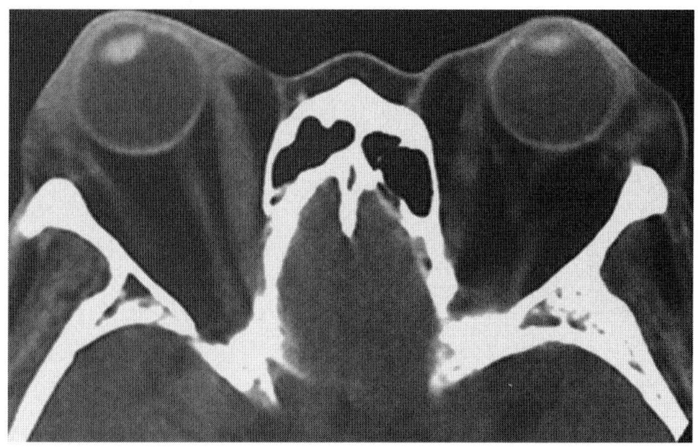

Figure 8C

1. List three causes of increased orbital fat; list the diagnosis of this case first.
2. Is this patient likely to have diminished visual acuity?
3. Can computed tomography (CT) or magnetic resonance imaging (MRI) be used to predict whether diminished visual acuity is likely in this condition? How is optic nerve compression (vascular compromise) treated in this condition?

Findings

A generalized, markedly increased fat content in both the intraconal and extraconal compartments of the orbits with enlargement of the extraocular muscles, some of which contain focal areas of low attenuation. The lacrimal glands are displaced because of the excessive accumulation of orbital fat. Because the orbital apices are not visible, protrusion of the orbital fat through the superior orbital fissure cannot be analyzed. Obvious bilateral proptosis is present as noted clinically.

Problem

Bilateral, chronic proptosis in an adult caused by an increased volume of orbital fat and enlargement of the extraocular muscles

Anatomy

A. Extraconal muscles (origin and insertion of each)
B. Extraconal orbital fat
C. Lacrimal gland (orbital and palpebral portions)

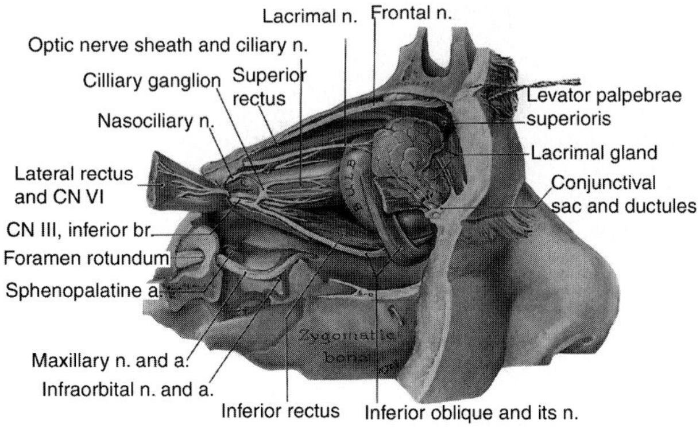

Figure 8D

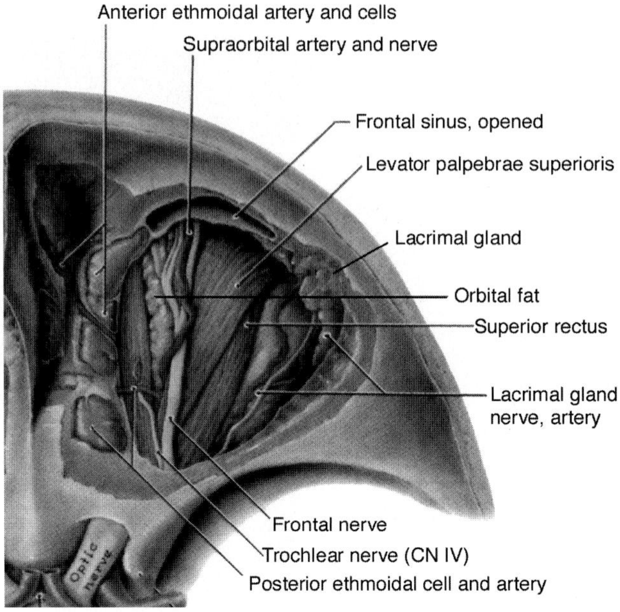

Figure 8E

Differential Diagnosis

1. For increased orbital fat: normal variation, obesity, steroid use, diabetes
2. For isolated muscle enlargement: myositis, pseudotumor, metastasis (if focal)

Diagnosis

Thyroid ophthalmopathy, Grave's disease, dysthyroid orbitopathy

Diagnostic Imaging Approach

A. Confirm presence and establish probable cause of proptosis.
B. Which muscles are enlarged? Are they diffusely enlarged or is there tapering of the origin and insertion? Are there "inflammatory" changes around muscles?
C. Is the volume of orbital fat abnormally increased? Does the fat protrude through the superior orbital fissure?
D. Are the tissue planes surrounding the optic nerve–sheath complex obliterated?

Clinical Points Of Importance And Supplemental Information

A. Complete obliteration of fat planes surrounding the optic nerve–sheath complex is associated with visual loss in 60% of cases. Protrusion of orbital fat 1 cm beyond the superior orbital fissure toward the middle cranial fossa has also been identified as a risk factor for compressive optic neuropathy.
B. Visual loss is believed to be caused by vascular compromise, congestion, or both, rather than direct optic nerve compression.
C. Imaging helps in planning and establishing the adequacy of surgical orbital decompression.
D. Dysthyroid ophthalmopathy does not necessarily correlate with abnormalities of thyroid function.
E. Increased signal intensity within involved muscles may help select patients who will respond favorably to steroid, immunosuppressive, or radiation management.
F. Focal low attenuation in the extraocular muscles on CT or evidence of focal fibrosis on MRI may indicate "burned out" muscle disease, which will not be responsive to medical management, or a primary muscle disease such as that seen in chronic progressive external ophthalmoplegia (CPEO). CPEO is believed to be a disease of mitochondrial dysfunction.

Answers To Questions

1. Grave's disease, steroid use, obesity
2. No, but it is possible.
3. Yes. Surgical decompression, radiation, or steroid use.

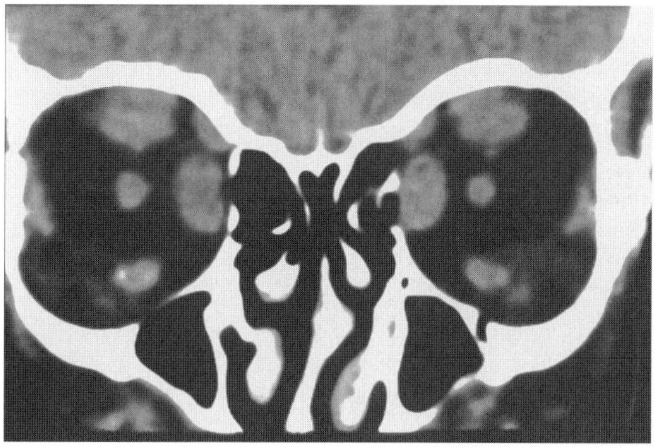

Figure 8F. Patient 1 with Grave's disease and visual loss before decompression, showing enlargement of the extraocular muscles bilaterally. Coronal computed tomography image.

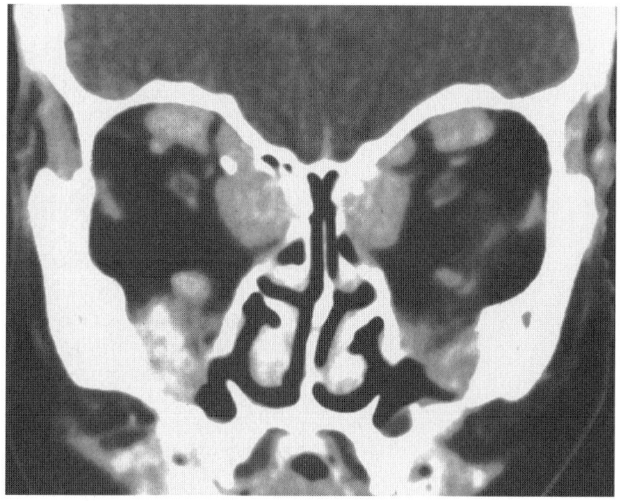

Figure 8G. Patient 1 with Grave's disease and visual loss after decompression with improved vision following the surgery. Coronal computed tomography image showing prolapse of the intraorbital contents into the subjacent maxillary sinus through the surgical defect in the orbital floor.

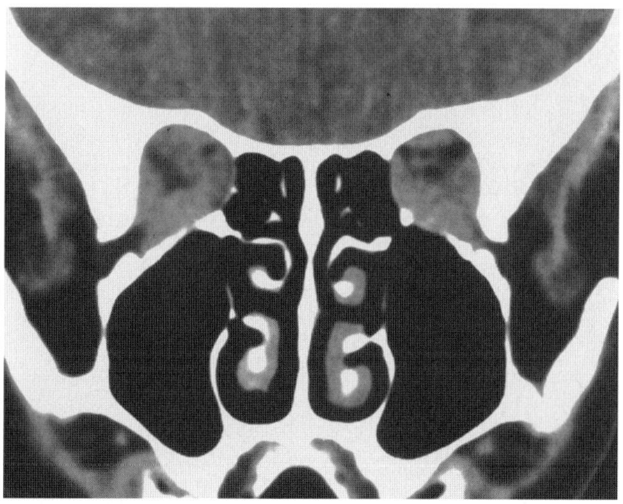

Figure 8H. Patient 1 with Grave's disease, visual loss, and only partial loss of fat planes near the orbital apex before decompression. Coronal computed tomography image.

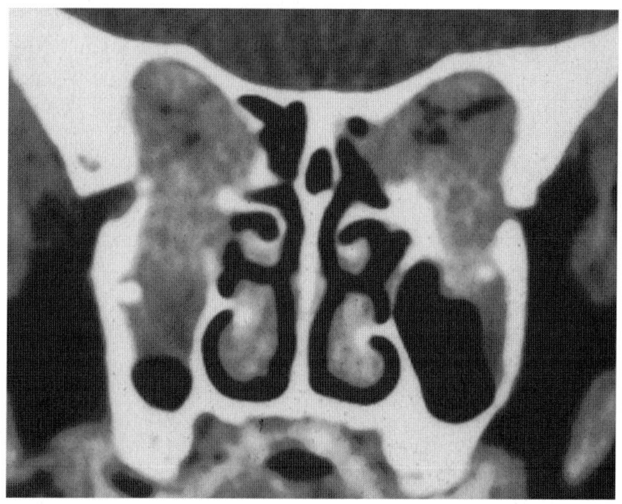

Figure 8I. Patient 1 with Grave's disease, visual loss, and only partial loss of fat planes. After decompression, the fat planes are essentially unchanged but a marked improvement of vision followed the surgery. Coronal computed tomography image.

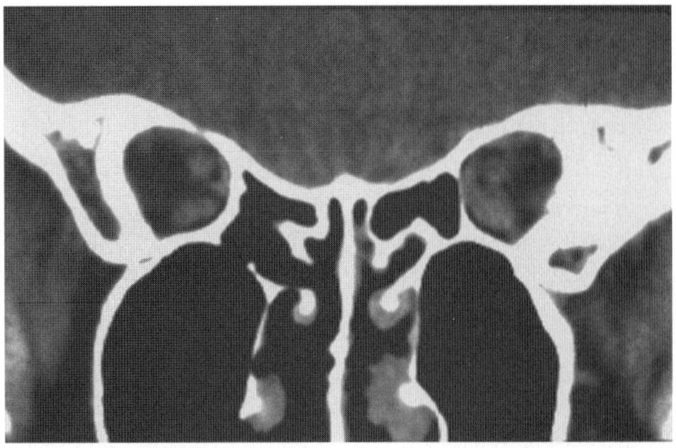

Figure 8J. Patient 2 with Graves disease and visual loss. Only minimal enlargement is seen of the extraocular muscles with other images showing rather marked increase in orbital fat content. Coronal computed tomography image.

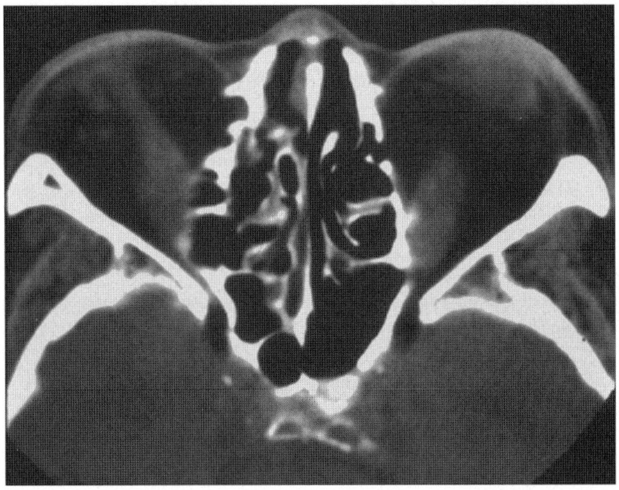

Figure 8K. Patient 2 with Grave's disease and excessive protrusion of fat through the orbital fissures at the orbital apex. The patient's visual loss improved following decompressive surgery. Axial computed tomography image.

CASE 9

Clinical History: A 50-year-old woman presents with pain and periorbital swelling on the right.

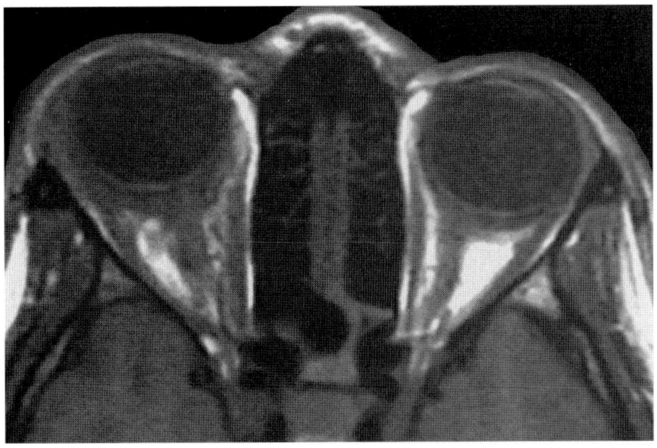

Figure 9A

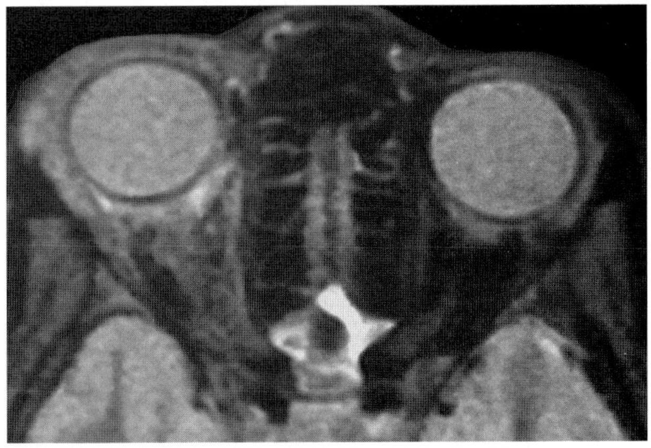

Figure 9B

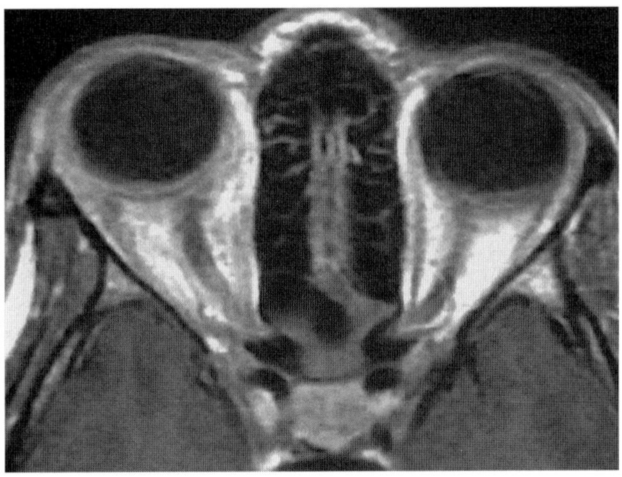

Figure 9C

1. What compartments or spaces of the eye and orbit are involved?
2. What diseases besides idiopathic orbital inflammatory syndrome (pseudotumor) result in such findings?
3. Name five subtypes of pseudotumor.

Findings

An enhancing, infiltrating process involving the periscleral regions bilaterally; the disease is much more prominent on the right where it also extends to involve the intraorbital fat. The STIR (short TI inversion recover) image strongly suggests that the Tenon's space is distended, at least on the right side.

Problem

Bilateral, infiltrating, likely inflammatory process affecting the sclera and Tenon's space

Anatomy

A. Eye: uveoscleral interface
B. Intraconal: Tenon's capsule and space and their relationship to the optic sheath

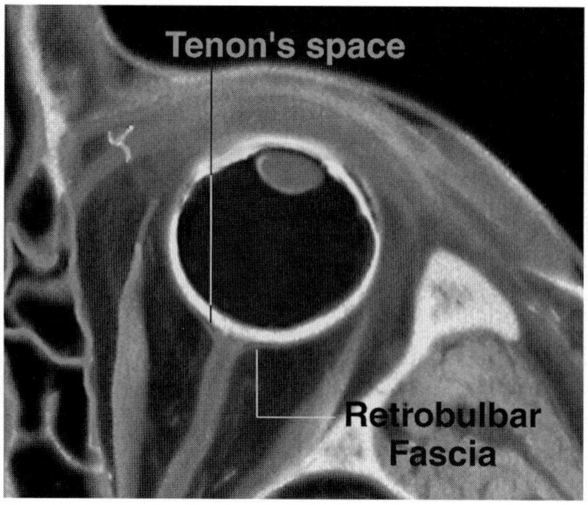

Figure 9D

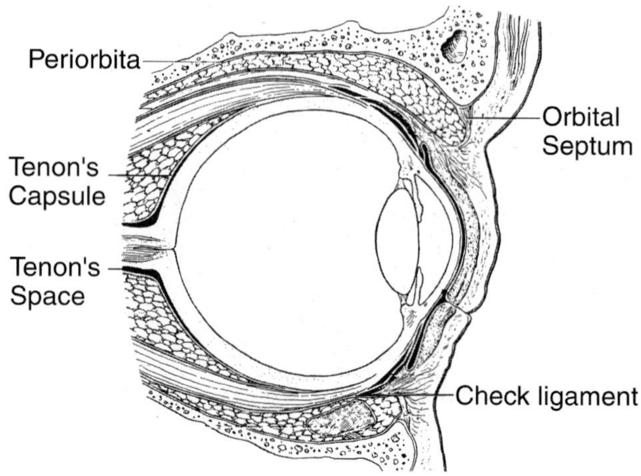

Figure 9E

Differential Diagnosis

Periscleritis associated with autoimmune disease; granulomatoses (e.g., Wegener's granulomatosis, sarcoid); Langerhans' cell histiocytosis; plasmacytosis; lymphoma, leukemia; infectious (e.g., syphilis)

Diagnosis

Idiopathic orbital inflammatory syndrome (i.e., pseudotumor): predominantly periscleritic or perineuritic variety

Diagnostic Imaging Approach

A. Well-circumscribed or infiltrating morphology?
B. Is the pathology intraconal, extraconal, or transcompartmental?
C. Unilateral or bilateral?
D. Associated findings
   1. Leptomeningeal, dural, sinonasal
E. Pseudotumor can be subclassified into five forms (they frequently overlap):
   1. Periscleritic
   2. Myositic
   3. Perineuritic
   4. Lacrimal (dacryoadenitis)
   5. Diffuse

Clinical Points Of Importance And Supplemental Information

A. Pseudotumor is almost always painful and unilateral.
B. When a pattern such as this is seen, suggest a workup for autoimmune diseases, Wegener's granulomatosis (antineutrophil cytoplasmic antibodies [ANCA]), and sarcoidosis (angiotensin-converting enzyme [ACE]) in your report.
C. Pseudotumor, granulomatoses, immune-mediated diseases, and lymphoma are indistinguishable, based solely on the imaging presentation, including the tendency for these processes to appear either of high or low signal compared with muscle on T2-weighted magnetic resonance imaging (MRI).
D. When such a disease process is hyperintense to muscle on T2-weighted images, this finding suggests a tendency for the process to be more responsive to immunosuppressive therapy. When hypointense to muscle on T2-weighted images, these processes have sometimes reached a more chronic, fibrotic stage.

Answers To Questions

1. Intraconal, extraconal, preseptal
2. Granulomatoses, histiocytoses, and so forth
3. Periscleritic, myositic, perineuritic, lacrimal (dacryoadenitis), diffuse

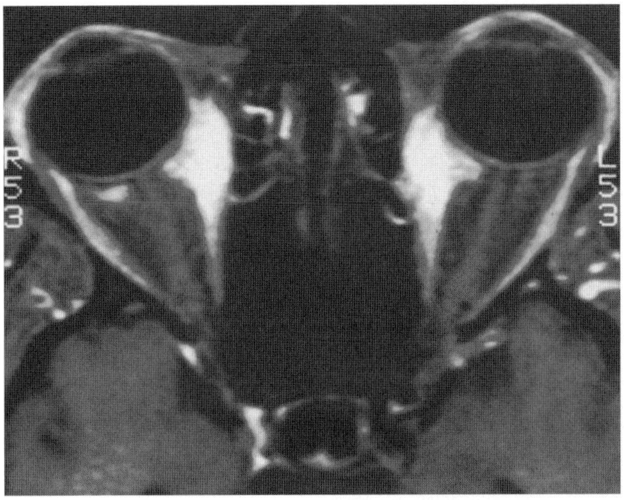

Figure 9F. Patient 1 with bilateral orbital sarcoidosis. T1-weighted, fat-suppressed image with contrast showing a transcompartmental (intra- and extraconal) mass surrounding the optic nerve on the both sides.

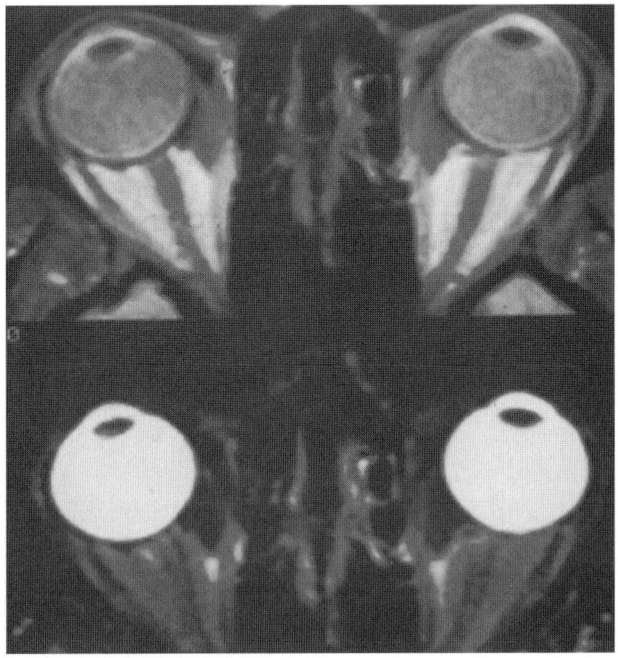

Figure 9G. Patient 1 with bilateral orbital sarcoidosis. Proton-density and T2-weighted images.

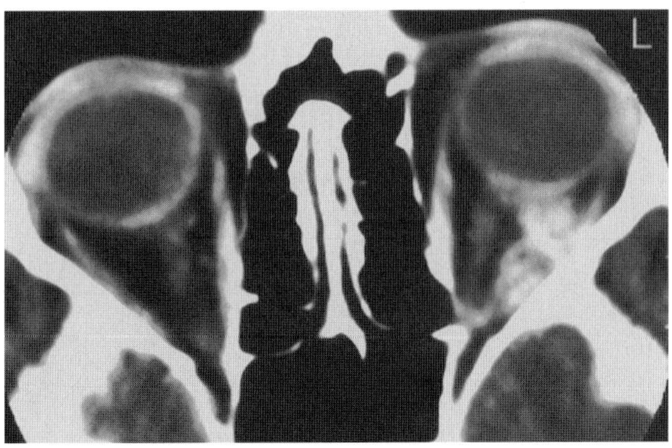

Figure 9H. Patient 2 with orbital pseudotumor. Computed tomography image showing a mixed perineuritic and myositic pattern.

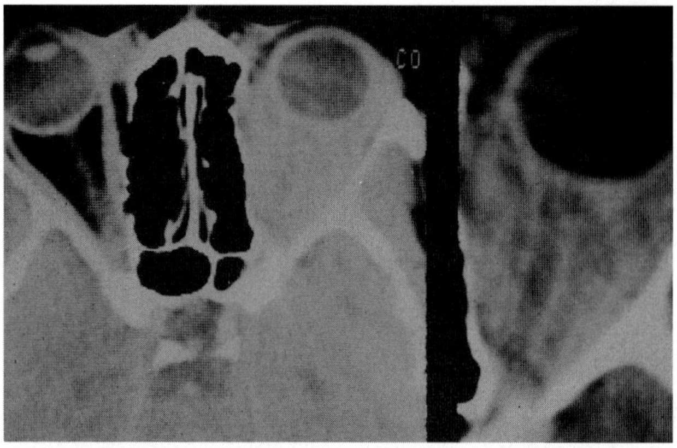

Figure 9I. Patient 3 with orbital pseudotumor. Computed tomography image showing a diffuse pattern.

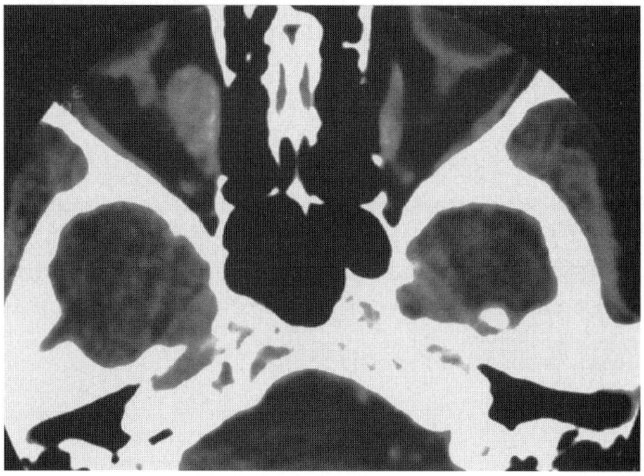

Figure 9J. Patient 4 with metastasis to the medial rectus muscle from an ovarian cancer in a patient presenting with ophthalmoplegia. Computed tomography image.

CASE 10

Clinical History: A 5-year-old presents with low-grade fever and acute, minimally painful proptosis.

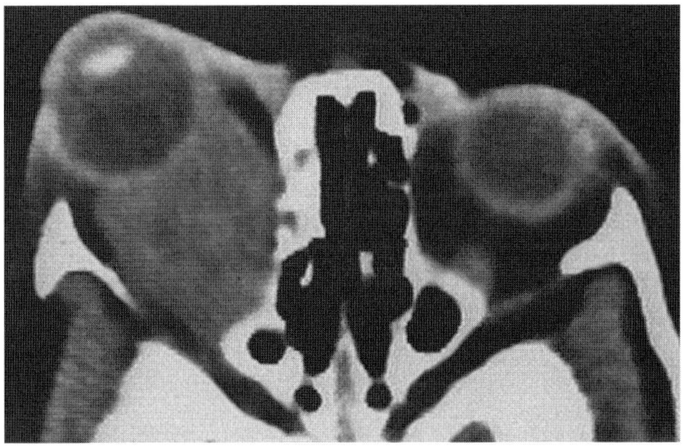

Figure 10A

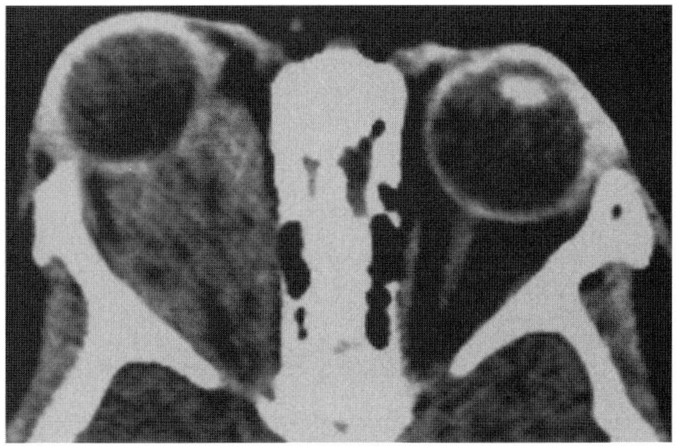

Figure 10B

1. Is the lesion intraconal, extraconal, or transcompartmental?
2. If the lesion were bilateral, how would it alter your differential diagnosis?
3. Give the one most likely diagnosis based on the imaging and clinical information.

Findings

Unilateral proptosis with a diffusely infiltrating, transcompartmental mass centered in the intraconal compartment of the orbit. The bones of the face, skull base, and sinonasal region appear normal so far as these areas are visualized and are presumed entirely normal for the purposes of discussion.

Problem

Child with potentially rapidly progressive proptosis and a transcompartmental, infiltrating orbital mass

Anatomy

A. Compartments of the orbit
   1. Extraconal
      a. Bone
      b. Subperiosteal
      c. Extraconal fat (peripheral orbital compartment)
   2. Intraconal

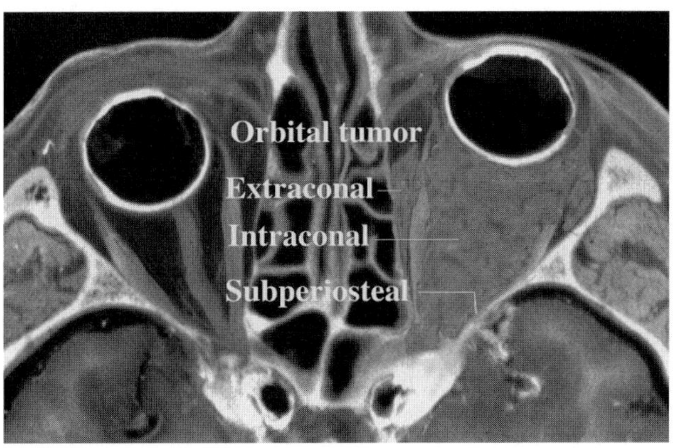

Figure 10C

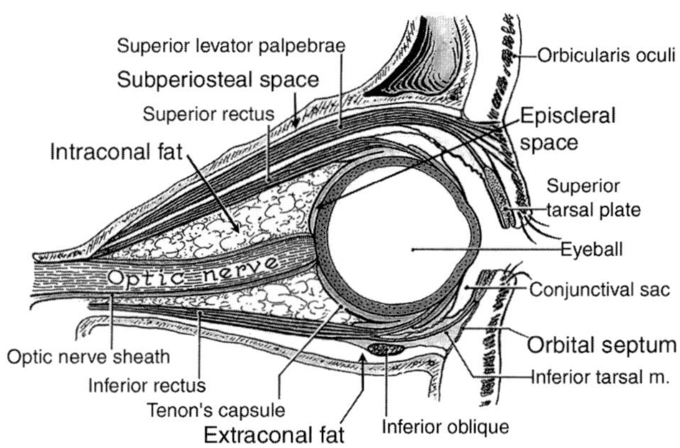

Figure 10D

Differential Diagnosis

Rhabdomyosarcoma, infiltrating "round cell" process (leukemia, lymphoma, poorly differentiated neoplasm, histiocytosis, or granulomatosis), pseudotumor

Diagnosis

Primary rhabdomyosarcoma of the orbit

Diagnostic Imaging Approach

A. Confirm presence and establish probable cause of proptosis.
B. Is the pathology intraconal, extraconal, or transcompartmental (origin and extent, if possible)?
C. Mass
   1. Focal or diffuse
   2. Unilateral or bilateral
   3. Margins
   4. Morphology
   5. Is there bone involvement or does the process arise from bone?

Clinical Points Of Importance And Supplemental Information

A. Exclude pyogenic sinonasal disease as a cause for the eye findings.
B. Rhabdomyosarcoma vs. bleed or inflammation in venolymphatic malformation are likely choices, based on history alone.
C. Granulocytic sarcoma (chloroma), lymphoma, and metastases (e.g., neuroblastoma) may be unilateral.
D. Pseudotumor is rare in young children as are Wegener's granulomatosis and sarcoidosis. Langerhans' cell histiocytosis should always be considered as a possible cause for infiltrating orbital masses in children, especially in cases of bone involvement.

Answers To Questions

1. Transcompartmental
2. Consider systemic diseases
3. Rhabdomyosarcoma vs. lymphoma

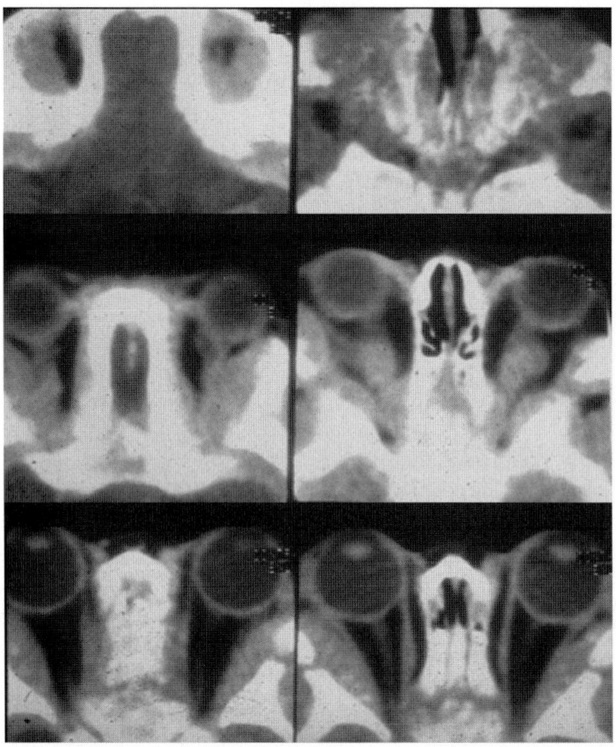

Figure 10E. Patient 1 with diffuse, bilateral leukemia, showing multifocal soft tissue masses diffusely involving both intraconal and extraconal spaces, subperiosteal space, and bony walls of the orbit on both sides. Computed tomography images.

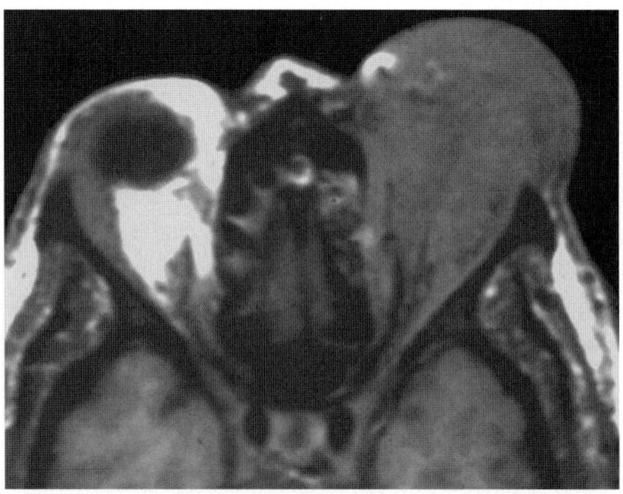

Figure 10F. Patient 2 with granulocytic sarcoma (focal leukemic mass). T1-weighted image without contrast showing a soft tissue mass involving the entire left orbit. Note the smaller mass on the right.

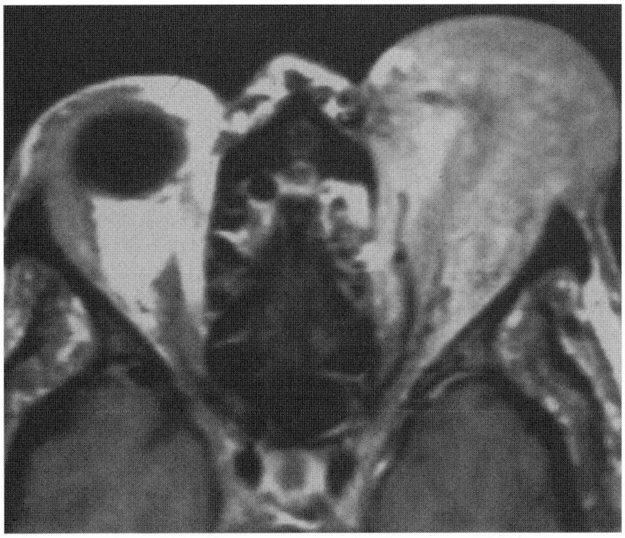

Figure 10G. Patient 2 with granulocytic sarcoma (focal leukemia). T1-weighted image with contrast. Note the smaller mass on the right.

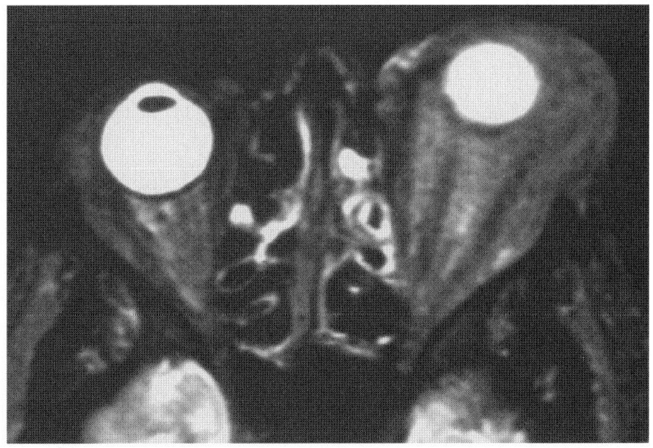

Figure 10H. Patient 2 with granulocytic sarcoma (focal leukemia). T2-weighted image.

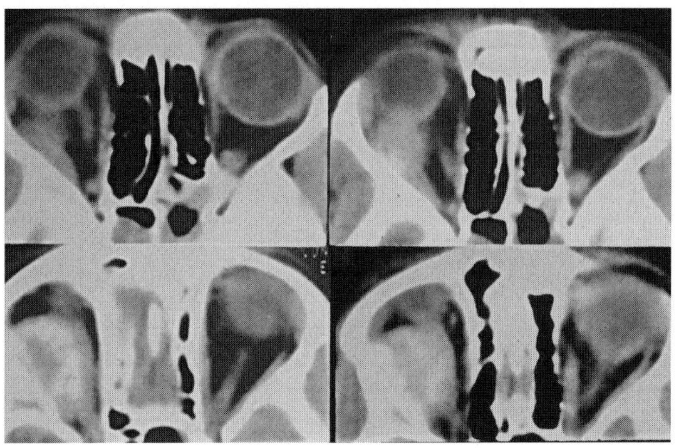

Figure 10I. Patient 3 with Ewing's sarcoma metastasis showing a calcified mass involving the right orbit.

CASE 11

Clinical History: A 26-year-old woman presents with a tender, slightly proptotic eye.

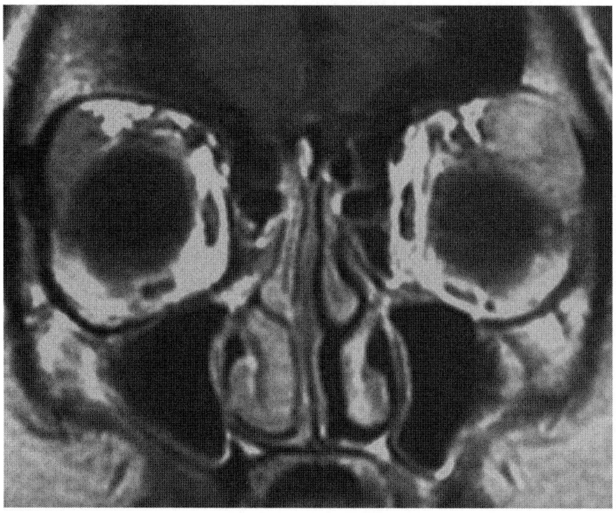

Figure 11A

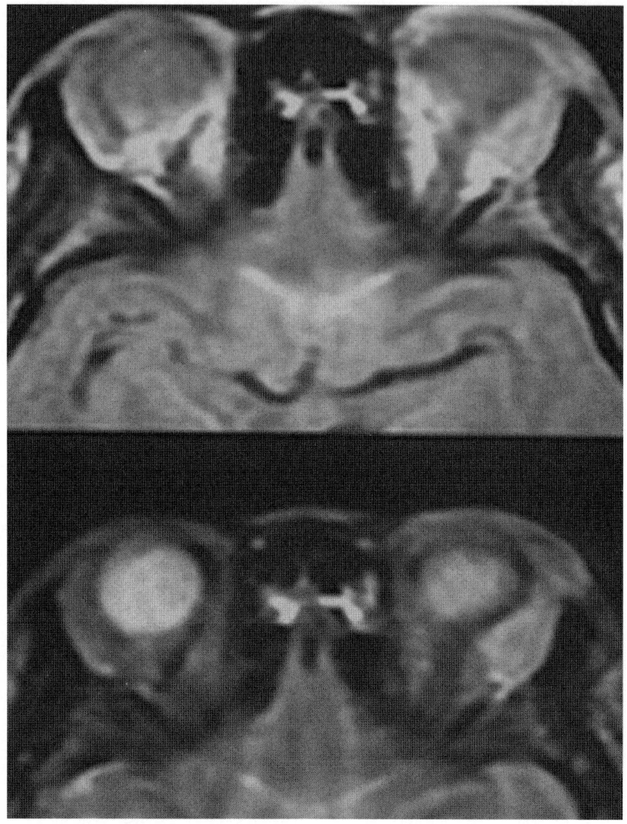

Figure 11B

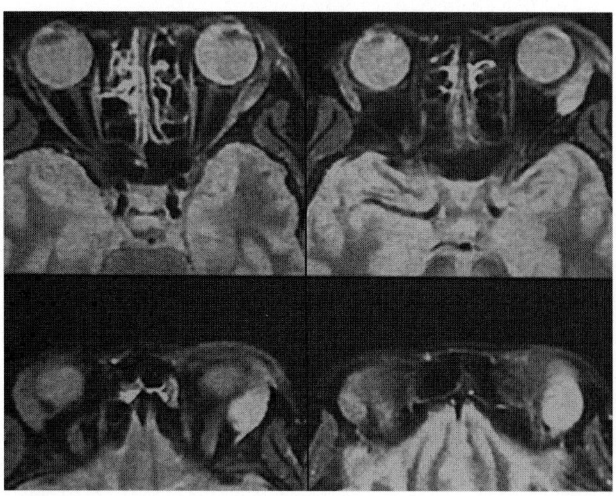

Figure 11C

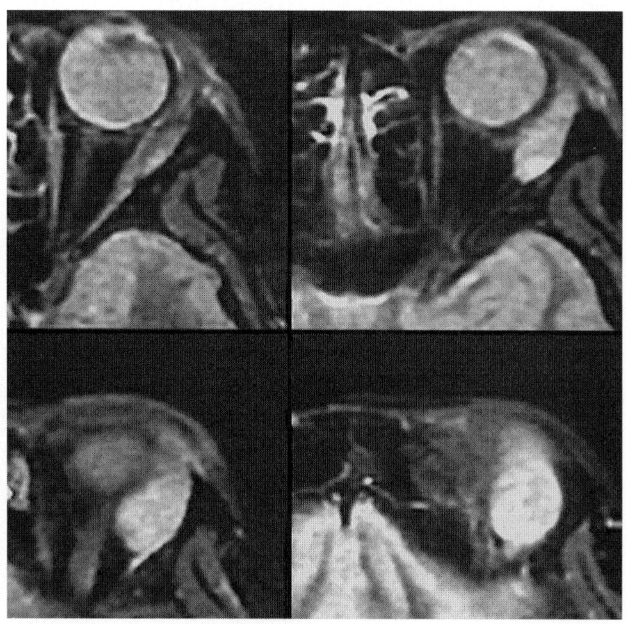

Figure 11D

1. Is the lesion intraconal, extraconal, or transcompartmental?
2. What structure is the focal point of the lesion?
3. List two neoplastic and three nonneoplastic lesions that might produce these findings. (For extra credit, add one additional lesion to each category.)
4. If the lesion were bilateral, how would it alter your list in question 3?

Findings

Inferomedial displacement of the eye by a mass that appears to be arising from and completely involving the left lacrimal gland. The mass involves both the orbital and palpebral portions of the gland. The disease process appears hyperintense to skeletal muscle on the density and T2-weighted pair of images, as well as the STIR images, and it enhances homogeneously. The margins of the mass are smooth. The remainder of the study is normal, showing the right lacrimal gland, bones, sinonasal region, and meninges to be normal so far as these areas are visualized. For the sake of discussion, findings on the remainder of the examination will be presumed to be entirely normal.

Problem

Inferomedial proptosis in a young adult caused by a mass in the upper outer quadrant of the orbit, apparently arising in and completely infiltrating the lacrimal gland.

Anatomy

A. Lacrimal gland (see Fig. 7E)
   1. Palpebral portion
   2. Orbital portion
B. Lacrimal drainage system
   1. Puncta, canaliculi
   2. Lacrimal sac
   3. Nasolacrimal duct
   4. Lacrimal bone and nasolacrimal canal

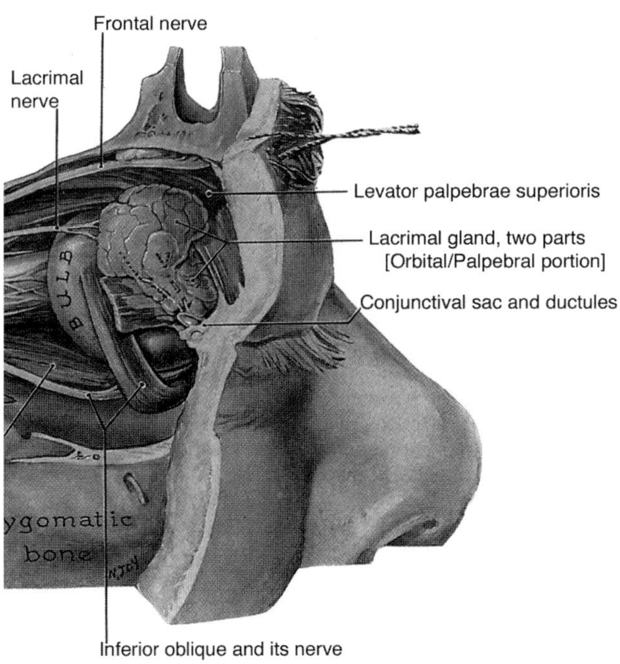

Figure 11E

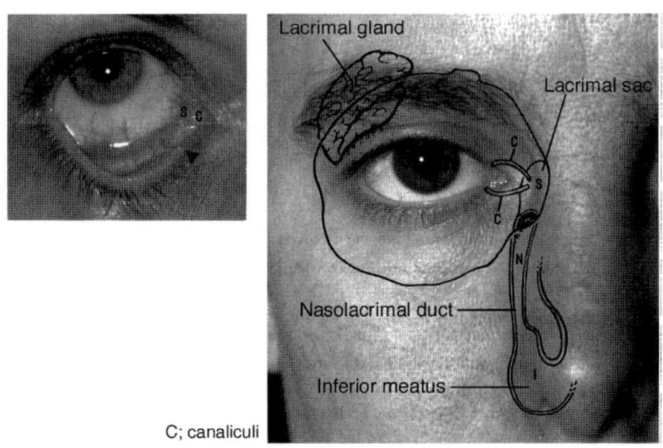

Figure 11F

Differential Diagnosis

1. Nonneoplastic: pseudotumor, sarcoidosis, infectious (viral) dacryoadenitis; immune-mediated dacryoadenitis or Sjögren's syndrome; dermoid, epidermoid
2. Neoplastic: epithelial (e.g., benign mixed tumor, adenoidcystic carcinoma, mucoepidermoid carcinoma), lymphoma
3. Bilateral disease favors systemic diseases (e.g., sarcoidosis, immune-mediated or Sjögren's syndrome, lymphoma)

Diagnosis

Sarcoidosis of the lacrimal gland

Diagnostic Imaging Approach

A. Intraconal, extraconal, or transcompartmental
B. Identify structure of origin (e.g., lacrimal gland, bone) and local extent
C. Unilateral, bilateral, or multifocal disease
D. Morphology of disease: margins, density or intensity, enhancement

Clinical Points Of Importance And Supplemental Information

A. Always consider lymphoma.
B. Malignant neoplasms are more common than benign neoplasms in the lacrimal gland, which is the expected trend because this is a modified minor salivary gland and in minor salivary glands the relative incidence of benign and malignant neoplasms is about equal.
C. Lacrimal gland disease is occasionally the first clinically obvious manifestation of an immune-mediated disease.
D. If benign mixed tumor can be anticipated, it is useful to suggest this to the surgeon so that the tumor capsule is not violated.
E. Signal intensity on T2-weighted images is nonspecific with regard to the differential diagnosis of disease processes such as sarcoidosis, lymphoma, and pseudotumor.

Answers To Questions

1. Extraconal
2. Lacrimal gland
3. Lymphoma, adenoidcystic carcinoma, pseudotumor, sarcoidosis, dacryoadenitis
4. Lymphoma, immune-mediated disease, sarcoidosis are most likely

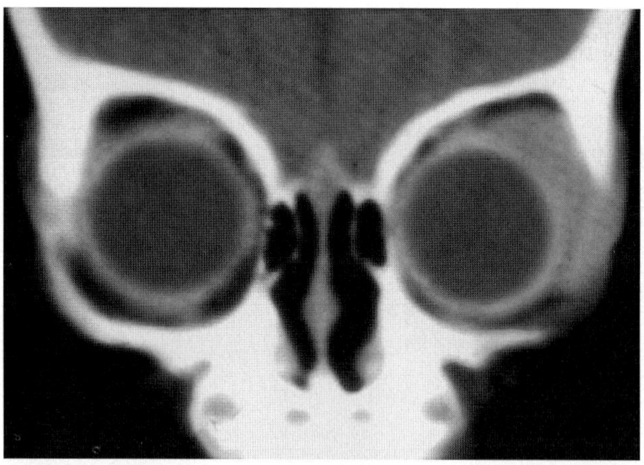

Figure 11G. Patient 1 with hemangioma of the lacrimal gland showing a mass centered in the superolateral aspect of the orbit on the left. Contrast-enhanced, coronal computed tomography image.

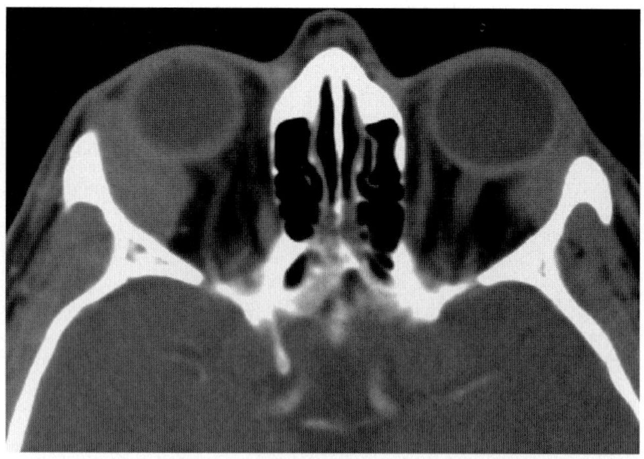

Figure 11H. Patient 2 with non-Hodgkin's lymphoma. Contrast-enhanced computed tomography image showing bilateral infiltration of the lacrimal gland.

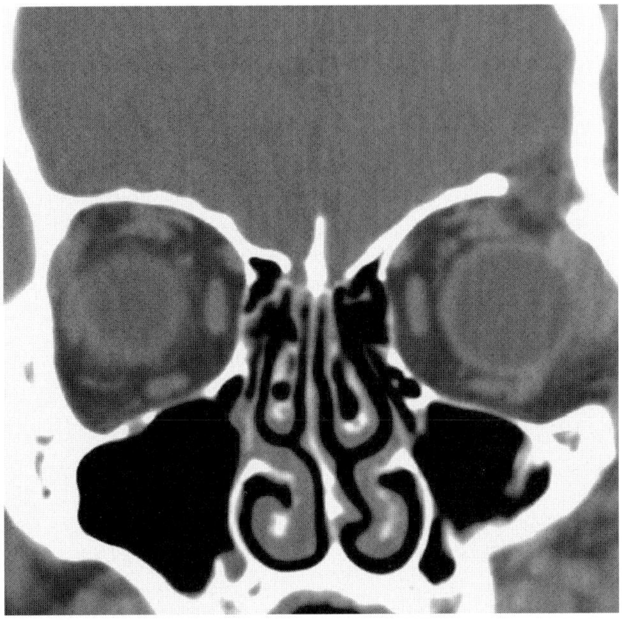

Figure 11I. Patient 3 with dermoid of the orbit. Computed tomography image at soft tissue window setting shows a focal mass involving the superolateral aspect of bony orbit, which is partially of fatty attenuation.

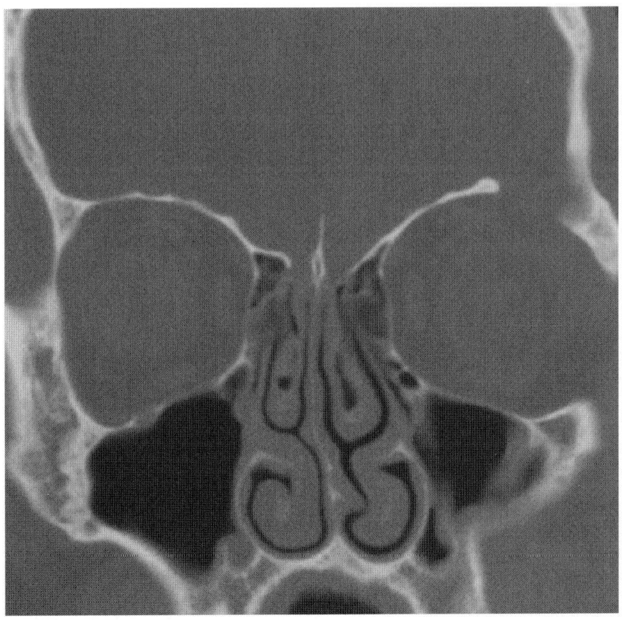

Figure 11J. Patient 3 with dermoid of the orbit. Computed tomography image at bone window setting shows well-defined focal defect at superolateral aspect of left orbit.

CASE 12

Clinical History: A 50-year-old man presents with proptosis.

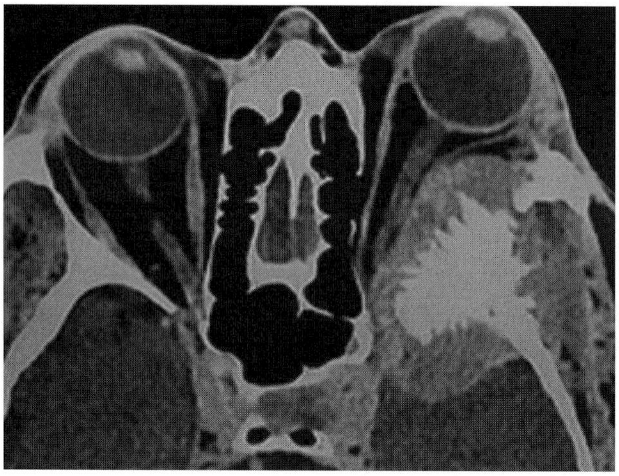

Figure 12A

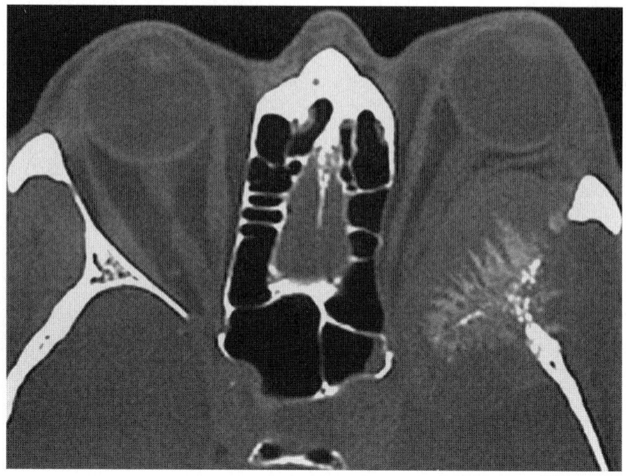

Figure 12B

1. Overall, is the mass intraconal, extraconal, or transcompartmental? Be as specific as possible about the site of origin.
2. List the diagnostic possibilities.

Findings

An apparently solitary mass centered in the greater wing of the sphenoid bone, resulting in marked proptosis of the left eye with an intracranial extradural or dural component, as well as a soft tissue component in the orbit and adjacent periorbital region. The mass enhances with contrast. A spiculated pattern of ossification or calcification that has a "sunburst" appearance is seen centrally.

Problem

Unilateral proptosis in a middle-aged adult caused by a lesion centered in the greater wing of the sphenoid bone

Anatomy

A. Orbital periosteum (review)
B. Greater wing of the sphenoid as it relates to:
   1. Orbit: superior and inferior orbital fissures
   2. Floor of the middle cranial fossa
   3. Squamous portion of the temporal bone

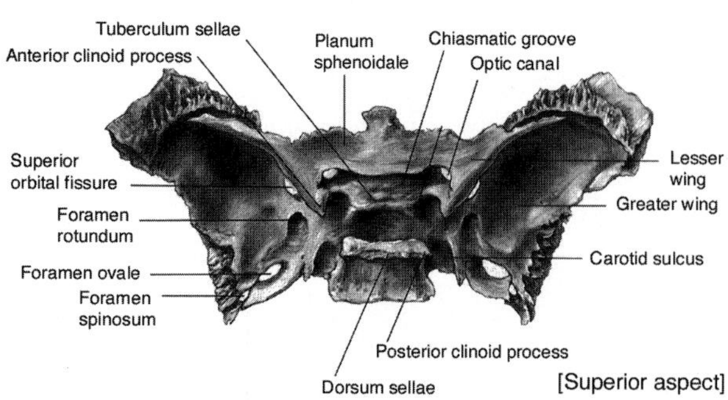

Figure 12C

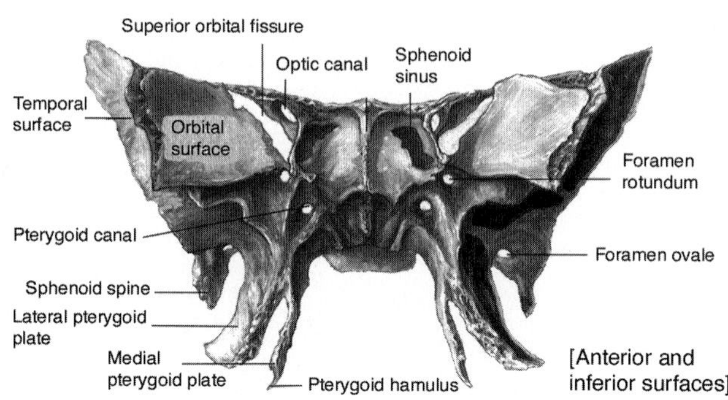

Figure 12D

Differential Diagnosis

Intraosseous meningioma, metastasis, osteogenic sarcoma

Diagnosis

Intraosseous meningioma of the greater wing of the sphenoid bone

Diagnostic Imaging Approach

A. Intraconal, extraconal, or transcompartmental
B. Identify specific site and structure of origin
C. Full extent
D. Morphology of disease: enhancement, matrix (osseous, chondroid, fibrous)

Clinical Points Of Importance And Supplemental Information

A. Intraosseous and *en plaque* meningiomas can be difficult to recognize. Failure to recognize their nature and the extent of bone involvement can lead to unnecessarily morbid attempts at gross total resection.
B. It can be difficult to distinguish fibrous dysplasia from intraosseus meningioma without both a magnetic resonance image (MRI) and computed tomography (CT) scan.
C. The greater wing of the sphenoid bone is the most common site of skull base metastasis.

Answers To Questions

1. Extraconal; originates from bone
2. Metastasis, meningioma, osteosarcoma

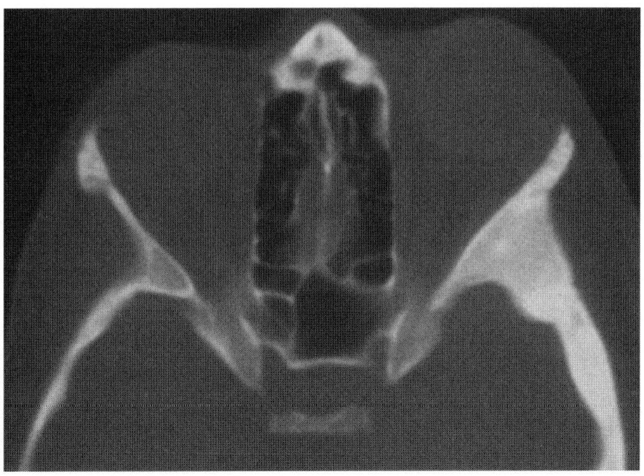

Figure 12E. Patient 1 with fibrous dysplasia. Computed tomography image at bone window setting, showing ground-glass pattern involving the lateral wall of orbit, greater wing of the sphenoid bone, and squamous portion of the temporal bone on the left with an "expanded" appearance.

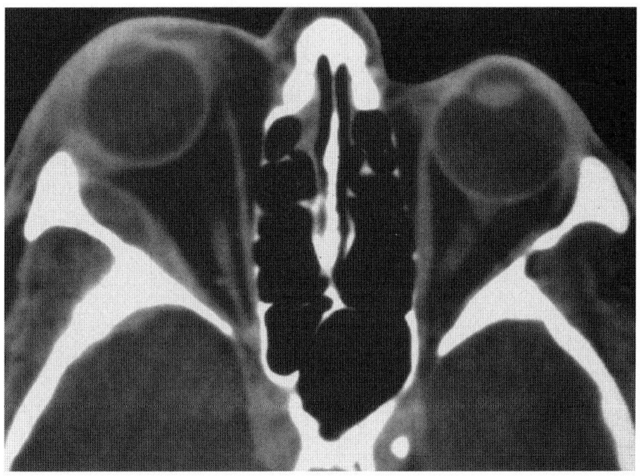

Figure 12F. Patient 2, with osteoblastic metastasis from carcinoma of the prostate, presents with proptosis. Contrast-enhanced computed tomography image showing a mass centered in the lateral wall of the orbit on the right, with dural thickening intracranially; involvement of the temporalis muscle externally; and extension into the subperiosteal space in the orbit.

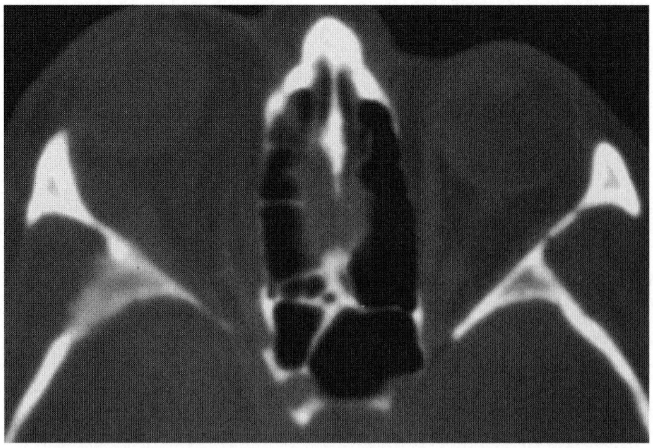

Figure 12G. Patient 2, with osteoblastic metastasis from carcinoma of the prostate, presents with proptosis. Computed tomography image at bone window setting.

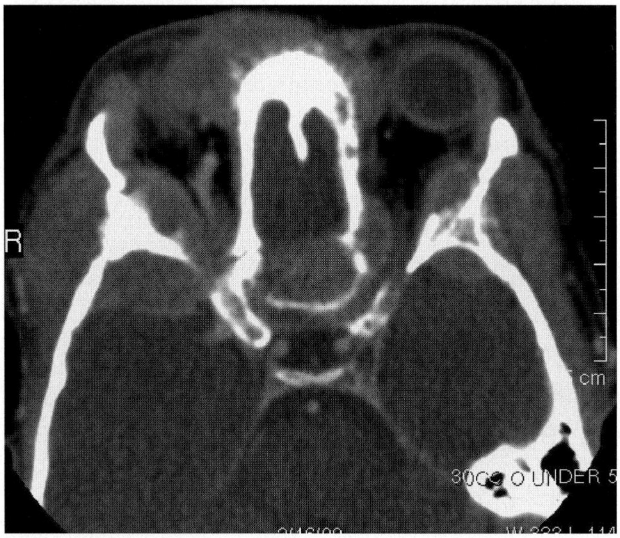

Figure 12H. Patient 3 with multiple bone metastases to the orbit from neuroblastoma. Contrast-enhanced computed tomography image.

CASE 13

Clinical History: A 20-year-old man presents with fever, proptosis, visual loss, and periorbital cellulitis.

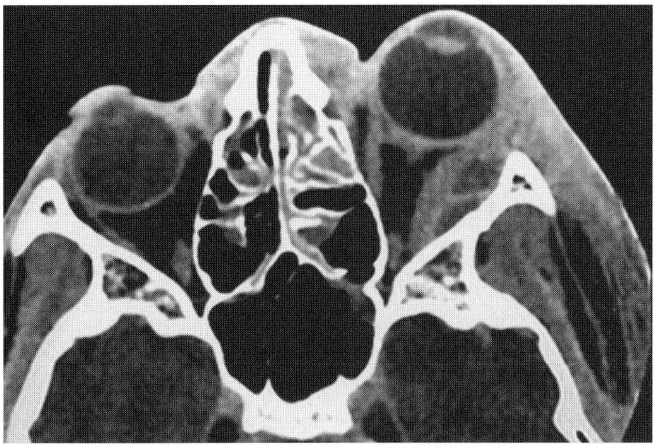

Figure 13A

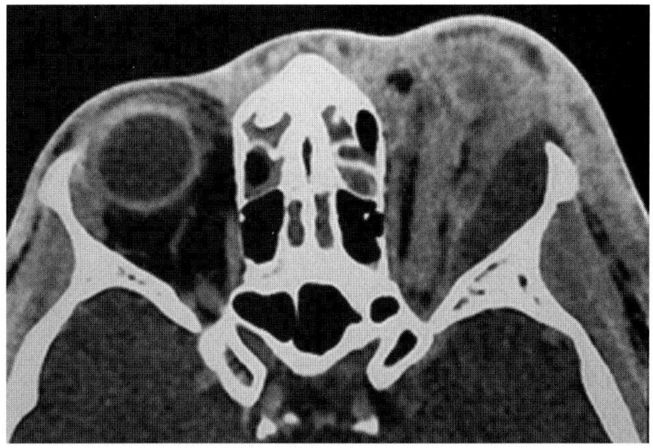

Figure 13B

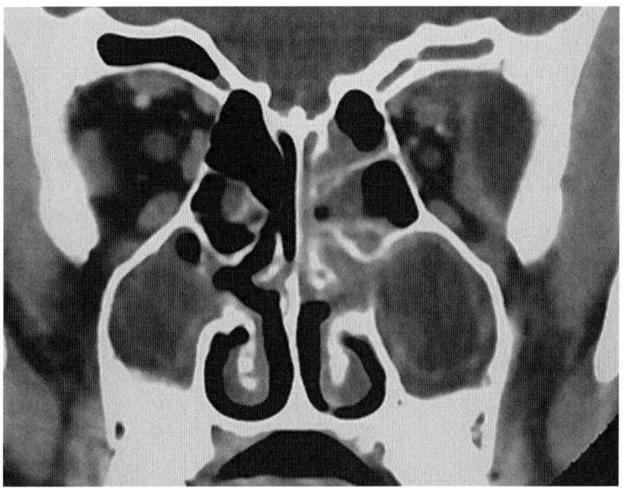

Figure 13C

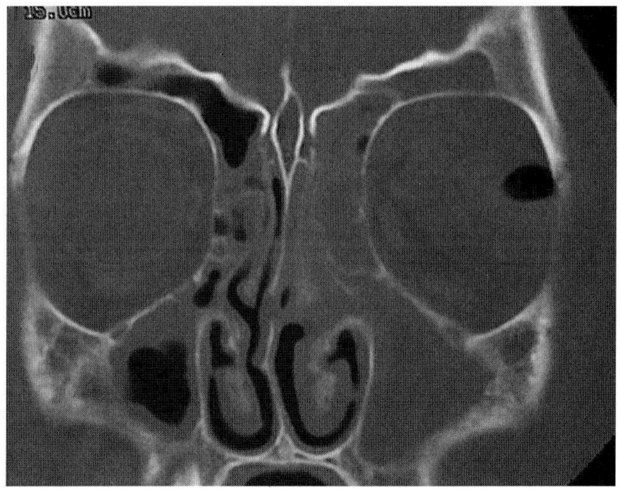

Figure 13D

1. What is the underlying cause of this abscess? Why is it in the lateral orbit?
2. What compartment(s) does the abscess involve?
3. What possible causes of the diminished visual acuity would you suggest to the ophthalmologist?

Findings

A subperiosteal, loculated, peripherally enhancing and gas-containing fluid collection in the superior lateral orbit. On the more superior axial section is seen a suggestion of the process extending into the muscle cone along its superior lateral margin. Obvious marked proptosis and thickening of the preseptal soft tissues are noted.

The coronal bone window view shows possible thinning of the bone between the most lateral aspect of the frontal sinus floor and the orbital soft tissues.

Diffuse mucoperiosteal thickening in the nasal cavity and sinuses that is worse on the left than the right

Problem

Periorbital cellulitis and proptosis in a young patient with postseptal orbital complications, all likely secondary to pyogenic sinonasal infection

Anatomy

A. Orbital septum
   1. Attachments
   2. Relationship to the eyelid
   3. Sites of "weakness"
B. Orbital periosteum
C. Tenon's capsule (space) and its relationship to the optic sheath
D. Orbital veins and their proximal and distal anastomoses

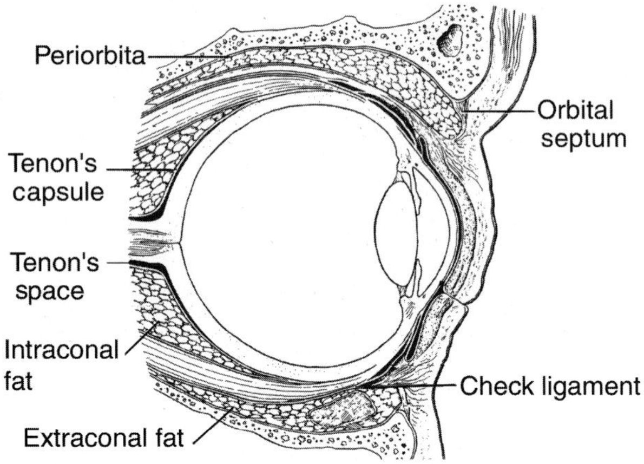

Figure 13E

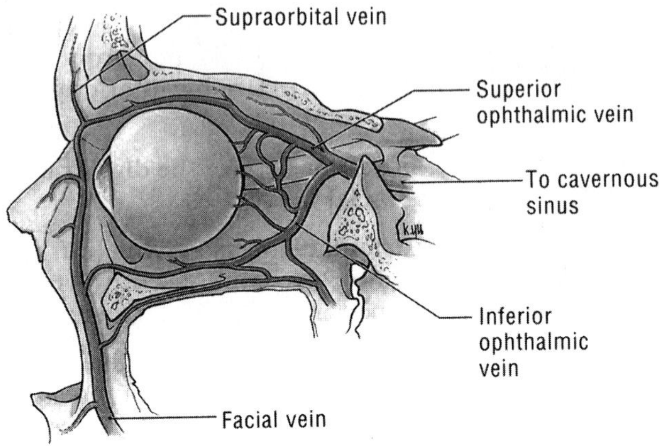

Figure 13F

Differential Diagnosis

Not applicable

Diagnosis

Preseptal cellulitis, with superolateral subperiosteal orbital abscess and probable intraconal extension of purulent material secondary to pyogenic sinusitis

Diagnostic Imaging Approach

A. Is there postseptal disease?
   1. Abscess vs. cellulitis
   2. Anatomic relationship to the causative pathology (e.g., purulent rhinosinusitis)
B. Any other complications?
   1. Ocular
   2. Optic nerve or sheath
   3. Intracranial
   4. Osteomyelitis

Clinical Points Of Importance And Supplemental Information

A. Determine whether the orbital abscess is in continuity with sinus disease to help plan the approach for drainage of the abscess or sinuses.
B. When vision is diminished, try to identify a specific cause, including tension orbit; intraconal extension with involvement of the optic nerve; septic thrombophlebitis within orbital veins or the cavernous sinus with secondary ischemic or congestive optic neuropathy; extension of sinonasal pathology to the orbital apex or optic canal, with compressive optic neuropathy.
C. Postseptal abscess will almost always be drained. Postseptal cellulitis may require sinus drainage as a part of management, but may also be controlled with antibiotic therapy alone.

Answers To Questions

1. Sinusitis. Direct spread from frontal sinus or thrombophlebitic spread
2. Extra and intraconal
3. Early tension orbit: vascular

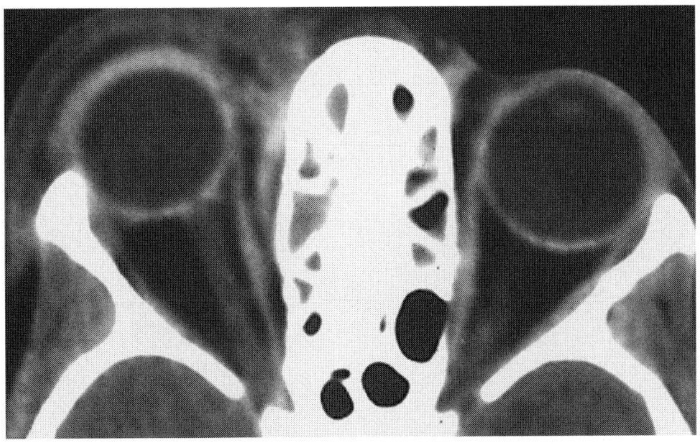

Figure 13G. Patient 1 with subperiosteal cellulitis (or early subperiosteal abscess), showing thickening of the periorbita, which contains a fluid attenuation area adjacent to the opacified ethmoid sinus on the right. Computed tomography image.

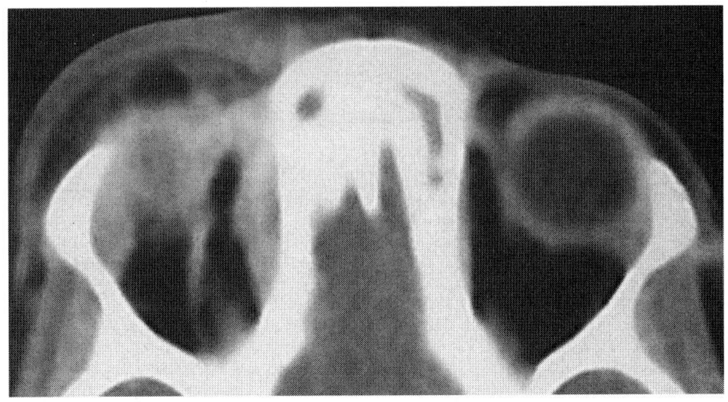

Figure 13H. Patient 1 with subperiosteal cellulitis (or early subperiosteal abscess). Computed tomography image superior to 13G.

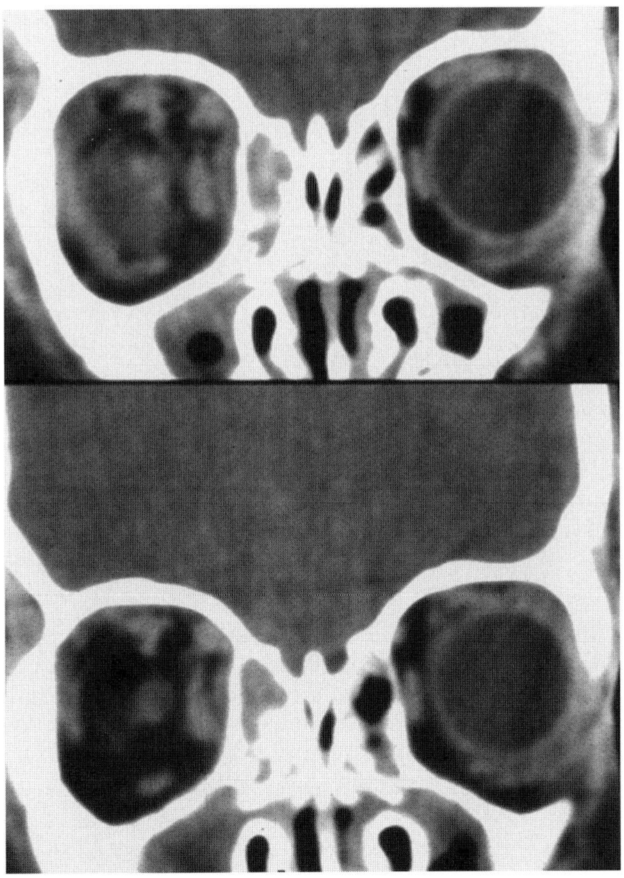

Figure 13I. Patient 1 with subperiosteal cellulitis (or early subperiosteal abscess). Coronal computed tomography images of same findings as in 13G and 13H.

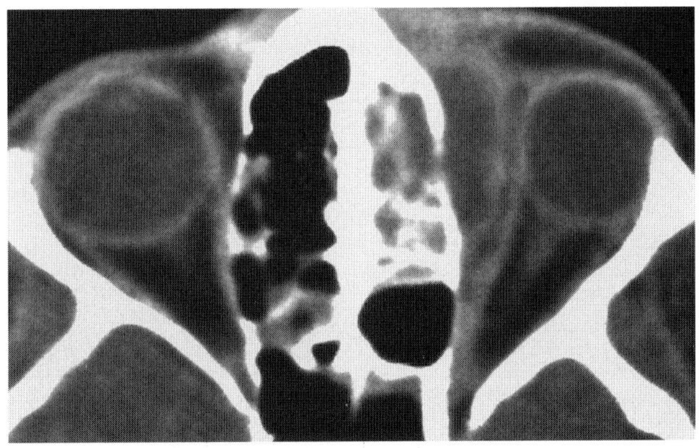

Figure 13J. Patient 2 with subperiosteal abscess as an orbital complication of ethmoid sinusitis, showing a fluid collection in the subperiosteal space along the medial wall of the orbit adjacent to the opacified ethmoid sinus on the left. Computed tomography image.

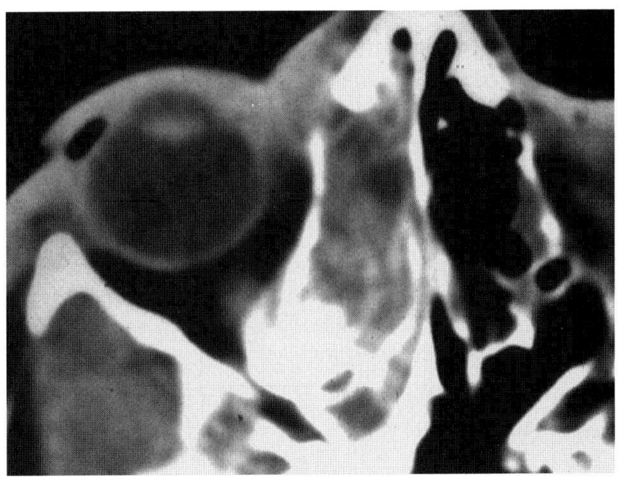

Figure 13K. Patient 3 with preseptal soft tissue swelling as a complication of sinusitis. Computed tomography image.

CASE 14

Clinical History: A 58-year-old woman presents with diminished visual acuity.

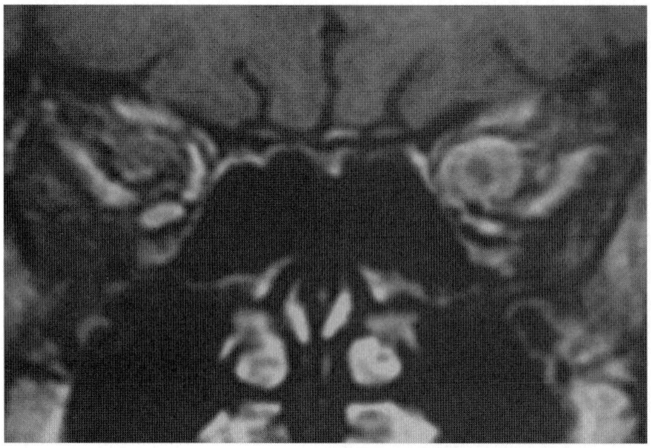

Figure 14A

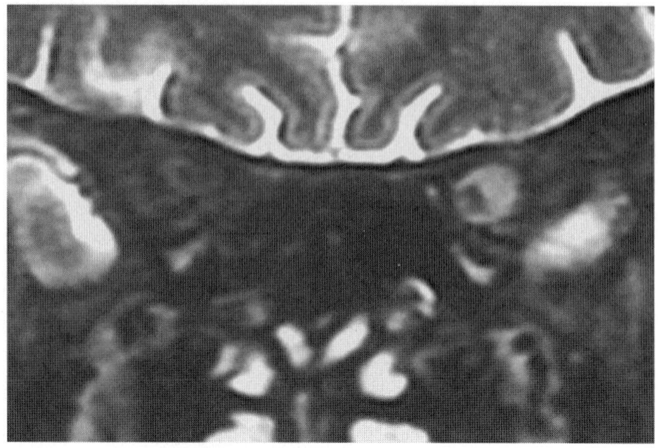

Figure 14B

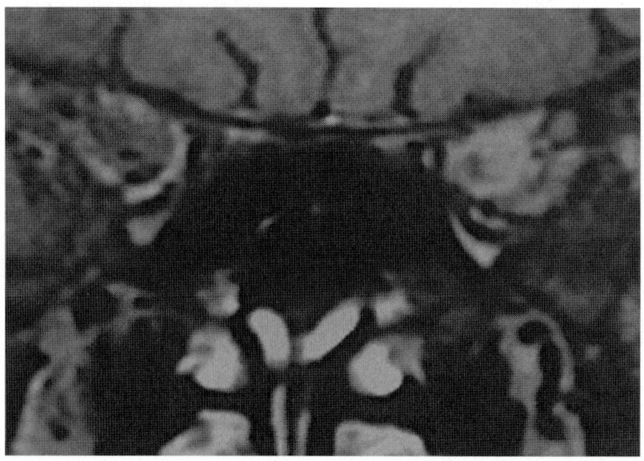

Figure 14C

1. Is the lesion intraconal or extraconal? From what structure does it most likely originate?
2. What magnetic resonance imaging (MRI) pulse sequences are used?
3. Give the most likely diagnosis. What will be a prime clinical consideration related to the extent of the lesion?

Findings

On both fat-suppressed, contrast-enhanced T1-weighted and T2-weighted images is seen a disease process within the optic sheath that surrounds an otherwise normal-appearing optic nerve. The abnormality enhances homogenously and has sharp margins; it is also markedly hyperintense to muscle on the T2-weighted images. Note that, although surrounded, the optic nerve is relatively normal.

Problem

Visual loss in a middle-aged woman caused by an intraconal mass most likely arising from the optic sheath

Anatomy

A. Optic nerve–sheath complex
   1. Nerve
   2. Sheath
   3. Subarachnoid space
B. Optic canal or tuberculum sella
C. Optic chiasma

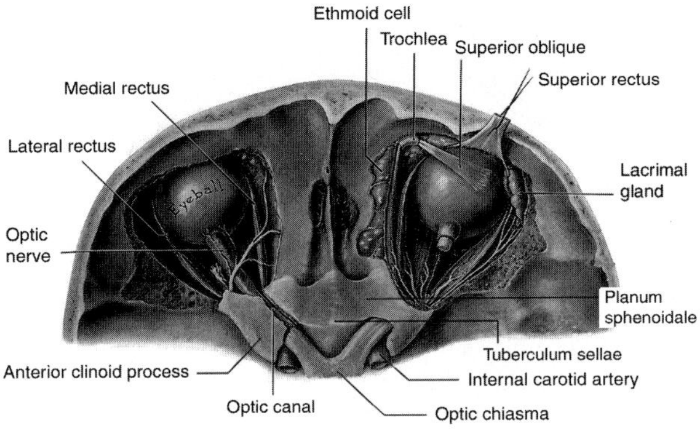

Figure 14D

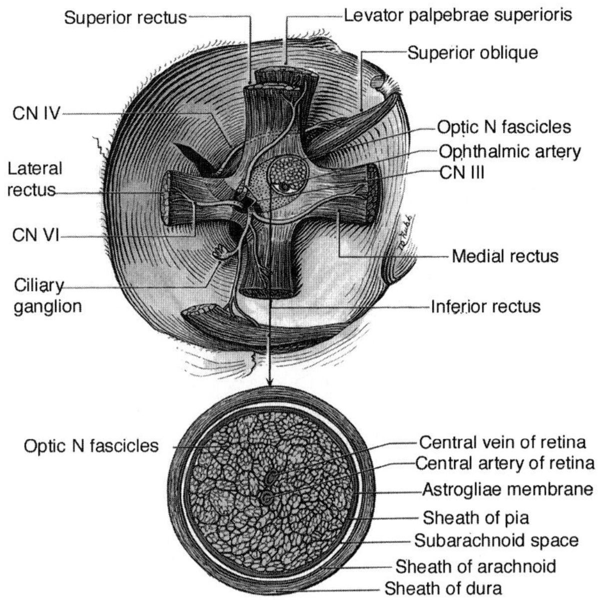

Figure 14E

Differential Diagnosis

Perineural processes arising in or secondarily extending to the optic sheath (which, for the most part, are diseases of the pia-arachnoid) including:

1. Pseudotumor
2. Meningeal carcinomatosis or lymphomatosis, or leukemic or plasma cell infiltration
3. Wegener's granulomatosis, sarcoidosis, Langerhans' cell histiocytosis
4. Infectious granulomatous process such as syphilis

Diagnosis

Optic sheath meningioma

Diagnostic Imaging Approach

A. Does the pathology arise from the sheath, nerve, within the subarachnoid space, or adjacent to the sheath (vector of sheath contact with the lesion)?
B. Extent
   1. Orbit
   2. Optic canal
   3. Chiasma
   4. Optic tracts or radiations
   5. Dural, leptomeningeal disease
C. Unilateral, bilateral, or multifocal
D. Morphology: infiltrative, discrete mass, enhancement, calcifications

Clinical Points Of Importance And Supplemental Information

A. Optic sheath meningiomas can be bulky and more infiltrative than in this case. They can involve the inner and outer aspects of the optic sheath. The conditions in the differential diagnosis given above usually have ill-defined margins and cause edema of the optic nerve or intraconal orbital fat adjacent to the optic sheath. Optic glioma is not included in differential diagnosis because the lesion is clearly not of the nerve.

B. The relationship of the lesion to the chiasma will always be of critical importance in therapeutic decisions.

C. MRI with and without fat suppression (FS) and with contrast is ideal for showing extent of the lesion. Very high spatial resolution is mandatory in evaluating optic nerve or sheath lesions.

Answers To Questions

1. Intraconal. Optic nerve sheath.
2. T1-weighted fat-suppression image with contrast; fast spin echo (FSE) T2-weighted, fat-suppression image
3. Optic sheath meningioma. Proximal spread toward the chiasma

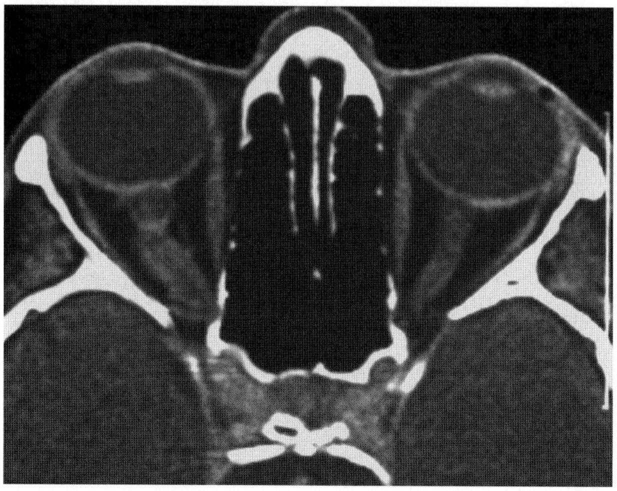

Figure 14F. Patient 1 with optic sheath meningioma showing an enhancing mass around the optic nerve on the right, representing "tram-track" appearance. Contrast-enhanced computed tomography image.

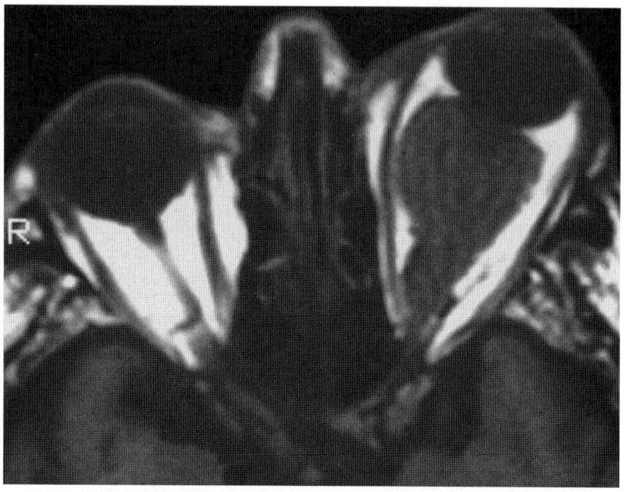

Figure 14G. Patient 2 with large optic sheath meningioma. T1-weighted image without contrast, showing a mass extending along the optic nerve sheath.

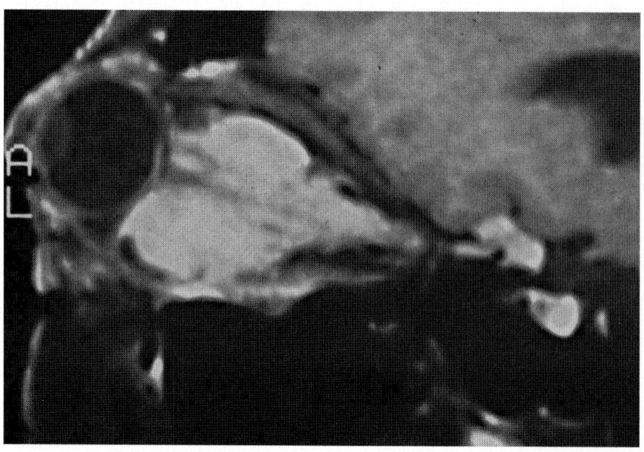

Figure 14H. Patient 2 with large optic sheath meningioma protruding to the cranial end of the optic canal. T1-weighed sagittal image with contrast.

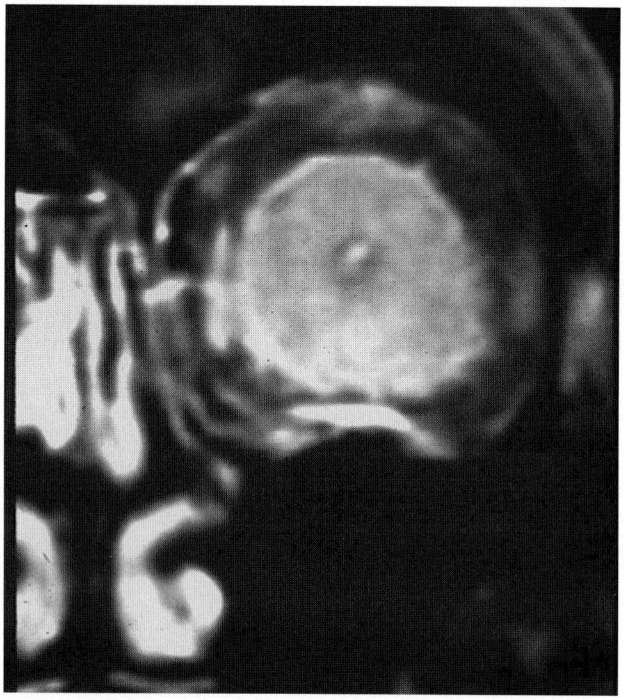

Figure 14I. Patient 2 with large optic sheath meningioma showing the effects of the compressive optic neuropathy on the nerve as it is encased by the tumor. Fat-suppressed, T1-weighted coronal image with contrast.

CASE 15

Clinical History: A 3-year-old child presents with diminished visual acuity.

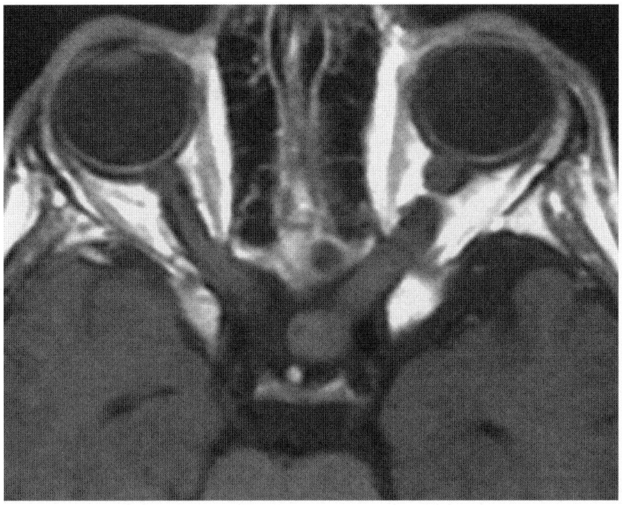

Figure 15A

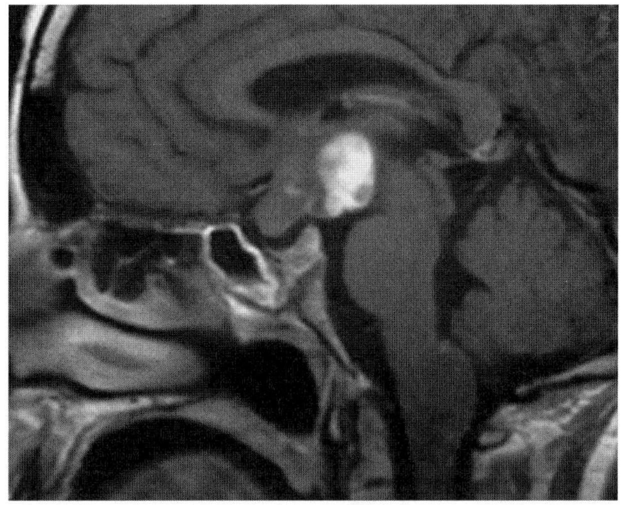

Figure 15B

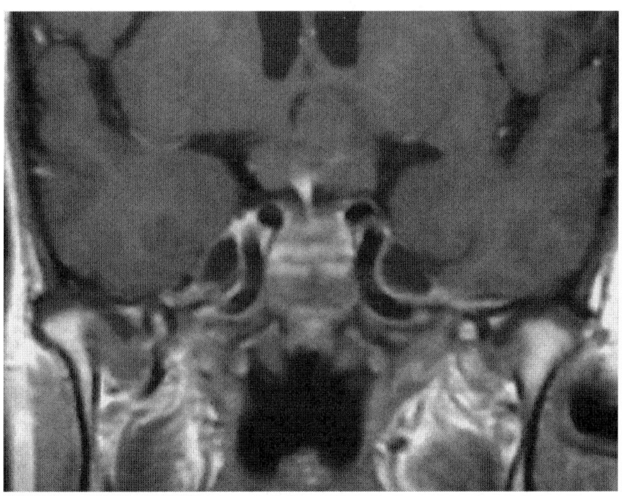

Figure 15C

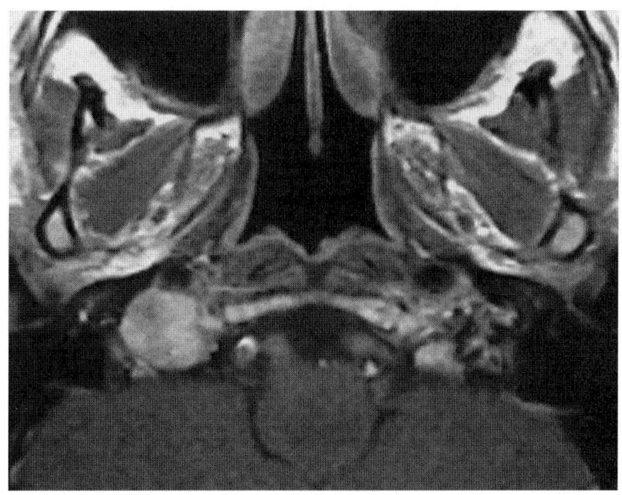

Figure 15D

1. What is the cause of the visual loss?
2. What overall disease process might be afflicting this child? Name four manifestations of this disease process.

Findings

The optic nerves and optic chiasma are enlarged by a mass that distorts or involves the adjacent hypothalamus and pituitary stalk. An enhancing mass is centered in the right jugular foramen. Other enhancing, extraaxial "nodules" are present just ventral to the upper medulla.

Problem

Bilaterally enlarged optic nerves, chiasma, tracts, and other extraaxial masses in a child with diminished visual acuity

Anatomy

Optic nerve (visual) pathways

1. Nerve globe junction
2. Orbital segment
3. Canalicular segment
4. Prechiasmatic segment and chiasm
5. Optic tracts and radiations
6. Visual cortex

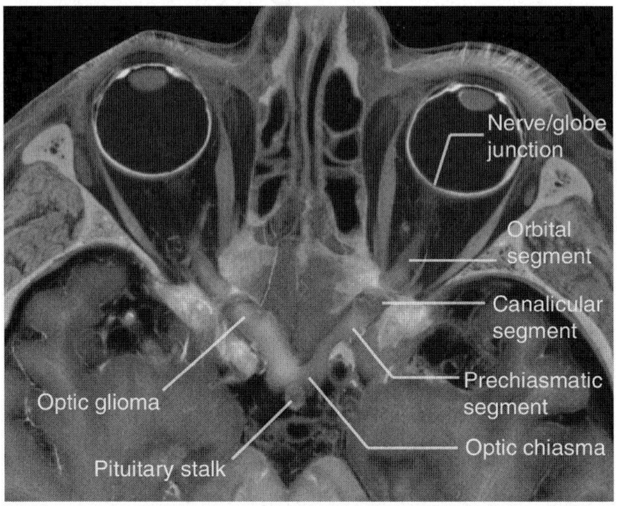

Figure 15E

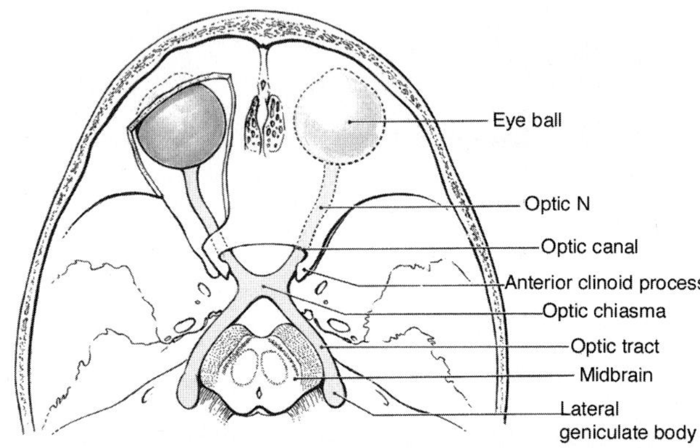

Figure 15F

Differential Diagnosis

1. If unilateral and relative subtle nerve enlargement, demyelinating disease (e.g., MS, ADEM); viral
2. If enhancement on surface of nerve, inflammatory or neoplastic, leptomeningeal or subarachnoid space process

Diagnosis

Bilateral optic gliomas with extension to chiasma, tracts, and along the optic radiation. Probable neurofibromas in the right jugular fossa, possibly involving the cisternal segments of the lower cranial nerves. All are manifestations of neurofibromatosis type 1 (NF1).

Diagnostic Imaging Approach

A. Does the pathology arise from the sheath, nerve, or within the subarachnoid space?
B. Extent of visual pathway involvement (nerve–eye junction to visual cortex.
C. Unilateral, bilateral, multifocal, leptomeningeal, or dural disease
D. Morphology: enhancement, infiltrative, intensity
E. Other findings (i.e., other stigmata of NF1)

Clinical Points Of Importance And Supplemental Information

A. In patients with optic gliomas, look for other manifestations of NF1.
B. Optic sheath ectasia can be a normal variant or a sign of subtle optic nerve sheath or subarachnoid space pathology.

Answers To Questions

1. Bilateral optic gliomas
2. NF1–prior case (see Clinical Points of Importance in Case 4)

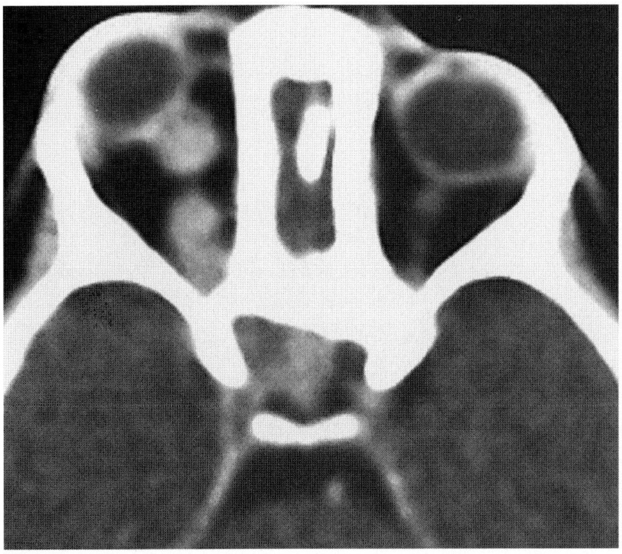 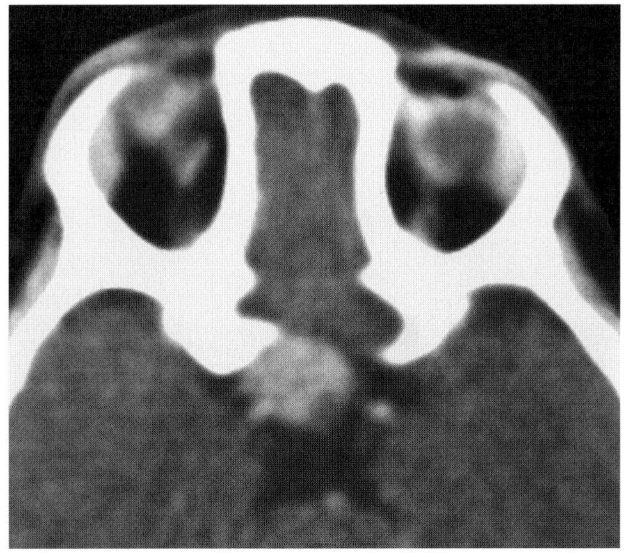

Figures 15G and **15H.** Patient 1 with an optic glioma extending through optic canal. Contrast-enhanced computed tomography image.

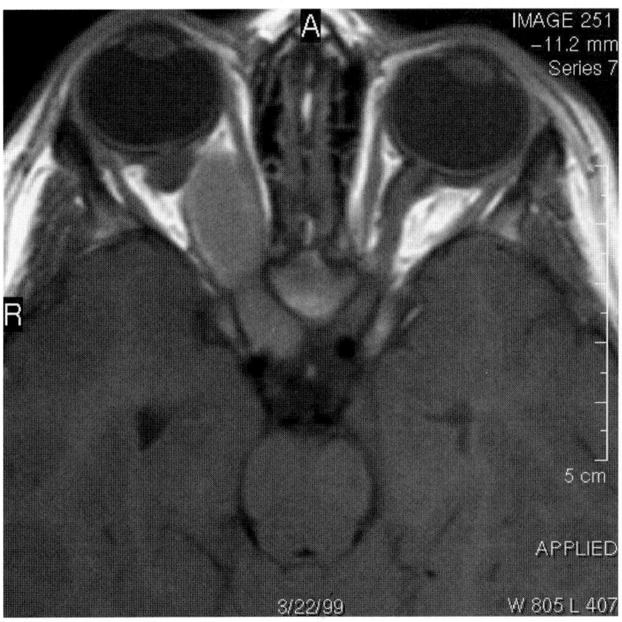

Figure 15I. Patient 2 with optic glioma. T1-weighted axial image with contrast showing tubular, enhancing mass along expected course of right optic nerve, extending intracranially through the optic canal.

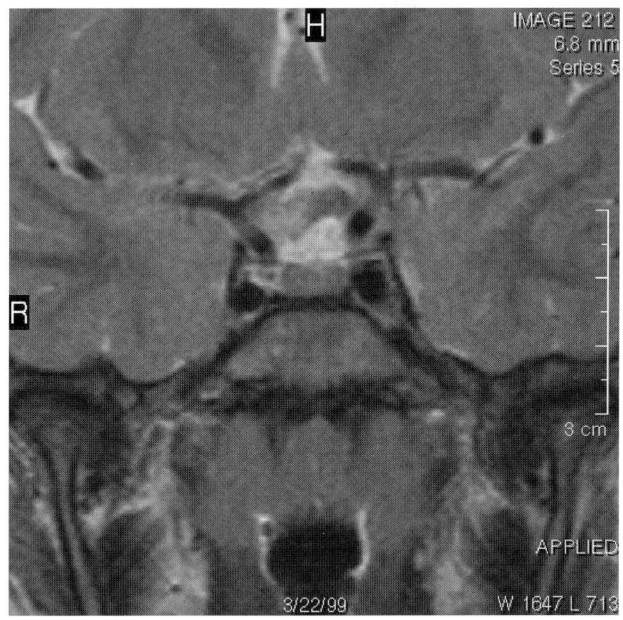

Figure 15J. Patient 2 with optic glioma. T2-weighted coronal image showing involvement of right half of the optic chiasma.

CASE 16

Clinical History: An 8-year-old girl presents with visual loss.

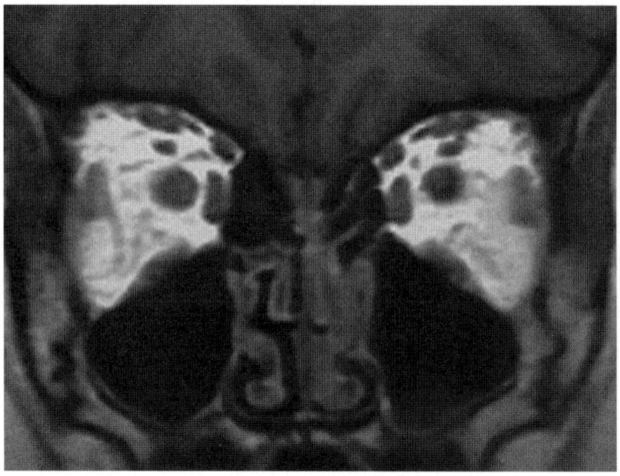

Figure 16A

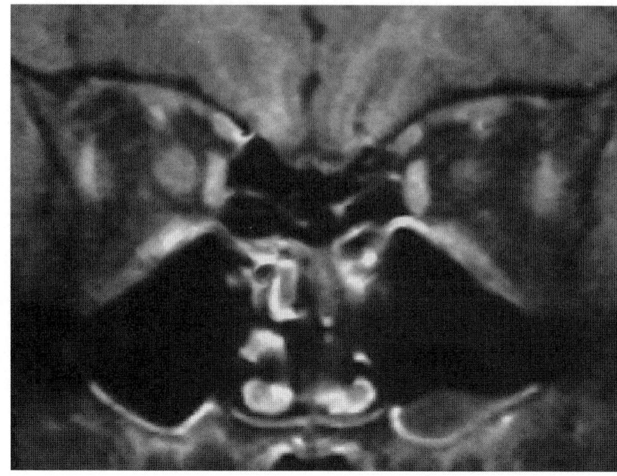

Figure 16B

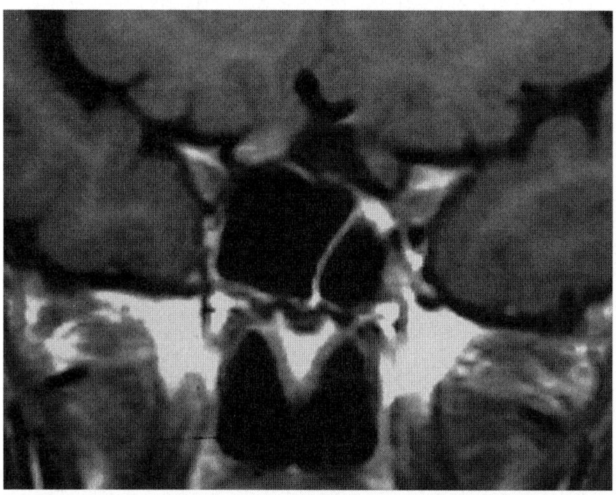

Figure 16C

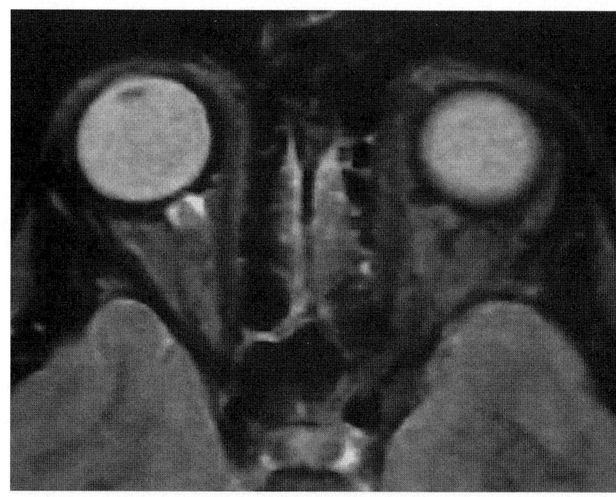

Figure 16D

1. What magnetic resonance imaging (MRI) technique is used in the second image?
2. List three diagnostic possibilities. If the patient were 30 years old, what would be the leading diagnostic possibility and what would you do to confirm it?

Findings

Unilateral thickening of the optic nerve on the right, which enhances after administration of paramagnetic contrast as best seen on fat-suppressed, T1-weighted image. The enhancement is visible at the prechiasmatic segment of the nerve as seen on the coronal image. Fat-suppressed, T2-weighted image shows a focal high intensity area at the right optic nerve–sheath junction because of trapping of cerebral spinal fluid in the distal optic sheath.

Problem

Acute, unilateral optic nerve enlargement and enhancement in a child with visual loss

Anatomy

Optic nerve–sheath complex: normal appearance on T1- and T2-weighted images with and without fat suppression.

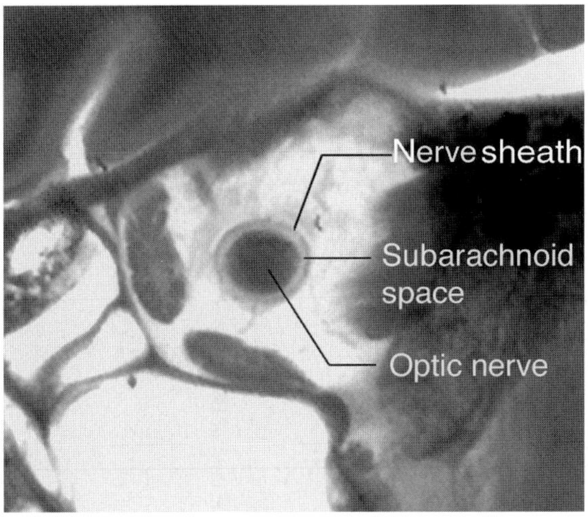

Figure 16E

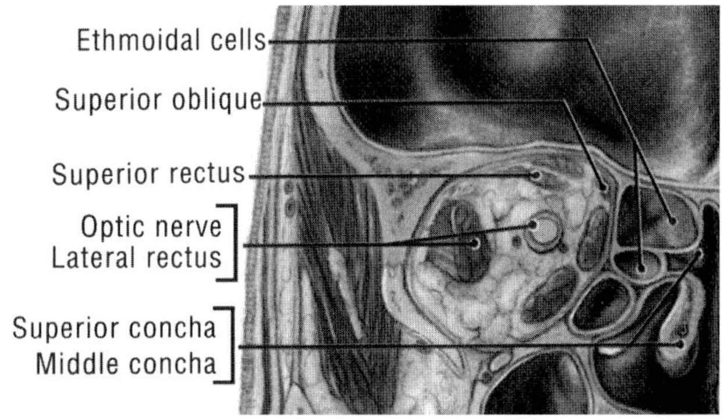

Figure 16F

Differential Diagnosis

Optic glioma, leptomeningeal disease with secondary nerve involvement, lesion compressing the nerve with secondary swelling.

Diagnosis

Optic neuritis: viral vs. demyelinating disease

Diagnostic Imaging Approach

A. Is the disease limited to the nerve?
B. Is the nerve enlarged and does it enhance?
C. Extent of involvement
D. Unilateral, bilateral, or multifocal disease
E. Associated findings: deep white matter, leptomeninges

Clinical Points Of Importance And Supplemental Information

A. Main point of imaging is usually to exclude "compressive lesion" and these are seen only in about 1% to 5% of patients who present for imaging.
B. High-resolution studies of the nerve are mandatory.
C. Protocols must include sequences that exclude demyelinating disease and leptomeningeal pathology with a high degree of confidence.
D. Follow-up MRI in 4 to 6 weeks (up to 3 months) will show resolution of swelling and separate this process from optic glioma.

Answers To Questions

1. Enhanced T1-weighted fat suppression image
2. Optic glioma, optic neuritis, leptomeningeal disease with secondary optic nerve involvement. Optic neuritis; perform T_2-weighted images through the entire brain and cervical spinal cord.

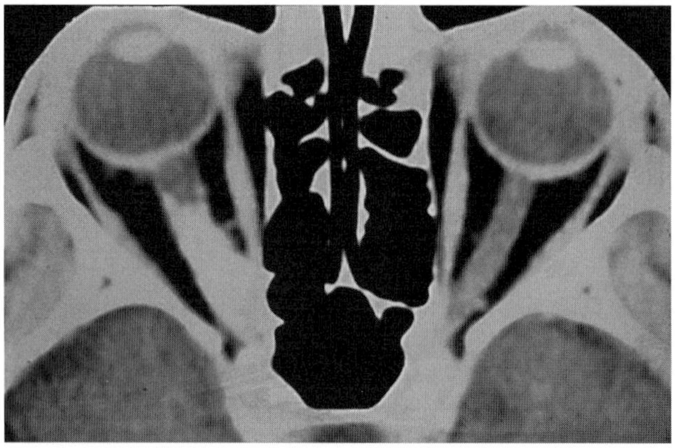

Figure 16G. Patient 1 with optic sheath meningioma, presenting as an enhancing mass along right optic nerve. Contrast-enhanced computed tomography image.

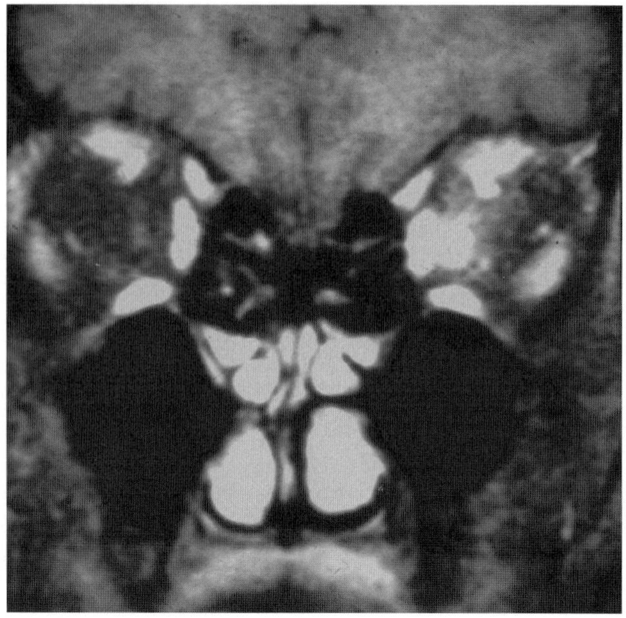

Figure 16H. Patient 2 with Wegener's granuloma, showing abnormal enhancement of thickened optic nerve–sheath complex and evidence of perioptic infiltration. T1-weighted, fat-suppression image with contrast.

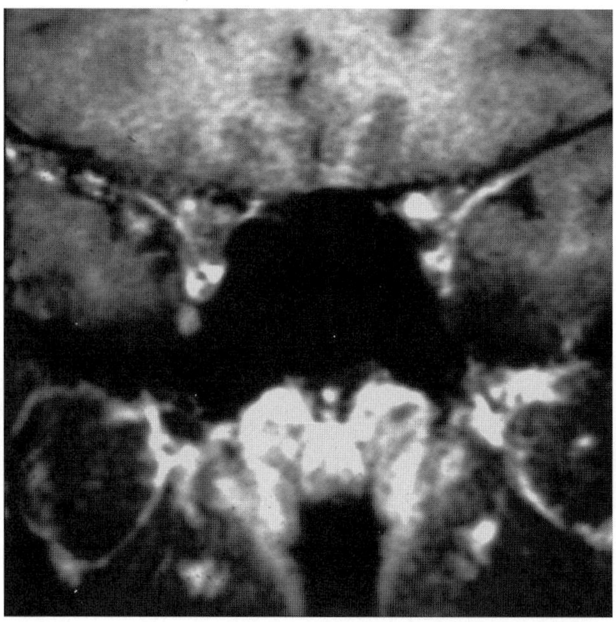

Figure 16I. Patient 2 with Wegener's granuloma, showing abnormal enhancement of thickened optic nerve–sheath complex within the optic canal. T1-weighted, fat-suppression image with contrast.

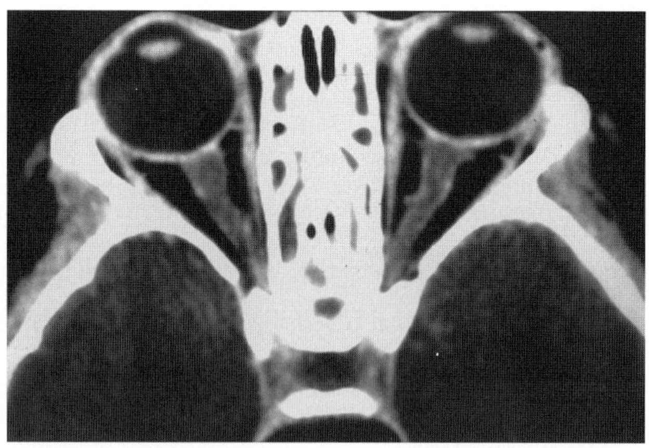

Figure 16J. Patient 3 with streptococcal meningitis. Contrast-enhanced computed tomography image showing abnormal enhancement of dura and nodular thickening of the optic sheath contour bilaterally.

CASE 17

Clinical History: A 45-year-old woman presents with bilateral ocular dysmotility and visual loss on the right.

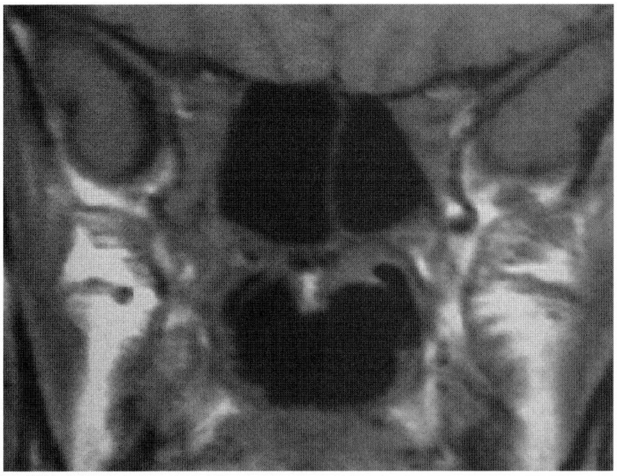

Figure 17A

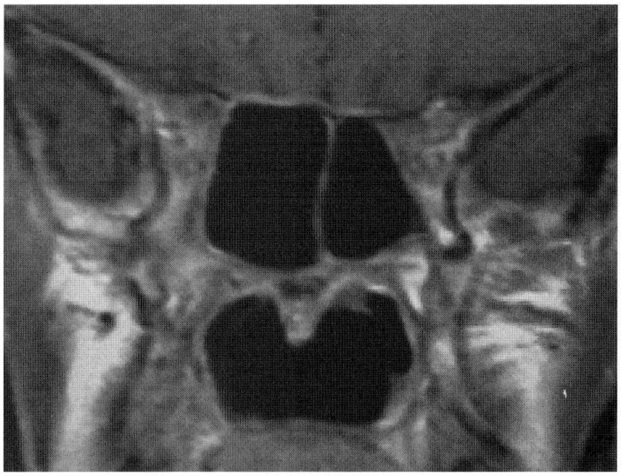

Figure 17B

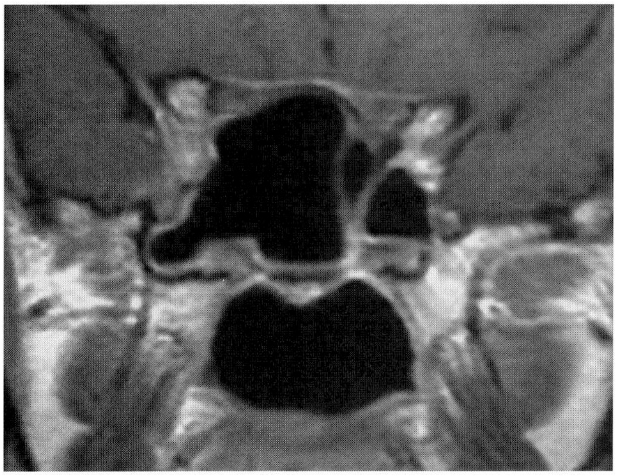

Figure 17C

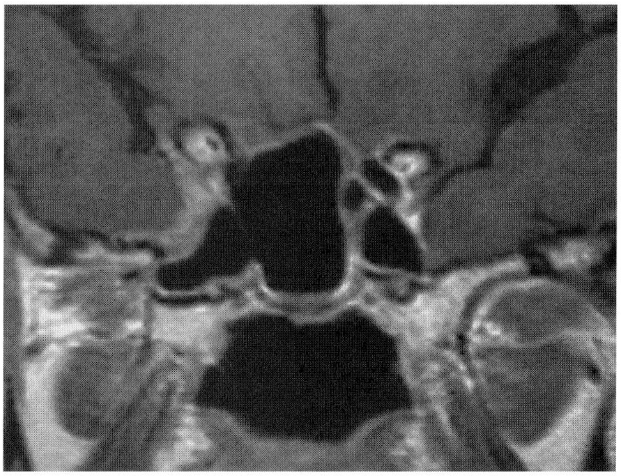

Figure 17D

1. List the normal contents of the superior and inferior orbital fissures.
2. Comparing the pre- and postcontrast coronal images, what is the major generic finding? Is the disease unilateral or bilateral?
3. List three categories of disease that could produce these findings. Name two laboratory studies that might help in evaluating this patient.

Findings

Comparing the pre- and postcontrast coronal T1-weighted images, enhancing tissue replaces the high intensity of normal fat within the both superior and inferior orbital fissures bilaterally. No frank destruction is seen of adjacent bony structures. Also note dural enhancement along the planum sphenoidale and around the optic sheath.

Problem

An infiltrating process involving both orbital apices

Anatomy

A. Superior orbital fissure
   1. Bony limits
   2. Contents (including cranial nerves)
B. Inferior orbital fissure
   1. Bony limits
   2. Contents (including cranial nerves)
C. Optic canal

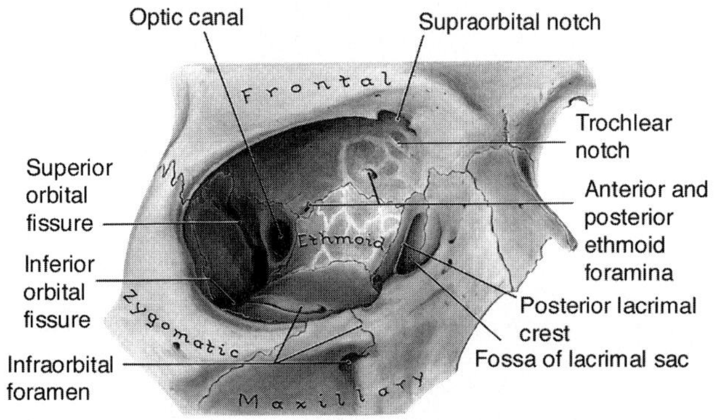

Figure 17E

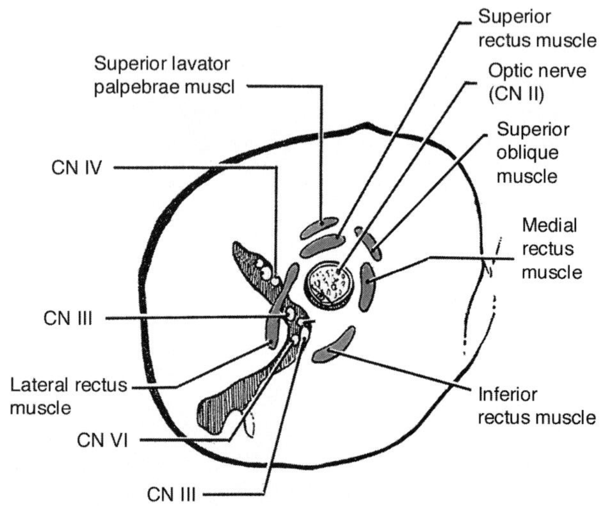

Figure 17F

Differential Diagnosis

1. Bilateral, infiltrative process favors systemic disease (e.g., sarcoid [angiotensin-converting enzyme (ACE)] Wegener's granulomatosis [antineutrophil cytoplasmic antibodies (ANCA)]; histiocytosis).
2. Neoplastic disease that might occur (depending on age): leukemia, lymphoma, plasmacytoma, and metastatic disease
3. In the absence of pain, pseudotumor is unlikely.
4. In diabetes, consider aspergillosis (for unilateral disease).

Diagnosis

Wegener's granulomatosis of the orbits

Diagnostic Imaging Approach

A. Consider the anatomic pathways of cranial nerves responsible for ocular motility from brainstem to each intraocular muscle–look for pathology along that pathway.
B. Consider where, anatomically, both vision and ocular motility might be disrupted by the same lesion.
C. Morphology of disease: focal mass, infiltrative
D. Unilateral, bilateral, or multifocal
E. Associated findings: bone, dural, leptomeningeal involvement

Clinical Points Of Importance And Supplemental Information

A. When infiltrative processes are present in this location, it is extremely important to mention Wegener's granulomatosis and sarcoidosis to clinicians so that appropriate laboratory studies are ordered. Wegener's granulomatosis requires prompt cyclophosphamide treatment for best results.
B. Always consider aspergillosis (fungus) in unilateral orbital apex disease, especially in diabetics.

Answers To Questions

1. Cranial nerves III–VI, fat small vessels
2. Obliteration of fat by tissue that enhances. Bilateral.
3. Neoplastic (lymphoma). Inflammatory granulomatosis (sarcoidosis–ACE; Wegener's granulomatosis–ANCA); infectious–fungus

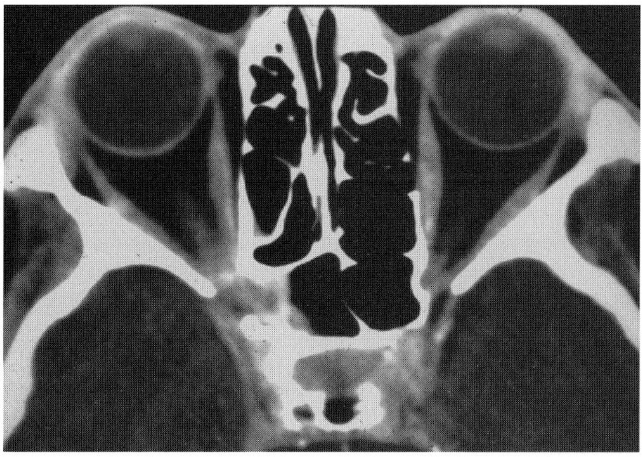

Figure 17G. Patient 1 with aspergillosis presenting as focal mass involving the left cavernous sinus and orbital apex. Contrast-enhanced computed tomography image.

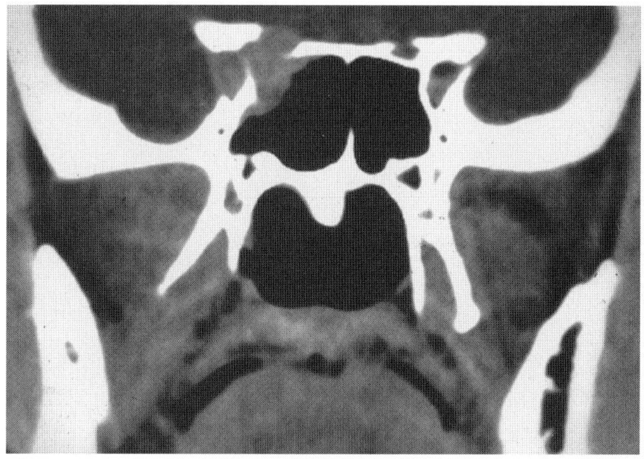

Figure 17H. Patient 1 with aspergillosis presenting as a destructive mass involving optic canal and superior orbital fissure. Contrast-enhanced, coronal computed tomography image.

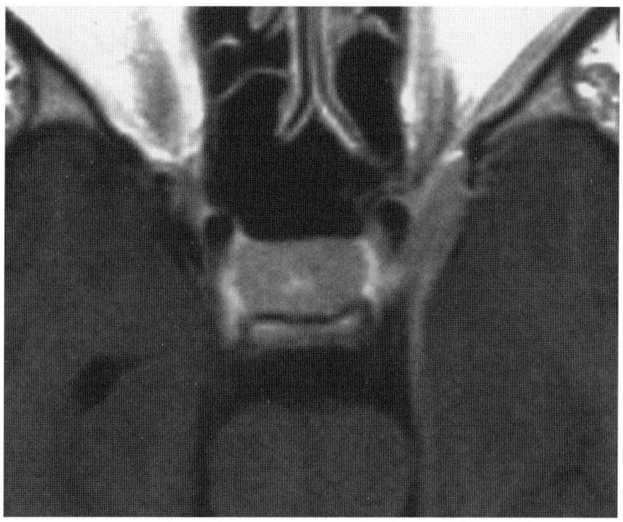

Figure 17I. Patient 2 with pseudotumor. T1-weighted axial image with contrast, showing widening of left cavernous sinus and enhancement of adjacent dura.

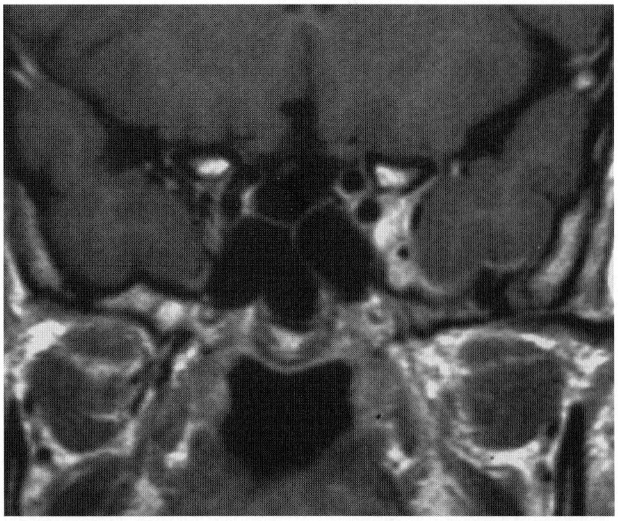

Figure 17J. Patient 2 with pseudotumor, showing infiltration of left cavernous sinus. T1-weighted coronal image with contrast.

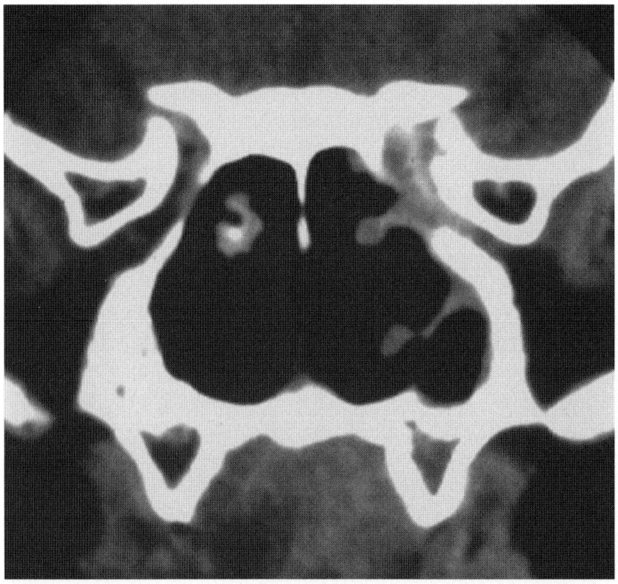

Figure 17K. Patient 3 with Wegener's granulomatosis. Contrast-enhanced computed tomography image, showing an infiltrative lesion involving orbital apex, inferior orbital fissure, and a region of sphenopalatine foramen on the left.

CASE 18

Clinical History: A 12-year-old with facial pain and ocular dysmotility.

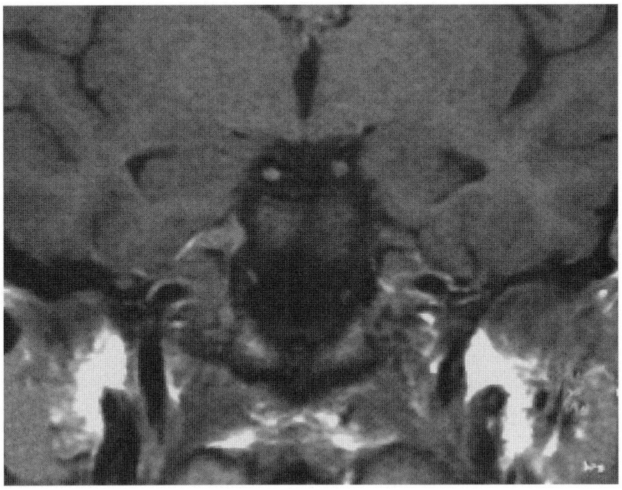

Figure 18A

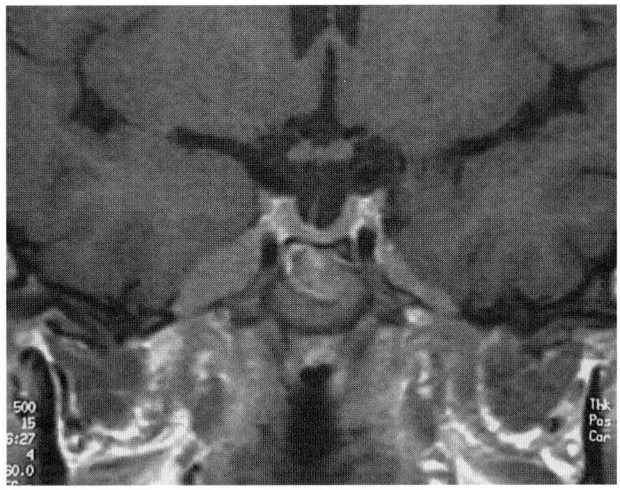

Figure 18B

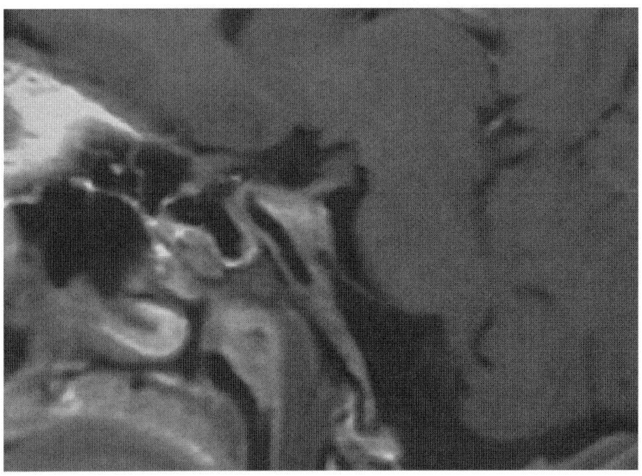

Figure 18C

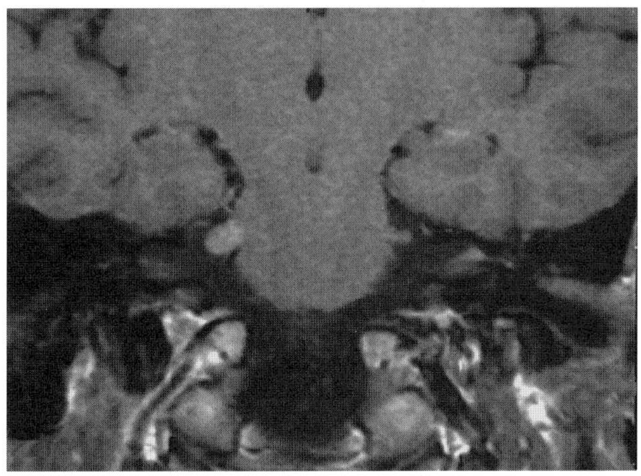

Figure 18D

1. List the cranial nerves that might cause these symptoms.
2. List two magnetic resonance imaging (MRI) signs that indicate a cranial nerve abnormality.
3. What is the radiologist's responsibility for study design in evaluating patients with possible cranial neuropathy?
4. What is the most likely diagnosis?

Findings

Abnormally enhancing tissue fills both trigeminal cisterns. The infiltrating process causes enlargement and enhancement of cranial nerves V, III, VI, and VII and/or VIII, as seen on various of the images submitted. In particular, note the spread along V3 below the skull base and on the sagittal view the VIth nerve as it goes from the pontomedullary junction to Dorello's canal as well as the IIIrd nerve in the suprasellar cistern on both the sagittal view and the coronal images.

Problem

Enlargement and abnormal enhancement of multiple cranial nerves in a pediatric patient with multiple cranial neuropathies

Anatomy

A. Review the entire course of cranial nerves III through VI from their brainstem nuclei to their end organ(s) considering:
   1. Position of cranial nerve nucleus in the brainstem
   2. Position of root entry (exit) zone on brain stem
   3. Cisternal segment
   4. Exit foramen and related vascular plexus
   5. Extracranial course and end organ(s)

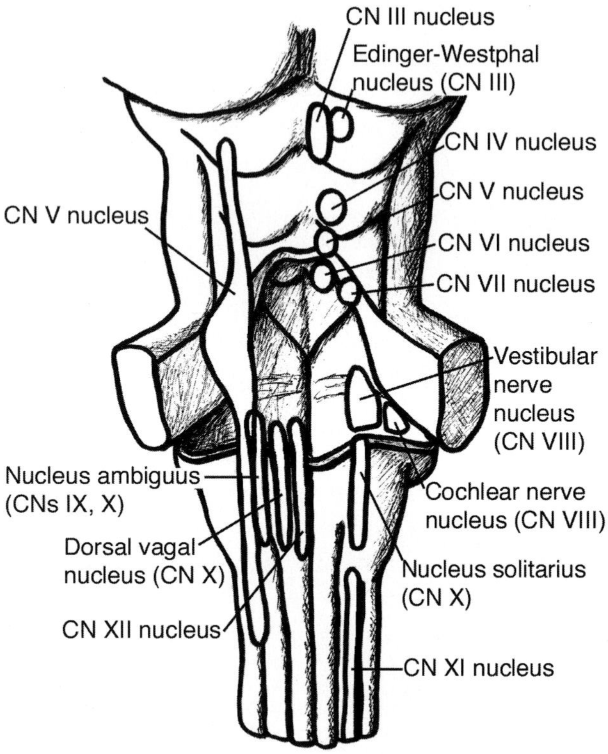

Figure 18E

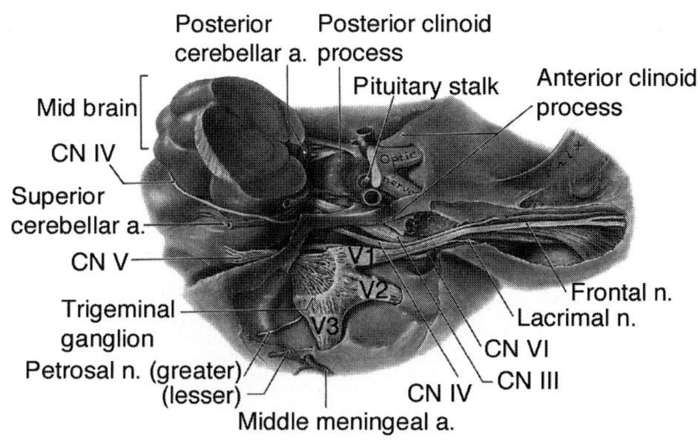

Figure 18F

Differential Diagnosis

None for the specific appearance and distribution seen here; however, carcinomatosis, leukemic infiltration, sarcoidosis, Wegener's granulomatosis, and infectious leptomeningitis might be considered.

Diagnosis

Lymphomatous infiltration of cranial nerves III through XII

Diagnostic Imaging Approach

A. Identify each cranial nerve at risk and its expected position and establish:
   1. If it is enlarged
   2. If it is enhancing abnormally (must be done from the nucleus of origin to the end organ)

Clinical Points Of Importance And Supplemental Information

A. Enhancement *around* a cranial nerve at or near its exit foramen is a normal variant.
B. Cranial nerve enhancement or enlargement is nonspecific and can be caused by inflammation or neoplasm.
C. A normal, excellent quality MRI does not exclude intrinsic cranial nerve pathology and does *not* replace cerebrospinal fluid sampling for detection of pathology of the subarachnoid space and meninges.
D. All cranial neuropathies must be studied from the site of origin of the cranial nerve in question to its end organ or distal site of innervation.

Answers To Questions

1. Cranial nerve III, IV, VI; V
2. Enlargement, enhancement
3. Study entire course of cranial nerve(s) in question from origin to distal sites of innervation.
4. Lymphoma

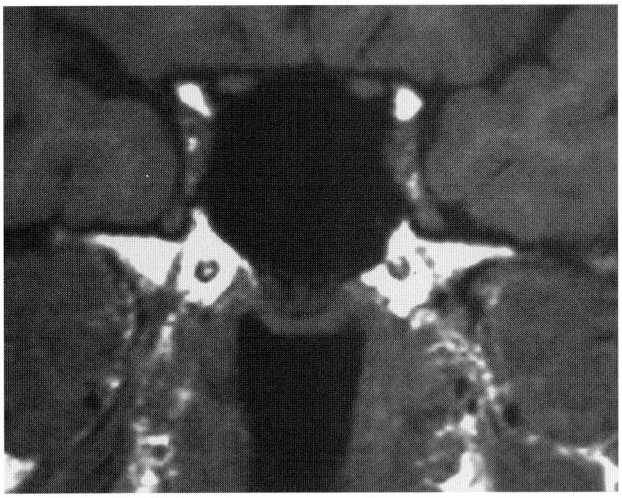

Figure 18G. Patient 1. T1-weighted image without contrast shows normal appearance of V2.

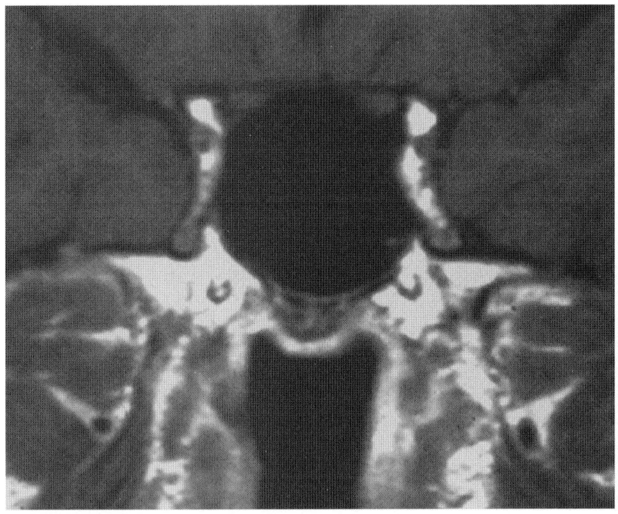

Figure 18H. Patient 1. T1-weighted image with contrast shows normal perineural enhancement around V2.

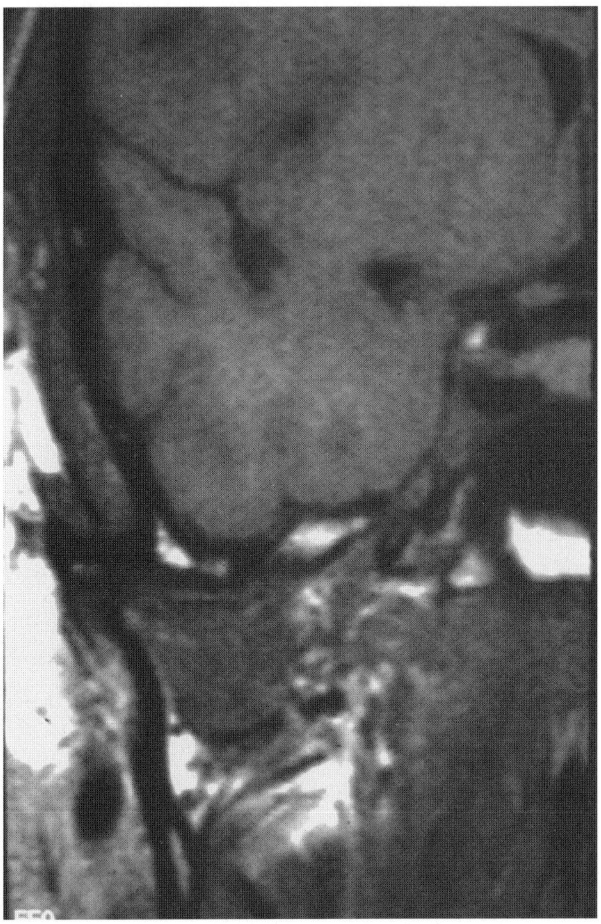

Figure 18I. Patient 2. T1-weighted image without contrast shows normal appearance of V3 at its origin from the trigeminal ganglion and through foramen ovale and upper masticator space.

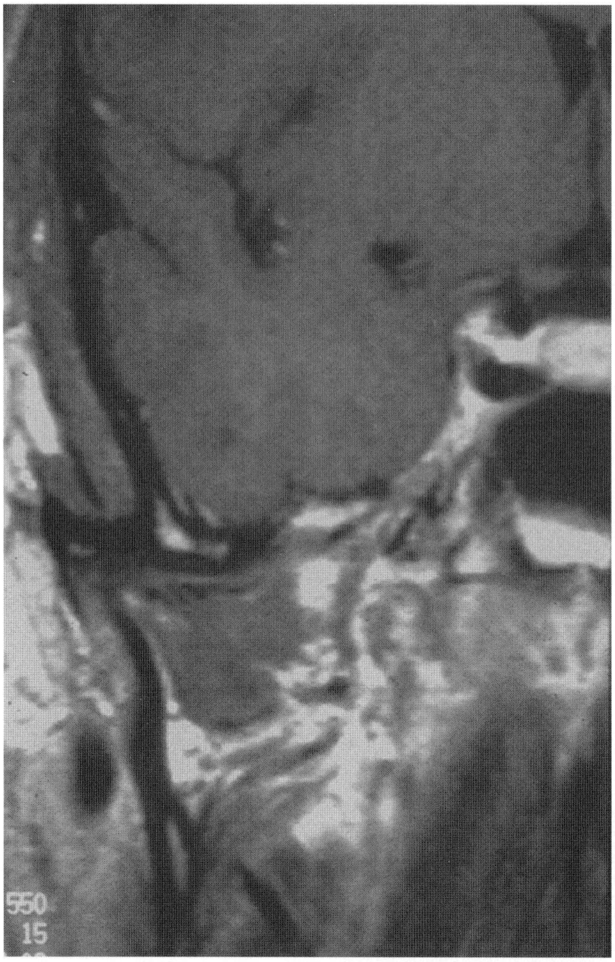

Figure 18J. Patient 2. T1-weighted image with contrast shows normal perineural enhancement around V3.

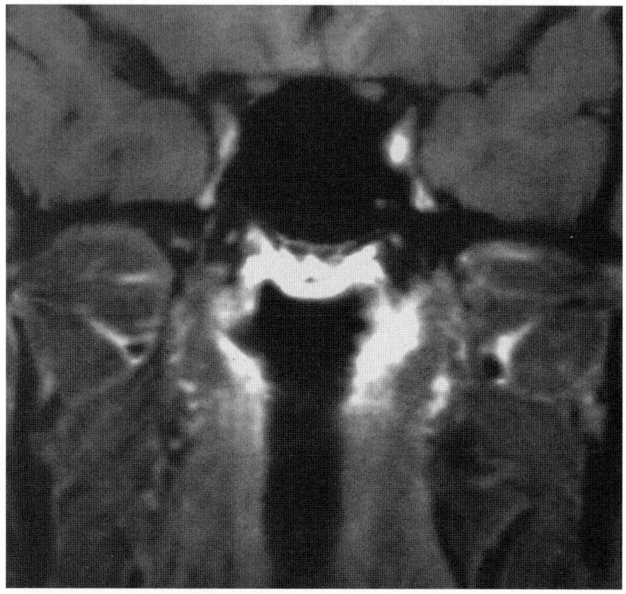

Figure 18K. Patient 3. T1-weighted, fat-suppression image with contrast, showing difficulty with frequency selective fat-suppression field distortion artifacts at the skull base when evaluating cranial nerves.

CASE 19

Clinical History: A 2-year-old presents with lethargy and multiple cranial nerve deficits.

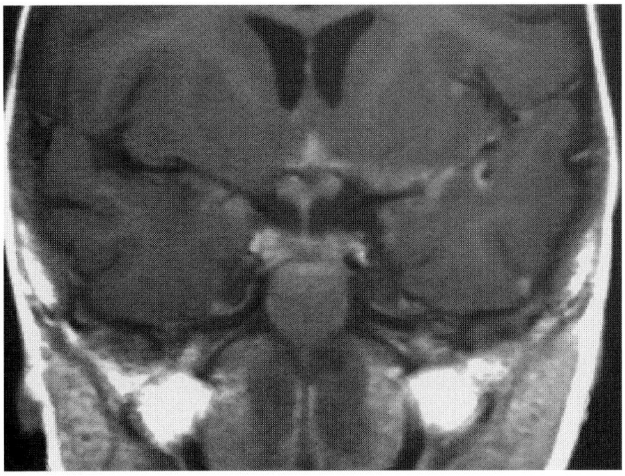

Figure 19A

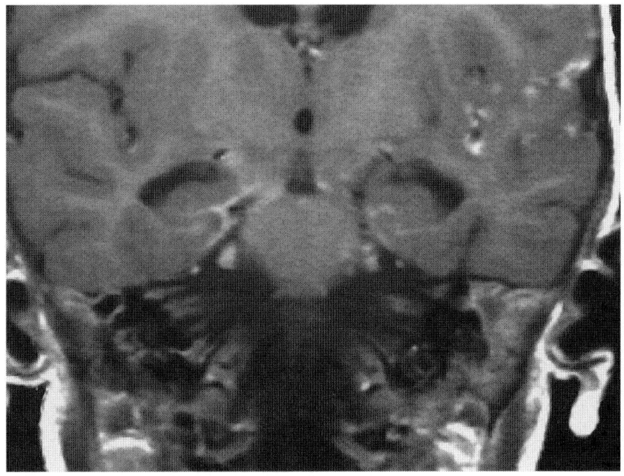

Figure 19B

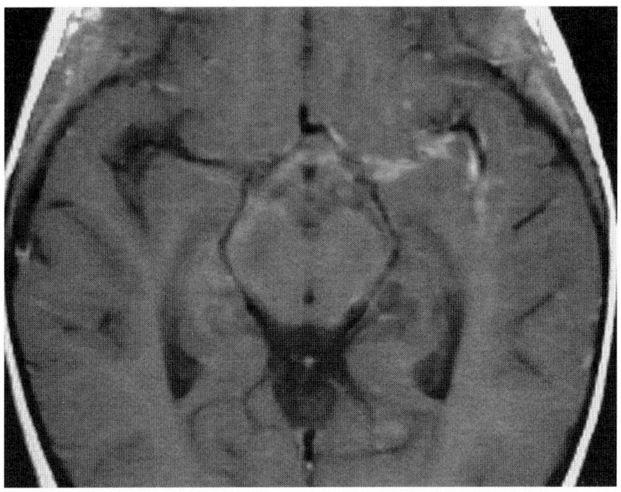

Figure 19C

1. Name the basic disease process.
2. List a differential diagnosis of at least three neoplastic and three nonneoplastic processes that might produce such findings. Rank the differential diagnosis according to the given age.
3. What would be the most likely diagnosis in a 35-year-old woman? A 70-year-old man?

Findings

Diffuse, predominantly basilar leptomeningeal enhancement pattern involving the course of some cranial nerves. In particular, note the Vth and VIIIth cranial nerve enhancement and thickening.

Problem

Diffuse, predominantly basilar meningeal enhancement with secondary cranial nerve enhancement in a young child

Anatomy

A. Detailed anatomy of cranial nerve V, from its root entry zone (REZ) to the trigeminal cistern
B. The relationship of meninges to cranial nerves, optic chiasm, and pituitary gland (see Fig. 4E)

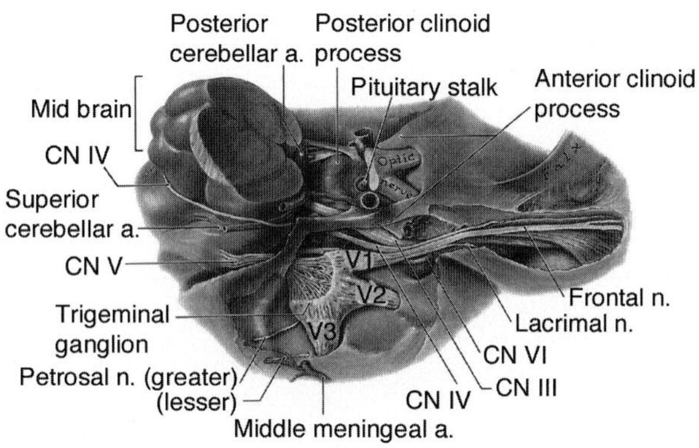

Figure 19D

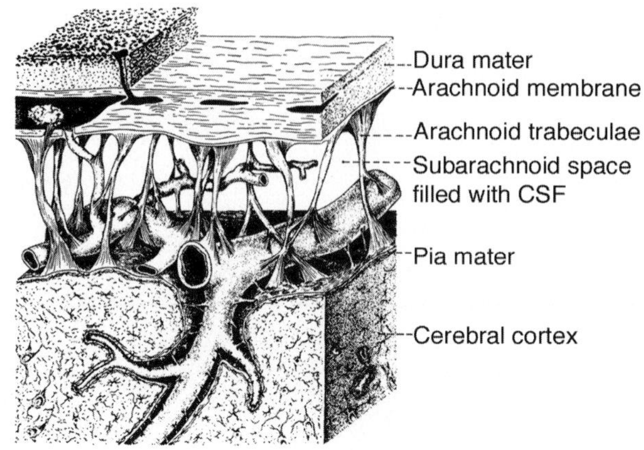

Figure 19E

Differential Diagnosis

1. Granulomatous diseases, infectious and noninfectious (e.g., tuberculosis, sarcoidosis, Wegener's granulomatosis)
2. Autoimmune arteritis; carcinomatosis; lymphomatosis; leukemia; seeding by a central nervous system tumor.

Diagnosis

Tuberculous meningitis with secondary cranial neuropathies

Diagnostic Imaging Approach

A. Evaluate the entire course of each cranial nerve in question, from nucleus of origin to REZ, cisternal segment, exit foramen, and extracranial course to end organ.
B. Evaluate basal cisterns
   1. Presence
   2. Abnormal enhancement of bordering brain (pia), arachnoid, or structures in cisterns (chiasma), and dura
C. Evaluate basal vascular spaces
D. Localized vs. diffuse disease
E. Distribution: basilar, diffuse, ventricles
F. Associated findings: hydrocephalus, infarct, venous and dural sinus thrombosis, empyema, subdural effusion

Clinical Points Of Importance And Supplemental Information

A. Timely recognition of subtle signs of disease can lead to earlier treatment.
B. A negative finding on magnetic resonance imaging does *not* exclude meningeal pathology or obviate the need for cerebrospinal fluid sampling.

Answers To Questions

1. Basilar meningitis
2. Neoplastic: leukemia, lymphoma, carcinomatosis. Nonneoplastic: granulomatosis or reticulocytosis, sarcoidosis, tuberculosis
3. Sarcoidosis. Carcinomatosis.

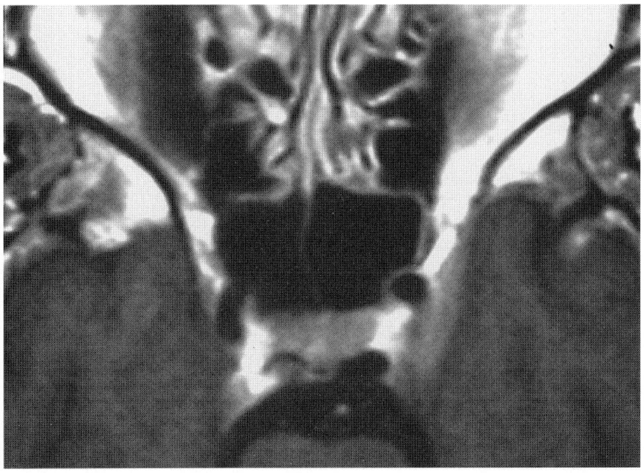

Figure 19F. Patient with cavernous sinus pseudotumor, showing thickening of left upper outer dura of the cavernous sinus. T1-weighted image with contrast.

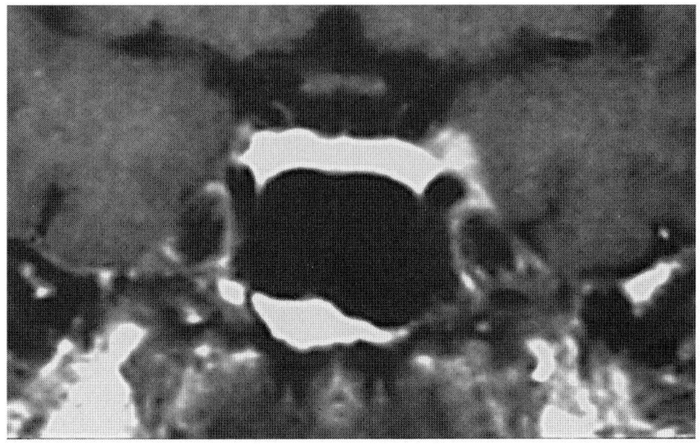

Figure 19G. Patient with cavernous sinus pseudotumor, showing enhancing mass mainly involving th area of the oculomotor nerve. T1-weghted coronal image with contrast.

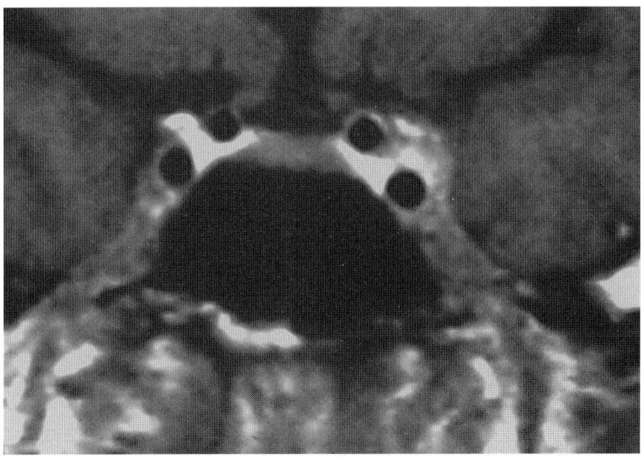

Figure 19H. Patient with cavernous sinus pseudotumor, showing enhancing mass adjacent superolateral to carotid siphon. T1-weghted coronal image with contrast.

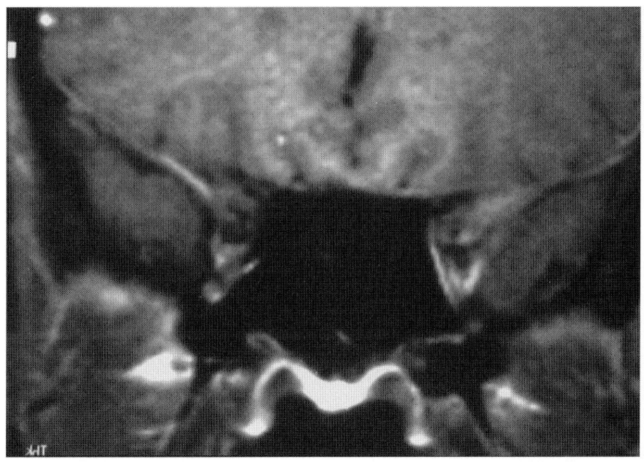

Figure 19I. Patient with cavernous sinus pseudotumor, showing abnormal enhancement of dura on the left, essentially following the oculomotor nerve and dura into the superior orbital fissure. T1-weighted coronal image with contrast at the level of orbital apex.

CHAPTER 2

CENTRAL SKULL BASE/ CAVERNOUS SINUS

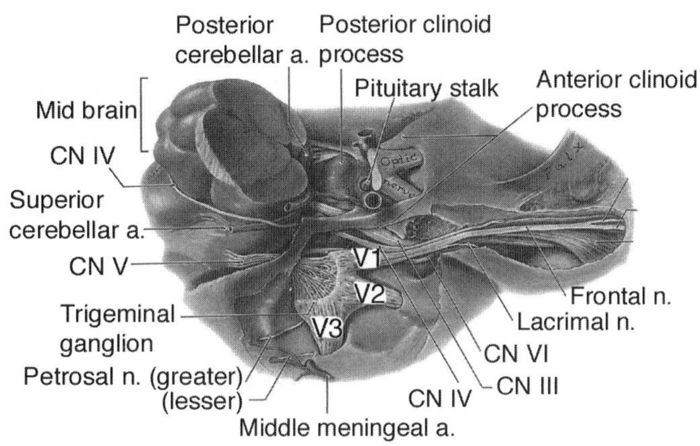

CASE 20

Clinical History: A 40-year-old woman presents with left hemifacial spasm.

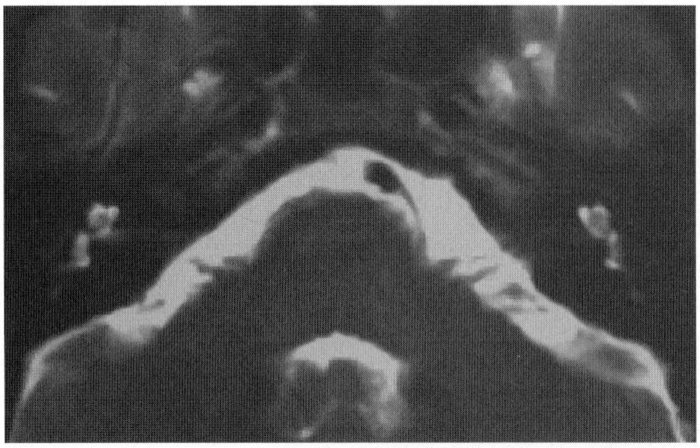

Figure 20A

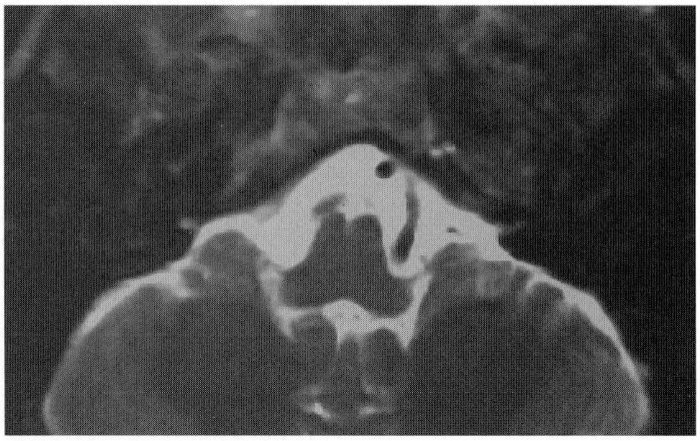

Figure 20B

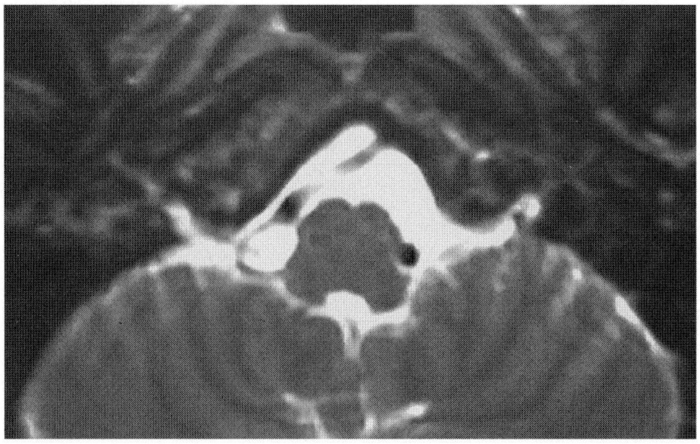

Figure 20C

1. Is the Vth or VIIth cranial nerve responsible for this symptom?
2. Are structural causes for hemifacial spasm likely or unlikely (<15% chance) to be identified on computed tomography (CT) or magnetic resonance imaging (MRI) studies?
3. What is the main purpose of imaging a patient with hemifacial spasm? Does this patient need a follow-up angiogram based on the MRI findings alone? Based on the clinical findings?

Findings

A tortuous left vertebral artery is directly impinging on the brainstem below the root entry zone of the left VIIth and VIIIth cranial nerves and the posterior inferior cerebellar artery is distorting the root entry zone (REZ) of the VIIth, VIIIth, or both nerves.

Problem

Tortuous vessels deforming the brainstem adjacent to and at the REZ of the lower cranial nerves.

Anatomy

A. Vertebral basilar system and major branches
B. Position of REZ of cranial nerves V–XII

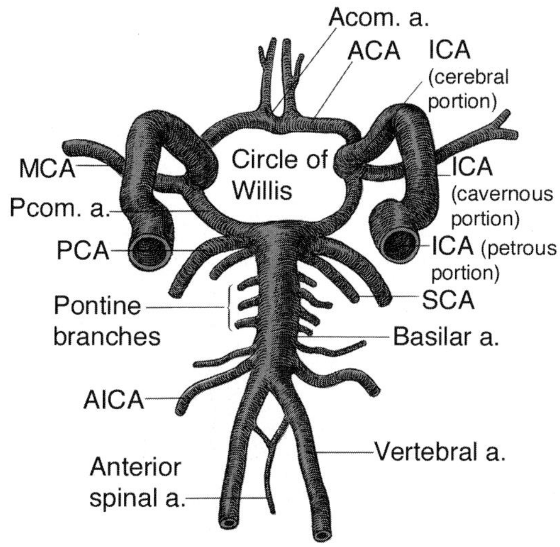

Figure 20D

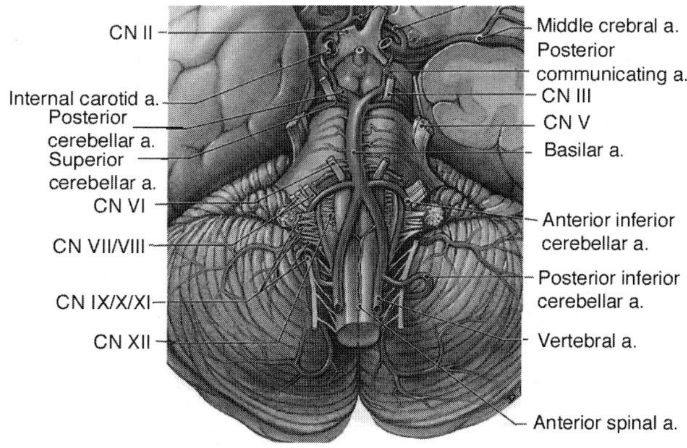

Figure 20E

Differential Diagnosis

Not applicable

Diagnosis

Normal: the history was invented

Diagnostic Imaging Approach

A. Identify tortuous vessels and their relationship to the brainstem
B. Look for evidence of edema or hemorrhage near the REZ
C. Exclude compression or other lesion involving the cranial nerve in question (e.g., hemifacial spasm–VIIth nerve)

Clinical Points Of Importance And Supplemental Information

A. Although a relationship seems to exist between symptoms (e.g., trigeminal neuralgia, hemifacial spasm) and the "macro" vascular findings, microvascular compression and the need for, or success of surgery (microvascular decompression) cannot be predicted by MRI, magnetic resonance angiography, or angiography alone.
B. Imaging with MRI (or CT) is done mainly to exclude compressive lesions (e.g., meningioma) rather than to confirm the likelihood of microvascular compression.

Answers To Questions

1. Cranial nerve VII
2. Unlikely (excluding those *suggestive* of microvascular compression)
3. To identify a causative lesion. No. No.

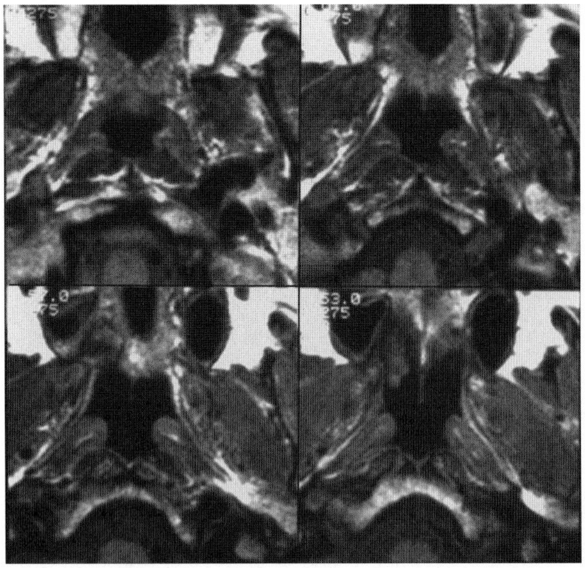

Figure 20F. Patient 1 with torturous internal carotid artery just below skull base in a position where it could "irritate" V3 and present as trigeminal neuralgia in the distribution of V3. T1-weighted axial images.

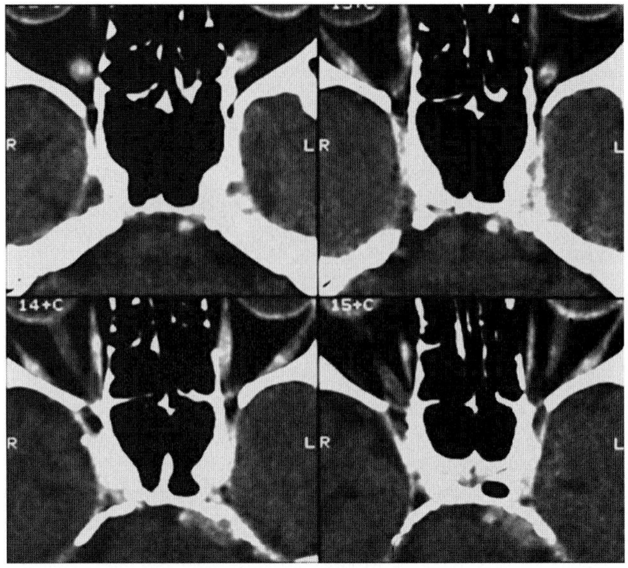

Figure 20G. Patient 2 with clival meningioma along the main trigeminal trunk at the petroclinoid ligament region. Presented as "trigeminal neuralgia." Contrast-enhanced CT images.

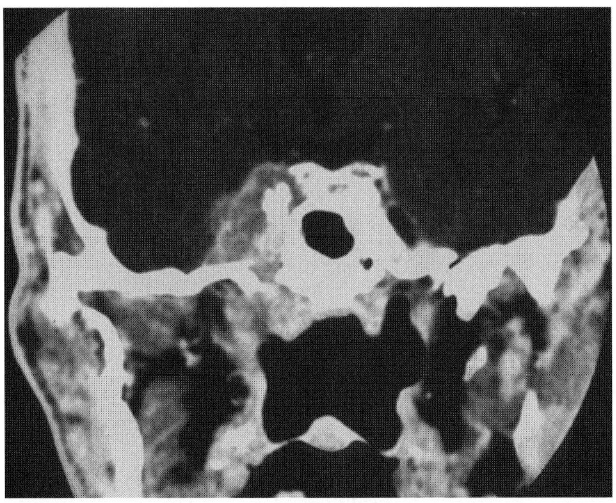

Figure 20H. Patient 3 with nasopharyngeal carcinoma extending into the cavernous sinus via petroclival fissure, presenting as "trigeminal neuralgia." Contrast-enhanced coronal CT image.

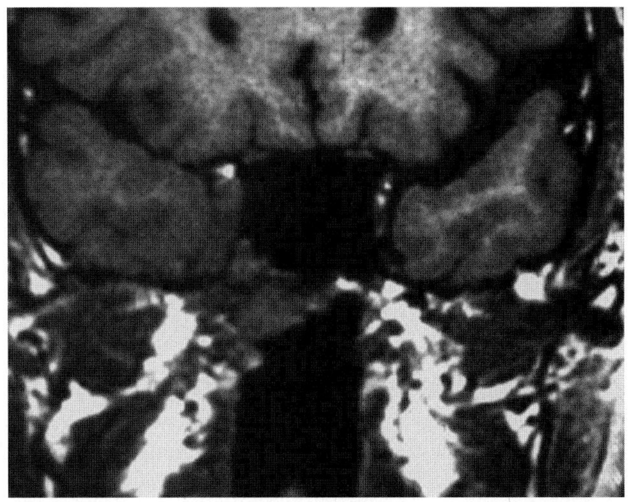

Figure 20I. Patient 3 with nasopharyngeal carcinoma extending into cavernous sinus via petroclival fissure. T1-weighted image without contrast, which originally was called a "meningioma" because the nasopharyngeal origin and skull base invasion were not recognized.

CASE 21

Clinical History: A 64-year-old woman presents with left-sided trigeminal neuralgia.

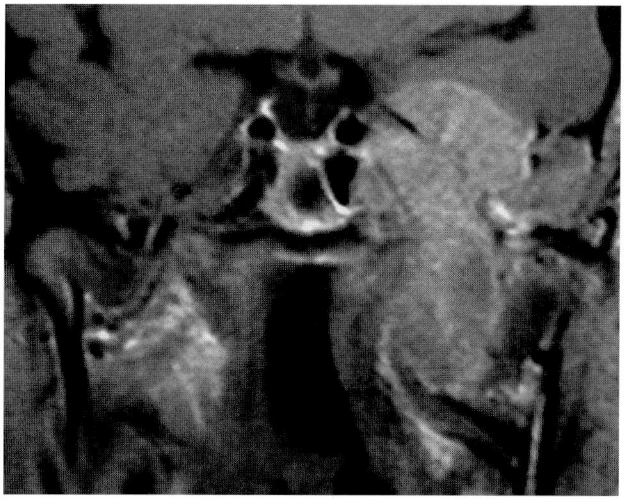

Figure 21A

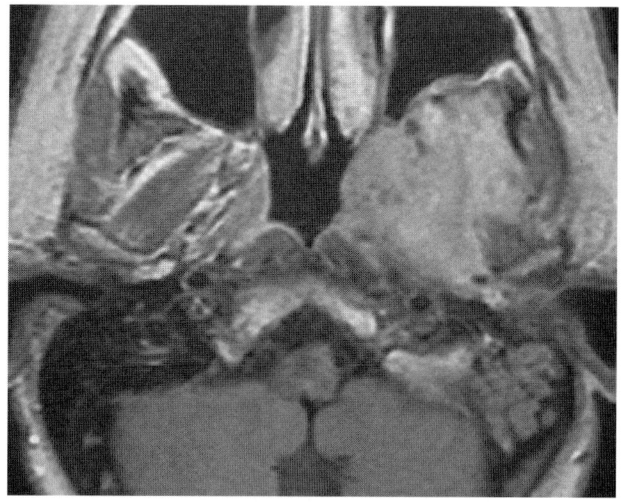

Figure 21B

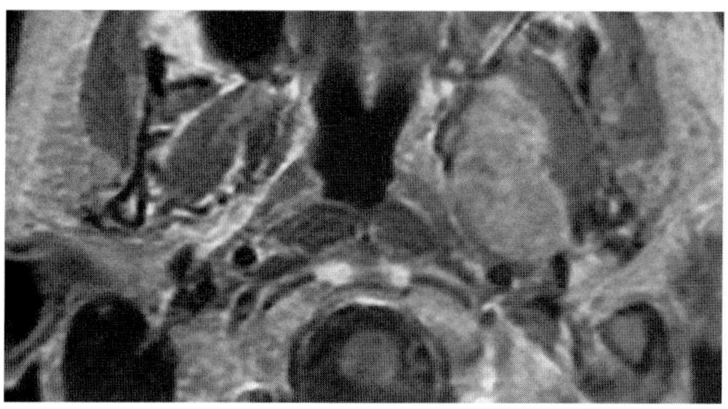

Figure 21C

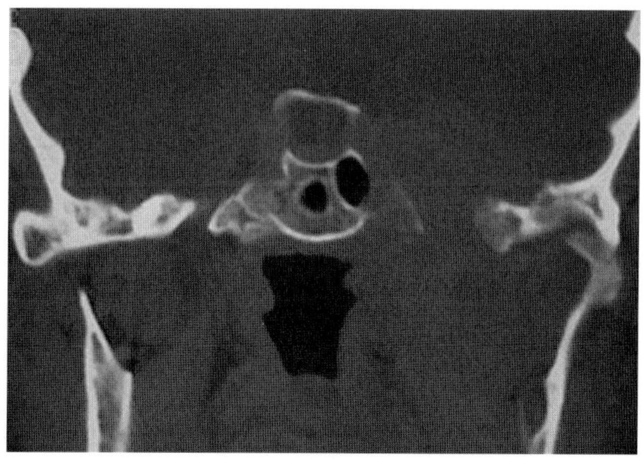

Figure 21D

1. What extracranial space(s) does the mass involve?
2. What is the "epicenter" of the lesion?
3. What are three possible diagnoses? Listing the one most likely first.

Findings

A homogeneously enhancing mass involves the left masticator space. The lesion spreads to within the left middle cranial fossa through the enlarged foramen ovale and directly involves the left cavernous sinus intracranially. Chronic remodeling in association with the mass is seen on a computed tomography (CT) scan of the skull base.

Problem

Mass involving the cavernous sinus, floor of the middle cranial fossa, and masticator space

Anatomy

A. Relationship of trigeminal cistern to (see Figs. 4E and19D)
   1. Cavernous sinus dura
   2. Trigeminal ganglion
   3. Divisions of cranial nerve V
B. Floor of the middle cranial fossa (composition or foramina)
C. Masticator space and extracranial course of V3 and middle meningeal artery

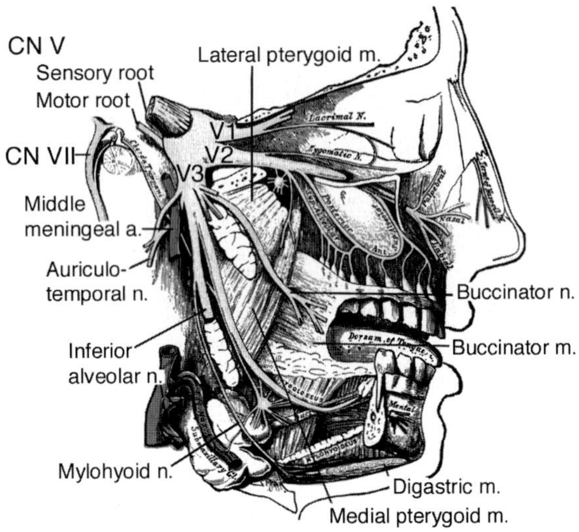

Figure 21E

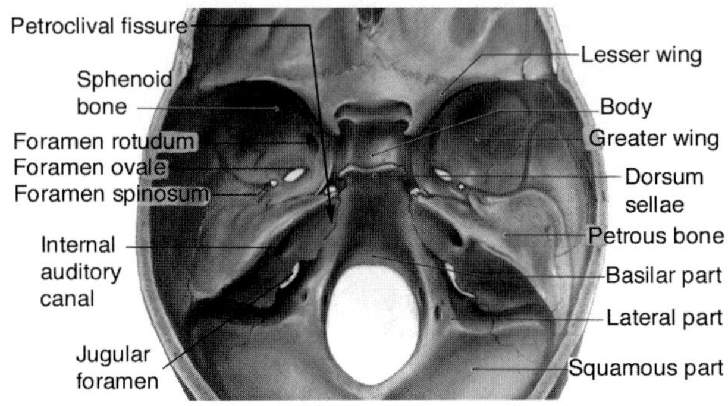

Figure 21F

Differential Diagnosis

Trigeminal schwannoma or neurofibroma, meningioma, hemangiopericytoma, sarcoma, metastasis

Diagnosis

Intracranial and extracranial meningioma

Diagnostic Imaging Approach

A. Identify the epicenter of the lesion to establish precise site or structure of origin
B. Evaluate vector of pathology (e.g., along dural surfaces, along cranial nerves)
C. Establish the relationship of the mass to critical surrounding structures (e.g., brain, carotid artery, cranial nerves)
D. Morphology of lesion
   1. Density or intensity, enhancement, flow voids, calcifications

Clinical Points Of Importance And Supplemental Information

A. It is essential to establish the relationship of the lesion in this location to the carotid and cavernous sinus to plan the surgical approach; CT and angiography are frequently required in addition to magnetic resonance imaging and magnetic resonance angiography.
B. CT-directed biopsy of masticator space lesions is safe and easy to perform. Cutting needles can be used if certain precautions are followed.

Answers To Questions

1. Masticator space
2. Foramen ovale region: "paracavernous"
3. Trigeminal schwannoma, transcranial meningioma, sarcoma

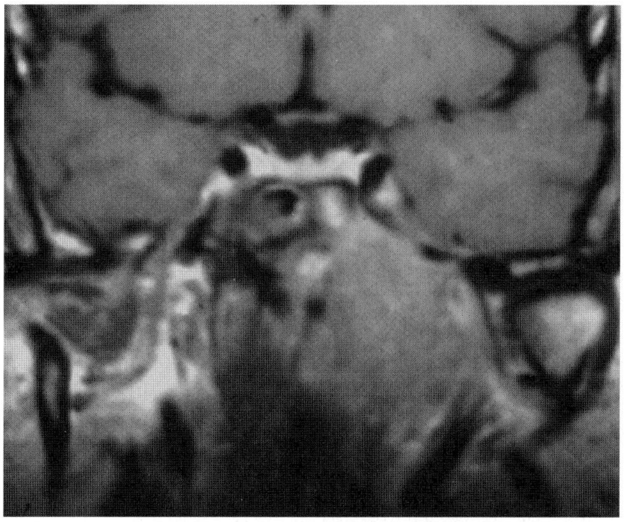

Figure 21G. Patient 1 with nasopharyngeal carcinoma directly involving the cavernous sinus with skull base destruction. T1-weighted coronal image with contrast.

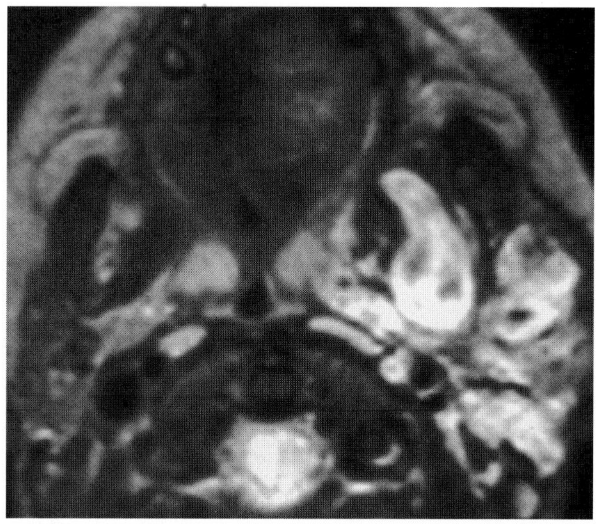

Figure 21H. Patient 2 with plexiform neurofibroma presenting as multinodular, high-intensity mass mainly involving the masticator, parapharyngeal, and parotid spaces. T2-weighted image.

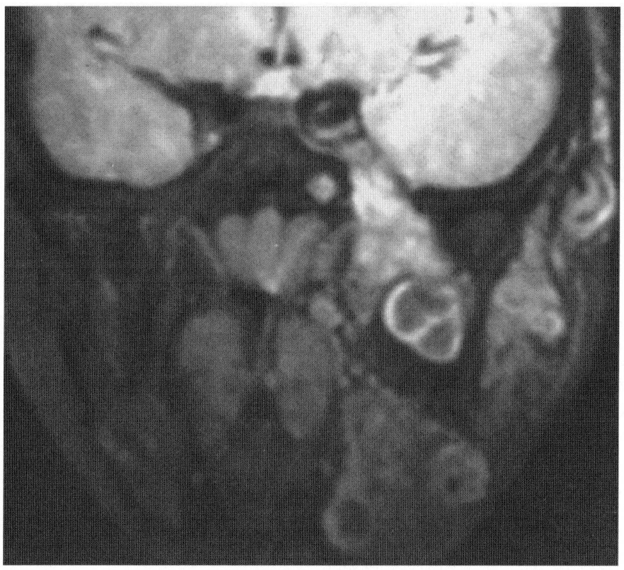

Figure 21I. Patient 2 with plexiform neurofibroma of the masticator space, extending intracranially along expected course of V3. T1-weighted fat-suppression image with contrast.

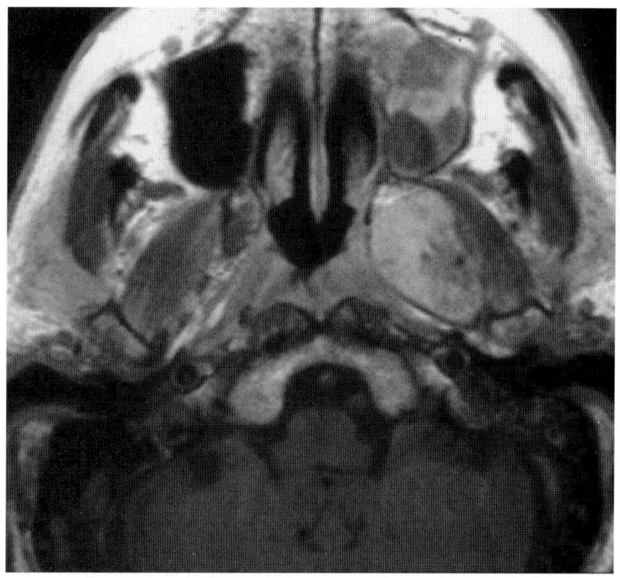

Figure 21J. Patient 3 with schwannoma of V3, presenting as a well-circumscribed mass centered in the expected location of V3 within the masticator space. T1-weighted image with contrast.

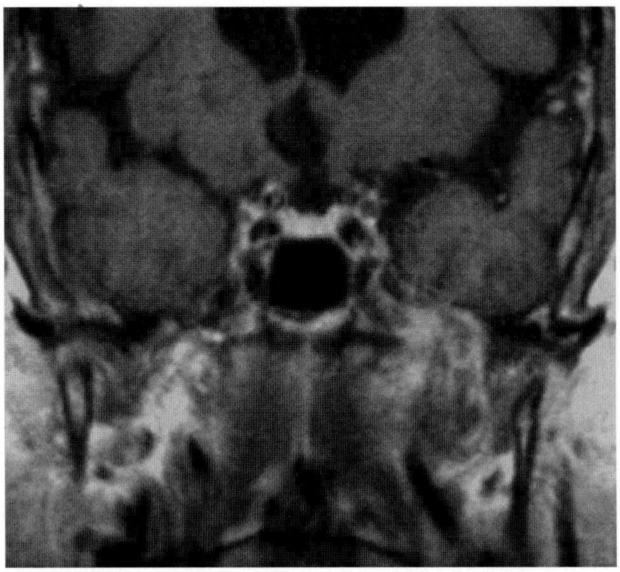

Figure 21K. Patient 3 with schwannoma of V3 involving the trigeminal ganglion. T1-weighted image with contrast.

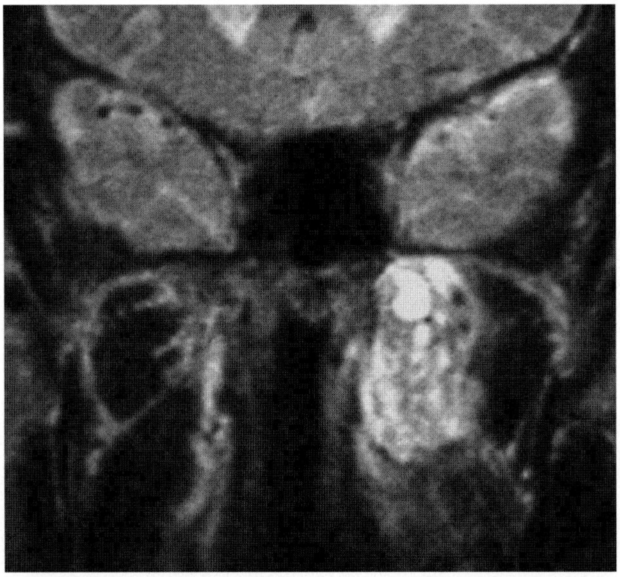

Figure 21L. Patient 3 with schwannoma of V3 manifested by a well-circumscribed, high-intensity mass containing several cystic areas. T2-weighted image.

CASE 22

Clinical History: A 54-year-old man presents with atypical, left-sided facial pain.

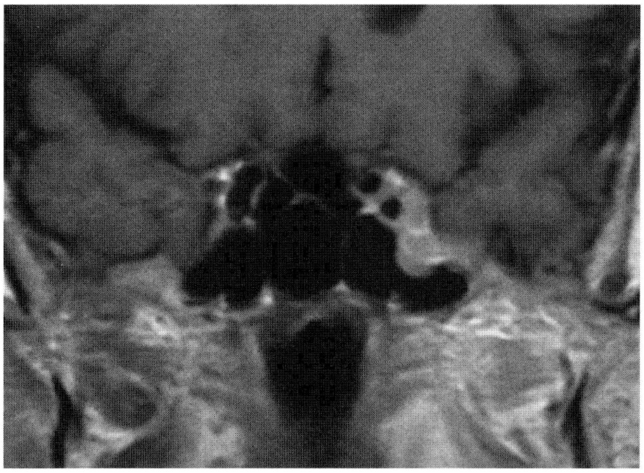

Figure 22A

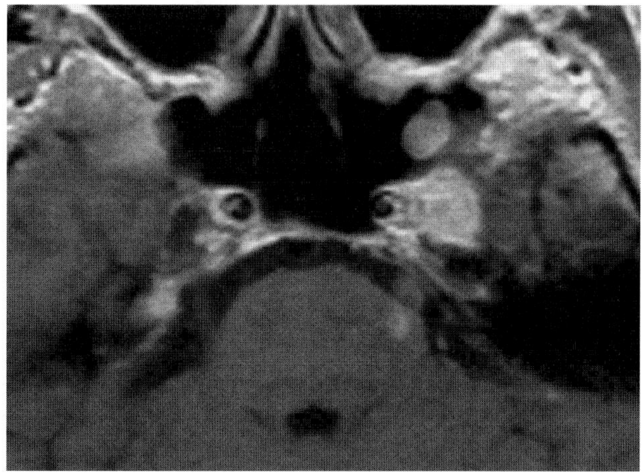

Figure 22B

1. What is atypical facial pain? When does it *require* imaging evaluation?
2. What portions of the trigeminal nerve are abnormal?
3. What are the radiologist's responsibilities in the design and interpretation of studies of patients with cranial neuropathy?

Findings

An enhancing, solid mass centered in the left trigeminal cistern. The lesion is contiguous along the second and third divisions of the left Vth cranial nerve as well as to the cisternal segment of the nerve posteriorly. The lesion also involves the root entry zone (REZ) of the trigeminal nerve at the belly of the pons.

Problem

Enlargement and abnormal enhancement of the trigeminal nerve in a patient with atypical, progressively worsening facial pain

Anatomy

A. Trigeminal nerve
   1. Ophthalmic division
   2. Maxillary division
   3. Mandibular division
   4. Trigeminal ganglion
   5. Cisternal segment and REZ

B. Muscles innervated by V3

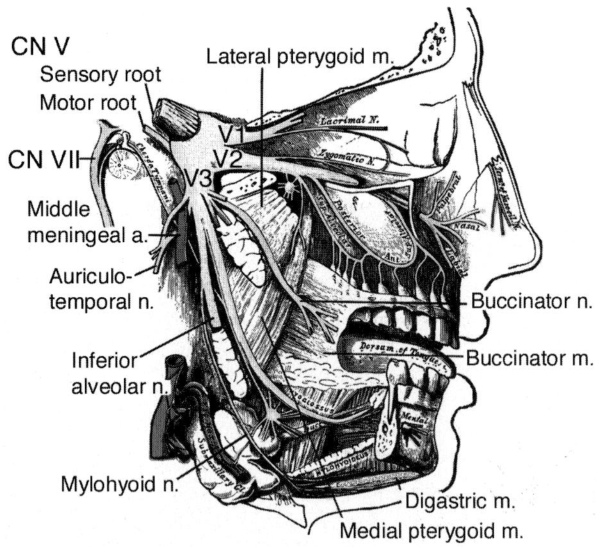

Figure 22C

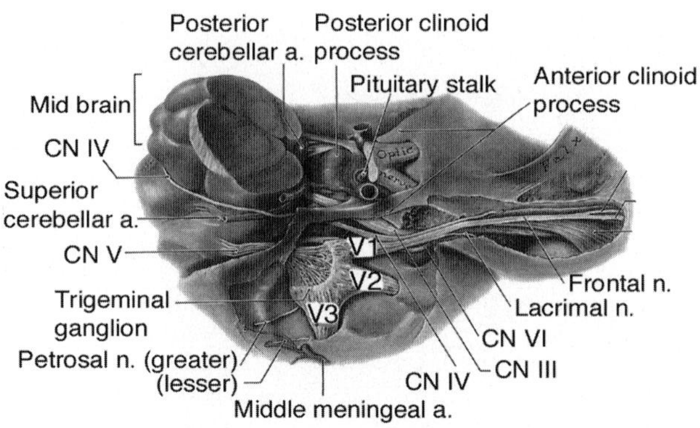

Figure 22D

Differential Diagnosis

Inflammatory vs. neoplastic cranial neuropathy

Diagnosis

Perineural spread of skin cancer along the infraorbital nerve to the trigeminal nerve (all major branches) and retrograde to its REZ

Diagnostic Imaging Approach

A. Trace all divisions of cranial nerve V, from the brainstem nucleus of origin to termination (end organ).
B. Identify enlargement, abnormal enhancement, or compressive pathology.
C. Identify manifestations of denervation atrophy in innervated muscles.
   1. Atrophy, fat replacement, if chronic
   2. Enhancement and enlargement, if acute

Clinical Points Of Importance And Supplemental Information

A. Perineural spread of skin cancer can occur long after the lesion has been removed. Whenever perineural spread is suspected radiographically, the patient must be asked if a skin lesion (in the appropriate location) has been removed.
B. Perineural spread can also be seen in recurrent mucosal carcinomas and is frequently identified at presentation in patients with adenoidcystic carcinoma.

Answers To Questions

1. When the pain does not behave like "tic." When symptoms worsen progressively
2. All three main divisions and the cisternal segment
3. To evaluate each symptomatic cranial nerve, *from its point of origin to its peripheral site of innervation*, as that peripheral site relates to the symptoms

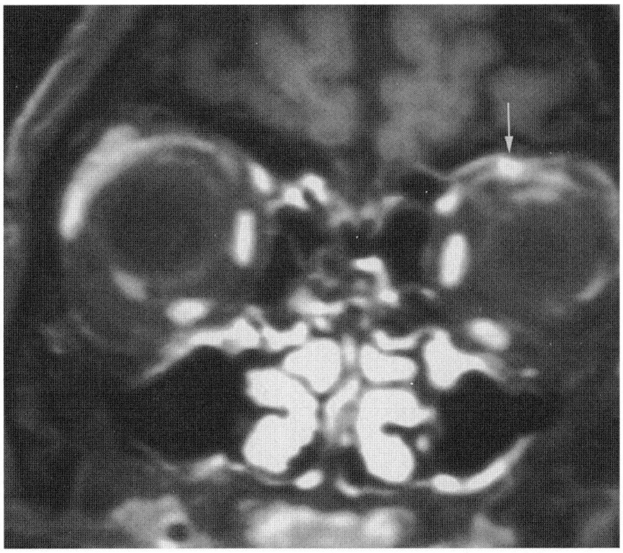

Figure 22E. Patient 1 with perineural tumor spread along V1 on the left. T1-weighted fat-suppression image with contrast.

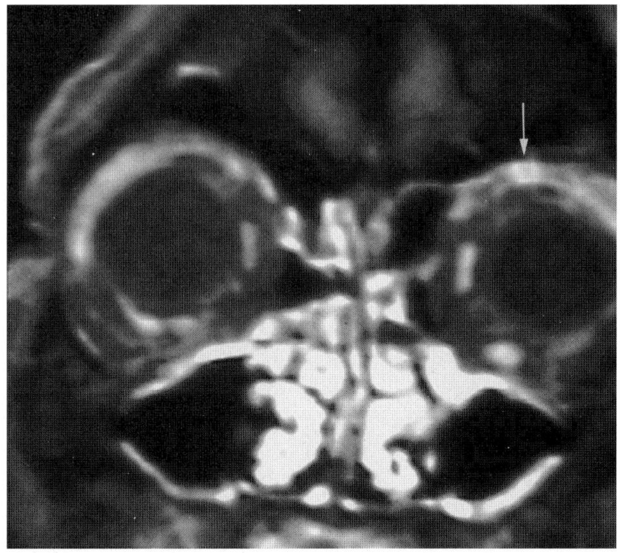

Figure 22F. Patient 1 with perineural tumor spread along V1 on the left. T1-weighted fat-suppression image with contrast slightly anterior to that in 22E.

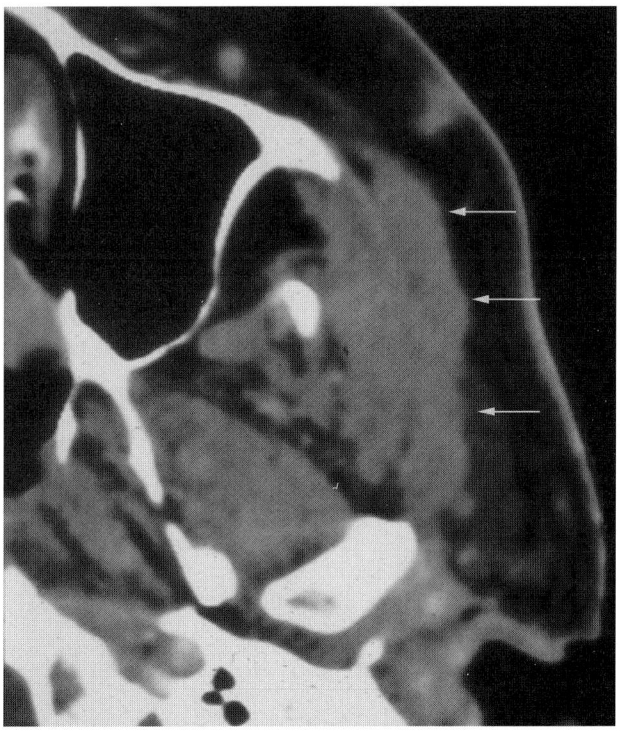

Figure 22G. Patient 2 with a perineural tumor spread along the buccal branch of the facial nerve, presenting as infiltrative soft tissue mass extending in anteroposterior direction just under superficial musculoaponeurotic layer and just lateral to the masseter muscle.

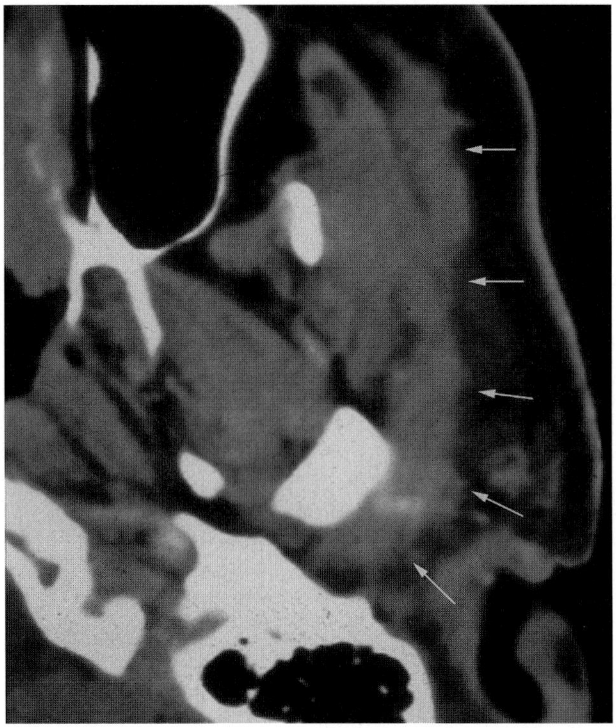

Figure 22H. Patient 2 with a perineural tumor spread along the facial nerve and auriculotemporal nerve (V3). Posteriorly, mass seen on 22F is contiguous with soft tissue mass around the posterior edge of the ascending ramus of mandible; this is the course of the auriculotemporal nerve.

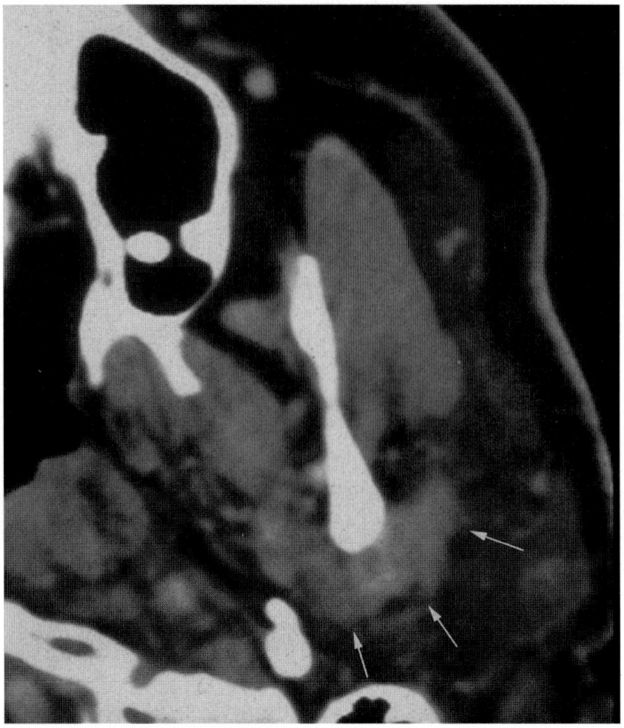

Figure 22I. Patient 2 with a perineural tumor spread along the facial nerve to the auriculotemporal nerve (V3), the infiltrating perineural mass wrapping around the posterior aspect of the mandibular condyle where the auriculotemporal nerve joins V3.

CASE 23

Clinical History: A 65-year-old man presents with left-sided facial pain and recent onset of diplopia.

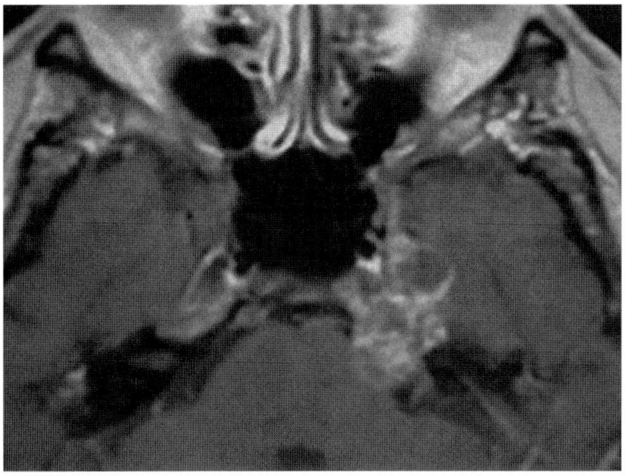

Figure 23A

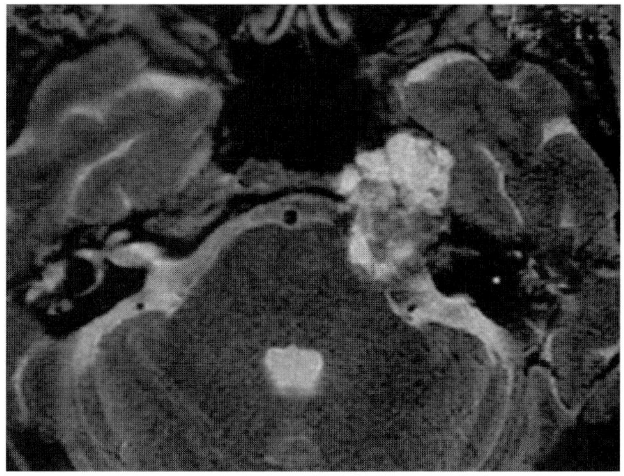

Figure 23B

1. Why does this patient have diplopia and facial pain?
2. Where is the lesion centered?
3. What is the most likely diagnosis? Does the T2-weighted image help in the differential diagnosis? Does the enhancement?

Findings

A high-intensity mass with a lobulated contour centered in the left petroclival fissure on T2-weighted images. Multiple septations are seen within the mass. Postcontrast T1-weighted image shows a rim-enhancement and ringlike enhancement of the lesion.

Problem

Mass involving the central skull base at the petroclival fissure, presenting with Vth and VIth cranial nerve deficits

Anatomy

A. Central skull base
   1. Petroclival fissure (see Fig. 21F)
   2. Clival vascular plexus
B. Cranial nerve V and trigeminal cistern
C. Cranial nerve VI and Dorello's canal

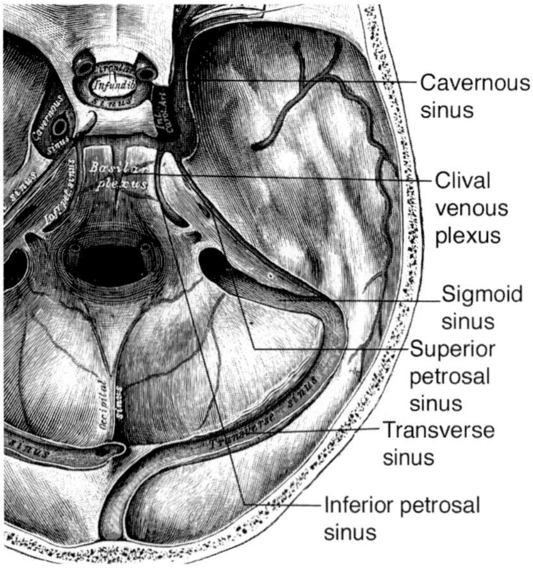

Figure 23C

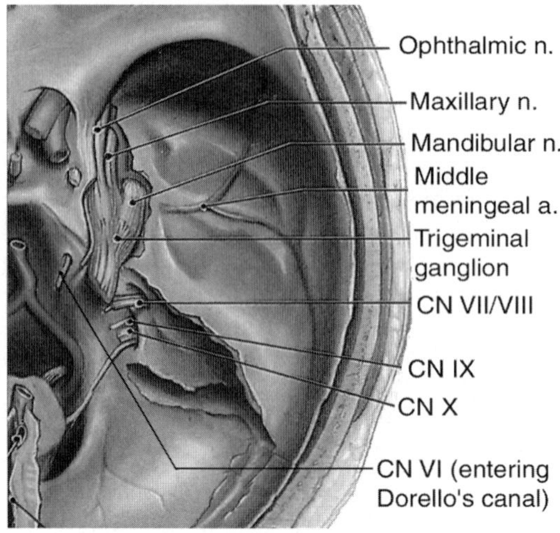

Figure 23D

Differential Diagnosis

Chordoma; chordoma, chondroid variant; chondrosarcoma; neurogenic tumor; meningioma (atypical); metastasis (rare); enhancing epidermoid (rarely seen after rupture or when it contains a coexisting carcinoma)

Diagnosis

Chordoma vs. chondrosarcoma of the central skull base

Diagnostic Imaging Approach

A. Identify epicenter of lesion and precise site or structure of origin.
B. Determine if vector of spread is along dura or particular cranial nerve.
C. Determine relationship of mass to carotid, cavernous sinus, or other adjacent critical anatomy.
D. Morphology of lesion
   1. Signal intensity, density, calcifications, flow voids, enhancement

Clinical Points Of Importance And Supplemental Information

A. It is essential *initially* to exclude aneurysm as a cause of any central skull base lesion.
B. The relationship of central skull base lesions to critical anatomy (e.g., carotid, cavernous sinus) is essential for treatment planning. This frequently requires computed tomography (CT) and angiography as well as magnetic resonance imaging and magnetic resonance angiography.

Answers To Questions

1. VIth and Vth cranial neuropathy
2. Petroclival
3. Chondrosarcoma. Yes; chondrosarcoma and chordoma are typically bright. Yes; lobulated enhancement pattern fairly typical as well.

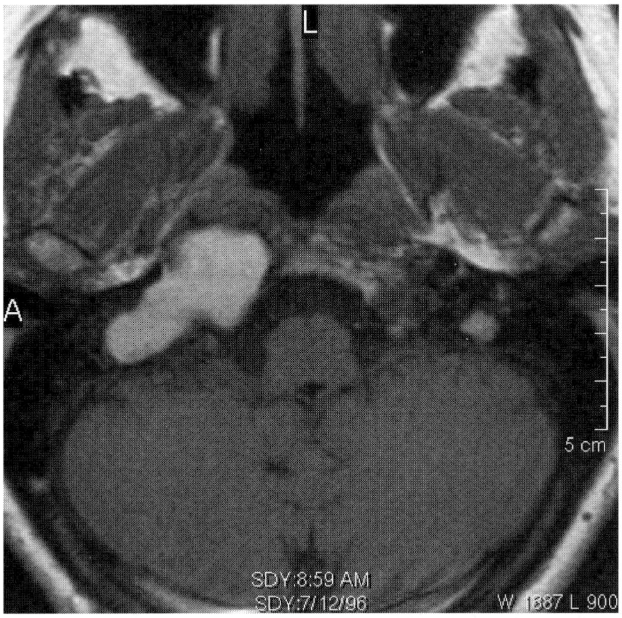

Figure 23E. Patient 1 with cholesterol granuloma. T1-weighted image without contrast, showing an expansile, high-intensity mass centered in the right petrous apex.

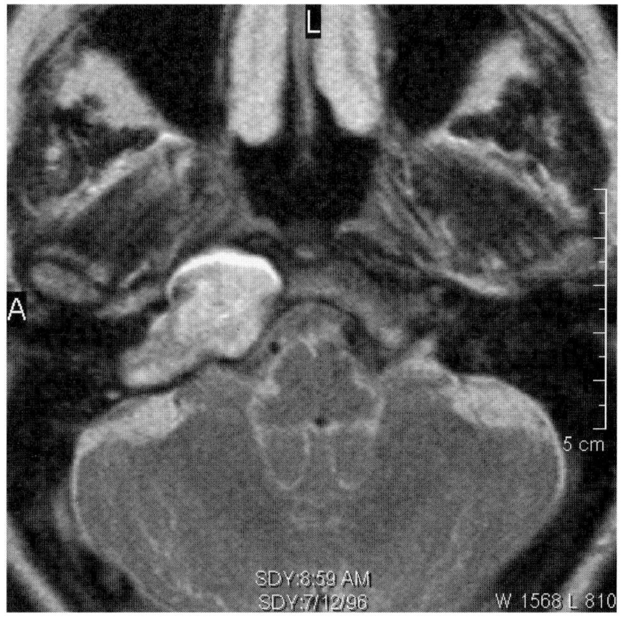

Figure 23F. Patient 1 with cholesterol granuloma. T2-weighted image.

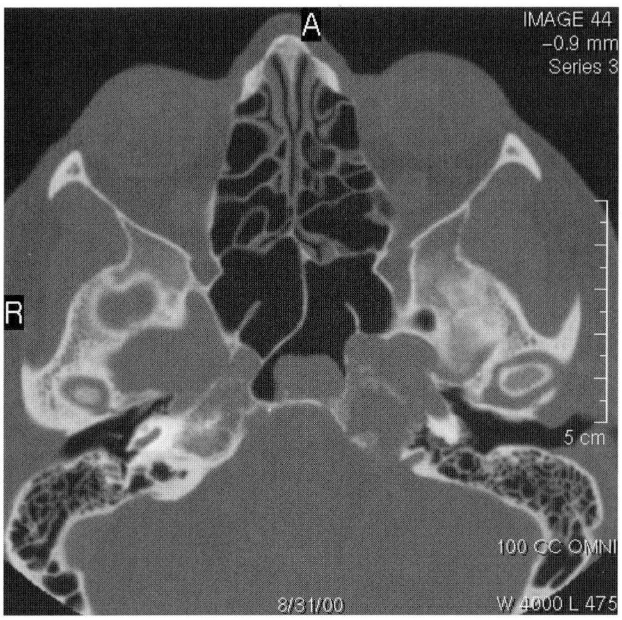

Figure 23G. Patient 2 with chondrosarcoma arising from petroclival fissure. Axial CT image at bone window setting shows destructive yet "expansile" mass with scattered mineralization centered in the left petrous apex.

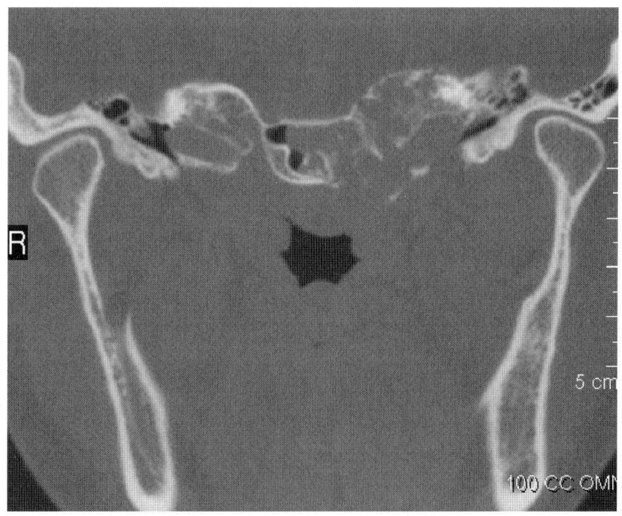

Figure 23H. Patient 2 with chondrosarcoma arising from petroclival fissure. Coronal CT image at bone window setting.

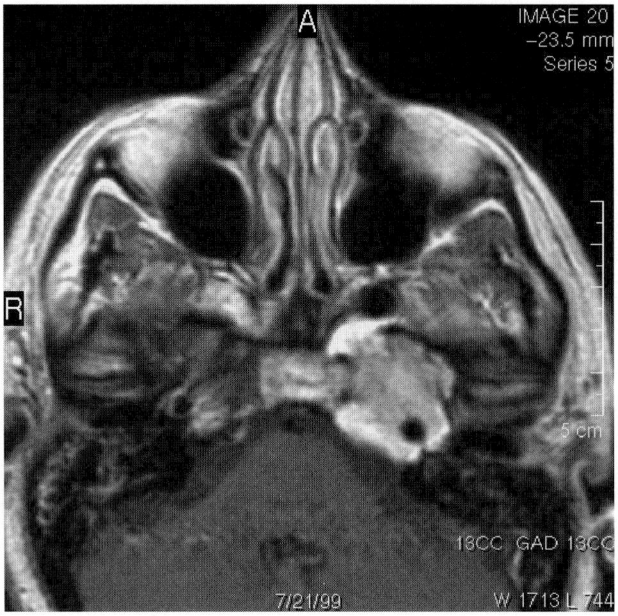

Figure 23I. Patient 3 with plasmacytoma of skull base. T1-weighted image with contrast, showing homogeneously enhancing mass involving the left petrous apex.

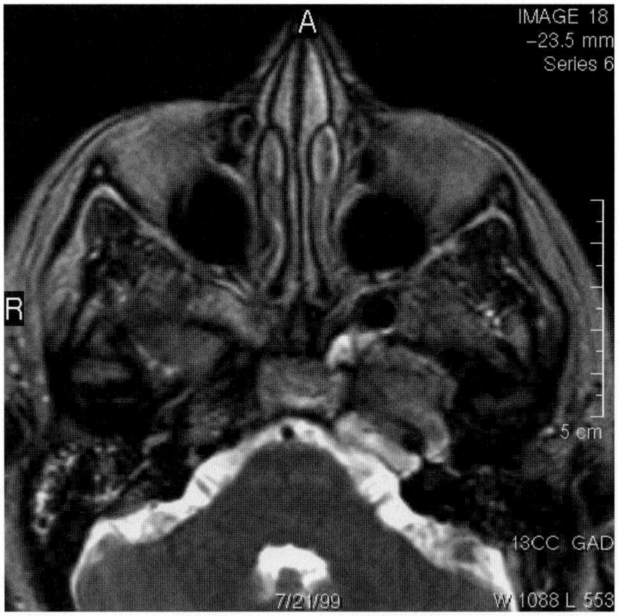

Figure 23J. Patient 3 with plasmacytoma of skull base. T2-weighted image showing relatively low-intensity mass (compared with the typical chondrosarcoma or chordoma) of the left petrous apex.

CASE 24

Clinical History: A 50-year-old man presents with chronic, progressive left-sided facial pain.

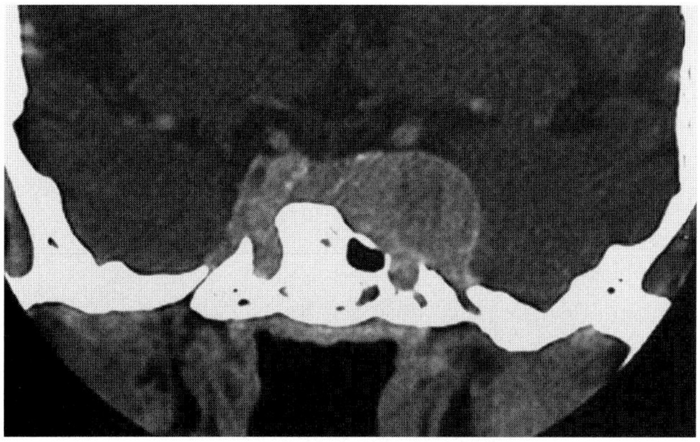

Figure 24A

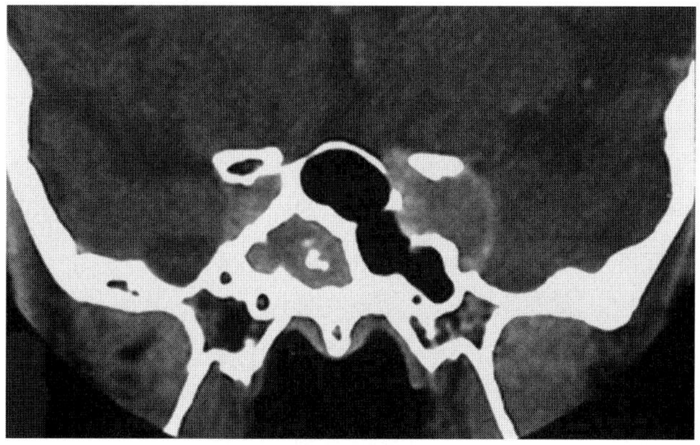

Figure 24B

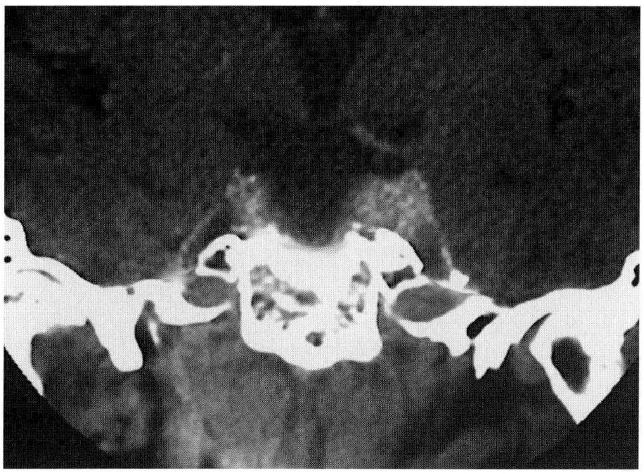

Figure 24C

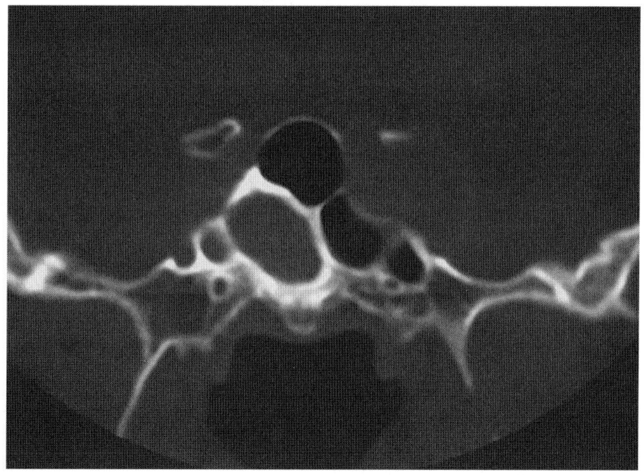

Figure 24D

1. Where is the lesion centered?
2. List the three most probable diagnoses in rank order of likelihood of occurrence and then significance (the first most likely, the second most significant).
3. What additional tests would you suggest and why?

Findings

A well-circumscribed mass centered in the left cavernous sinus with pressure erosion of the sella turcica and the left posterior clinoid process. The lesion homogeneously enhances on postcontrast computed tomography (CT) image. The integrity of the left trigeminal cistern is maintained. The concomitant, chronic sphenoid sinusitis with fungal colonization may be ignored.

Problem

An enhancing cavernous sinus region mass causing trigeminal nerve symptoms

Anatomy

A. Cavernous segment of the internal carotid artery
   1. Segments
   2. Main branches
   3. Relationship to adjacent cranial nerves and venous sinusoids

B. Trigeminal cistern, ganglion and major divisions in the cavernous sinus region

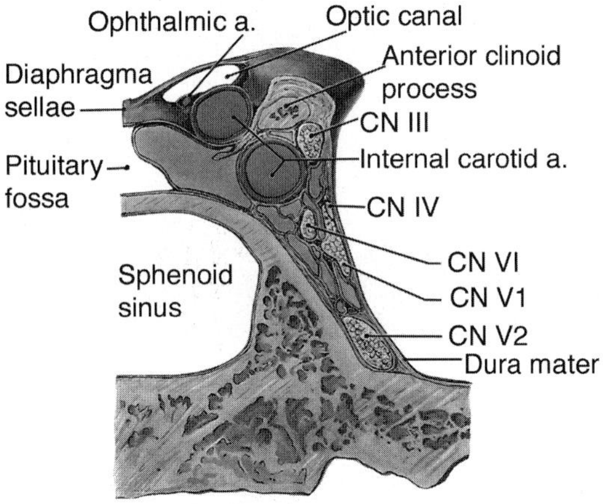

Figure 24E

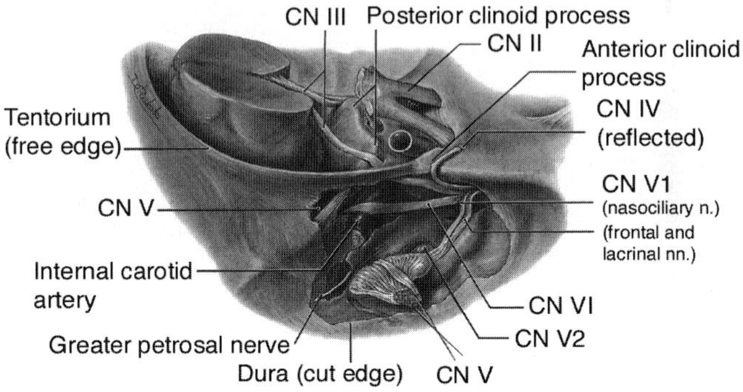

Figure 24F

Differential Diagnosis

Aneurysm, meningioma, neurogenic tumor, hemangioma (rare), metastasis, lymphoma

Diagnosis

Cavernous carotid artery aneurysm

Diagnostic Imaging Approach

A. *First*, exclude aneurysm or other vascular lesion (e.g., cavernous-carotid [CC] fistula) as a cause.

B. Establish vector of lesion: along dura, along a cranial nerve, nonspecific.

C. Consider source besides cavernous sinus region (e.g., pituitary gland, sphenoid bone or sinus, perineural or direct extension of nasopharyngeal cancer).

D. Morphology of lesion
   1. Signal intensity or density, flow voids, enhancement, calcification (curvilinear)

Clinical Points Of Importance And Supplemental Information

A. A patient with deficits of all divisions of the trigeminal nerve frequently has a structural lesion within the cavernous sinus as an explanation for the pain.

B. Any discrete, enhancing mass in the cavernous sinus should be considered an aneurysm until proved otherwise.

Answers To Questions

1. Cavernous sinus
2. Occurrence: meningioma, aneurysm, schwannoma. Significance: aneurysm, meningioma, schwannoma
3. Computed tomographic angiogram, magnetic resonance angiography, angiography to avoid inadvertent (uniformed) arterial injury

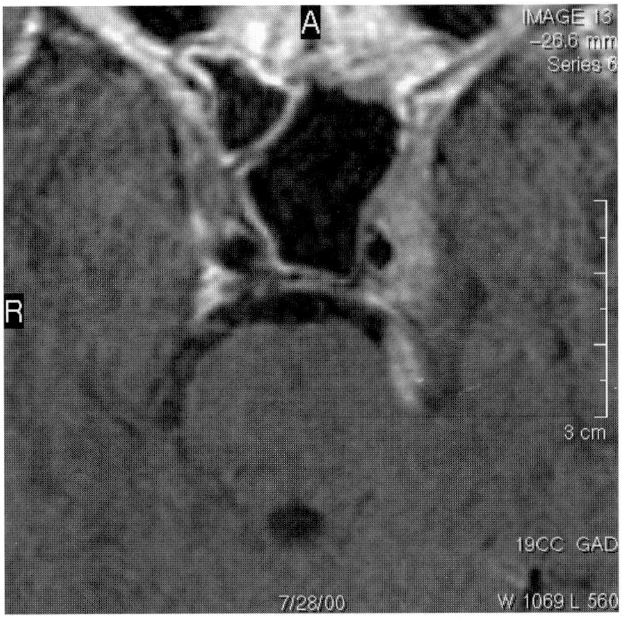

Figure 24G. Patient 1 with skin carcinoma. T1-weighted axial image with contrast, showing perineural tumor spread along cranial nerve V, which involves proximal V2, trigeminal ganglion, and cisternal segment and reaches the root entry zone without obvious pontine invasion.

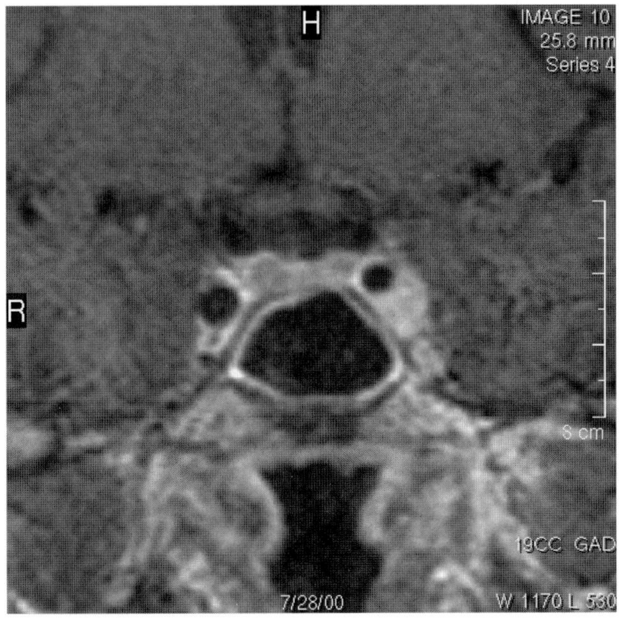

Figure 24H. Patient 1 with skin carcinoma. T1-weighted coronal image with contrast at level of cavernous sinus, showing lobulated enhancing mass along expected course of cranial nerves in the outer dura of the cavernous sinus.

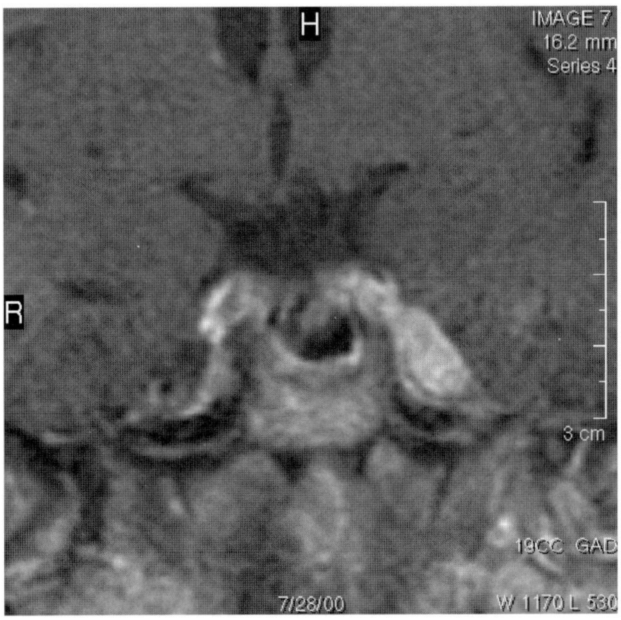

Figure 24I. Patient 1 with skin carcinoma. T1-weighted coronal image posterior to 24 hours, showing the mass to fill the trigeminal cistern.

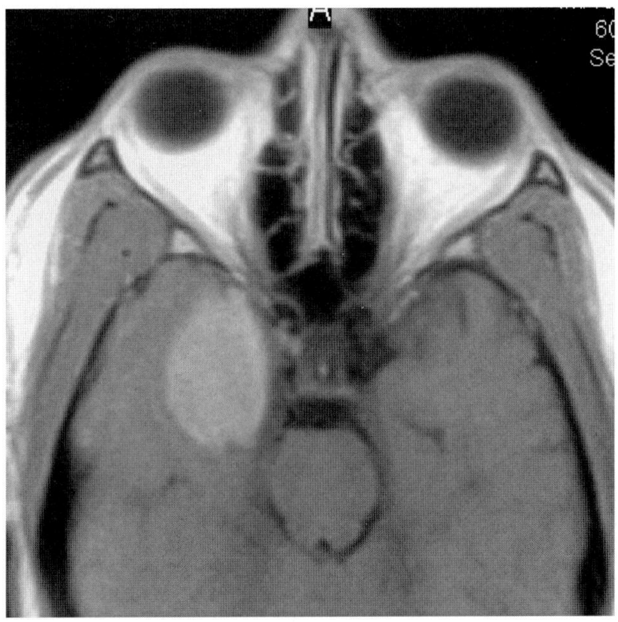

Figure 24J. Patient 2 with meningioma. T1-weighted transverse image with contrast, showing homogeneously enhancing mass lateral to the right cavernous sinus.

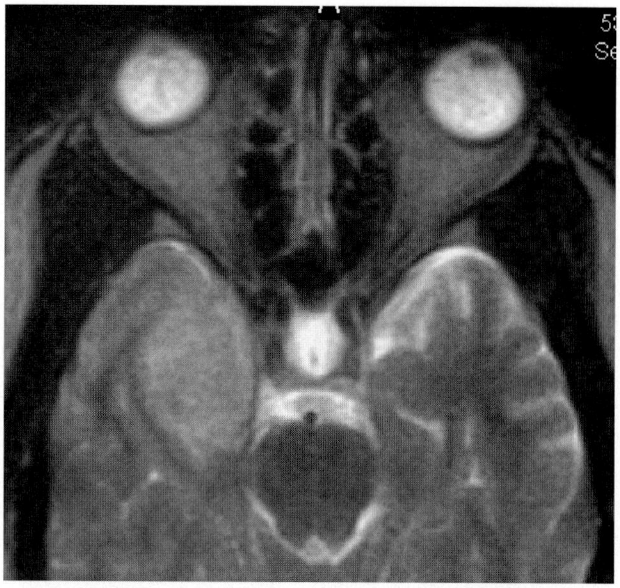

Figure 24K. Patient 2 with meningioma. T2-weighted transverse image showing mass as slightly hyperintense to brain.

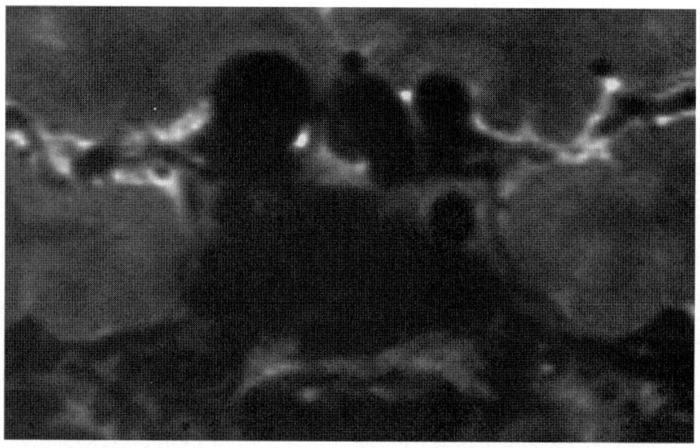

Figure 24L. Patient 3 with multiple aneurysms. T2-weighted coronal image, showing multiple aneurysm probably arising from the internal carotid artery and its branches.

CASE 25

Clinical History: A 28-year-old psychiatric patient presents with facial pain.

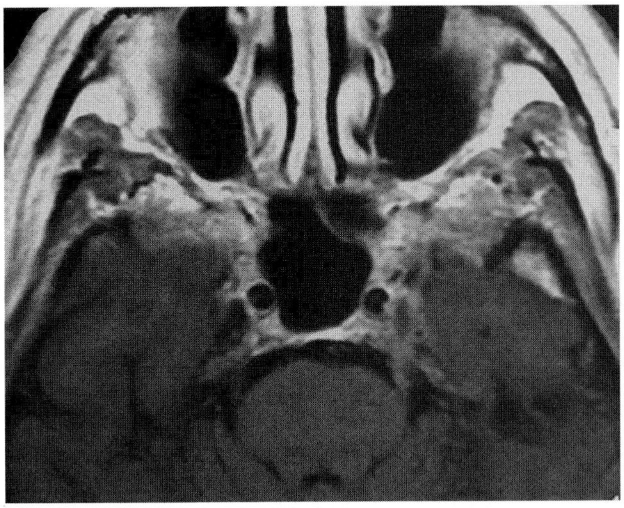

Figure 25A

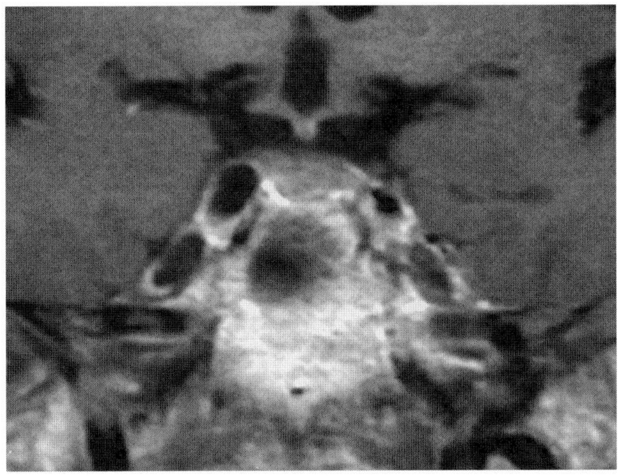

Figure 25B

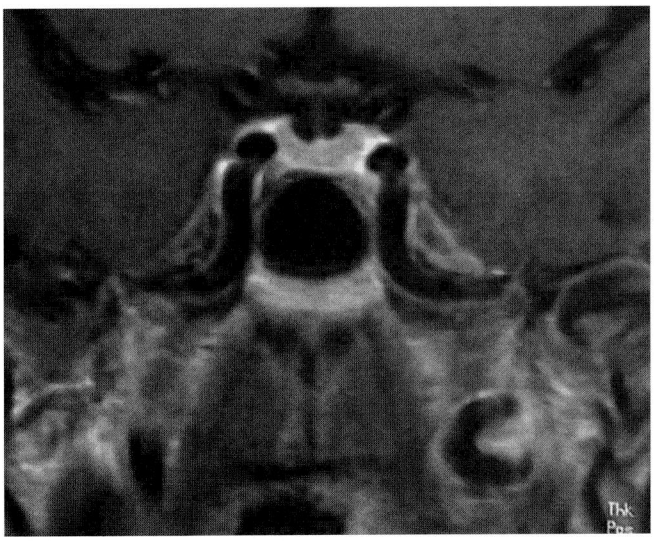

Figure 25C

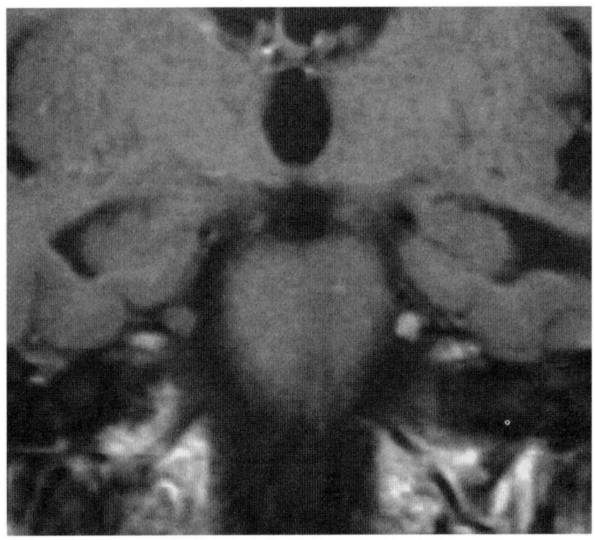

Figure 25D

1. What specific parts of the trigeminal nerve are abnormal? How are they abnormal?
2. What else would you like to evaluate?
3. List 3 neoplastic and three nonneoplastic etiologies for the clinical and MRI findings.

Findings

T1-weighted MRI after contrast administration show abnormal enhancement and thickening of cisternal segment of the left trigeminal nerve, including the segment of the nerve in the trigeminal cistern. The enhancement seems to be centered in and around the trigeminal ganglion.

Problem

Abnormal enhancement of the trigeminal ganglion rootlets and trigeminal nerve in an adult with acute facial pain

Anatomy

A. Trigeminal cistern
B. Trigeminal ganglion
C. Trigeminal nerve

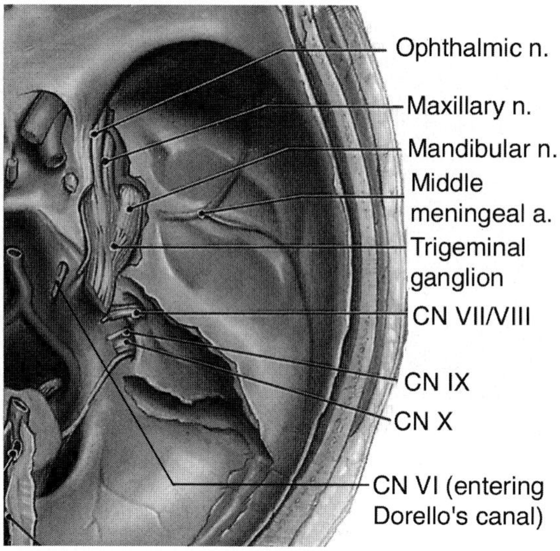

Figure 25E

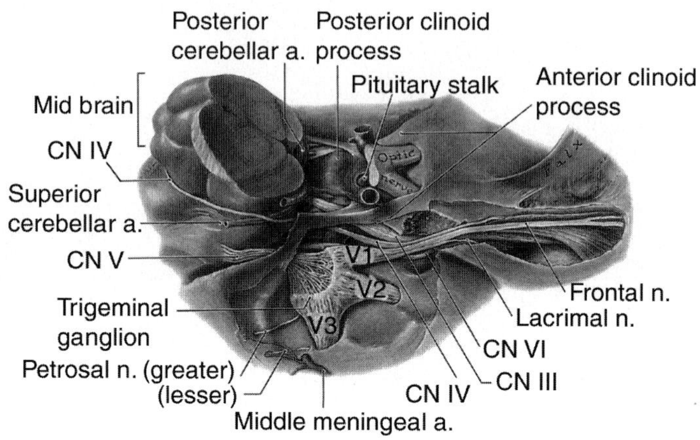

Figure 25F

Differential Diagnosis

1. Inflammatory enhancement: viral (e.g., herpes trigeminus), syphilis; when disease is not strictly confined to the nerve, consider sarcoidosis, Wegener's granulomatosis, pseudotumor.
2. Neoplastic: neurogenic tumor, perineural spread of cancer, lymphoma

Diagnosis

Herpes trigeminus

Diagnostic Imaging Approach

A. Trace all branches of the trigeminal nerve from the periphery to the ganglion and nerve. Identify enlargement or abnormal enhancement and portions of the trigeminal nerve that are involved.
B. Is this isolated disease or part of a generalized process involving other nerves or meninges?
C. Are there any associated mass lesions or brain involvement?

Clinical Points Of Importance And Supplemental Information

A. Cranial nerve enhancement must first be differentiated from *normal* perineural enhancement. If abnormal, it is nonspecific. Inflammatory enhancement is usually caused by a reaction of latent viral infections and will resolve in 6 weeks to 3 months.
B. Always consider perineural spread of cancer as a possible cause and diligently search for appropriate history or a primary tumor.

Answers To Questions

1. Cisternal segment, rootlets. Enlarged, enhancing.
2. Distal course of divisions
3. Neoplastic: perineural spread of carcinoma, lymphoma, neurogenic. Nonneoplastic: viral neuritis, sarcoidosis, Wegener's granuloma.

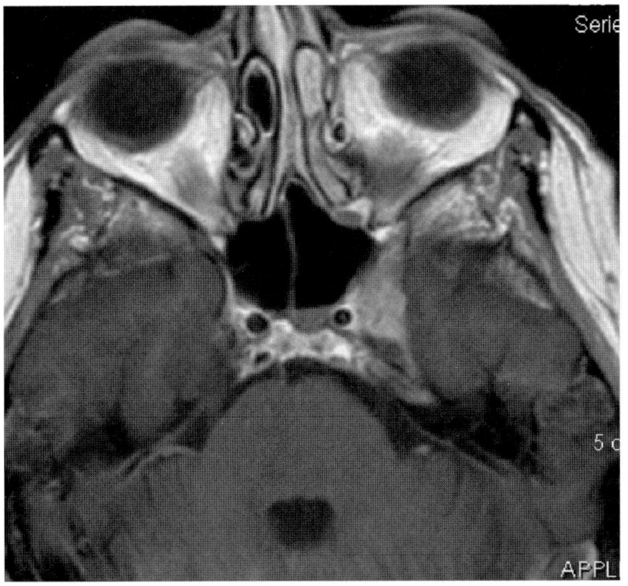

Figure 25G. Patient 1 with poorly differentiated carcinoma of parotid gland. T1-weighted axial image with contrast, showing enhancing mass along lateral aspect of left cavernous sinus caused by perineural tumor spread along cranial nerve V3.

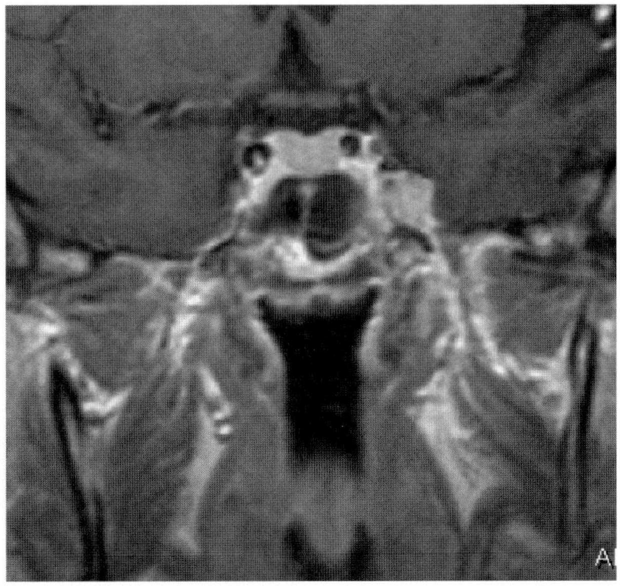

Figure 25H. Patient 1 with poorly differentiated carcinoma of parotid gland. T1-weighted coronal image with contrast, showing enhancing mass in the area of left cavernous sinus just above the foramen ovale.

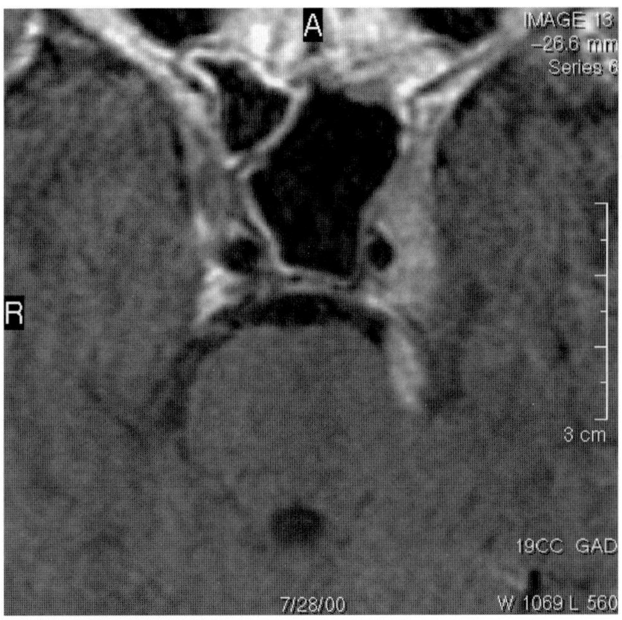

Figure 25I. Patient 2 with skin cancer. T1-weighted axial image with contrast, showing thickening and abnormal enhancement of cisternal segment of left cranial nerve V and cavernous sinus representing perineural tumor spread that reaches the root entry zone of cranial nerve V.

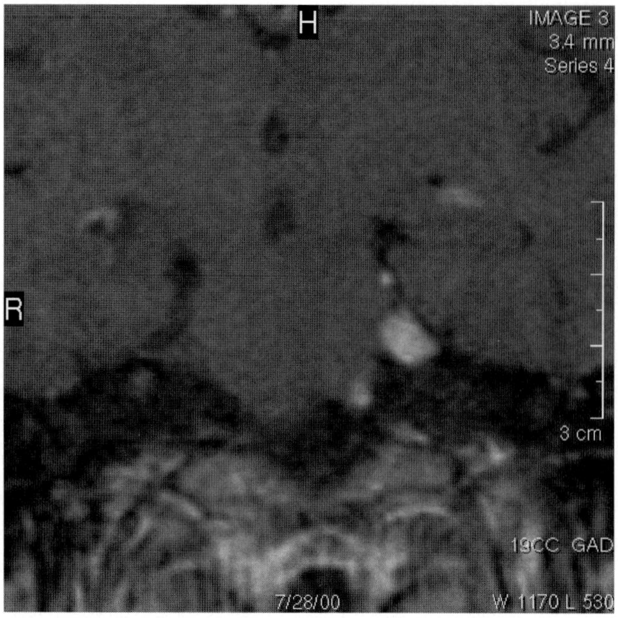

Figure 25J. Patient 2 with skin cancer. T1-weighted coronal image with contrast, showing perineural tumor spread along left cranial nerves III, IV, and VI, manifested by thickening and abnormal enhancement.

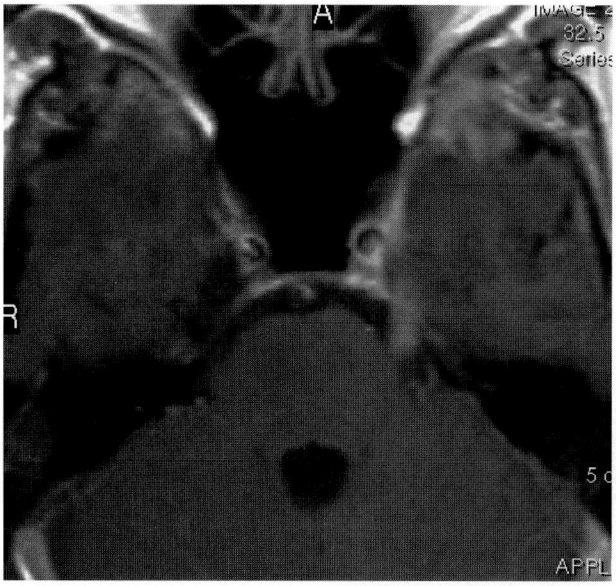

Figure 25K. Patient 3 with "neurotropic" lymphoma. T1-weighted axial image with contrast, showing thickening and abnormal enhancement of cisternal segment of left cranial nerve V and cavernous sinus.

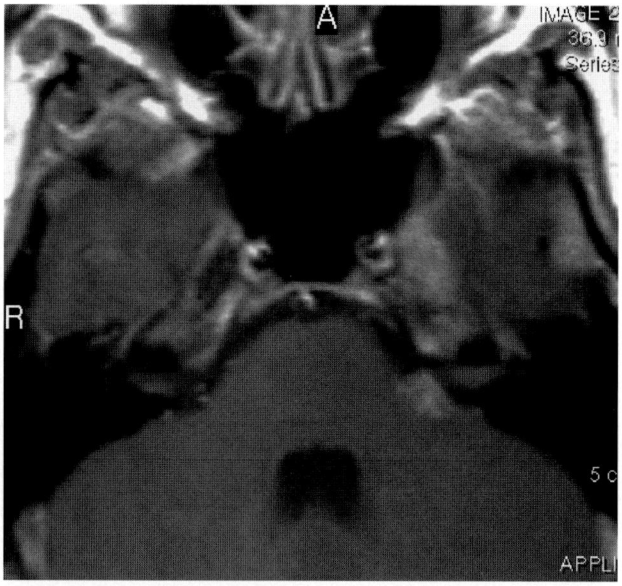

Figure 25L. Patient 3 with "neurotropic" lymphoma. T1-weighted axial image with contrast inferior to 25K, showing enhancing mass filling trigeminal cistern and another enhancing mass in the left cerebellopontine angle, which is contiguous with the left internal auditory canal, and labyrinthine portion, anterior genu, and proximal tympanic segment of the facial canal.

CHAPTER 3

TEMPORAL BONE / POSTERIOR FOSSA

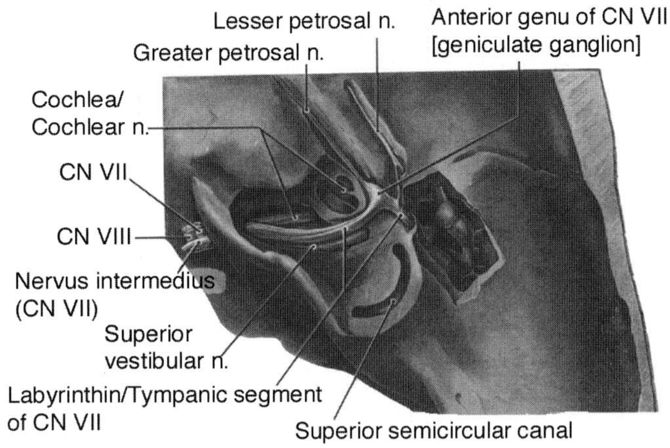

CASE 26

Clinical History: A 40-year-old man presents with fever, headaches, and multiple cranial nerve deficits.

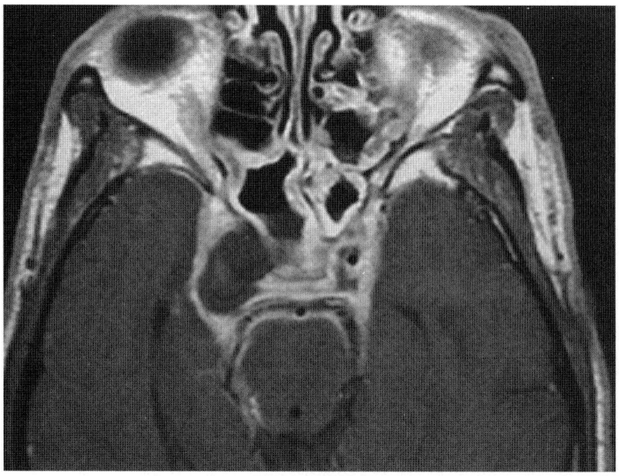

Figure 26A

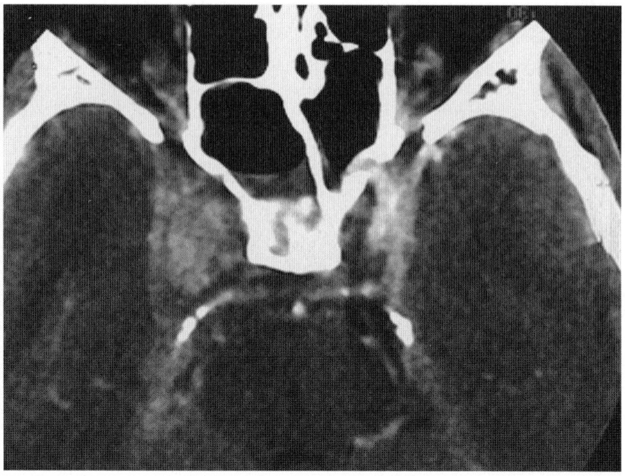

Figure 26B

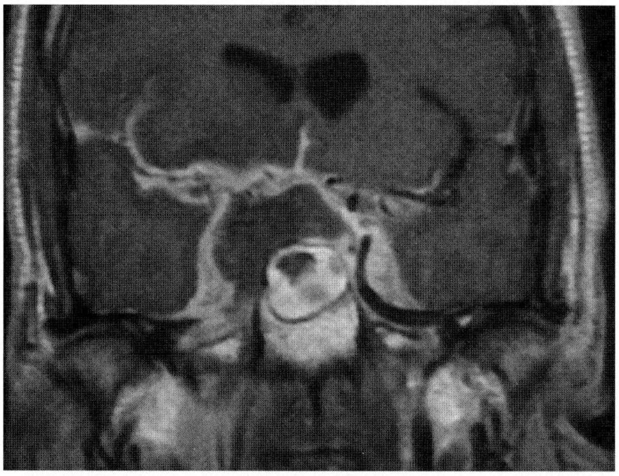

Figure 26C

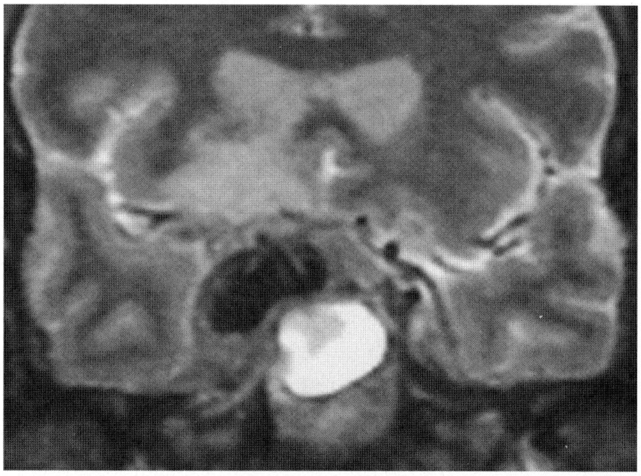

Figure 26D

1. Is the basic disease process inflammatory or neoplastic?
2. Where did the disease originate?
3. List four specific likely secondary diagnoses (i.e., extensions of the primary disease process).

Findings

Irregular mucoperiosteal thickening and an air-fluid level in the sphenoid sinus. An extraaxial "cystic" mass is present in the right paracavernous area and the suprasellar cistern on postcontrast, T1-weighted image. It is seen as an area of flow void on T2-weighted image, which suggests its being an aneurysm. Enhancement of the lesion on postcontrast computed tomography (CT) suggests an infected aneurysm. Postcontrast images also show extensive meningeal enhancement.

Problem

Inflammatory mass centered in the sphenoid sinus, with intracranial involvement and multiple cranial nerve deficits

Anatomy

A. Basisphenoid (see Fig. 21F)
   1. Sphenoid sinus
   2. Upper clivus
B. Cavernous sinus
   1. Dural relationships
   2. Carotid artery segments
C. Clival vascular plexus

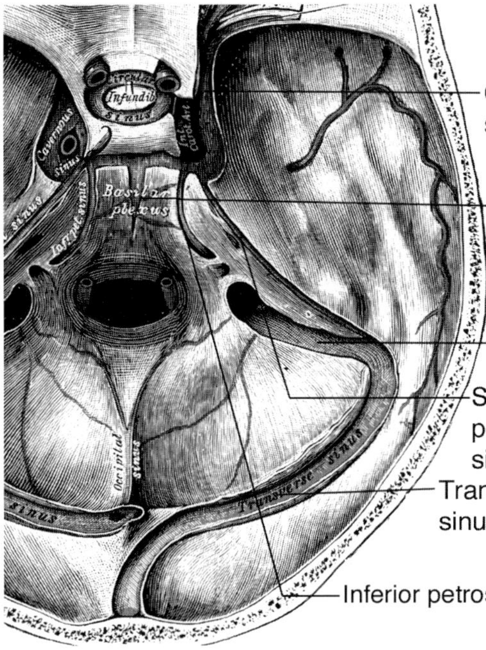

Figure 26E

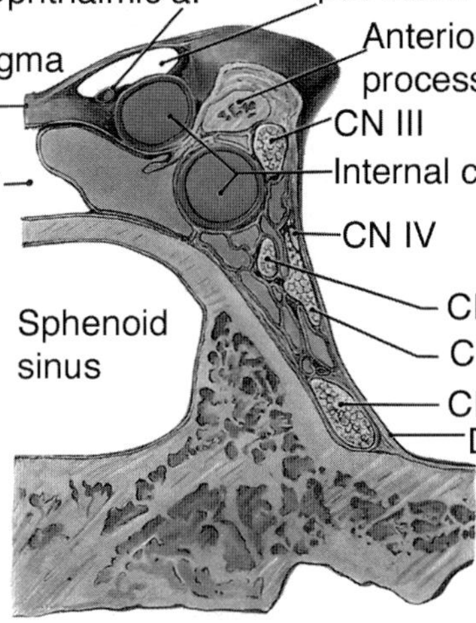

Figure 26F

Differential Diagnosis

None

Diagnosis

Sphenoid sinus pyomucocele, with dural phlegmon, subdural empyema, fulminant pyogenic meningitis, and septic cavernous carotid aneurysm

Diagnostic Imaging Approach

A. Recognize inflammatory morphology.
B. Establish origin of inflammatory pathology.
C. Search for complications on the basis of pathophysiology or anatomy:
   1. Thrombophlebitis, direct extension, meningeal, subarachnoid space, hydrocephalus, herniation

Clinical Points Of Importance And Supplemental Information

Intracranial complications of extracranial infections must be anticipated and recognized promptly by using high resolution imaging techniques; such action helps avoid the fatal situation illustrated by this case.

Answers To Questions

1. Inflammatory
2. Sphenoid sinus
3. Septic cavernous carotid artery aneurysm, left cavernous sinus thrombosis, pyogenic meningitis, subdural empyema

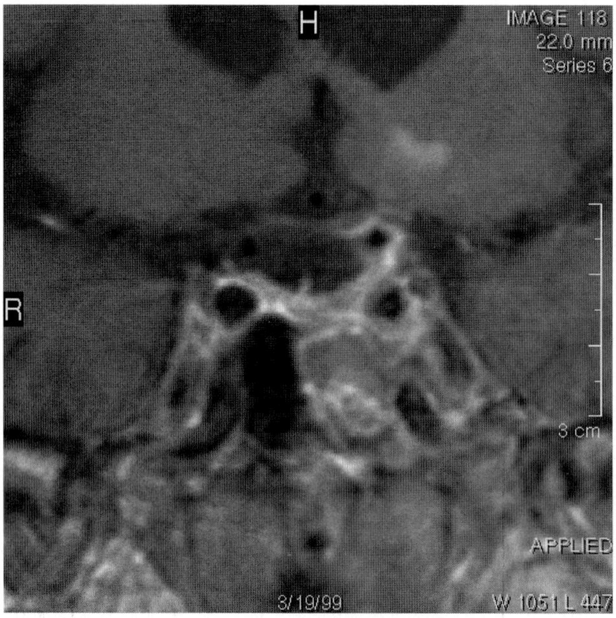

Figure 26G. Patient 1 with invasive fungal sinusitis. T1-weighted coronal image with contrast, showing enhancing tissue in left-sided sphenoid sinus, which is contiguous with enhancing tissue around the clinoid segment of the left internal carotid artery. Irregular enhancement of adjacent brain representing infarction caused by vascular invasion.

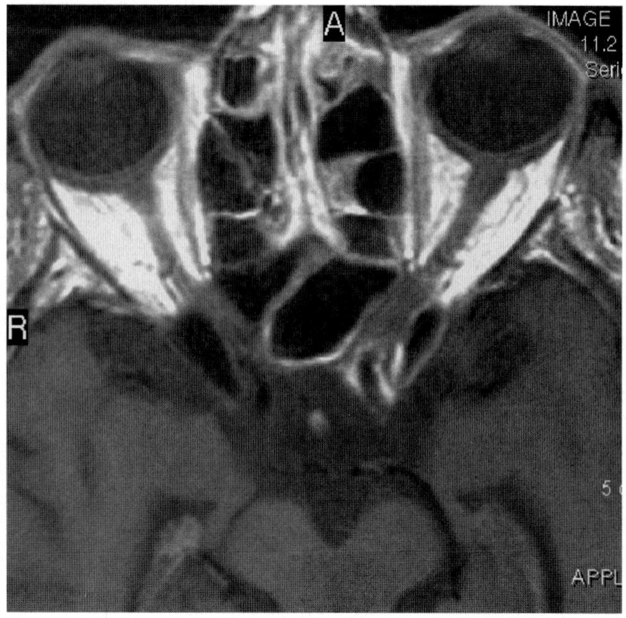

Figure 26H. Patient 1 with invasive fungal sinusitis. T1-weighted axial image with contrast, showing abnormally enhancing tissue surrounding the clinoid segment of the left internal carotid artery.

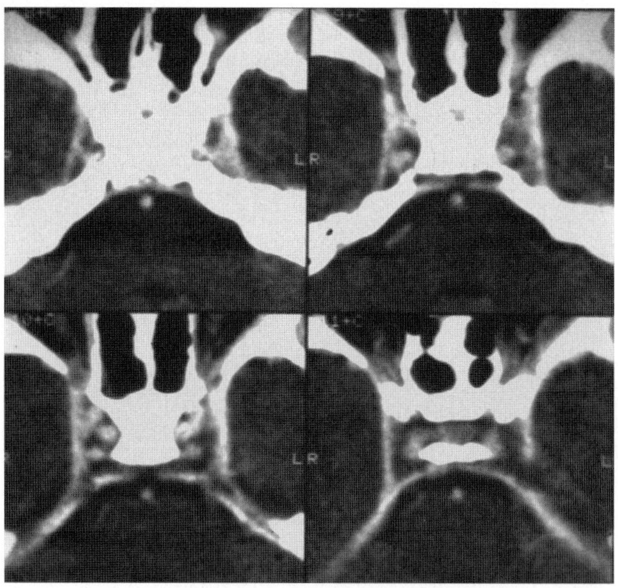

Figure 26I. Patient 2 with sinusitis and "frozen eyes." Contrast-enhanced computed tomography image, showing multiple filling defects in the cavernous sinus on each side, strongly suggestive of cavernous sinus thrombosis extending into the left superior petrosal sinus and clival venous plexus.

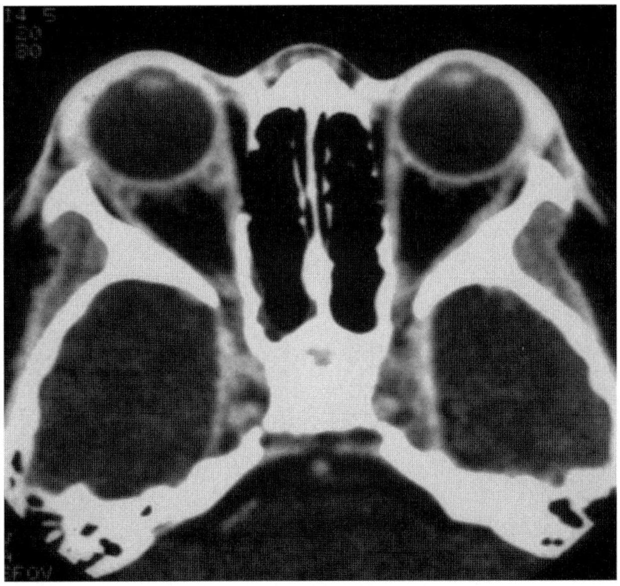

Figure 26J. Patient 2 with sinusitis and "frozen eyes," showing deficit of normal, diffuse enhancement of both cavernous sinuses, suggestive of cavernous sinus thrombosis. The defects highlight the enhanced cavernous segment of the internal carotid arteries.

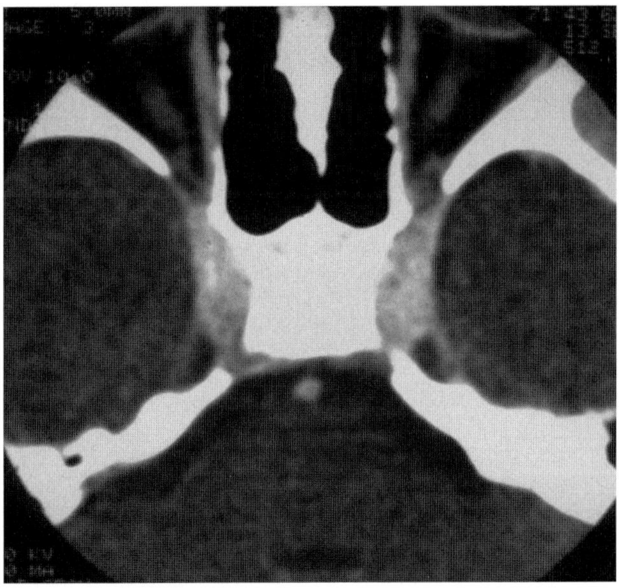

Figure 26K. Patient 2 with sinusitis and "frozen eyes." Contrast-enhanced computed tomography image 2 weeks after 26I, showing complete resolution of cavernous sinus thrombosis.

CASE 27

Clinical History: A 42-year-old man presents with acute onset of peripheral facial nerve palsy.

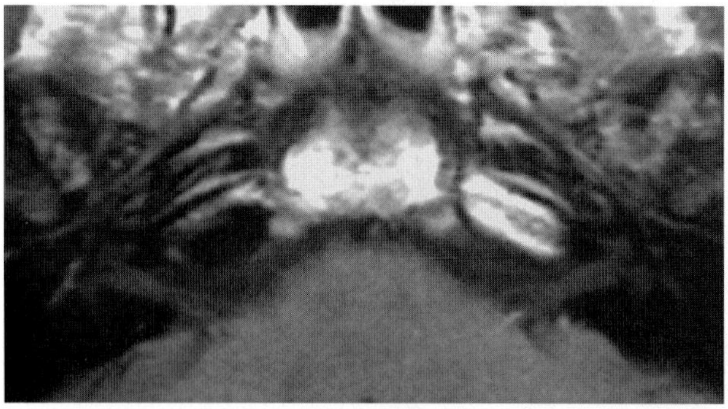

Figure 27A

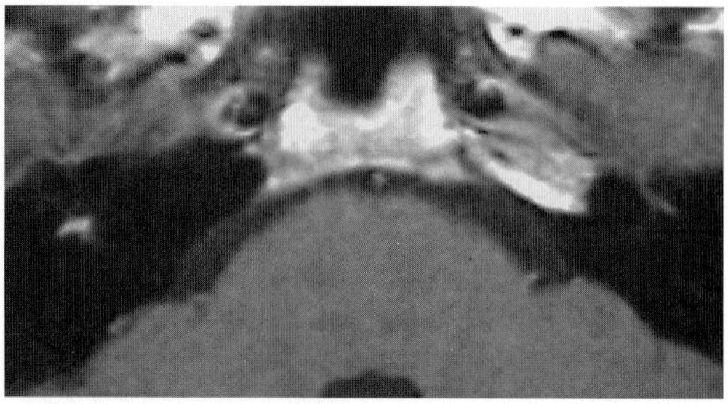

Figure 27B

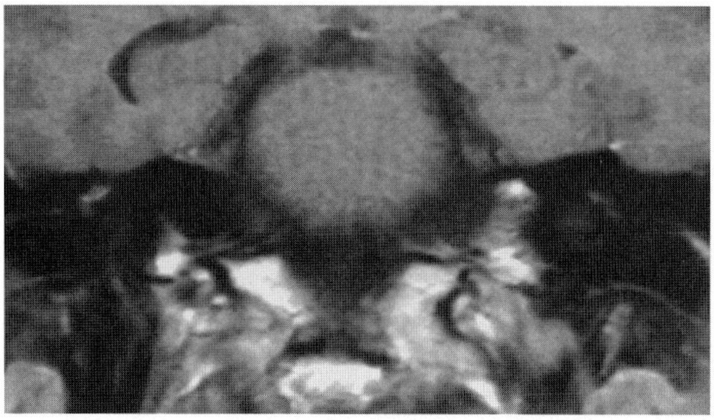

Figure 27C

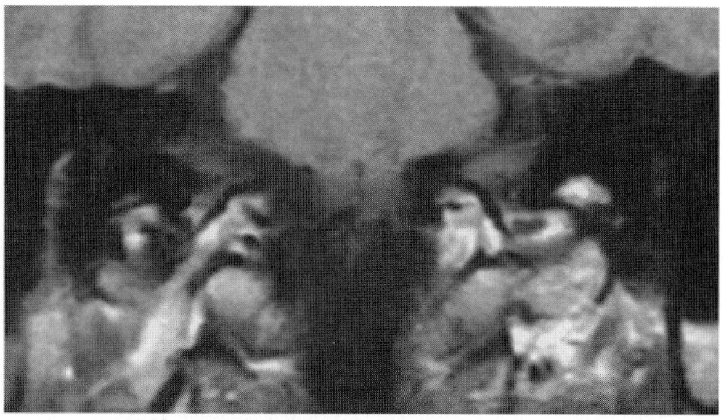

Figure 27D

1. Is the study abnormal? What is "Bell's" palsy?
2. Was the study necessary?
3. List two diagnostic criteria for declaring a cranial nerve abnormal. List one common normal variation seen along cranial nerves as they exit the skull.

Findings

Abnormal enhancement of the anterior genu, tympanic segment, posterior genu, and mastoid segment of the right facial nerve.

Problem

Abnormal enhancement of the facial nerve in an adult with acute onset of peripheral facial nerve palsy

Anatomy

A. Facial nerve on magnetic resonance imaging (MRI), including normal perineural enhancement
   1. Labyrinthine segment
   2. Anterior genu
   3. Tympanic segment
   4. Posterior genu
   5. Descending segment

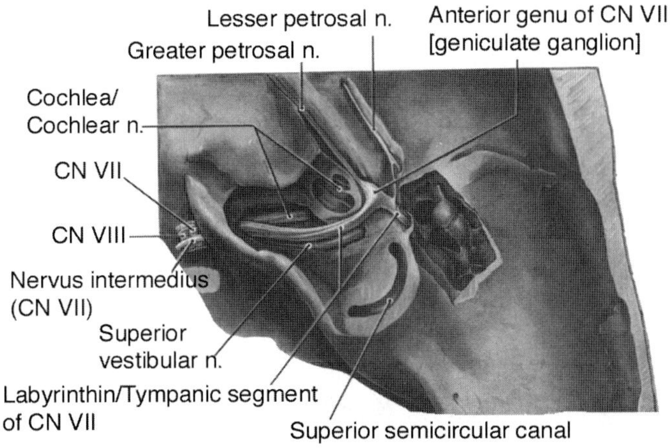

Figure 27E

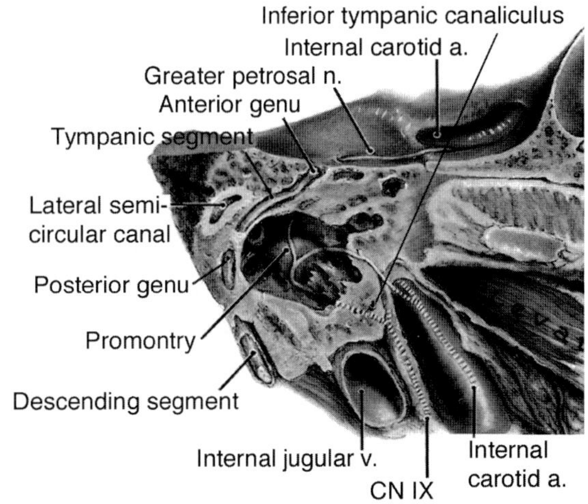

Figure 27F

Differential Diagnosis

Viral or granulomatous neuritis, perineural spread of cancer (i.e., skin, parotid, adenoid cystic carcinoma), neurogenic tumor, hemangioma

Diagnosis

Inflammatory enhancement of the facial nerve—probably viral

Diagnostic Imaging Approach

A. Trace the entire course of the facial nerve from its nucleus to the end organ; look for enlargement, abnormal enhancement, or a compressive lesion.
B. Remember, proximal enlargement or enhancement of the nerve can reflect retrograde spread from a more peripheral source of disease.

Clinical Points Of Importance And Supplemental Information

A. Acute onset of peripheral facial nerve palsy is almost always caused by viral neuritis. Of these cases, 80% will resolve in 4 to 6 weeks. These cases do not require a MRI study at initial presentation except in unusual circumstances (e.g., pediatric age group, associated neurologic deficits).
B. All nonresolving acute palsies and all slow or "stuttering" onset palsies *must* be studied. The *entire* nerve must be studied in all cases.
C. Always consider retrograde spread of skin cancer as a possible cause and ask for a history of possible skin lesion removal.
D. Facial weakness is sometimes the initial presentation of demyelinating disease.

Answers To Questions

1. Yes. Acute onset of a peripheral facial palsy.
2. Probably not
3. Enlargement or enhancement. Perineural enhancement related to normal vascular plexus.

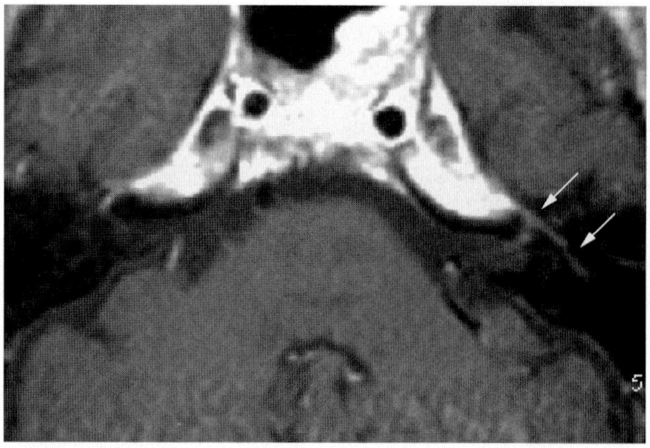

Figure 27G. Patient 1 with "neurotropic" non-Hodgkin's lymphoma. T1-weighted image with contrast, showing asymmetric enhancement of labyrinthine segment, anterior genu, and tympanic segment of left facial nerve.

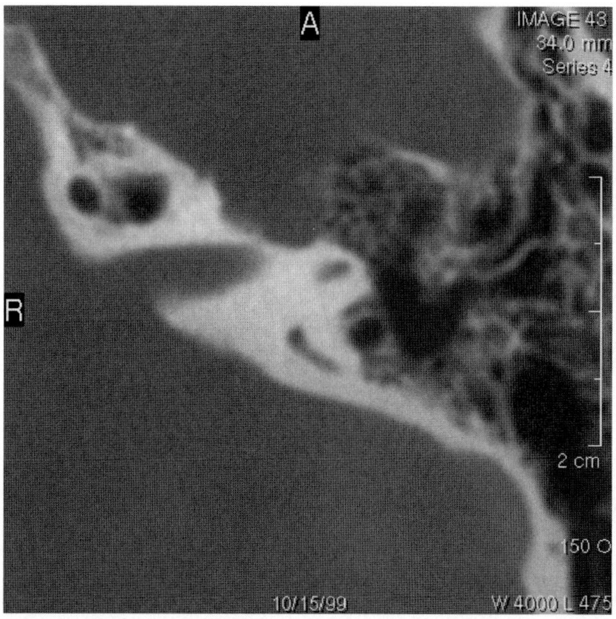

Figure 27H. Patient 2 with schwannoma of facial nerve. Computed tomography (CT) showing focal bone destruction centered in the expected position of anterior genu of left facial nerve.

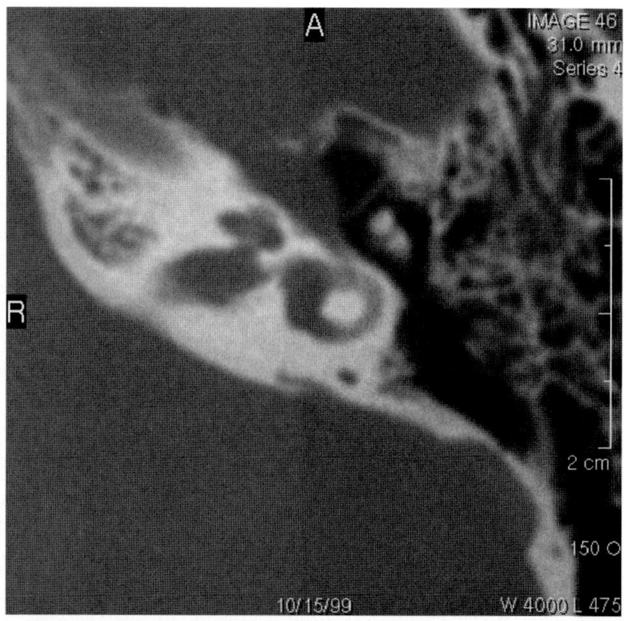

Figure 27I. Patient 2 with schwannoma of facial nerve. CT image inferior to 27H, showing enlargement of proximal tympanic portion of the facial canal, with tapering into a relatively spared distal part of that segment.

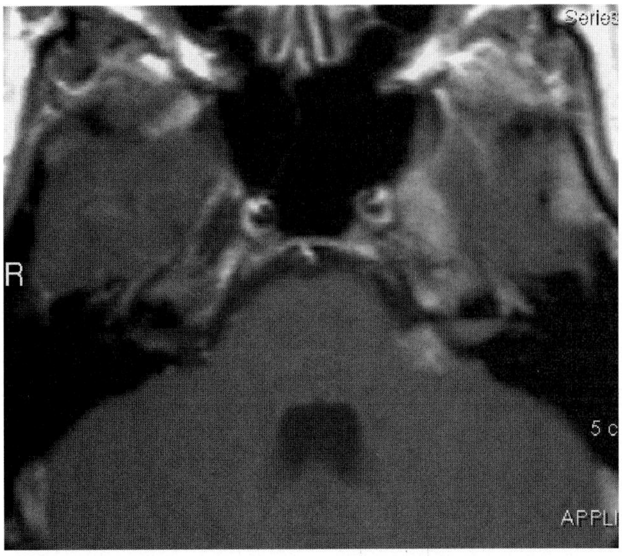

Figure 27J. Patient 3 with "neurotropic" lymphoma. T1-weighted axial image with contrast, showing enhancing mass filling trigeminal cistern and another enhancing mass in the left cerebellopontine angle, which is contiguous with left internal auditory canal, and labyrinthine portion, anterior genu, and proximal tympanic segment of the facial canal.

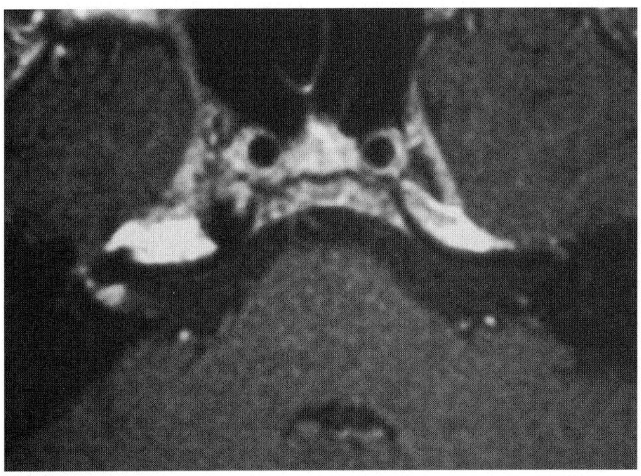

Figure 27K. Patient 4 with Masson's vegetant intravascular hemangioepithelioma. T1-weighted axial image with contrast, showing enhancing mass in the fundus of the right internal auditory canal and smaller enhancing nodules in the labyrinthine segment and anterior genu of the right facial canal, which was surgically proved.

CASE 28

Clinical History: A 22-year-old man presents with enlargement of the external ear (pinna) and hearing loss. Facial nerve function is normal.

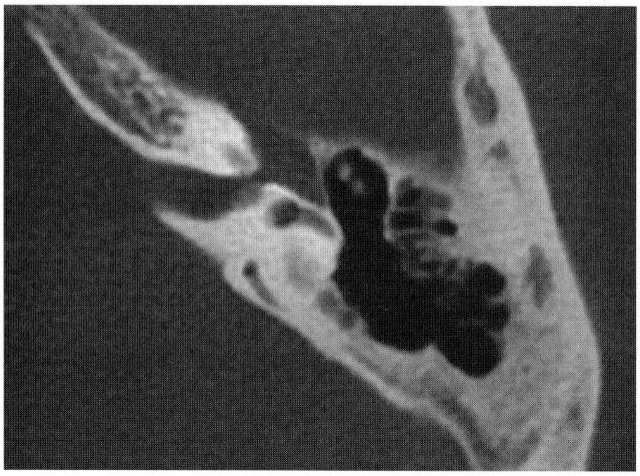

Figure 28A

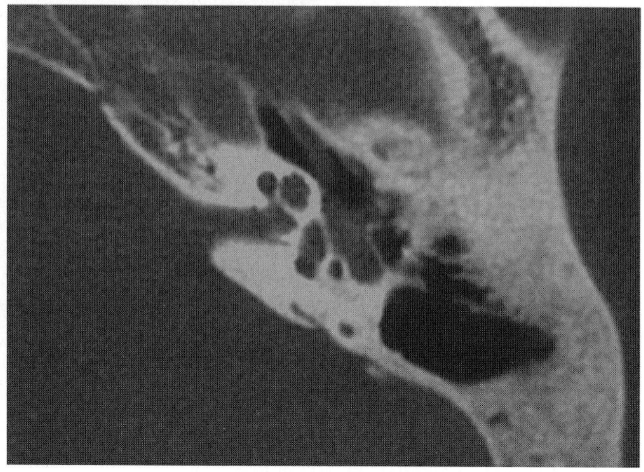

Figure 28B

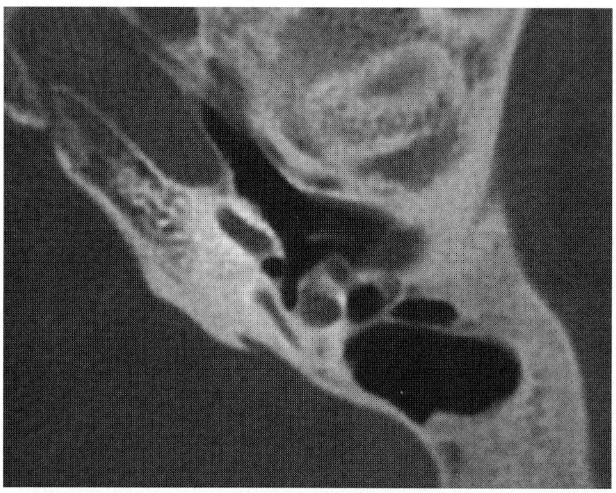

Figure 28C

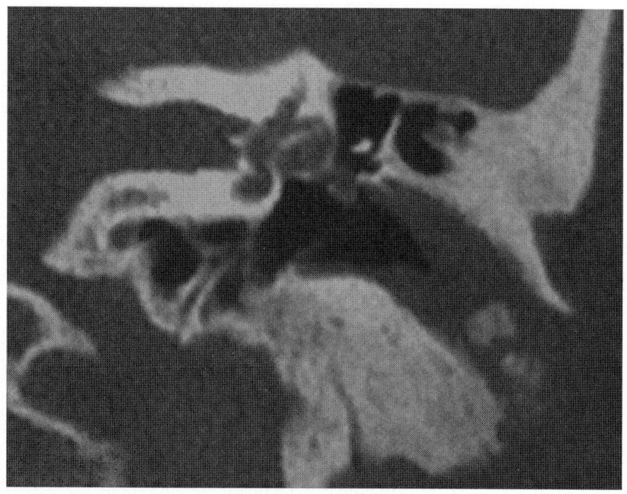

Figure 28D

1. Is the mass intrinsic or extrinsic to the facial nerve?
2. Is magnetic resonance imaging (MRI) necessary to establish the diagnosis? What is the diagnosis (be as specific as you can)?
3. Do patients with gradual onset of peripheral facial nerve dysfunction need to be imaged?
4. List all structures (areas) that must be studied when evaluating the facial canal.

Findings

Enlargement of the left facial nerve canal involving the labyrinthine segment, anterior genu, tympanic segment, posterior genu, and mastoid segment. An excessive soft tissue partly fills the left external auditory canal.

Problem

Gross enlargement of the facial nerve and its branches associated with a dysmorphic ear

Anatomy

Facial nerve: from anterior genu to and within parotid gland, including its major branches proximal to and within the parotid gland

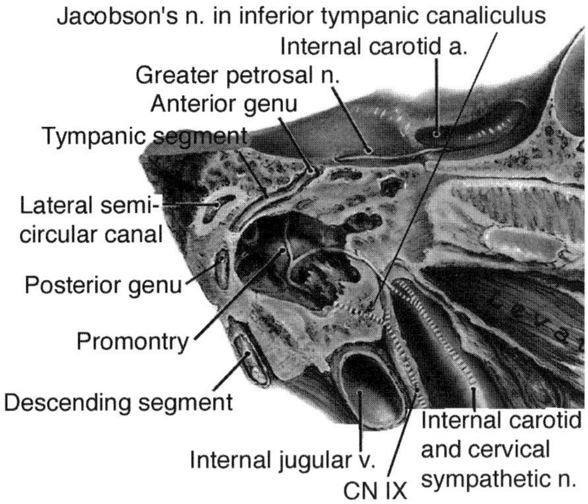

Figure 28E

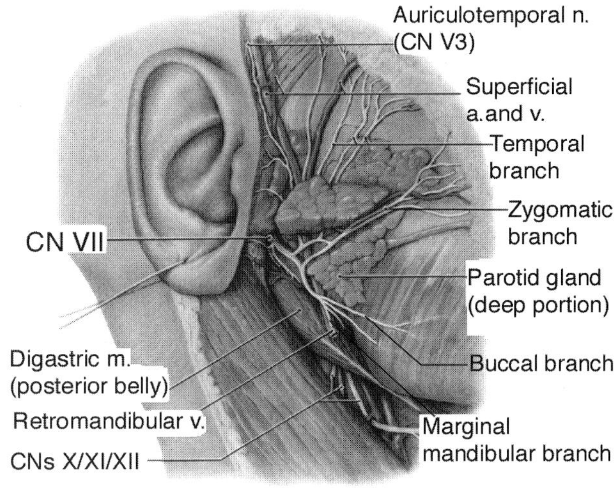

Figure 28F

Differential Diagnosis

None

Diagnosis

Plexiform neurofibroma of the facial nerve and its peripheral branches

Diagnostic Imaging Approach

A. Evaluate the temporal bone systematically:
   1. External auditory canal, middle ear, mastoid
   2. Facial nerve
   3. Inner ear, petrous apex, internal auditory canal

B. Try to establish cause for hearing loss.

C. Evaluate for associated abnormalities.

Clinical Points Of Importance And Supplemental Information

A. Plexiform neurofibromata are frequently asymptomatic.

B. Neurofibromatosis is often not a clinically obvious diagnosis until suggested by imaging study findings.

Answers To Questions

1. Intrinsic
2. No. Plexiform neurofibroma of the facial nerve.
3. Virtually always
4. Labyrinthine segment, Bill's bar, anterior genu, greater superficial petrosal nerve, tympanic segment, second genu, descending segment, stylomandibular foramen

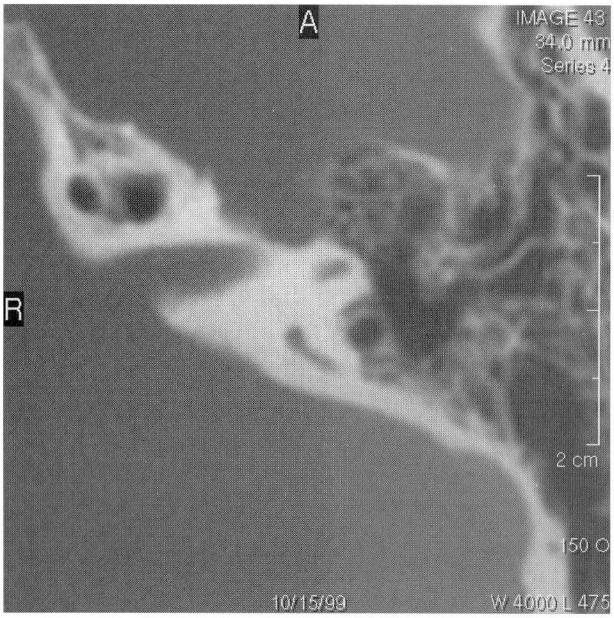

Figure 28G. Patient 1 with schwannoma of the facial nerve. Computed tomography image showing focal bone destruction centered in the expected position of the anterior genu of the left facial nerve.

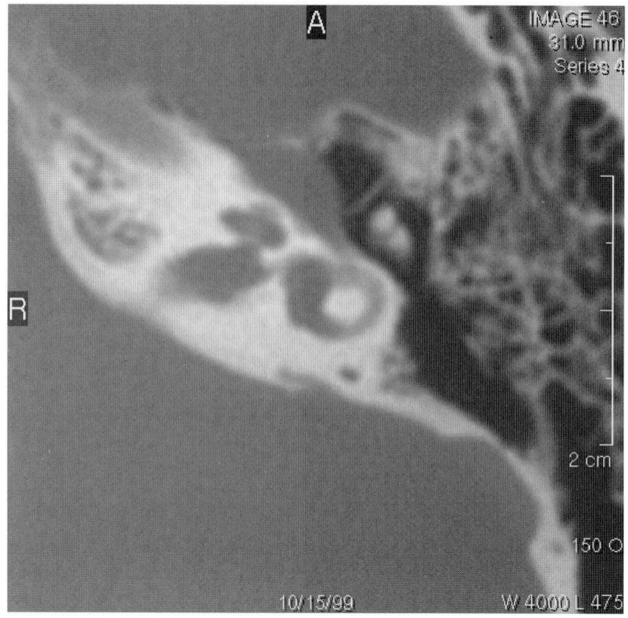

Figure 28H. Patient 1 with schwannoma of facial nerve. Computed tomography image inferior to 28G, showing enlargement of proximal tympanic portion of facial canal tapering into relatively spared part of that segment.

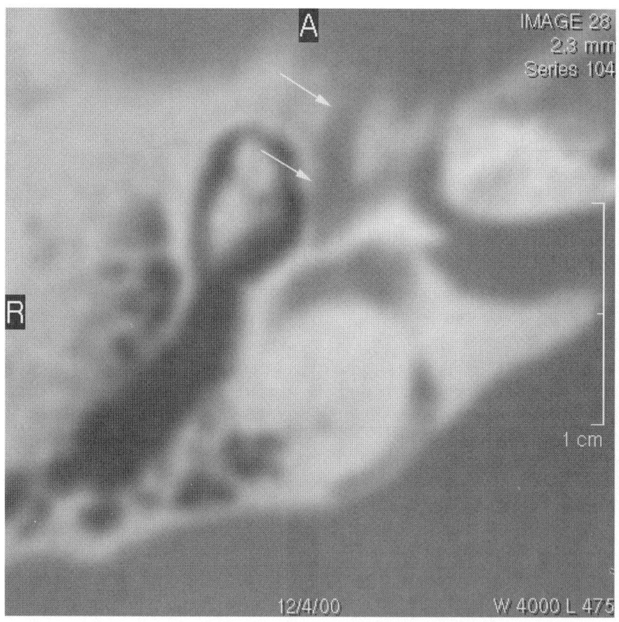

Figure 28I. Patient 2 with persistent stapedial artery. Axial computed tomography image, showing tubular area of radiolucency along the proximal tympanic segment of facial canal.

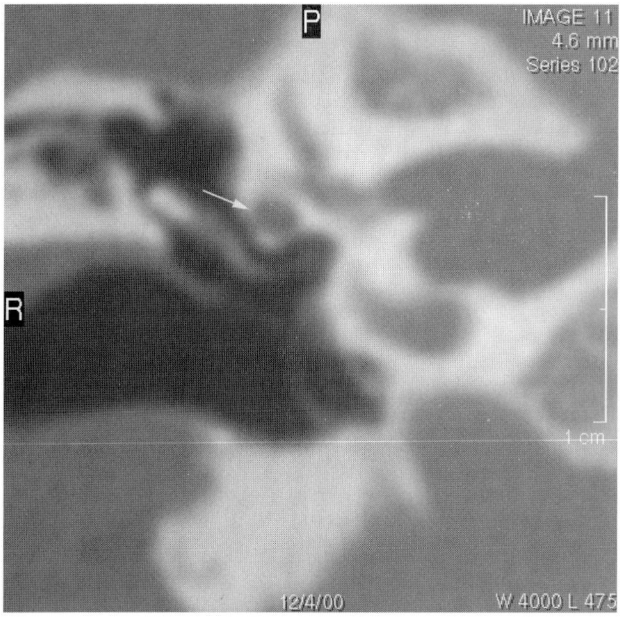

Figure 28J. Patient 2 with persistent stapedial artery. Coronal computed tomography image, showing enlargement of tympanic segment of facial canal just above oval window niche.

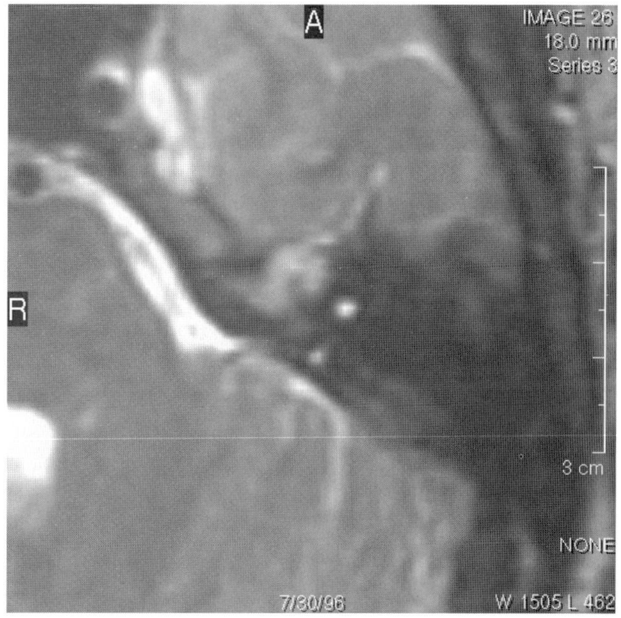

Figure 28K. Patient 3 with hemangioma of facial nerve. T2-weighted axial image, showing high-intensity mass centered just above the anterior genu of left facial nerve (this area enhanced with intravenous contrast [not shown]).

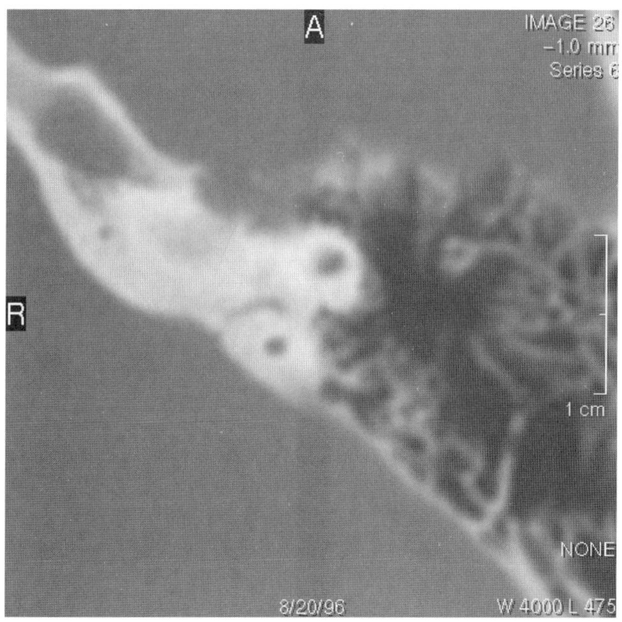

Figure 28L. Patient 3 with schwannoma of facial nerve. Computed tomography image of the temporal bone to correlate with the magnetic resonance image in 28K and other similar cases.

CASE 29

Clinical History: A 29-year-old woman presents with headaches and multiple cranial nerve deficits.

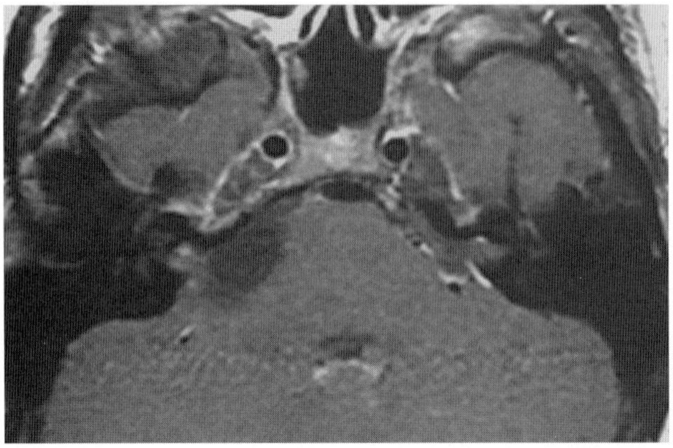

Figure 29A

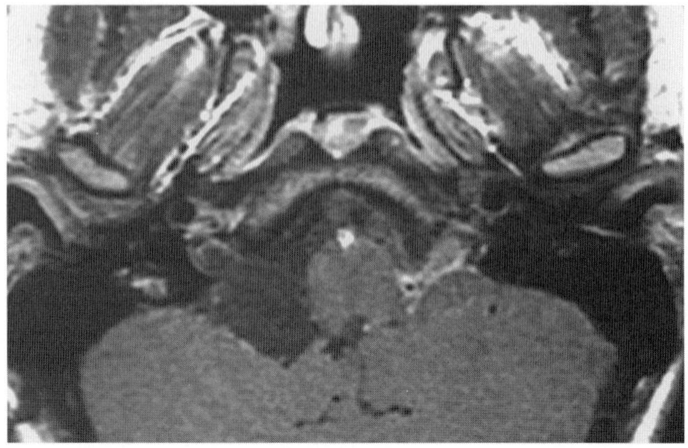

Figure 29B

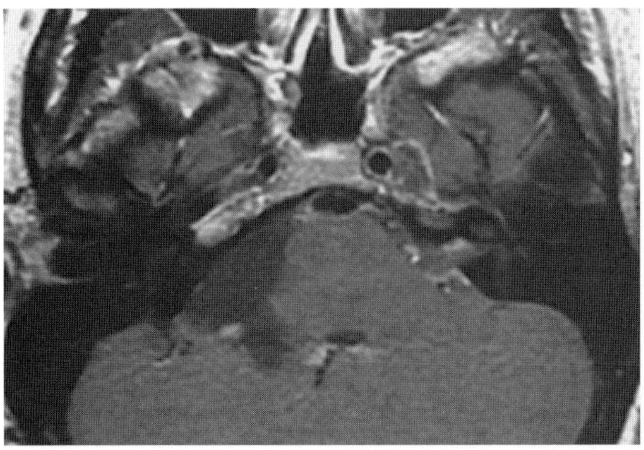

Figure 29C

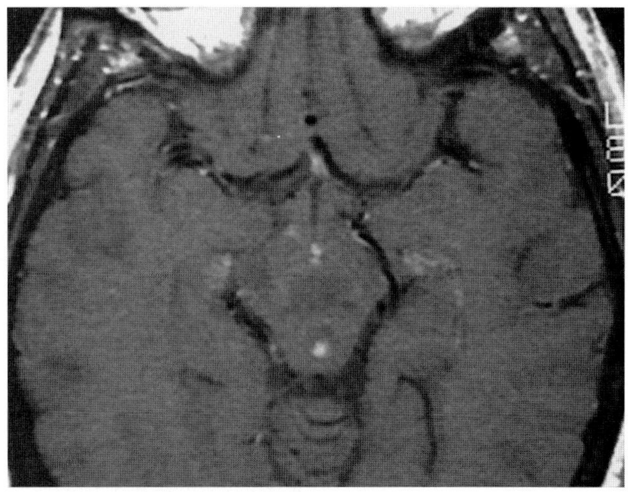

Figure 29D

1. There are two related diagnoses: list both.
2. Predict which cranial nerves are abnormal.

Findings

A loculated cystic mass without enhancing solid component in the right cerebellopontine (CP) angle, distorting the adjacent lower pons and an inferomedial aspect of the right cerebellar hemisphere. Abnormal enhancement surrounds the right VIIth and VIIIth cranial nerves and the other lower cranial nerves as the latter traverse the cisterns to enter the jugular fossa on each side. Also diffuse and nodular enhancement is seen in the cisterns and the cerebral aqueduct.

Problem

A nonenhancing CP angle mass associated with nodular enhancement throughout the cisterns and along multiple the cranial nerves

Anatomy

A. Posterior fossa cisterns
B. Cranial nerves V–XII: their cisternal course and exit foramina

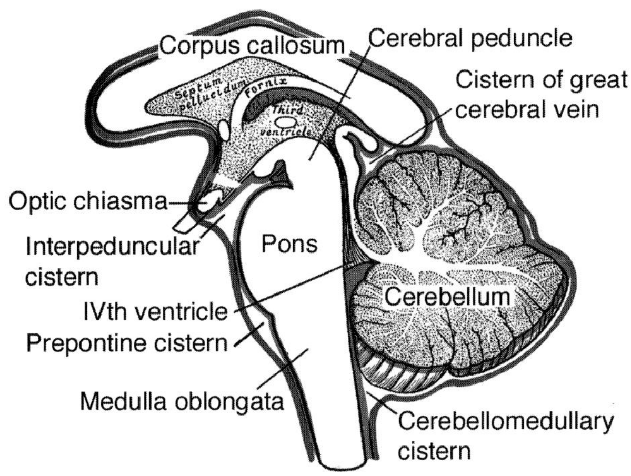

Figure 29E

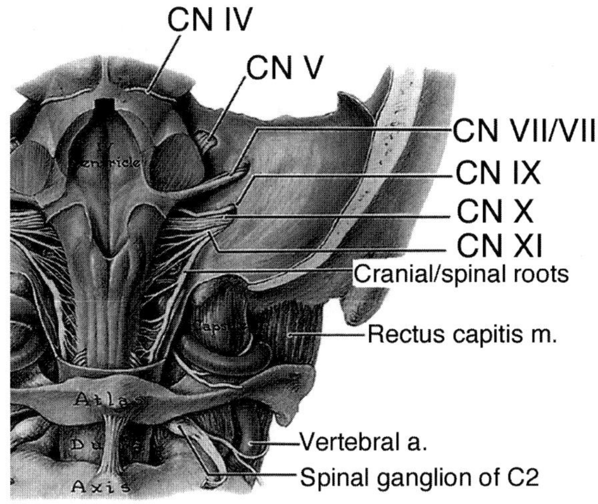

Figure 29F

Differential Diagnosis

None

Diagnosis

Ruptured epidermoid with "chemical" arachnoiditis and secondary cranial nerve deficits.

Diagnostic Imaging Approach

A. With regard to CP angle mass, they should be divided into three categories:
   1. Nonenhancing with fluidlike characteristics (e.g., epidermoid or arachnoid cyst)
   2. Enhancing focal
   3. Meningeal or subarachnoid space pattern
B. With regard to cranial nerve deficits, evaluate dura and pia arachnoid (subarachnoid space) for focal, multifocal diffuse disease.
C. Look for complications (e.g., hydrocephalus).

Clinical Points Of Importance And Supplemental Information

Recognition of such findings and possible complications (i.e., hydrocephalus, herniation) helps plan approach (i.e., lumbar puncture in this case could have led to clinical deterioration).

Answers To Questions

1. Ruptured CP angle epidermoid and meningitis (arachnoiditis)
2. Cranial nerves V, VII, VIII, IX–XII

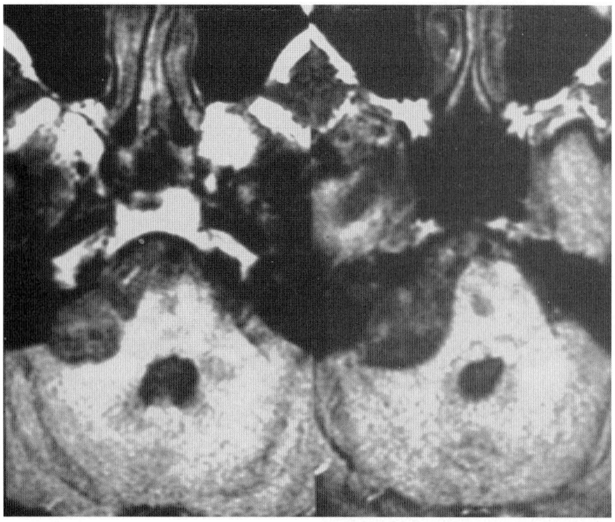

Figure 29G. Patient 1 with epidermoid, showing cystic mass with internal inhomogeneity centered in the right cerebellopontine angle, distorting adjacent lower pons and cerebellum–T1-weighted axial image.

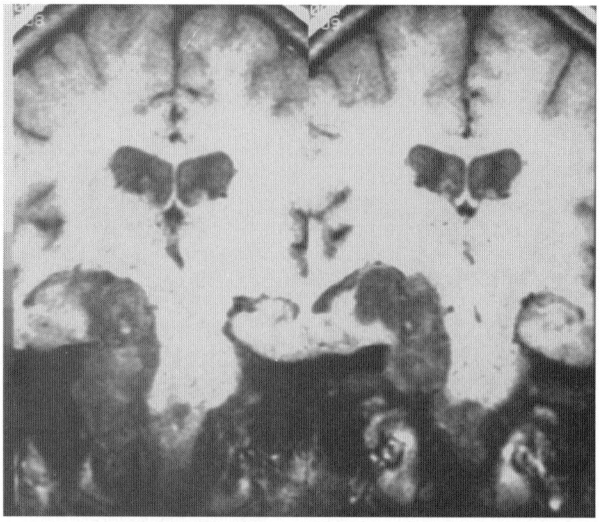

Figure 29H. Patient 1 with epidermoid in the right right cerebellopontine angle crossing the incisura–T1-weighted coronal image.

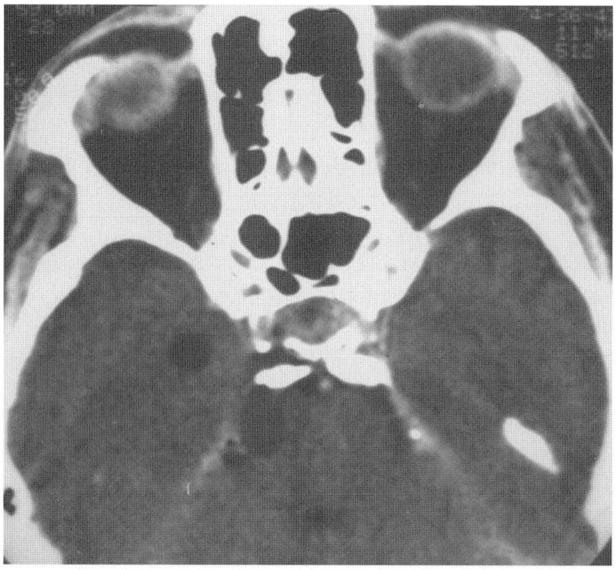

Figure 29I. Patient 2 with ruptured epidermoid. Contrast-enhanced CT image showing loculated cystic mass in the right upper cerebellopontine angle and another cystic mass of probable fat-density in medial aspect of the right temporal lobe.

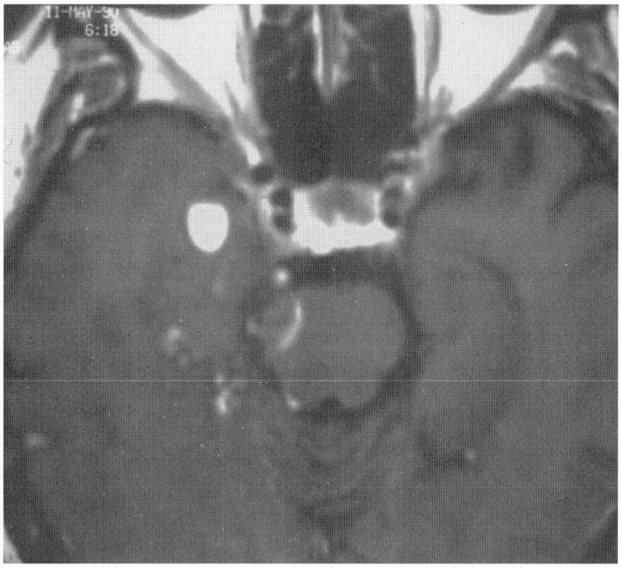

Figure 29J. Patient 2 with ruptured epidermoid–T1-weighted axial image with contrast showing high intensity mass (consistent with "fat") in the medial aspect of the right temporal lobe and multiple small high intensity foci in the prepontine cistern and parahipocammpal gyrus.

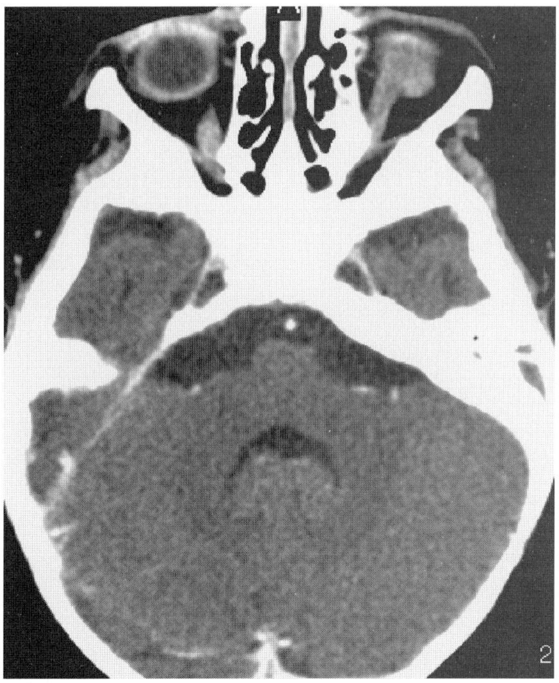

Figure 29K. Patient 3 with tuberculous basilar meningitis, showing loculated fluid collections in the prepontine cistern and bilateral upper cerebellopontine angle distorting the adjacent pons and cerebellum. Axial computed tomography image with contrast.

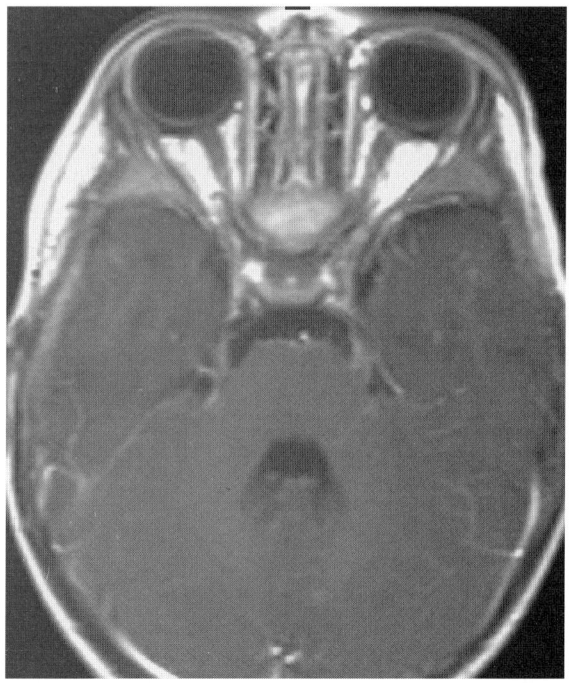

Figure 29L. Patient 3 with tuberculous basilar meningitis, showing diffuse leptomeningeal enhancement around the trigeminal nerves and ventral aspect of the pons. T1-weighted axial image with contrast—this is a case of infectious meningitis, which can be compared with the effects of chemical meningitis.

CASE 30

Clinical History: A 44-year-old woman presents with dizziness. A contrast-enhanced computed tomography (CT) image shows the mass enhanced. A proton density-weighted magnetic resonance image (MRI) at the same level as the CT is available.

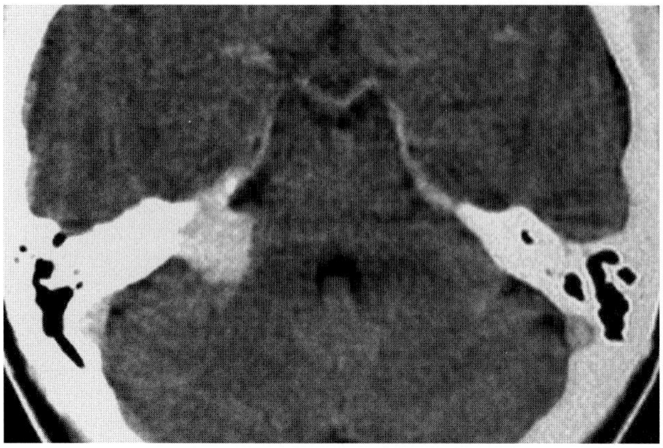

Figure 30A

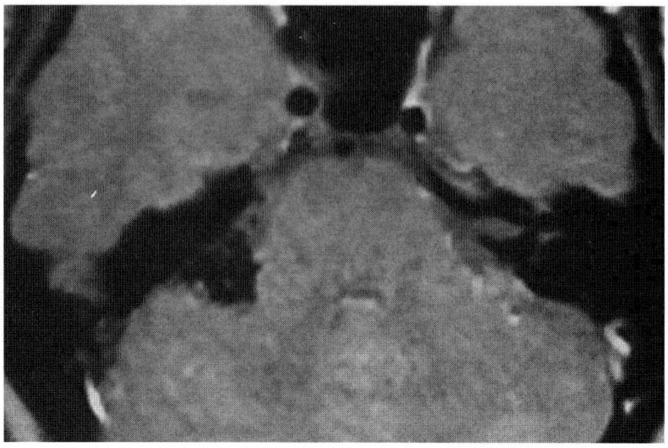

Figure 30B

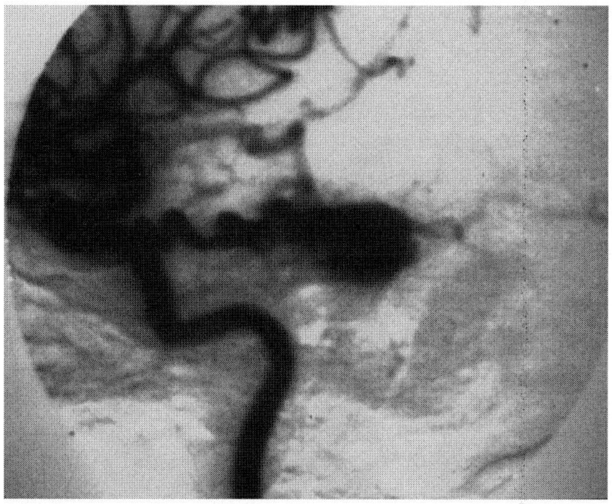

Figure 30C

1. List five possible causes of an enhancing cerebellopontine (CP) angle mass. Two must be nonneoplastic.
2. What is your diagnosis? Are any other studies necessary?

Findings

A homogeneously enhancing extraaxial mass in the right CP angle cistern on postcontrast CT image. A proton density-weighted image depicts the lesion as a cluster of multiple, small areas of signal void; some of them are isolated from a main cluster.

Lateral view of the arterial phase of the right internal carotid angiography reveals dilated abnormal vessels at expected area of the CP angle.

Problem

A discrete, enhancing CP angle mass producing vestibular symptoms in a middle-aged woman.

Anatomy

A. Contents of the CP angle
   1. Cranial nerves VII, VIII
   2. Anterior inferior cerebellar artery (AICA) and branches
   3. Petrosal vein
   4. Dura or arachnoid, subarachnoid space
   5. Brainstem, flocculus, cerebellum
B. Superior and inferior petrosal sinuses

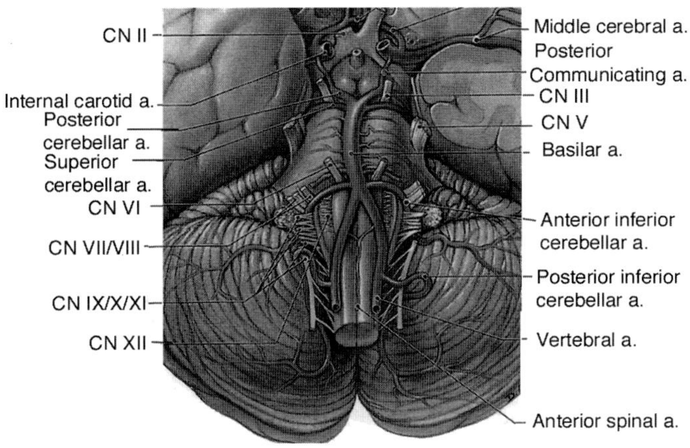

Figure 30D

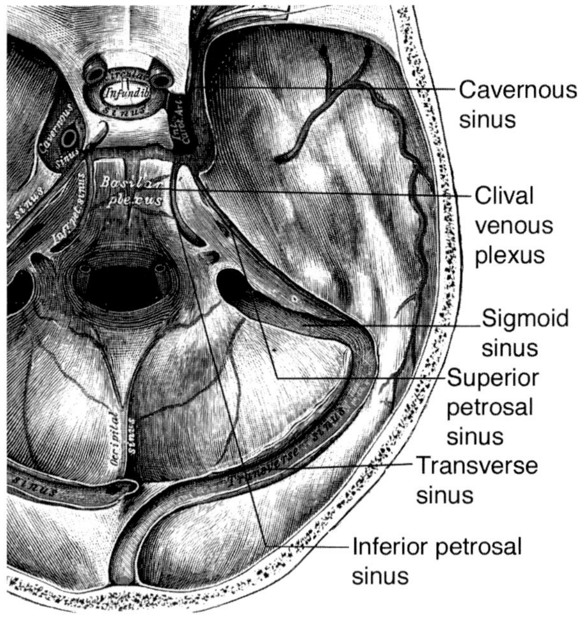

Figure 30E

Differential Diagnosis

1. Nonneoplastic: aneurysm (vascular malformation), inflammatory disease (syphilis, sarcoid), idiopathic pachymeningitis
2. Neoplastic: acoustic schwannoma, meningioma, metastasis, lymphoma, exophytic brainstem tumor
3. Tumoral and arachnoid cysts may be seen with some schwannomas and meningiomas.

Diagnosis

Dural vascular malformation with associated aneurysm

Diagnostic Imaging Approach

A. Cerebellopontine angle masses should be divided into three basic categories:
   1. Nonenhancing, fluidlike
   2. Discrete enhancing mass
   3. Meningeal or subarachnoid space pattern
B. Always exclude aneurysm or other vascular abnormalities as a possibility in cases of an enhancing mass (flow voids, other flow artifacts, enlarged associated vessels).
C. Observe associated findings (e.g., dural enhancement, spread to internal auditory canal).

Clinical Points Of Importance And Supplemental Information

A. Although rare, aneurysm or vascular malformation must always be excluded as the cause of an enhancing CP angle mass.
B. CT may be necessary to evaluate aeration of the petrous bone around the internal auditory canal and the proximity of the jugular bulb to the internal auditory canal before surgery. This is easily done with noncontrast axial sections.

Answers To Questions

1. Schwannoma, meningioma, metastasis, arteriovenous malformation (AVM), aneurysm
2. Aneurysm or AVM. Magnetic resonance angiography, angiogram.

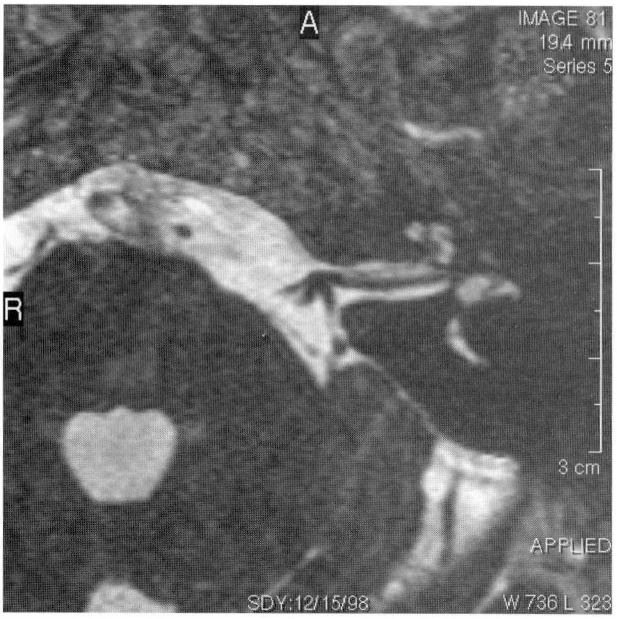

Figure 30F. Patient 1 showing prominent anterior inferior cerebellar artery vascular loop in the cerebellopontine angle, with impingement on the vestibulocochlear nerve in a patient with left-sided vestibular symptoms.

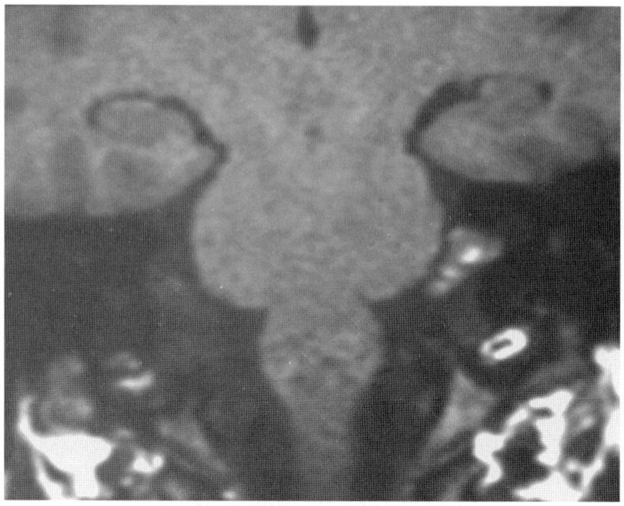

Figure 30G. Patient 2 with vascular malformation, showing focal areas of inhomogeneously high intensity in the left cerebellopontine angle. T1-weighted coronal image with contrast.

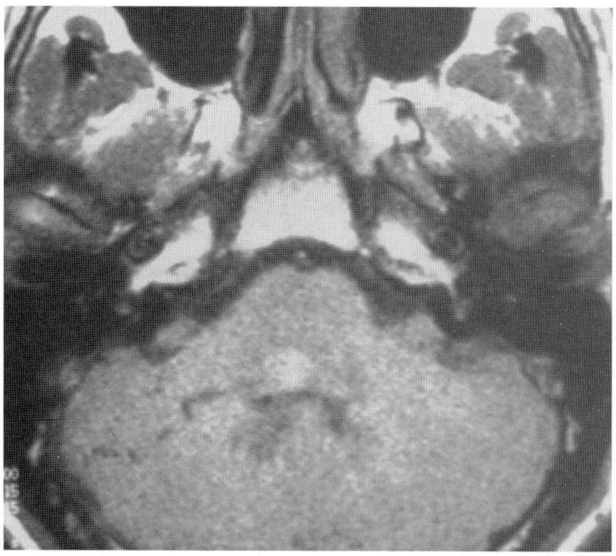

Figure 30H. Patient 3 with venous angioma, showing focal area of enhancement in dorsal aspect of the lower pons subjacent to the floor of the fourth ventricle with a flow-void from, and associated anomalous vein going into, the right cerebellar hemisphere. T1-weighted axial image with contrast.

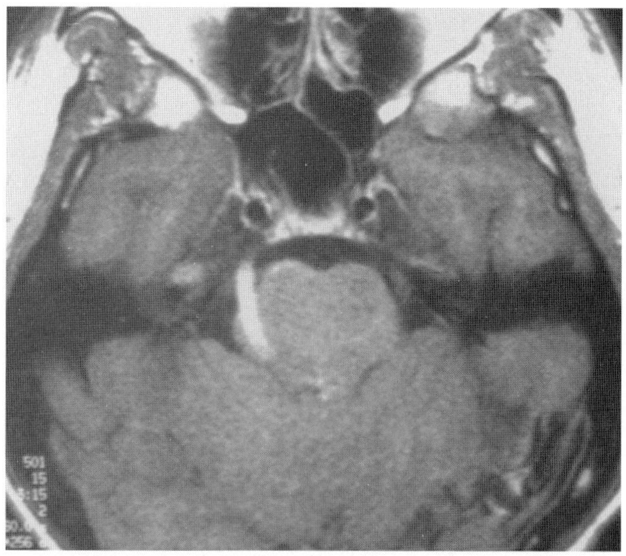

Figure 30I. Patient 3 with venous angioma. T1-weighted axial image with contrast cephalad to 30H, showing large draining vein traversing the right cerebellopontine angle.

CASE 31

Clinical History: A 51-year-old woman presents with hearing loss.

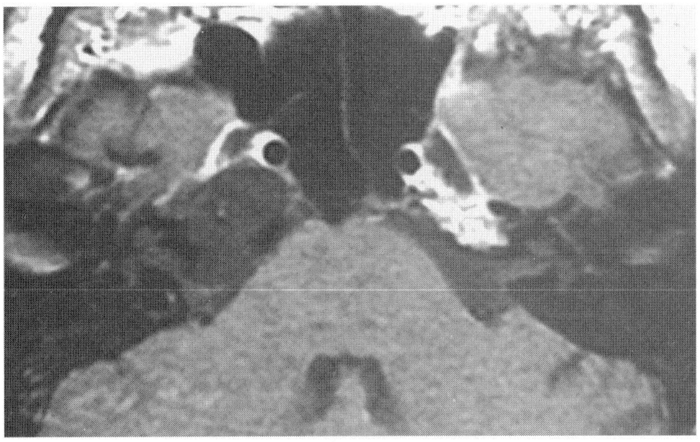

Figure 31A

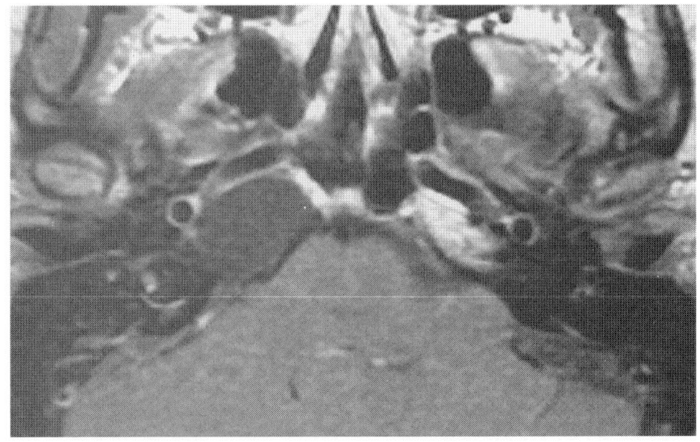

Figure 31B

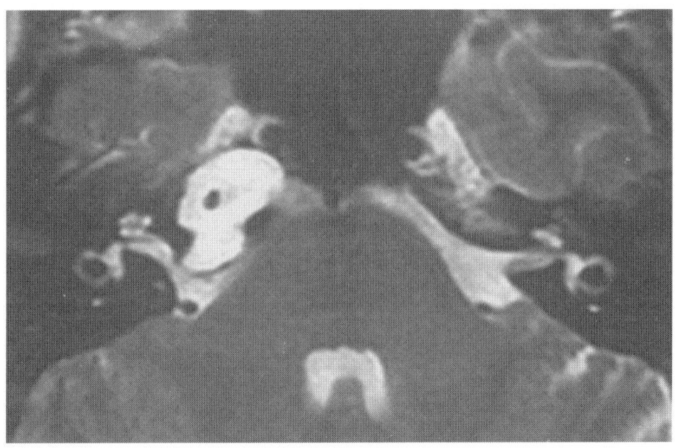

Figure 31C

1. List five lesions that commonly (realizing that petrous apex lesions are all relatively uncommon) involve the petrous apex and indicate the most likely diagnosis.
2. Does magnetic resonance imaging (MRI) help in establishing the correct diagnosis? What is your degree of confidence in the diagnosis?
3. If the periphery of the mass or the dura enhanced, would it change your diagnosis?
4. What normal anatomic variant is present?

Findings

An expansile, unilocular cystic mass involving the right petrous apex. Postcontrast image shows no enhancement of the lesion. The signal intensity of the lesion is slightly higher than the cerebrospinal fluid on both T1- and T2-weighted images. Although remodeling of the anterior wall of the right internal auditory canal is identified, the right inner ear itself is anatomically normal. The right jugular bulb protrudes as high as the middle ear cavity as an incidental normal variation.

Problem

"Expansile" mass of the petrous apex in a middle-aged woman with hearing loss

Anatomy

A. Petrous apex: normal variations in:
   1. Contents
   2. Air cell development
B. Carotid canal
C. Jugular bulb

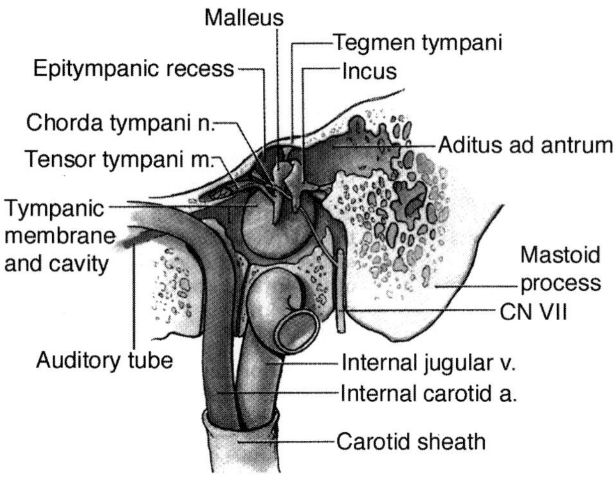

Figure 31D

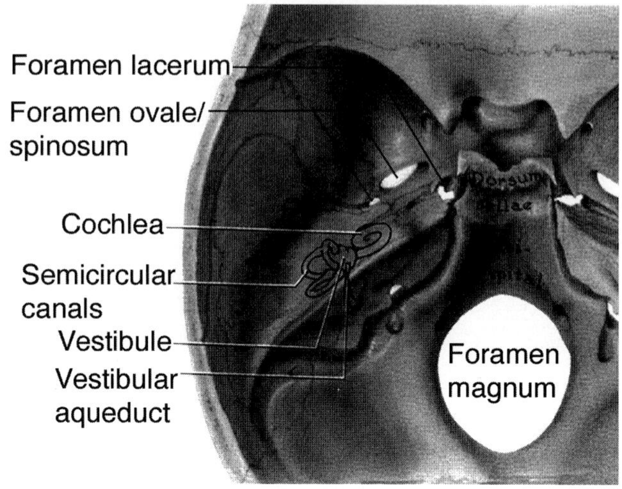

Figure 31E

Differential Diagnosis

Epidermoid (dermoid), cholesterolosis (cholesterol granuloma), mucocele (pyomucocele), chordoma (chondroid variant and chondrosarcoma), aneurysm, aneurysmal bone cyst

Diagnosis

Epidermoid tumor of the petrous apex, with secondary deformity of the internal auditory canal and a jugular diverticulum (normal variant)

Diagnostic Imaging Approach

A. Establish that the mass is centered within the petrous apex (i.e., as opposed to petroclival fissure, cavernous sinus or trigeminal cistern, dura).
B. Exclude aneurysm as a possible cause.
C. Morphology: margins, intensity (T1 or T2), flow voids, calcifications, enhancement
D. Look for associated findings: dural enhancement, meningeal or subarachnoid space abnormality.

Clinical Points Of Importance And Supplemental Information

A. Inconsequential mucosal thickening and secretions within petrous apex air cells is commonly seen on MRI. Assessing the need for computed tomography or follow-up in these patients is problematic.
B. Differentiating between an epidermoid and cholesterosis can affect the surgical approach.
C. Uncomplicated epidermoids and cholesterosis do not enhance. Enhancement of a petrous apex fluid-filled cavity, especially in cases of a dural phlegmon, strongly suggests a pyomucocele or at least the presence of petrous apicitis.

Answers To Questions

1. Epidermoid, cholesterolosis, mucocele, chondrosarcoma, cancer invasion, aneurysm. Epidermoid most likely in this case.
2. Yes. High.
3. Yes, pyomucocele.
4. High jugular bulb with a diverticulum

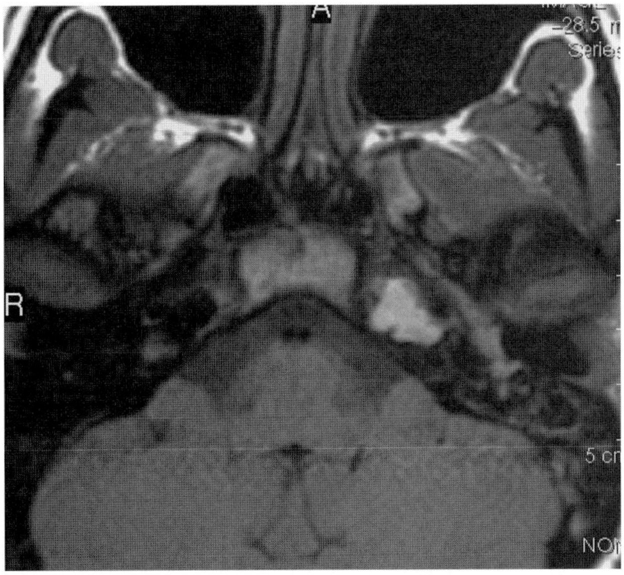

Figure 31F. Patient 1 with cholesterol granuloma, showing lobulated, minimally expansile mass of high intensity in the left petrous apex. T1-weighted axial image without contrast.

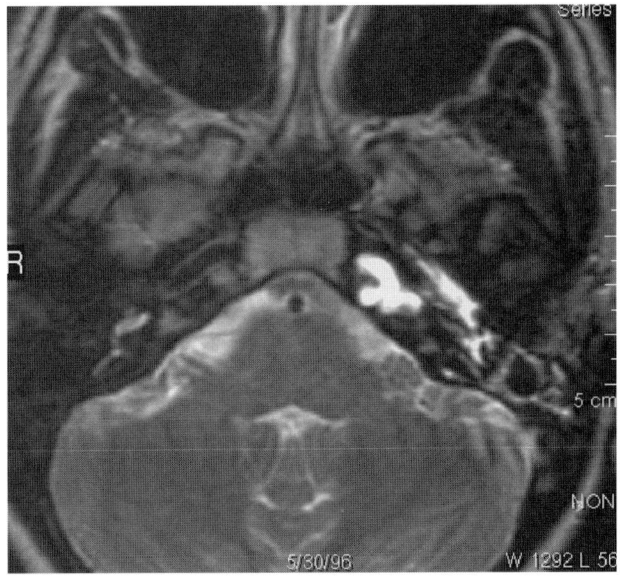

Figure 31G. Patient 1 with cholesterol granuloma. The mass reveals high intensity on T2-weighted axial image.

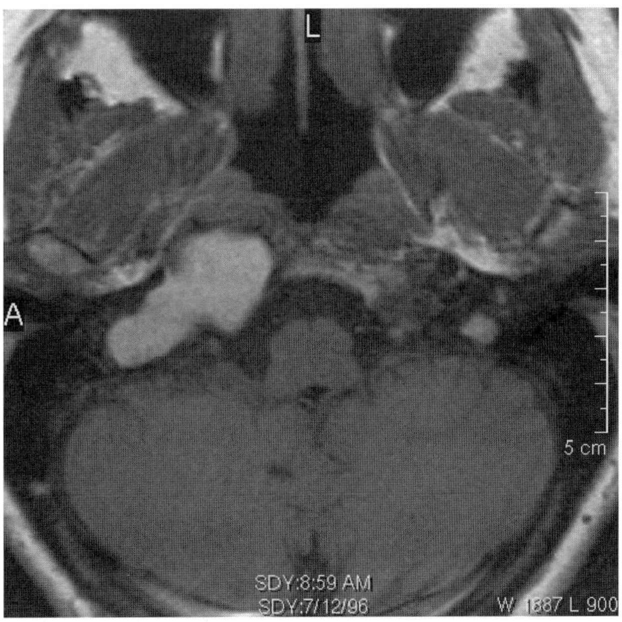

Figure 31H. Patient 2 with cholesterol granuloma, showing an expansile, high-intensity mass involving the right petrous apex. T1-weighted axial image without contrast.

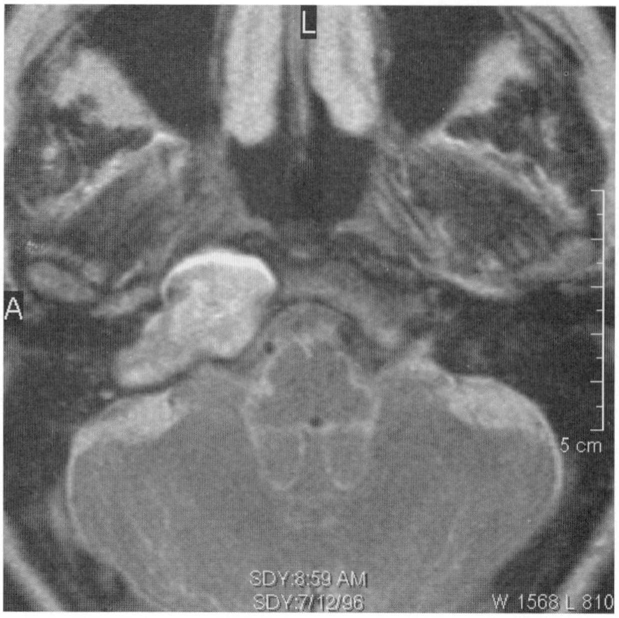

Figure 31I. Patient 2 with cholesterol granuloma. The mass is relatively dark on T2-weighted axial image (when compared with 31G). If this were equivalent to cerebrospinal fluid on a T2 weighted, it could also represent an epidermoid-type lesion.

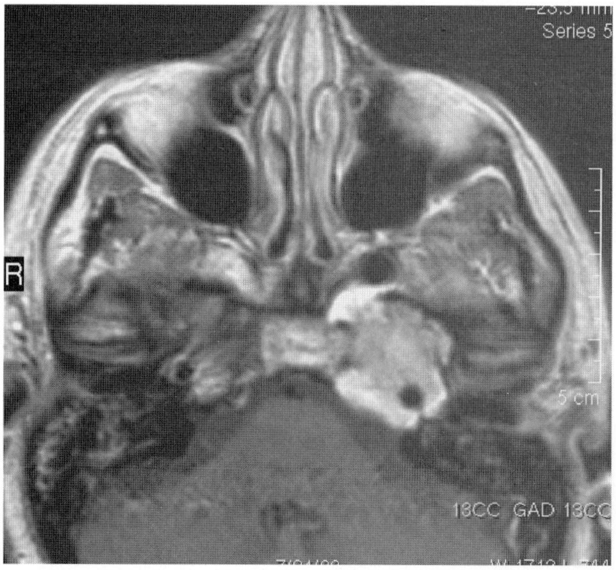

Figure 31J. Patient 3 with plasmacytoma of the skull base. T1-weighted image with contrast, showing homogeneously enhancing mass involving the left petrous apex.

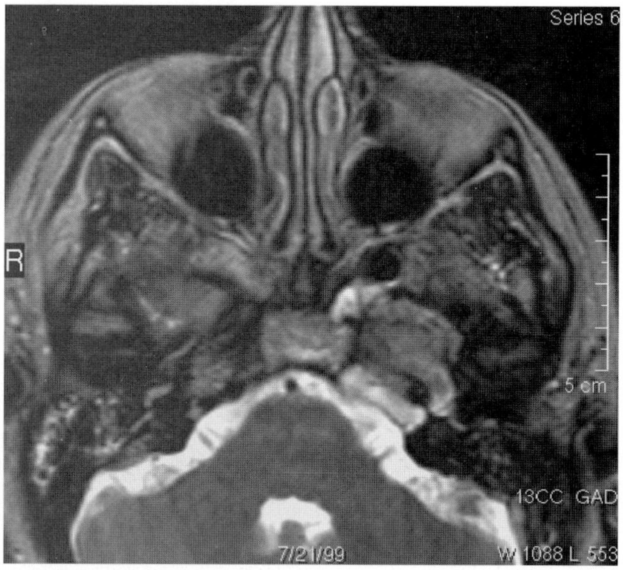

Figure 31K. Patient 3 with plasmacytoma of the skull base. T2-weighted image showing relatively low-intensity mass of left petrous apex.

CASE 32

Clinical History: A 6-year-old girl presents with ear pain, fever, and a mass in the mastoid region.

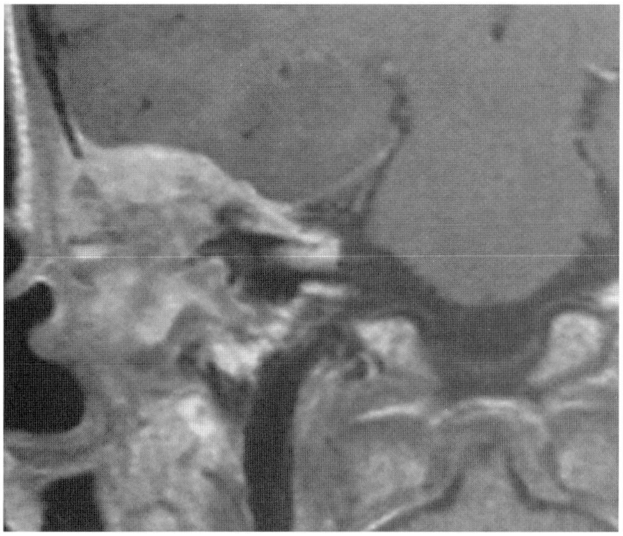

Figure 32A

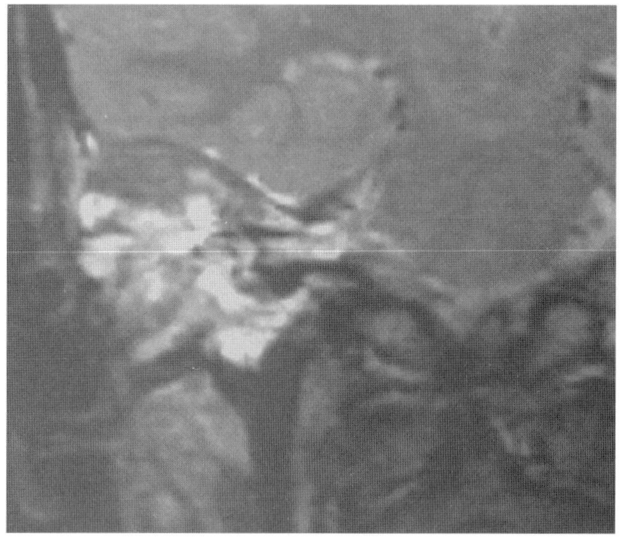

Figure 32B

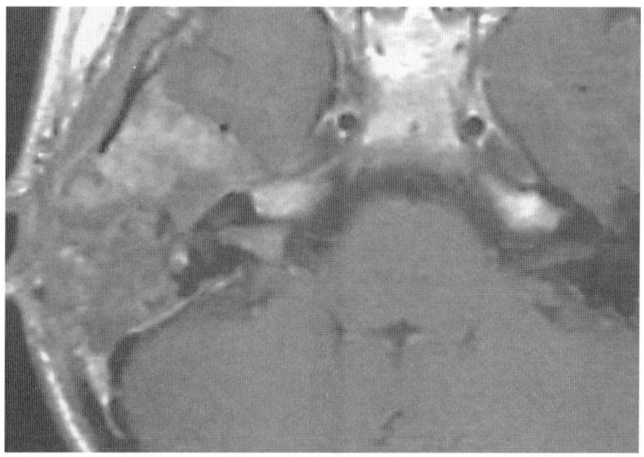

Figure 32C

1. List three possible diagnoses and indicate which is the most likely.
2. How will the diagnosis be established?

Findings

A diffuse, infiltrating mass, mainly involving the mastoid, tympanic, and petrous portions of the right temporal bone. The lesion inhomogeneously enhances. It extends directly into the middle cranial fossa and forms an extraosseous epidural mass in the fossa and displaces the right temporal lobe. Although distortion of the right temporal lobe and localized dural involvement are noted, no frank intraaxial involvement is seen.

Problem

Diffuse, infiltrating mass of the mastoid and petrous portions of the temporal bone, with dural involvement, in a young child.

Anatomy

A. Define the mastoid and petrous portions of the temporal bone and the important structures each encompasses:
   1. Middle ear and inner ear
   2. Carotid canal
   3. Jugular fossa
   4. Sigmoid sinus or superior and inferior petrosal sinuses

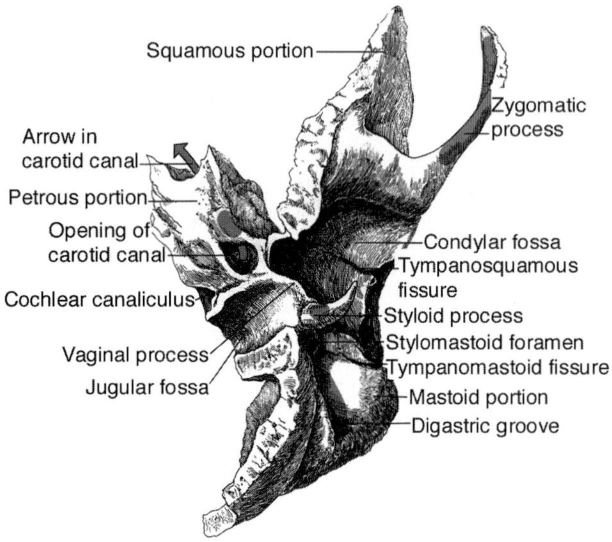

Figure 32D

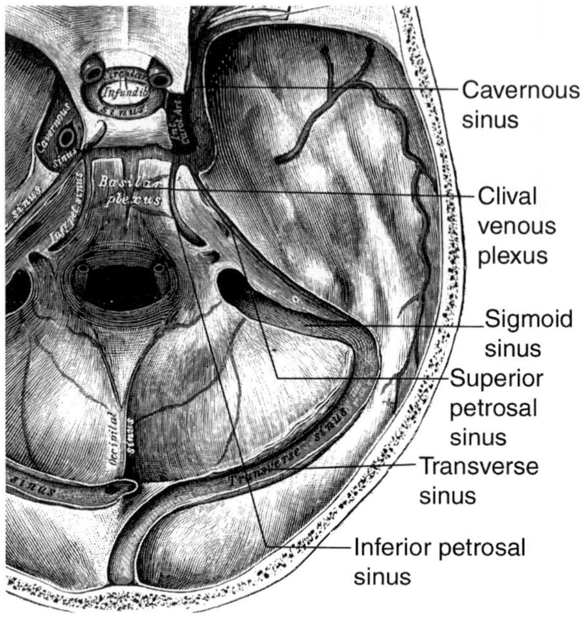

Figure 32E

Differential Diagnosis:

Rhabdomyosarcoma, lymphoma or leukemia, Langerhans' cell histiocytosis (eosinophilic granuloma), pyogenic or other infectious mastoiditis with petrous apicitis

Diagnosis

Rhabdomyosarcoma of the temporal bone, with intracranial extension limited to the dura

Diagnostic Imaging Approach

A. What portions of the temporal bone are primarily involved with the disease process? Is there an identifiable site or cause of origin?
B. Is the disease morphology suggestive of inflammatory or infectious disease or neoplasm?
C. Identify sites of contiguous spread and possible complications (e.g., meningeal or subarachnoid space spread, venous sinus thrombus, infectious aneurysm).

Clinical Points Of Importance And Supplemental Information

A. Imaging must immediately distinguish between pyogenic disease and other possibilities, if at all possible.
B. Diagnosis almost always requires biopsy. Try to use imaging to select an area most likely to produce diagnostic material (i.e., site of disease process vs. reactive mucosal disease in the mastoid).

Answers To Questions

1. Rhabdomyosarcoma, Langerhans' cell histiocytosis, lymphoma, mastoiditis. Rhabdomyosarcoma most likely.
2. Mastoidotomy or ectomy and biopsy

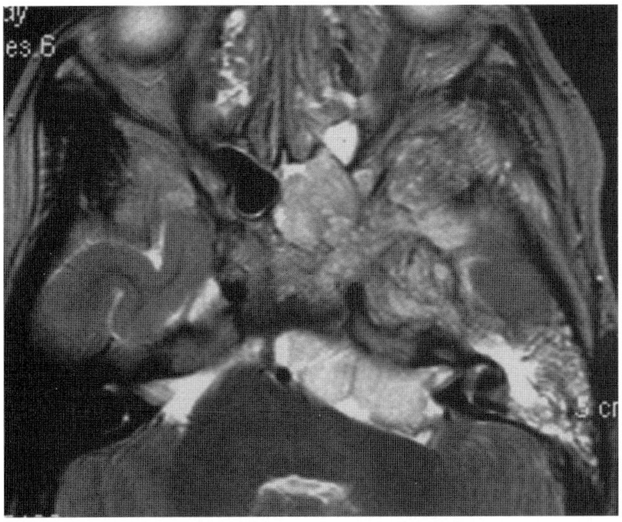

Figure 32F. Patient (pediatric) 1 with undifferentiated sarcoma involving the petrous bone, showing lobulated high-intensity mass extensively invading the petrous apex and body of the sphenoid. Fluid in the mastoid air cells and middle ear is caused by eustachian tube obstruction. T2-weighted axial image.

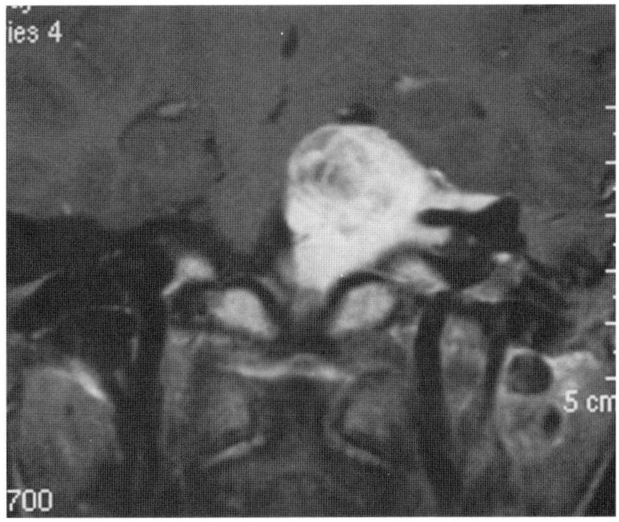

Figure 32G. Patient (pediatric) 1 with undifferentiated sarcoma involving the petrous bone. T1-weighted axial image with contrast, showing inhomogeneously, enhancing extraaxial mass also in the left cerebellopontine angle extending into the internal auditory canal and along the dural surface of the middle cranial fossa.

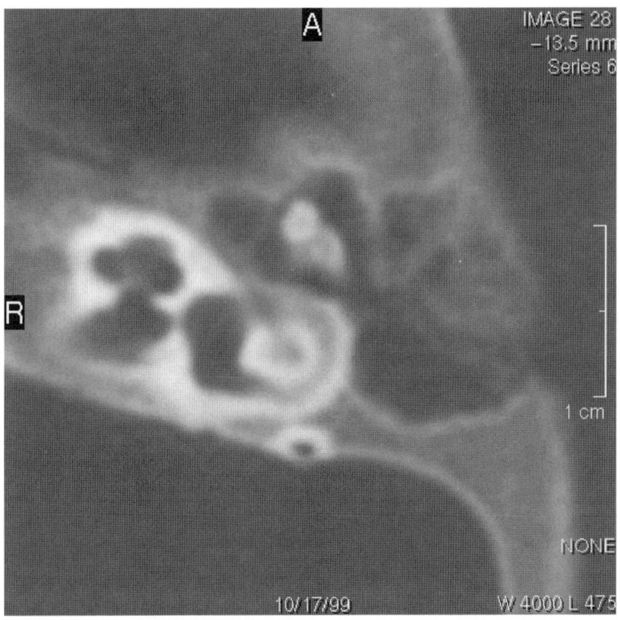

Figure 32H. Patient 2 with coalescent mastoiditis, showing mucosal thickening throughout the middle ear and mastoid air cells, with disruption of the outer cortex of the mastoid part of the temporal bone. Computed tomography axial image.

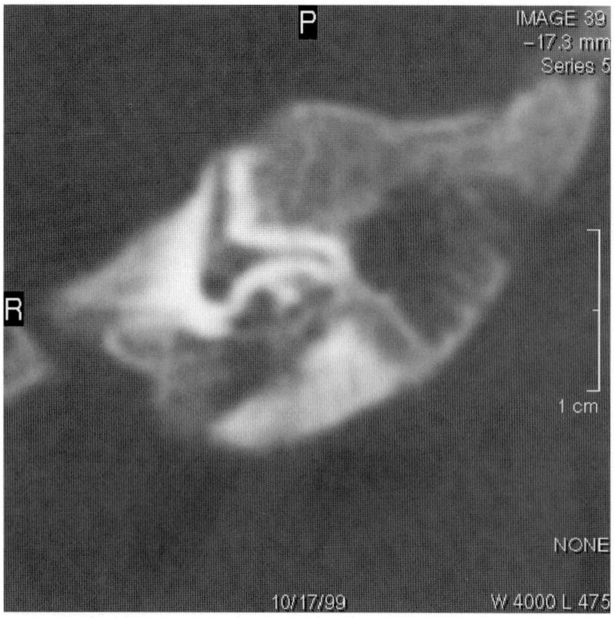

Figure 32I. Patient 2 with coalescent mastoiditis. Coronal computed tomography image also showing mucosal thickening of the mastoid cells and disruption of the outer cortex.

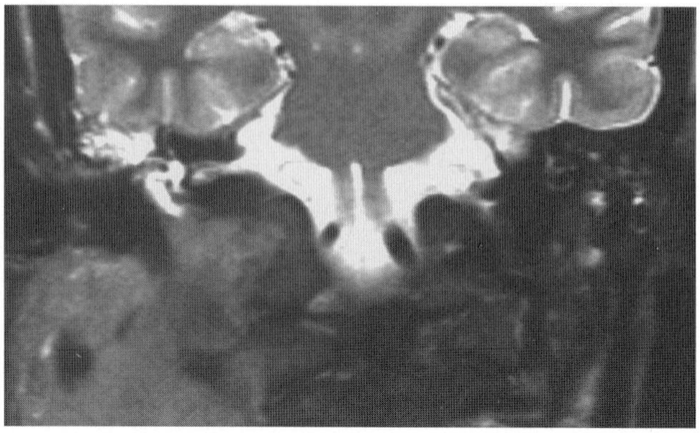

Figure 32J. Patient 3 with malignant lymphoma involving the temporal bone, showing a soft tissue mass centered below the skull base, with direct invasion of the undersurface of the right temporal bone. T2-weighted coronal image.

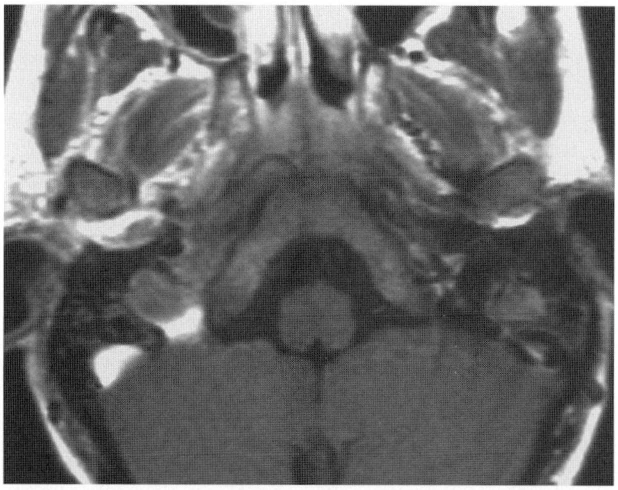

Figure 32K. Patient 3 with malignant lymphoma involving the temporal bone. T1-weighted axial image, with contrast showing mass lesion involving the undersurface of the right temporal bone and extending into the jugular foramen.

CASE 33

Clinical History: A 41-year-old woman presents with headaches, low-grade fever, and acute onset of VIth cranial nerve palsy. She had a suboccipital craniotomy at another institution for what was believed to be a tumor of the cerebellopontine angle; no intradural abnormality was seen and the procedure was terminated.

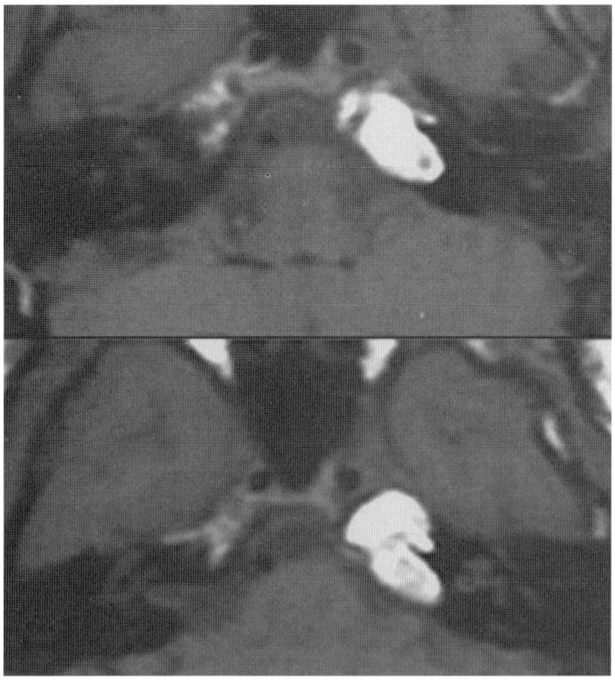

Figure 33A

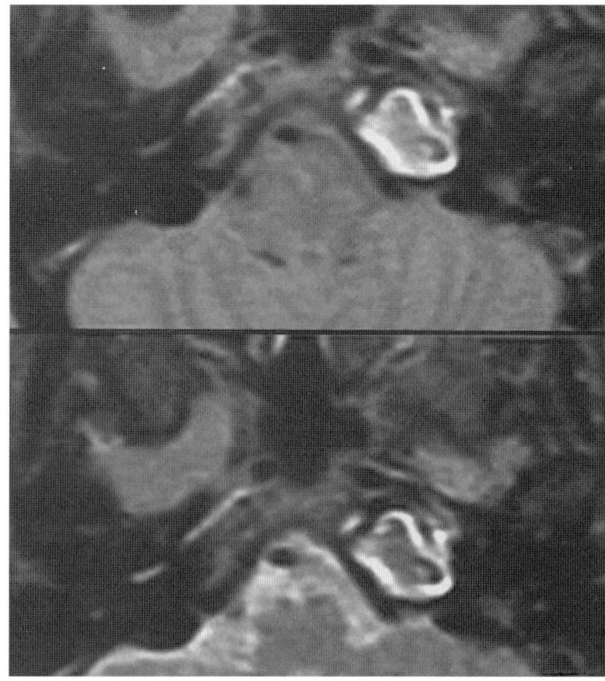

Figure 33B

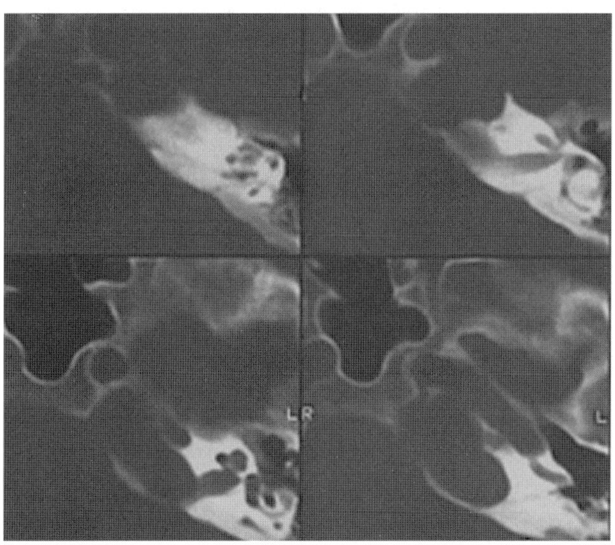

Figure 33C

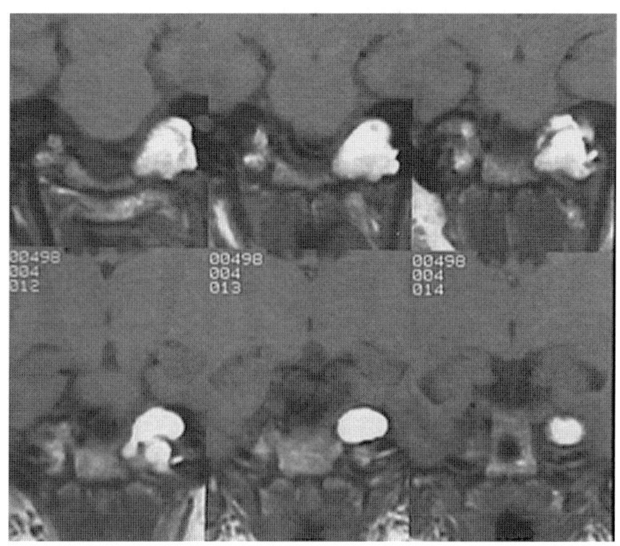

Figure 33D

1. Where is the pathology centered? Specify the diagnosis.
2. How do the magnetic resonance imaging (MRI) findings help with the differential diagnosis?
3. Can you explain the *acute* VIth nerve deficit?
4. How can this be treated? Can anything more be done to help plan the treatment?

Findings

An expansile mass centered *not* in the left petroclival fissure but in the left petrous apex. The high intensity of the lesion on T1-weighted image and mixed appearance on T2-weighted image suggest an episode of intralesional hemorrhage in a subacute phase. Computed tomography (CT) imaging shows the smooth remodeling of bone that is consistent with a slowly progressive growth pattern.

Problem

"Expansile" mass of the petrous apex causing an acute VIth cranial nerve palsy

Anatomy

A. Cranial nerve VI:
   1. Root entry zone (REZ)
   2. Cisternal segment
   3. Dorello's canal
B. Petrous apex
   1. Normal variation in mineralization, marrow content, and aeration
   2. Petrous apex air cell development

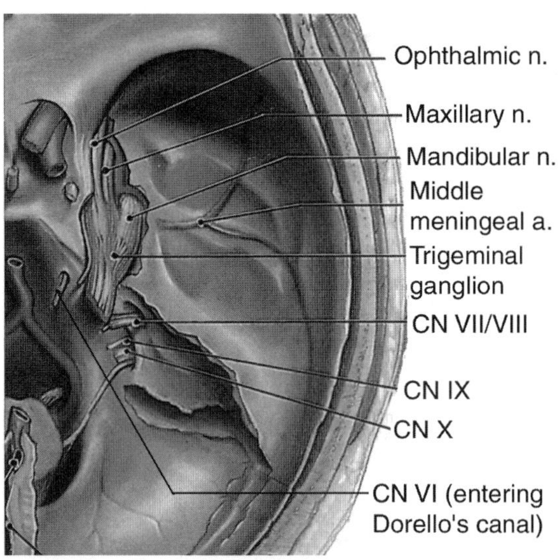

Figure 33E

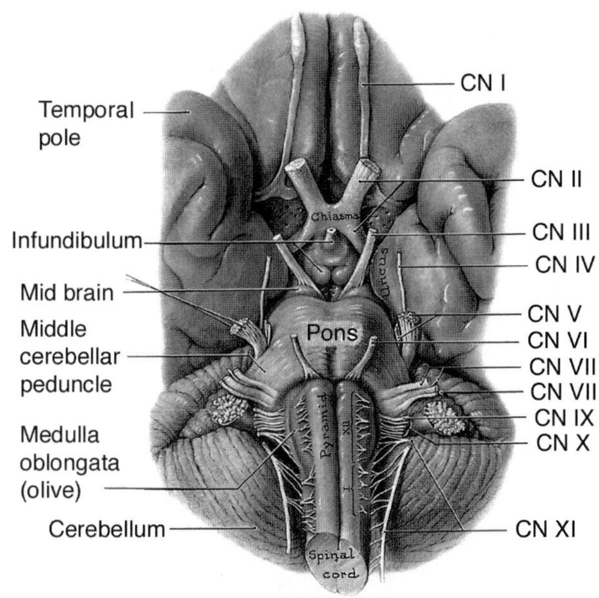

Figure 33F

Differential Diagnosis

Cholesterolosis (cholesterol granuloma), epidermoid (dermoid), mucocele (pyomucocele), chondroma (chondroid variant, chondrosarcoma), aneurysm, aneurysmal bone cyst

Diagnosis

Cholesterolosis of the petrous apex with recent hemorrhage is likely responsible for the acute VIth nerve palsy.

Diagnostic Imaging Approach

A. Confirm that the disease process is centered within the petrous apex rather than the adjacent petroclival fissure, cavernous sinus, trigeminal cistern, or dura.
B. Exclude aneurysm as a possibility.
C. Morphology: intensity (T1 or T2), blood products, flow voids, enhancement, margins, calcifications
D. Look for associated findings or complications: dural enhancement, meningeal or subarachnoid space abnormality.

Clinical Points Of Importance And Supplemental Information

A. Pathophysiology of cholesterolosis is cyclical mucosal inflammation, obstruction, and secondary hemorrhage within the petrous apex air cells.
B. Inconsequential mucosal thickening and secretions within the petrous apex air cells are commonly seen on MRI. The possibility of progression to cholesterolosis exists. A need for follow-up of minimal changes is difficult to determine.
C. Disease will be drained via a mastoid surgical approach if a safe transmastoid route to the petrous apex can be identified.

Answers To Questions

1. Petrous apex. Cholesterolosis
2. Identify blood products that reveal the correct diagnosis
3. Acute bleed into medial cystic component adjacent to Dorello's canal
4. Transmastoid drainage. CT to identify the safest air cell tract to follow

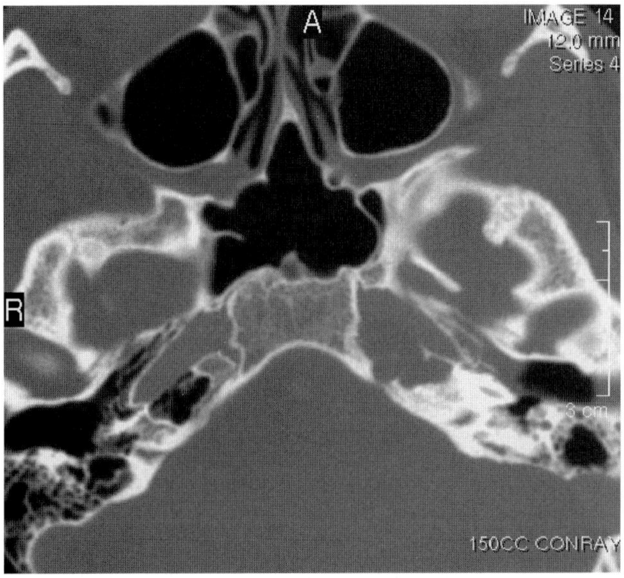

Figure 33G. Patient 1 with cholesterol granuloma, showing a somewhat expansile lesion centered in the left petrous apex with dehiscence of the medial wall of the carotid canal. Computed tomography axial image.

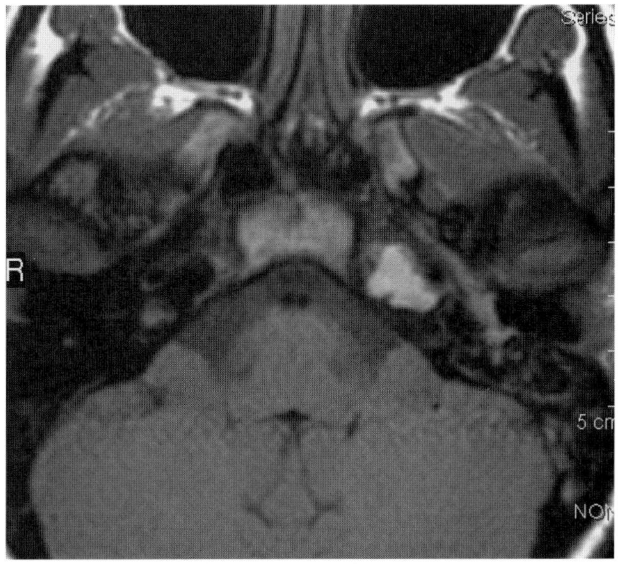

Figure 33H. Patient 1 with cholesterol granuloma, showing loculated, high intensity mass in the left petrous apex. T1-weighted axial image without contrast.

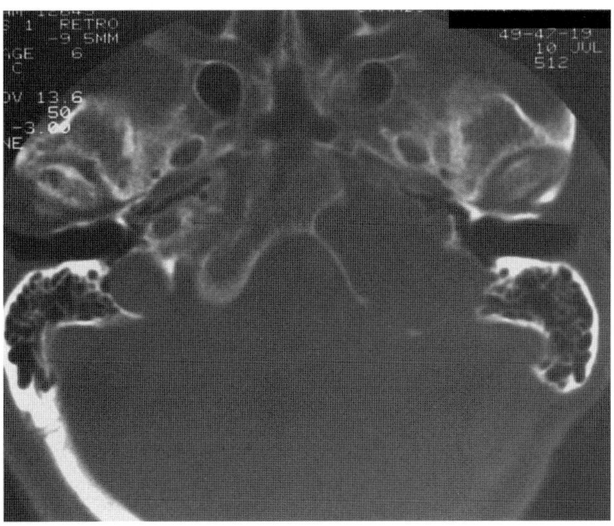

Figure 33I. Patient 2 with schwannoma involving the petrous apex, showing an expansile mass centered in the petrous apex with dehiscence of the cortex in the posterior aspect of the carotid canal. Axial computed tomography image at the bone window setting.

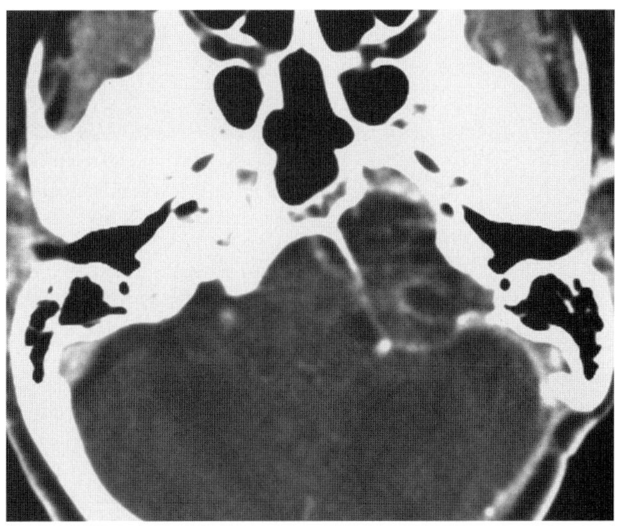

Figure 33J. Patient 2 with schwannoma involving the petrous apex, showing inhomogeneous internal architecture of the mass more typical of a neurofibroma. Axial computed tomography image at the soft tissue window setting.

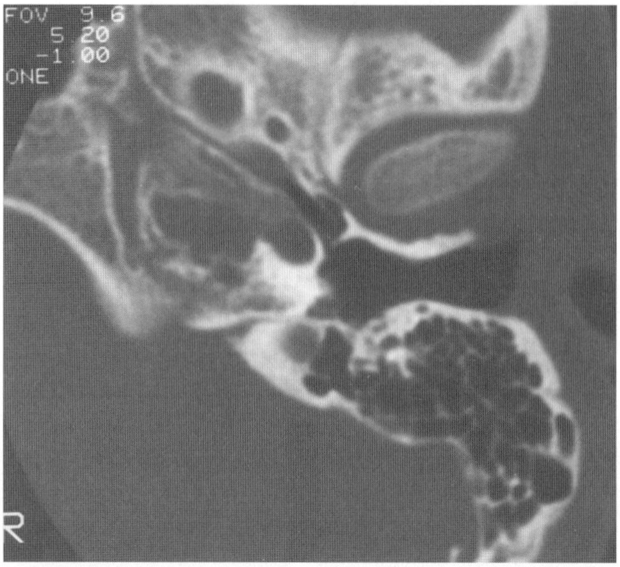

Figure 33K. Patient 3 with early cholesterol granuloma showing opacified air cell in the petrous apex with early "expansion" of the air cell(s) and deminerlization of the carotid canal. Axial CT image at bone window setting.

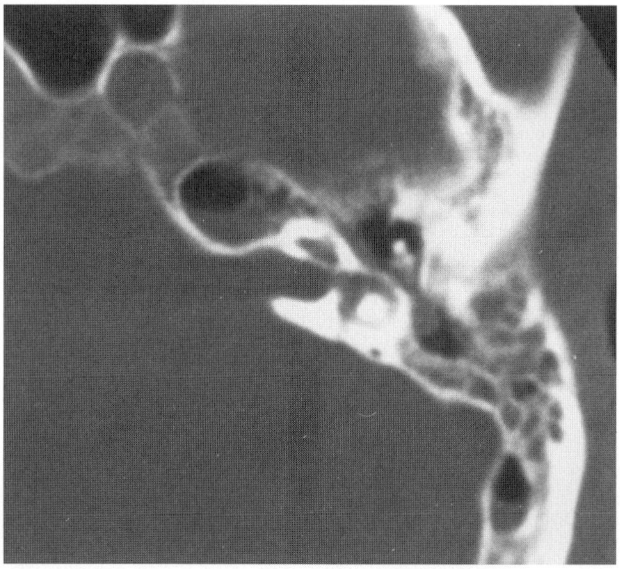

Figure 33L. Patient 4 with petrous apex air cells showing a possible air-fluid level and mucosal thickening similar to that in the mastoid air cells. Such findings are common in asymptomatic patients and have little risk for progressing to cholestrol garnauloma. Depending on the situation and the patient's wishes, these findings can be followed with imaging.

CASE 34

Clinical History: A 26-year-old man presented with *pulse-synchronous s*innusitus. A mass was seen behind his left tympanic membrane. History and physical examination were otherwise normal.

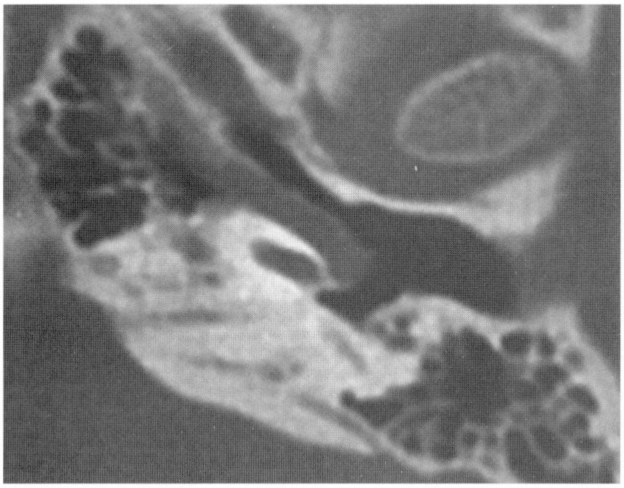

Figure 34A

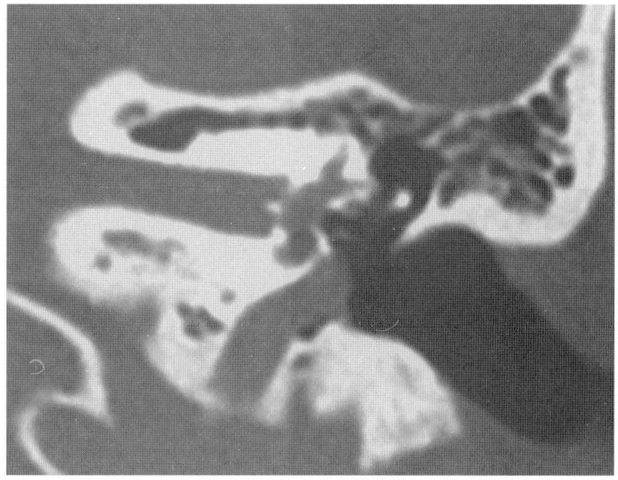

Figure 34B

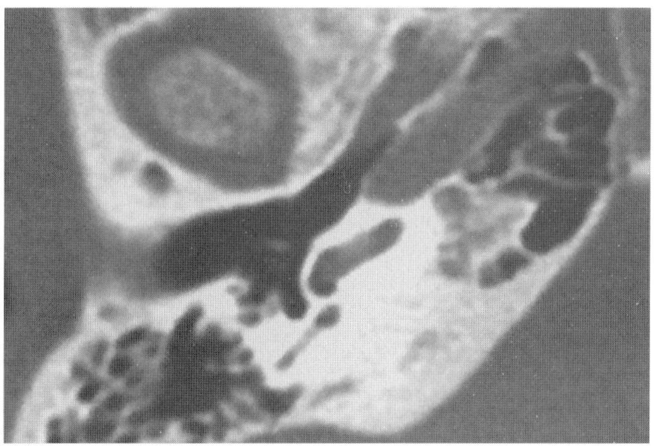

Figure 34C

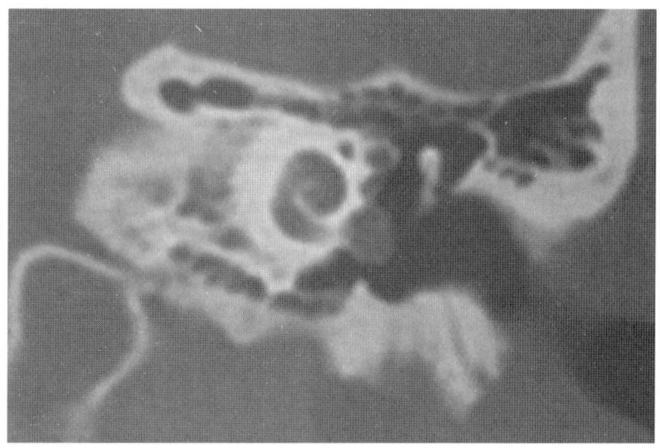

Figure 34D

1. Is a noncontrast temporal bone computed tomography (CT) study adequate for the evaluation of this patient?
2. Given the history and physical findings, list the three most likely diagnoses. Based on this patient's CT study, which one of those is the correct diagnosis?
3. How would you evaluate a patient with *pulsatile* tinnitus and no evidence of a middle ear mass?

Findings

A soft tissue density mass protruding into the hypo- and mesotympani of the left middle ear cavity. It is directly contiguous with the carotid canal. The proximal portion of the tympanic portion of the left facial nerve canal is enlarged because of the presence of a persistent stapedial artery.

Problem

Pulse synchronous tinnitus with a visible middle ear mass

Anatomy

A. Relevant to pulsatile tinnitus and middle ear mass
   1. Carotid canal: all segments
   2. Jugular bulb
   3. Inferior tympanic canaliculus (canal for Jacobson's nerve) (see 27F)
   4. Promontory
B. Relevant to persistent stapedial artery
   1. Anterior genu and tympanic segment of facial canal (see 27E)
   2. Semicanal for tensor tympani muscle
   3. Foramen ovale and spinosum (see 21F)

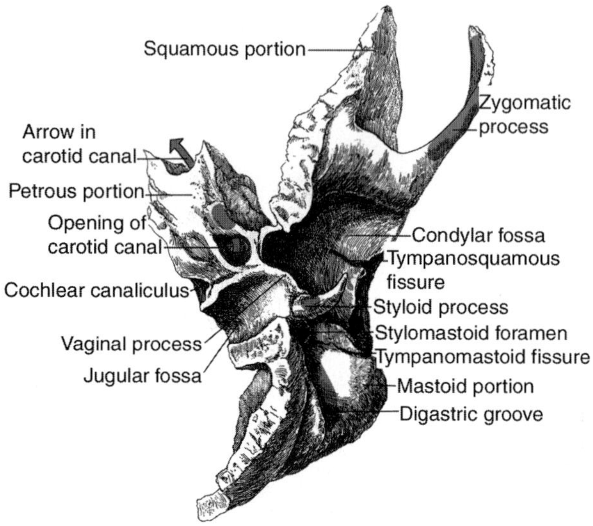

Figure 34E

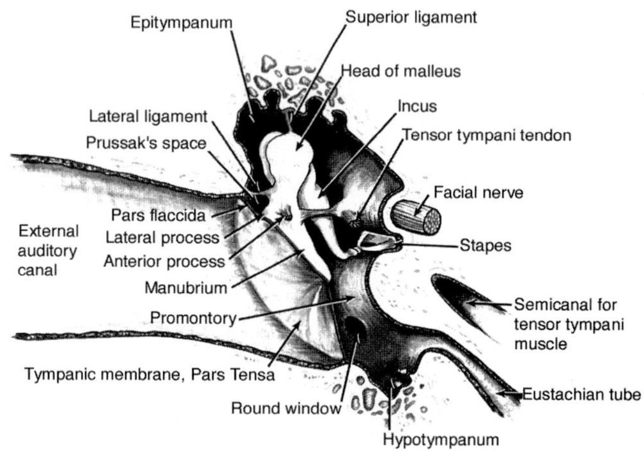

Figure 34F

Differential Diagnosis

1. Common: aberrant carotid; high (dehiscent) jugular bulb (fossa); glomus tympanicum or superior extension of glomus jugulare types of paragangliomas
2. Uncommon or rare: carotid aneurysm, encephalocele, vascular phase of otosclerosis

Diagnosis

Aberrant carotid artery with a persistent stapedial artery

Diagnostic Imaging Approach

(All Can Be Done On Noncontrast CT)

A. Relevant to pulsatile tinnitus and middle ear mass, identify:
   1. Carotid canal and artery
   2. Jugular bulb and vein
   3. Bony margins of each structure for position and erosion
   4. Middle ear mass or "opacification"
   5. Bone erosion between carotid canal and jugular fossa
B. Relevant to persistent stapedial artery, determine:
   1. Presence of an aberrant carotid or foramen spinosum
   2. Whether the proximal tympanic segment of facial canal is enlarged

Clinical Points Of Importance And Supplemental Information

A. Patients must have adequate radiologic evaluation before middle ear is explored.
B. Pulsatile tinnitus *without* a visible mass in the middle ear requires a much longer list of differential considerations and must be evaluated with detailed magnetic resonance imaging MRI or MR angiography (MRA) or high resolution, dynamic CT and, sometimes, conventional angiography.

Answers To Questions

1. Yes
2. Aberrant carotid artery, high jugular bulb, glomus tympanicum. Aberrant carotid artery is the correct diagnosis.
3. Contrast-enhanced CT, MRI, or both in the axial and coronal planes, including the entire brain inferiorly through and the carotid bifurcations with MRA (possibly including magnetic resonance venography); possibly, conventional angiography to follow, depending on clinical suspicion.

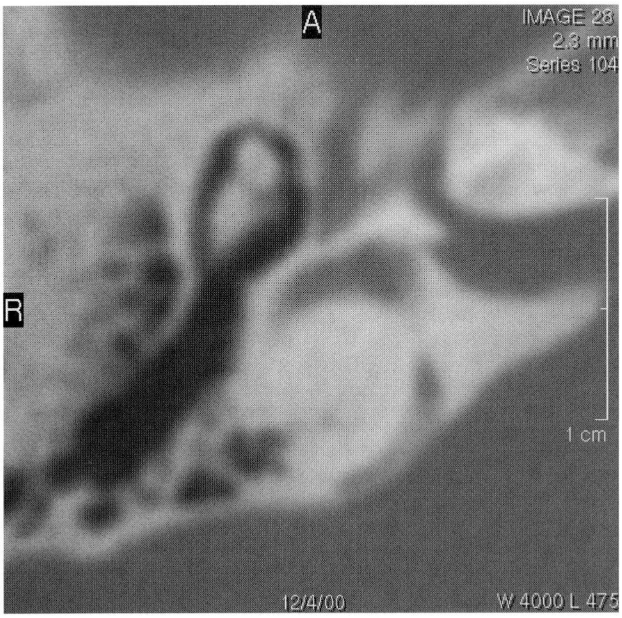

Figure 34G. Patient 1 with persistent stapedial artery. Axial computed tomography image showing the canal of the persistent artery entering the proximal tympanic segment of facial canal.

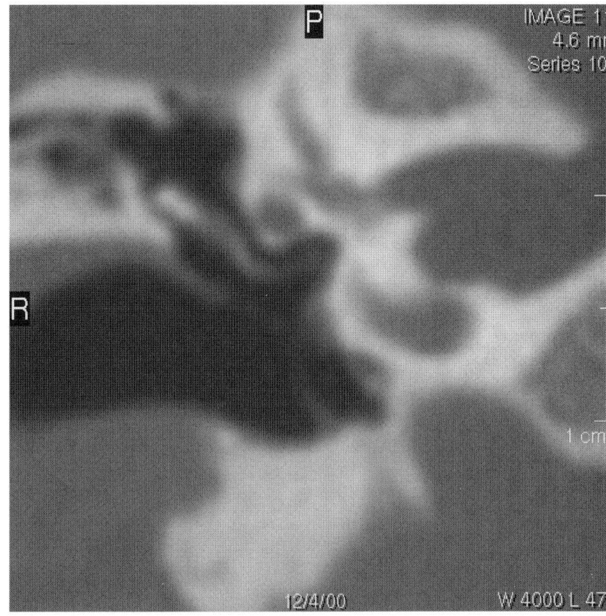

Figure 34H. Patient 1 with persistent stapedial artery. Coronal computed tomography image showing enlargement of the tympanic segment of the facial canal caused by the persistent artery coursing with the nerve over a short distance.

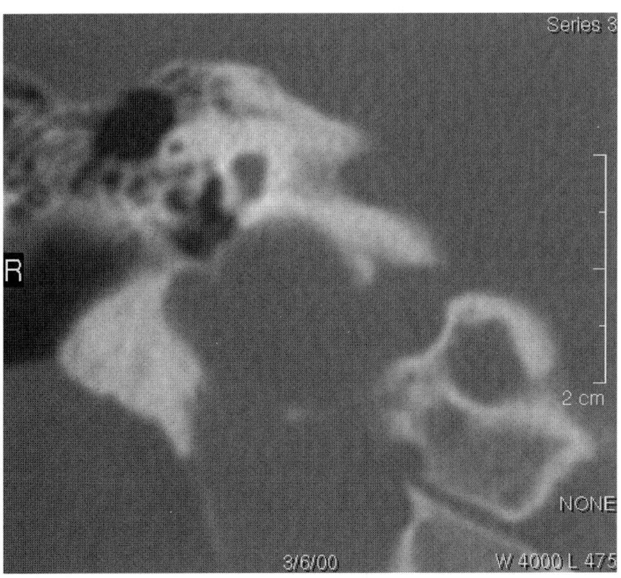

Figure 34I. Patient 2 with jugular diverticulum. Coronal computed tomography image showing small projection arising from the lateral aspect of the right jugular bulb—this and the high jugular bulb without a diverticulum are common normal variations of the jugular bulb anatomy that sometimes bulge into the inferior aspect of the hypotympanum.

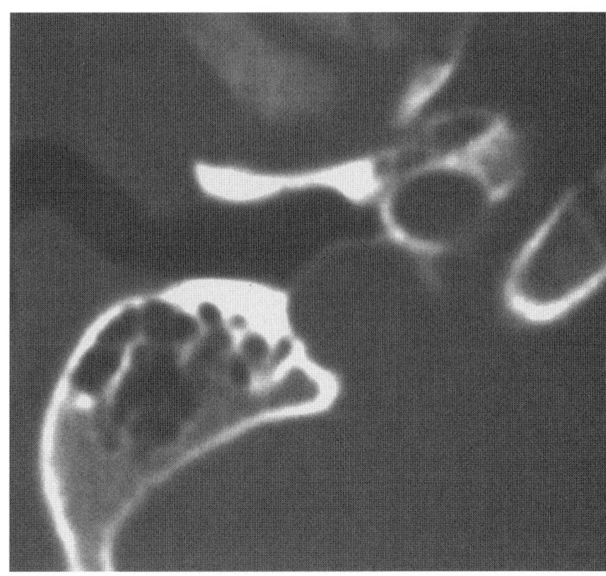

Figure 34J. Patient 3 with high jugular bulb. Axial computed tomography image at bone window setting, showing jugular bulb protruding into the posterior aspect of the hypotympanum.

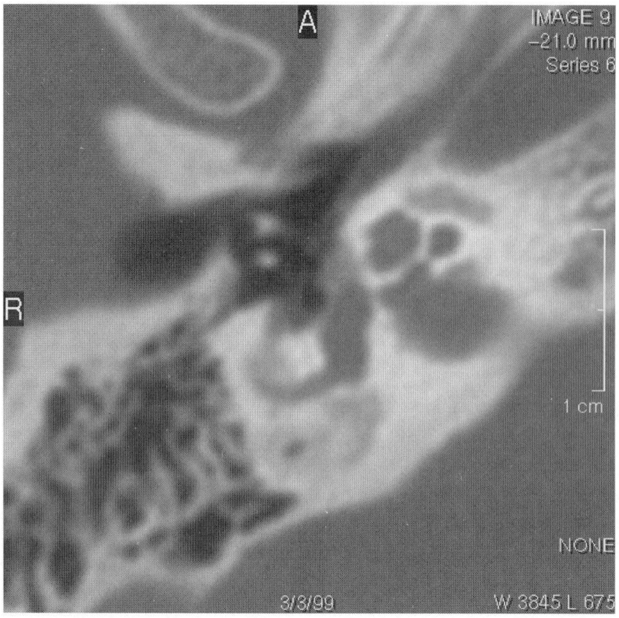

Figure 34K. Patient 4 with otosclerosis causing tinnitus. Axial computed tomography of the right temporal bone, showing areas of abnormal demineralization and bony productive changes in the fissula antefenestram and around cochlea and semicircular canals.

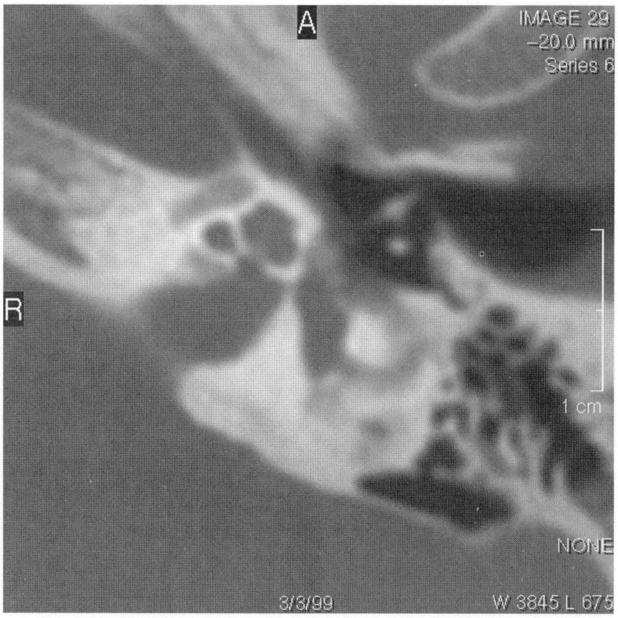

Figure 34L. Patient 4 with otosclerosis causing tinnitus. Axial computed tomography of the left temporal bone, also showing similar change with the opposite side (see 34K).

CASE 35

Clinical History: A 60-year-old woman presents with epistasis, fever, and Horner's syndrome.

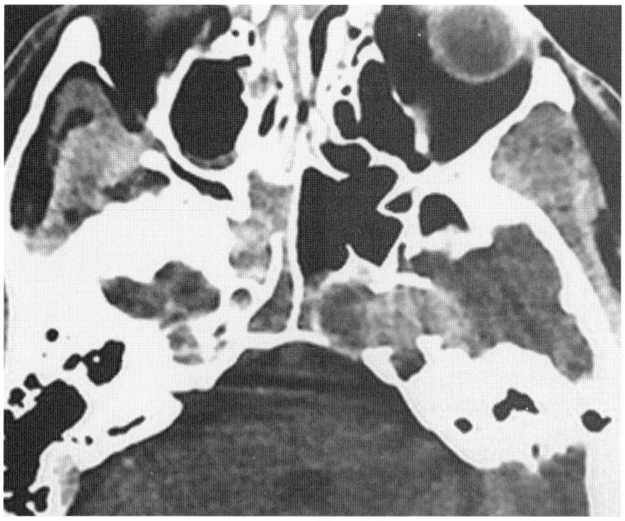

Figure 35A

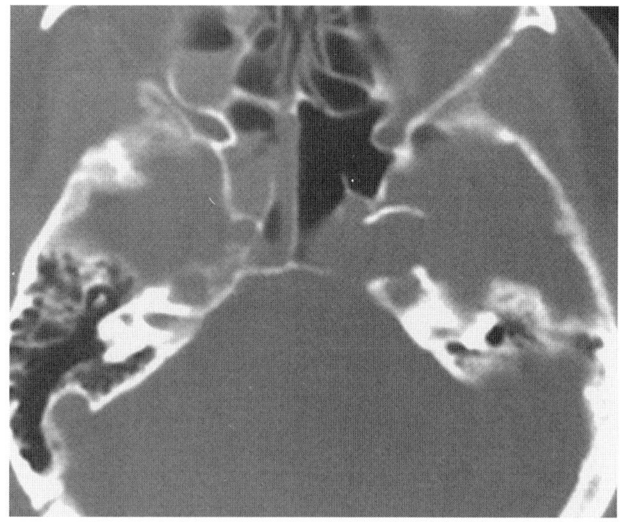

Figure 35B

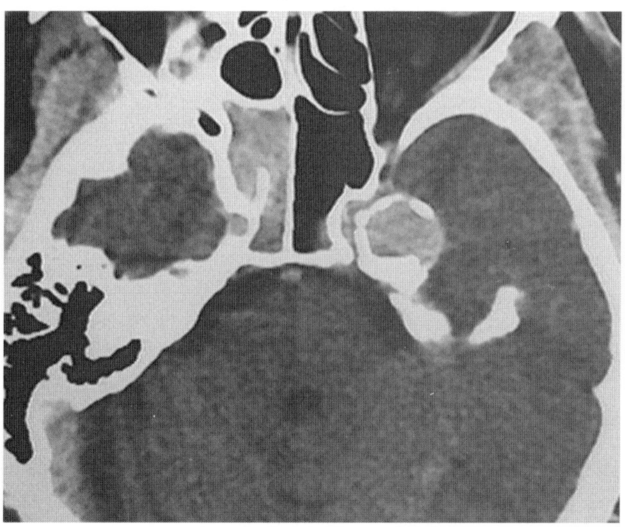

Figure 35C

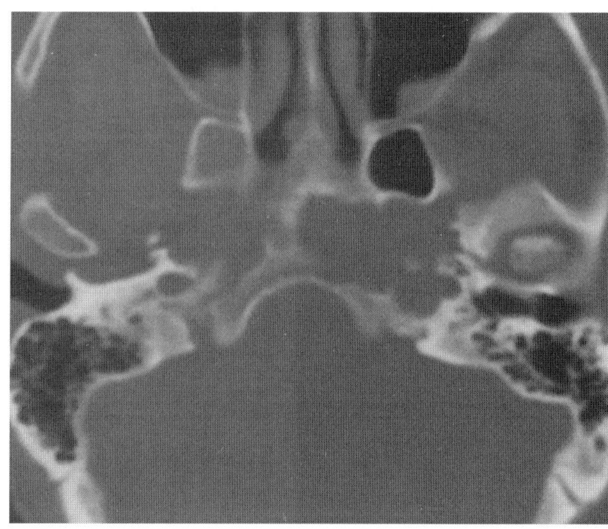

Figure 35D

1. Where is the lesion centered?
2. Why, anatomically speaking, does the patient have neurologic deficits related to the cervical sympathetics?
3. Are additional studies necessary for diagnosis? For management?

Findings

An expansile mass with remodeling of the carotid canal wall involves the left petrous apex. A portion of the lesion enhances as much as the opposite normal internal carotid artery and another nonenhancing portion is seen. A curvilinear calcification not related to surrounding bone surrounds part of the mass. Findings within the sphenoid sinus are noncontributory.

Problem

"Expansile" mass of the petrous apex, probable sphenoid sinusitis and sympathetic plexus neuropathy

Anatomy

A. Carotid canal and artery
B. Relationship of carotid artery and cervical sympathetic plexus
C. Normal variations in the relationship of the cavernous segment of the internal carotid artery to the sphenoid sinus (see 35L)

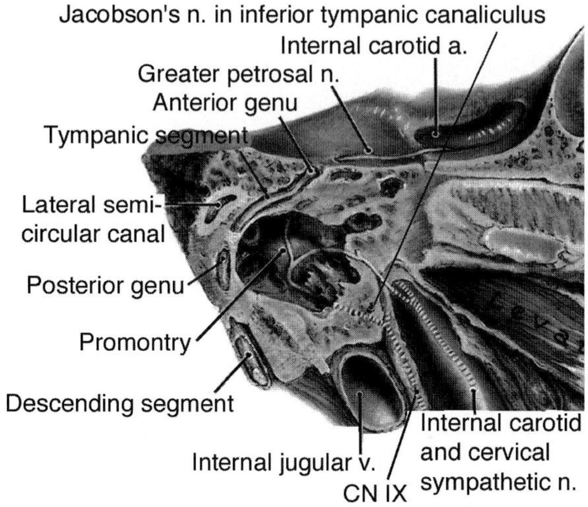

Figure 35E

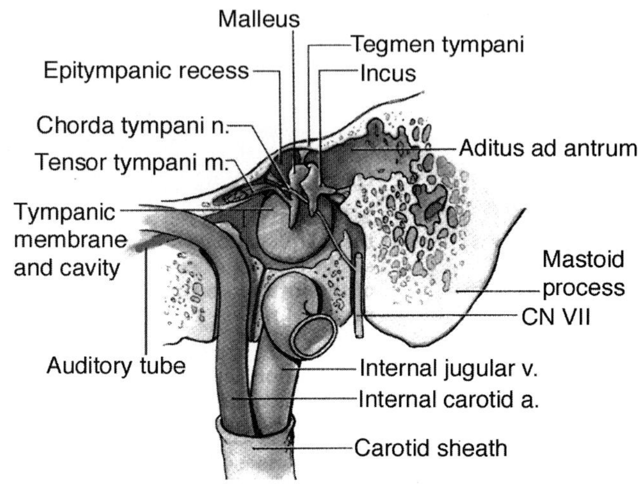

Figure 35F

Differential Diagnosis

None, once an aneurysm is properly identified—generically; cholesterosis or other expansile masses were initially in the differential diagnosis.

Diagnosis

Sphenoid sinusitis with petrous and cavernous carotid artery aneurysm causing Horner's syndrome

Diagnostic Imaging Approach

A. Confirm that the mass is centered in the petrous apex rather than the adjacent cavernous sinus, petroclival fissure, or trigeminal cistern.
B. Exclude aneurysm as a cause or complication of the mass:
   1. Target sign (computed tomography [CT]), flow void or artifacts (magnetic resonance angiography [MRA])
   2. Look for blood products: completely or nearly completely thrombosed aneurysms may have no or little evidence of flow, respectively.
   3. Trace the contour of the carotid canal diligently: look for curvilinear calcifications (CT).
C. Identify sites of contiguous extension, possible causes (sinusitis, dissection) and complications (thromboembolic).

Clinical Points Of Importance And Supplemental Information

A. Completely thrombosed aneurysms are usually suspected and sometimes finally diagnosed on the basis of imaging (as opposed to angiography).
B. The cervical sympathetics are intimately associated with the carotid artery throughout the neck and especially within the carotid canal. Any patient with Horner's syndrome must have the entire distribution of the cervical sympathetics studied.
C. Some carotid artery dissections can be diagnosed and managed solely on the basis of MR imaging , MRA, or CT findings.

Answers To Questions

1. Petrous apex or carotid canal
2. Because the cervical sympathetics run with the carotid artery plexus at the skull base
3. MRA or CTA. Angiography with test carotid occlusion.

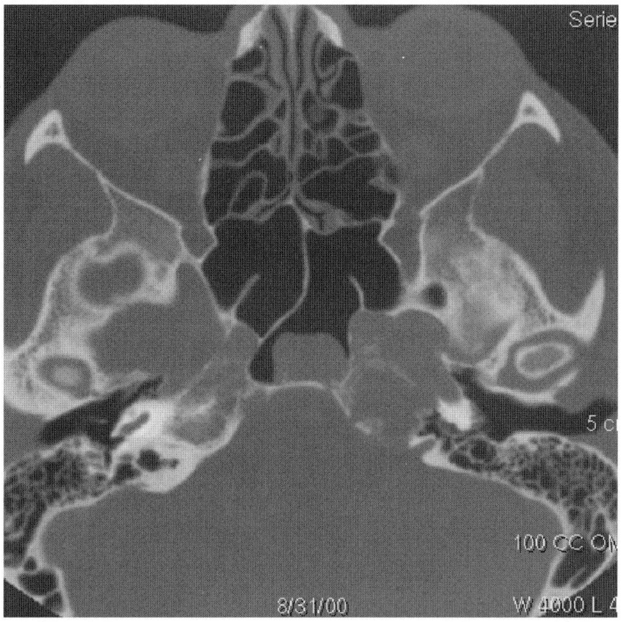

Figure 35G. Patient 1 with chondrosarcoma arising from a petroclival fissure. Axial computed tomography image at bone window setting showing destructive yet "expansile" mass with scattered mineralization centered in left petrous apex.

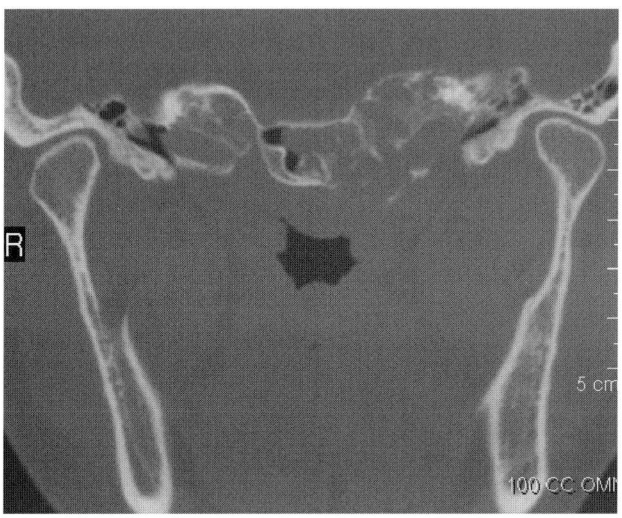

Figure 35H. Patient 1 with chondrosarcoma arising from a petroclival fissure. Coronal computed tomography image at bone window setting.

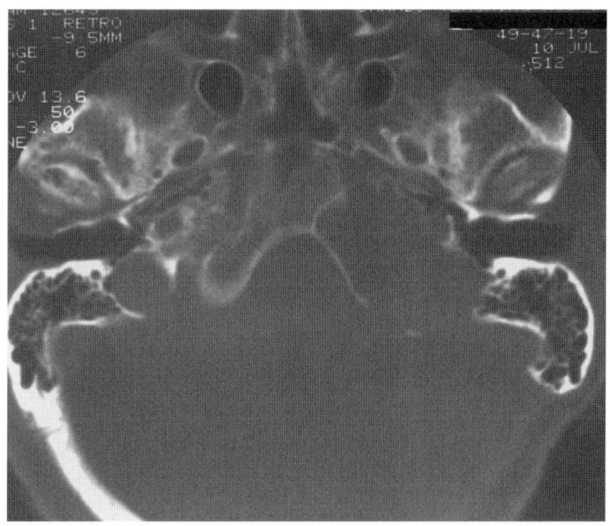

Figure 35I. Patient 2 with schwannoma involving the petrous apex, showing an exspansile mass centered in the petrous apex with dehiscence of cortex in the posterior aspect of the carotid canal–axial CT image at bone window setting.

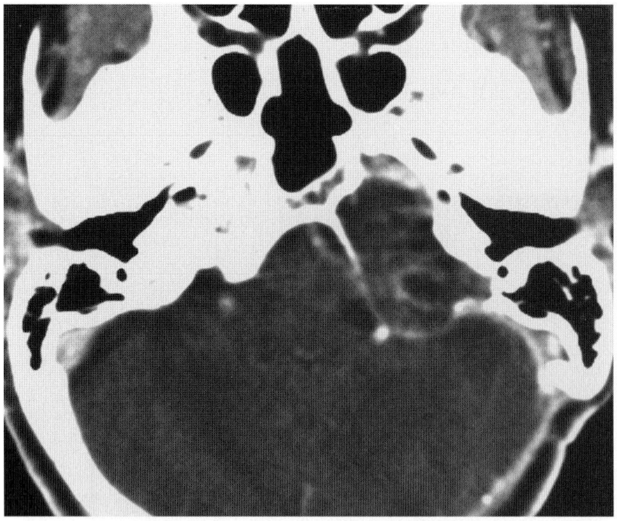

Figure 35J. Patient 2 with schwannoma involving the petrous apex, showing inhomogeneous internal architecture of the mass that is more typical of a neurofibroma. Axial computed tomography image at soft tissue window setting.

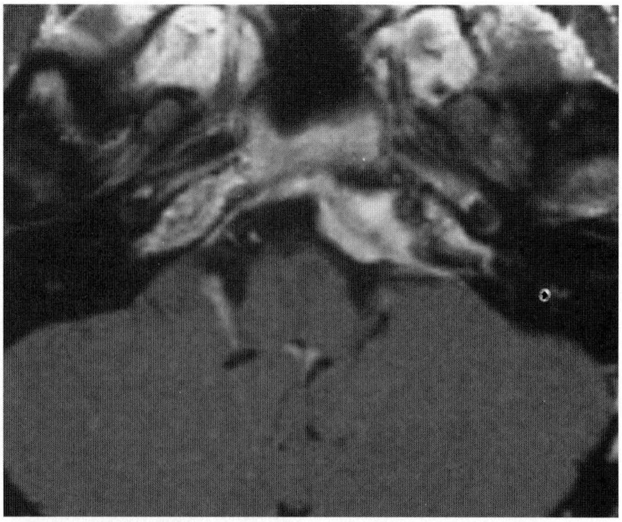

Figure 35K. Patient 3 with meningioma, showing homogeneously enhancing, extraaxial mass along the posterior aspect of the left petrous bone and clivus. The meningioma is partially intraosseous—the intraosseous feature is an important treatment consideration.

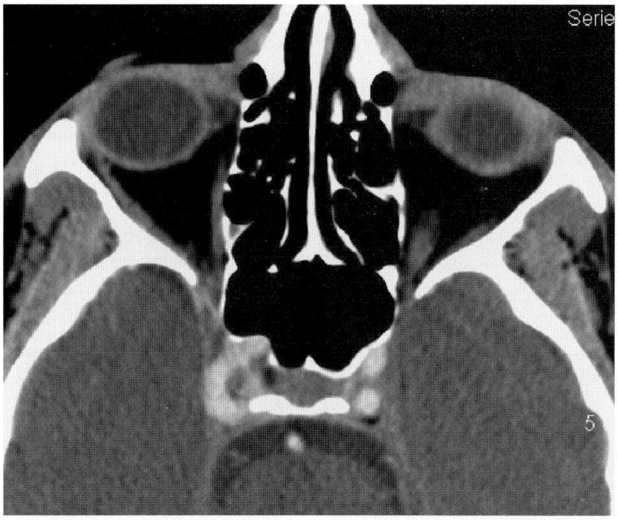

Figure 35L. Patient 4, showing the clinoid segment of both internal carotid arteries deeply indenting into the aerated sphenoid sinus and anterior clinoid processes as a normal anatomic variation.

CASE 36

Clinical History: A 15-year-old girl presents with hearing loss.

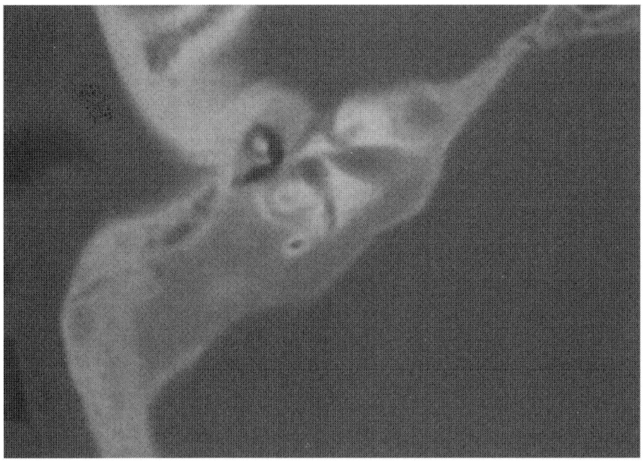

Figure 36A

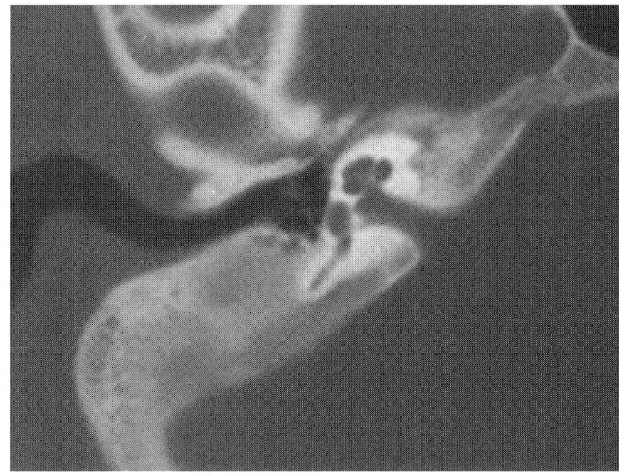

Figure 36B

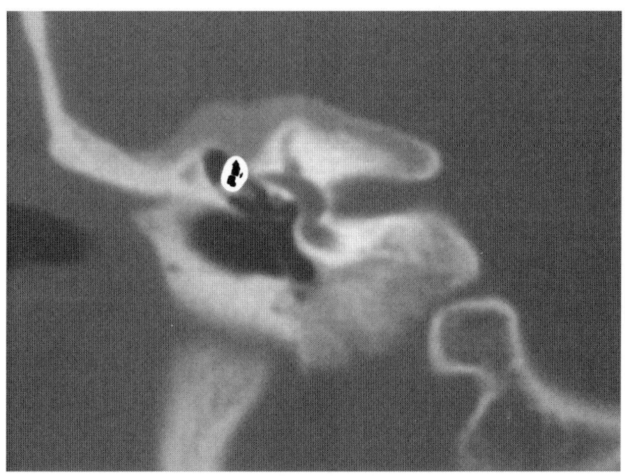

Figure 36C

1. Is the hearing loss more likely conductive or sensorineural?
2. List two developmental and one acquired disease that might show similar findings.

Findings

Normal differentiation between the cortex and medullary space is lost in the "expanded" appearing right temporal bone. Diffuse ground-glass pattern involves the bone but spares part of the otic capsule. The epitympanum and sinus tympani are somewhat "encroached upon" by the productive bony process.

Problem

Primary bony abnormality of the mastoid and petrous portions of the temporal bone, producing hearing loss in a child.

Anatomy

A. Identify the limits of the mastoid and petrous portions of the temporal bone.
B. What is the otic capsule?
C. Explain the variable appearance of the normal petrous apex on computed tomography (CT) and magnetic resonance (MR) images.

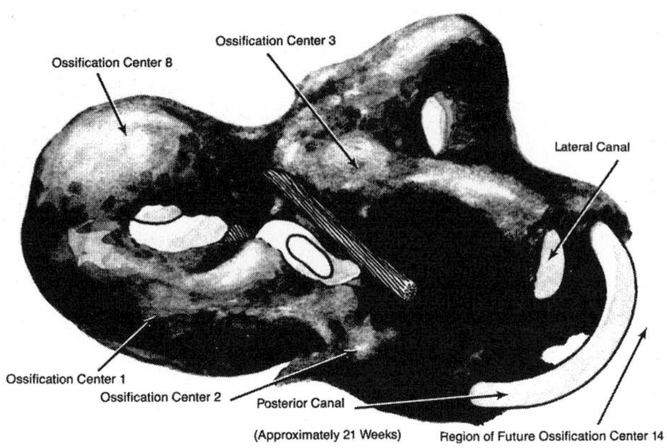

Ossification of the otic capsule at 21 weeks

Figure 36D

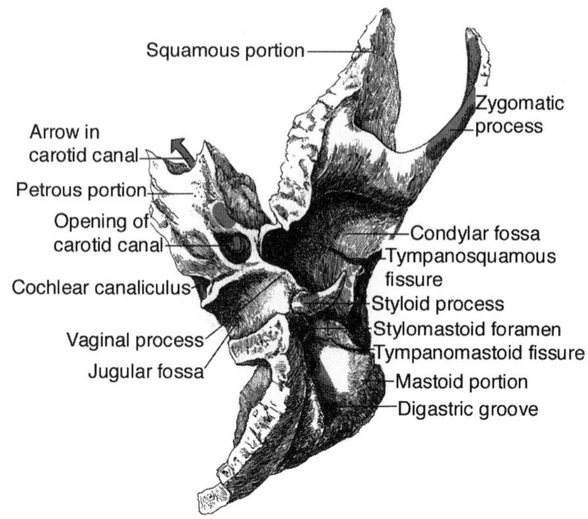

Figure 36E

Differential Diagnosis

None really. However, interesting to consider osteopetrosis, reactive bone caused by healed histiocytosis, or *en plaque* meningioma; intraosseous meningioma. It is very difficult to consider metastasis, lymphoma, and so on with such a benign appearance. Findings are too homogeneous and the patient's age is wrong for Paget's disease.

Diagnosis

Fibrous dysplasia of the temporal bone

Diagnostic Imaging Approach

A. Is the local abnormality of bone focal, multifocal, or diffuse? Is the disease process monostotic or polyostotic?
B. Are the changes reactive or caused by primary bone pathology?
C. Is there a pattern of "expansion" within the affected bone(s)?
D. Osteolytic, osteoblastic, or mixed?
E. Matrix: osteoid, chondroid, fibrous?
F. What structures are secondarily involved (e.g., otic capsule, ossicles, foramina, internal auditory canal)?

Clinical Points Of Importance And Supplemental Information

A. Patients may have conductive hearing loss in the absence of physical findings or history that suggests a cause.
B. High resolution CT frequently provides the answer. Meticulous technique is required; the standard for good temporal bone technique is consistent visualization of the stapes suprastructure.

Answers To Questions

1. Conductive
2. Fibrous dysplasia, osteopetrosis (not really), healed histiocytosis

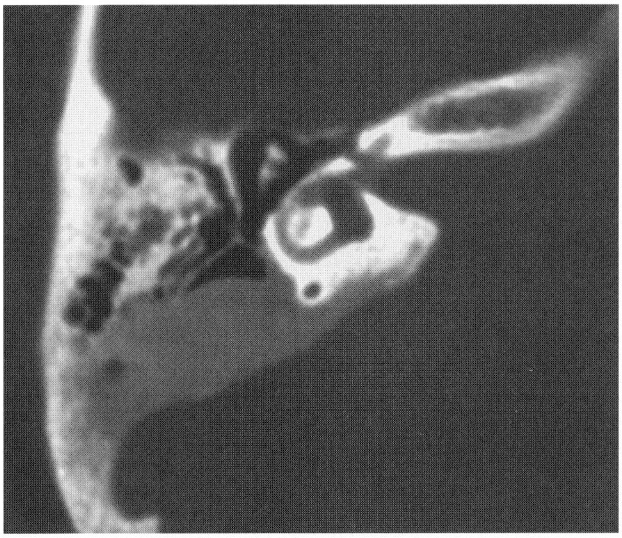

Figure 36F. Patient 1 with fibrous dysplasia of the temporal bone, showing a ground-glass pattern involving the posterior aspect of the petrous, tympanic, and mastoid bones with "expandable" appearance. Axial computed tomography image.

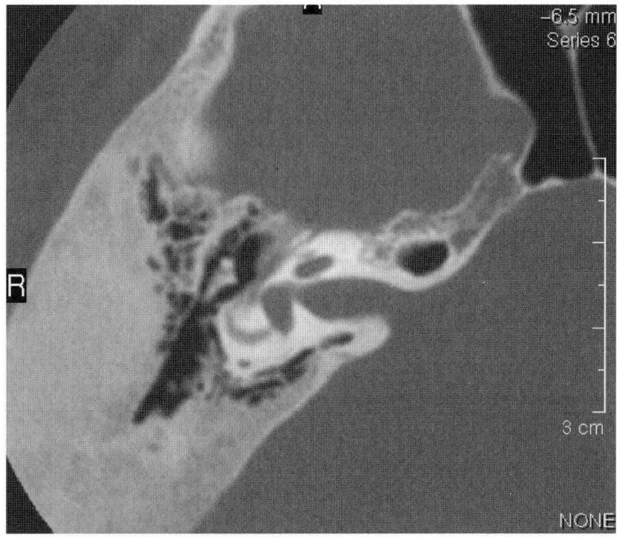

Figure 36G. Patient 2 with fibrous dysplasia of the skull with the ground-glass pattern involving the mastoid portion of the temporal bone while sparing the otic capsule. Axial computed tomography image.

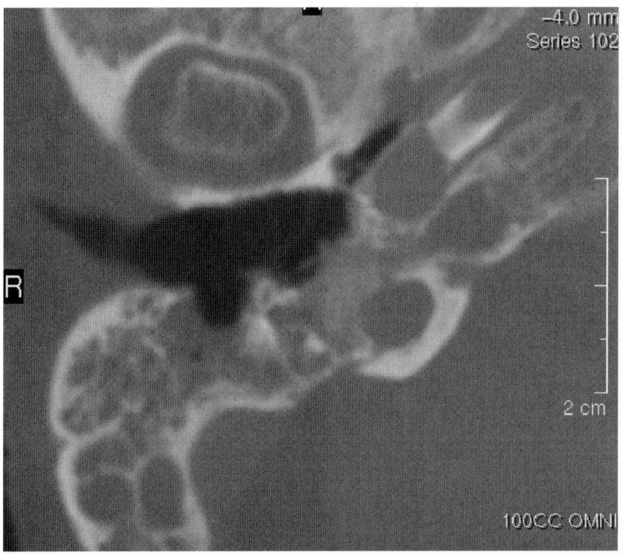

Figure 36H. Patient 3 with radionecrosis of the temporal bone, showing fragmentation, bone erosion, and sclerosis involving the mastoid and petrous portions of the temporal bone.

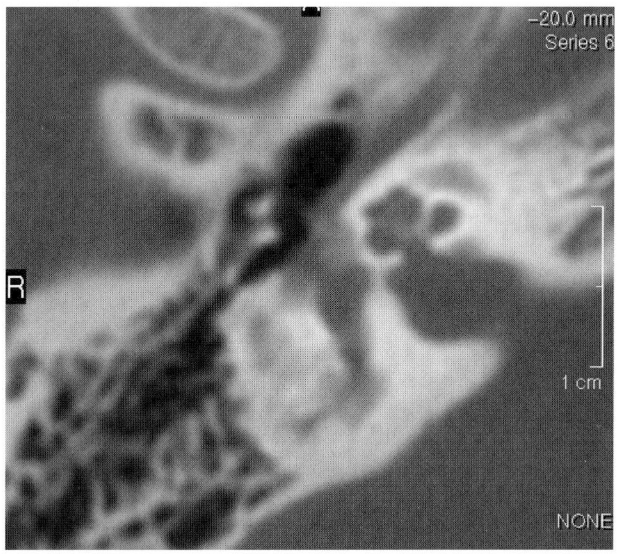

Figure 36I. Patient 4 with relatively early otosclerosis, showing areas of radiolucency in the otic capsule bone at the fissula antefenestram and around the cochlea, vestibule, and semicircular canals that are consistent with the osteolytic phase of otosclerosis.

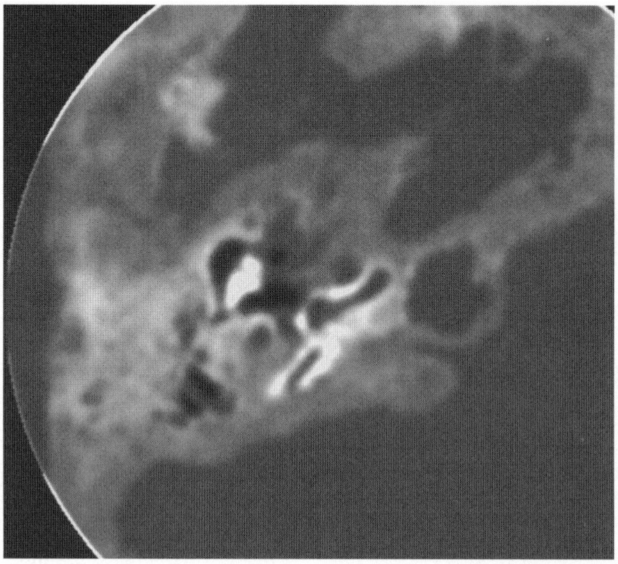

Figure 36J. Patient 5 with Paget's disease involving the temporal bone, showing diffuse expansion of the temporal bone with loss of normal internal architecture, which partially involves the otic capsule. Axial computed tomography image at bone window setting.

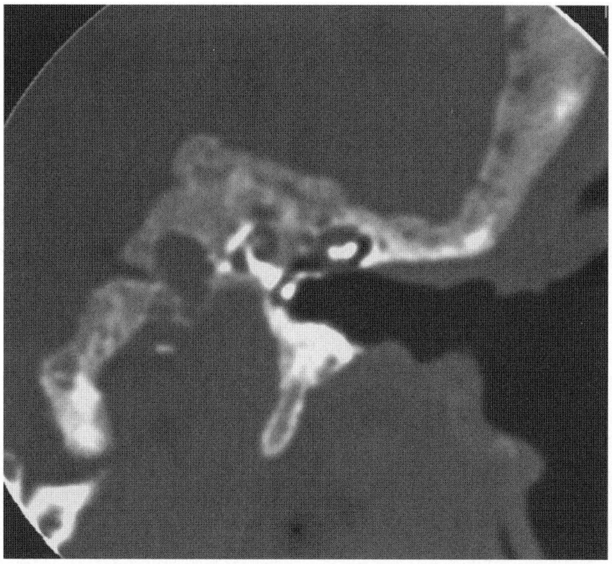

Figure 36K. Patient 5 with Paget's disease involving the temporal bone. Coronal computed tomography image at bone window setting.

CASE 37

Clinical History: An 8-year-old boy presents with bilateral, external auditory canal atresia. The left ear cannot be reconstructed. The parents strongly desire reconstruction of the right ear.

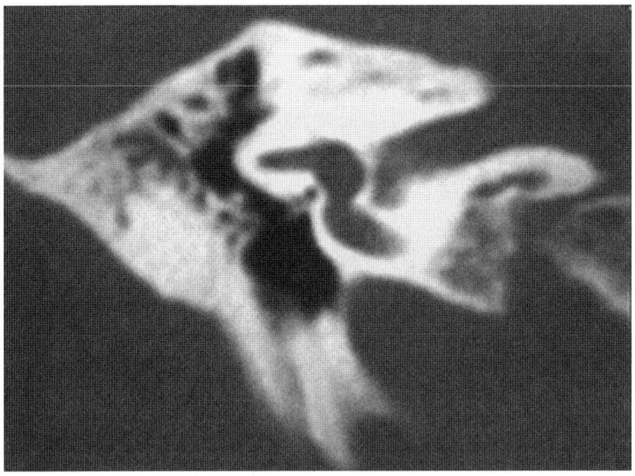

Figure 37A

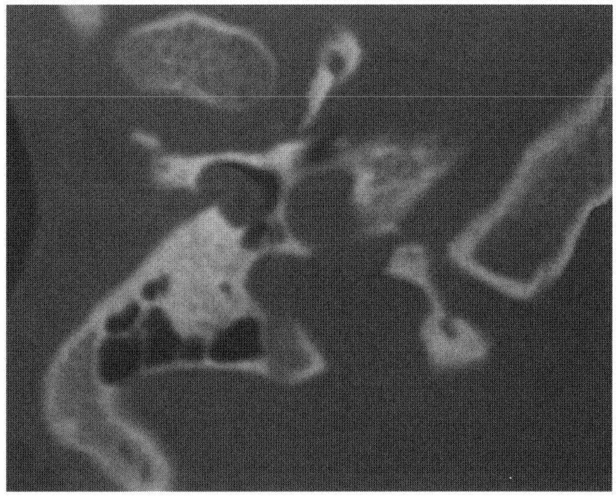

Figure 37B

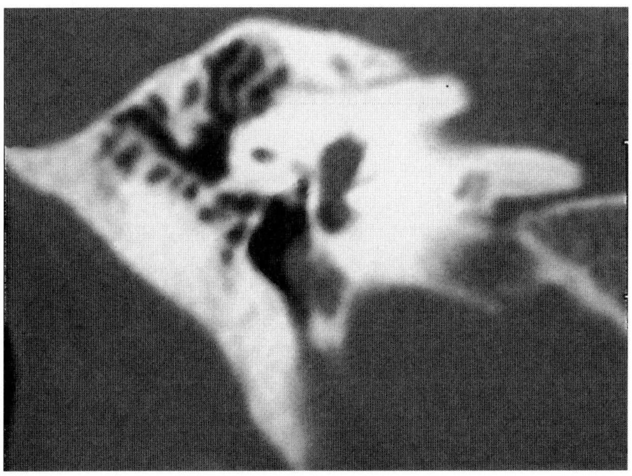

Figure 37C

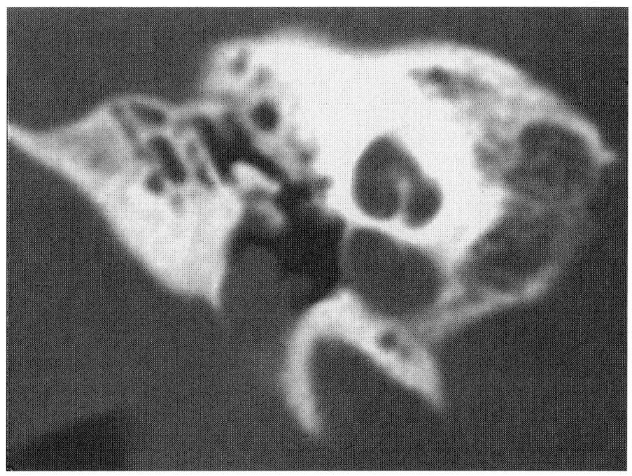

Figure 37D

1. List the most important factors for predicting successful reconstruction.
2. Where is the facial nerve?
3. This patient needs a follow-up study in about 1 year. Why?

Findings

An external auditory canal atresia. The oval window is severely stenotic without a normally developed stapes. The facial nerve canal (tympanic portion) is squarely in the tiny oval window niche. The middle ear cavity, which is poorly developed, contains a lobulated soft tissue mass.

Problem

External auditory canal narrowing, with related middle ear anomalies. Is the ear suitable for reconstruction?

Anatomy

A. External auditory canal
   1. Bony cartilaginous junction
   2. Tympanic ring
B. Middle ear
   1. Ossicles (especially stapes suprastructure and foot plate)
   2. Oval window niche
   3. Tympanic segment of the facial nerve

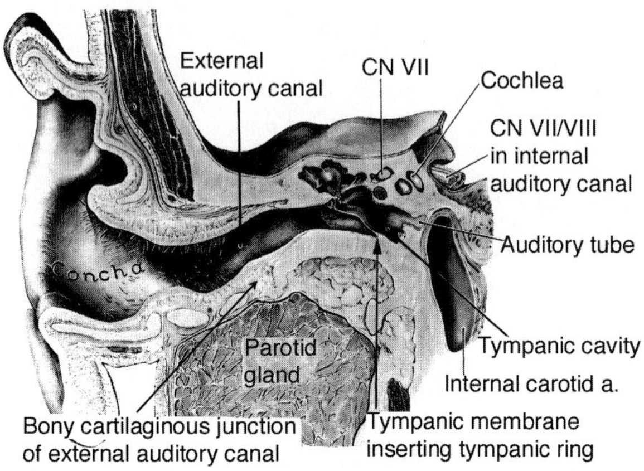

Figure 37E

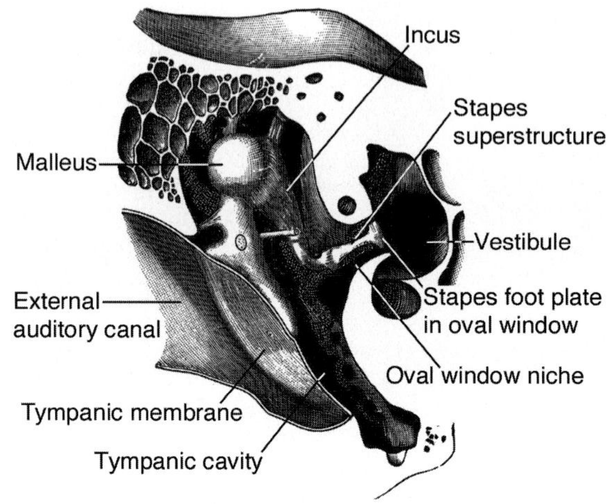

Figure 37F

Differential Diagnosis

Not applicable

Diagnosis

External auditory canal stenosis, with associated anomalous development of the stapes; severe coarctation of the oval window; and aberrant course of the facial nerve (i.e., crossing the severely narrowed oval window niche).

Diagnostic Imaging Approach

A. Evaluate the conductive loss by following the course of a sound stimulus to the inner ear:
   1. Pinna
   2. External canal: stenotic, atretic, thickness of atretic plate
   3. Tympanic cavity: size, aeration, presence of congenital cholesteatoma
   4. Ossicles
   5. Oval window niche
B. Clearly establish the course of the facial nerve.
C. Associated findings: mastoid development, sigmoid plate status, position of carotid artery and jugular veins

Clinical Points Of Importance And Supplemental Information

A. The most important determinants for success of middle ear reconstruction are the status of the stapes and oval window niche and the size of the middle ear cavity. An anomalous course of the facial nerve sometimes precludes surgery in an otherwise suitable patient.
B. An associated congenital cholesteatoma must be excluded in all cases of external and middle ear anomalies. If discrete masses are identified in the middle ear or mastoid, they should be followed radiographically at appropriate intervals if the ear is not explored and repaired.

Answers To Questions

1. Size of the middle ear cavity, status of the stapes and oval window, position of the facial nerve
2. Right over the diminutive oval window
3. Possible congenital cholesteatoma on axial CT image, so that patient needs follow-up CT in one year.

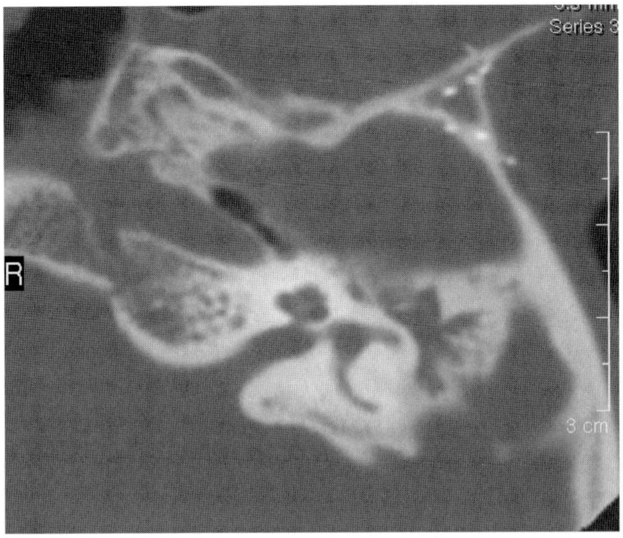

Figure 37G. Patient 1 with developmental abnormality of the first branchial arch apparatus, showing erosive mucosal thickening (probably congenital cholesteatoma) in the middle ear and minimally developed mastoid. Axial computed tomography image.

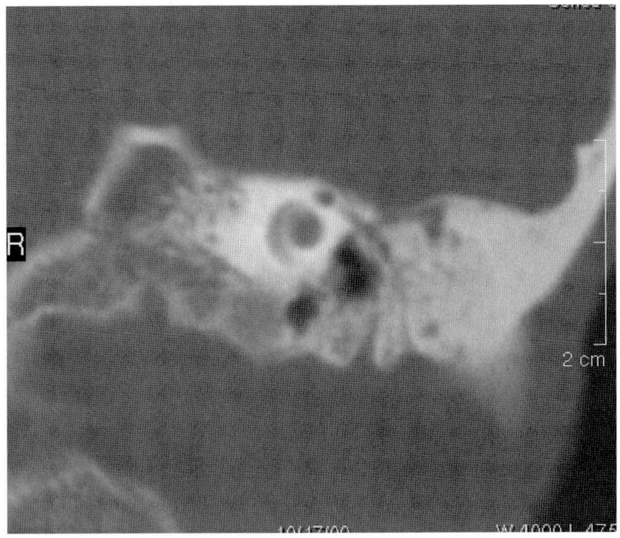

Figure 37H. Patient 1 with developmental abnormality of the first branchial arch apparatus, showing an unusually anterior position of the mastoid descending portion of the facial canal.

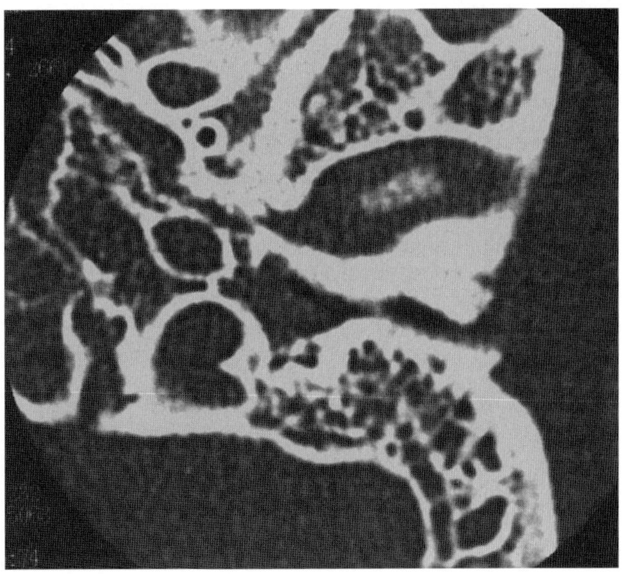

Figure 37I. Patient 2 with exostosis of bony external auditory canal (surfer's ear), showing narrowness of the normally developed bony portion of the external auditory canal caused by mature bony reactive changes. Axial computed tomography image at bone windows.

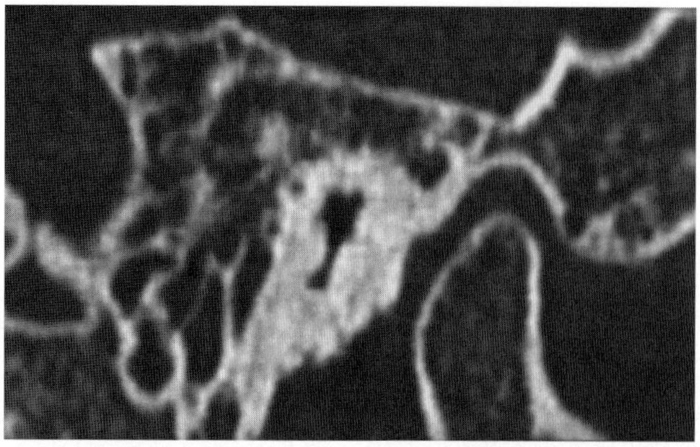

Figure 37J. Patient 2 with exostosis of the bony external auditory canal (surfer's ear). Sagittal image from multireformatted reconstruction, also showing marked narrowness of the bony portion of external auditory canal.

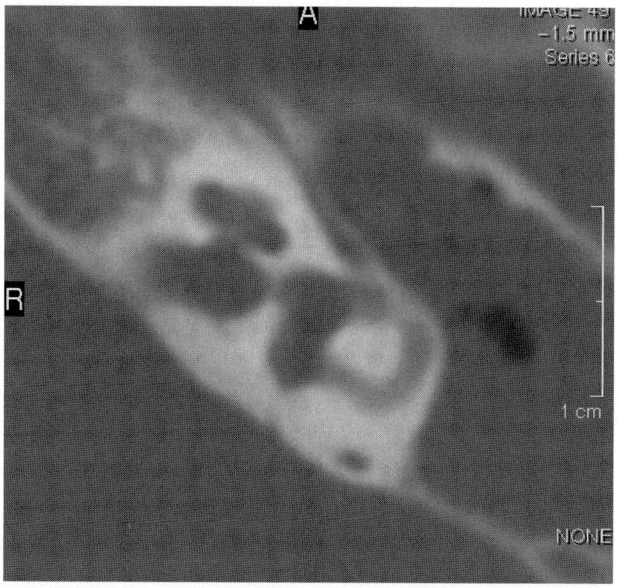

Figure 37K. Patient 3 with very advanced congenital cholesteatoma, showing marked mucosal thickening with almost complete erosion of the malleus head and body and short process of the incus. Its congential nature can be determined only with appropriate history in such an advanced state. Axial computed tomography image.

CASE 38

Clinical History: A 6-year-old girl presents with conductive hearing loss and a visible middle ear mass. The otolaryngologist thinks it looks like a cholesteatoma, but the tympanic membrane is entirely normal and the patient has no history of otomastoiditis.

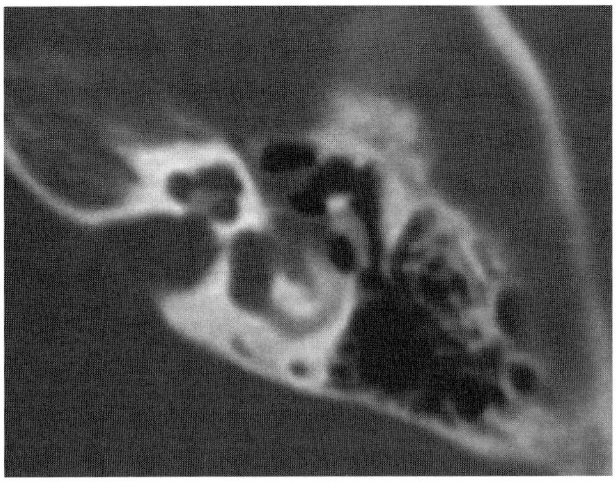

Figure 38A

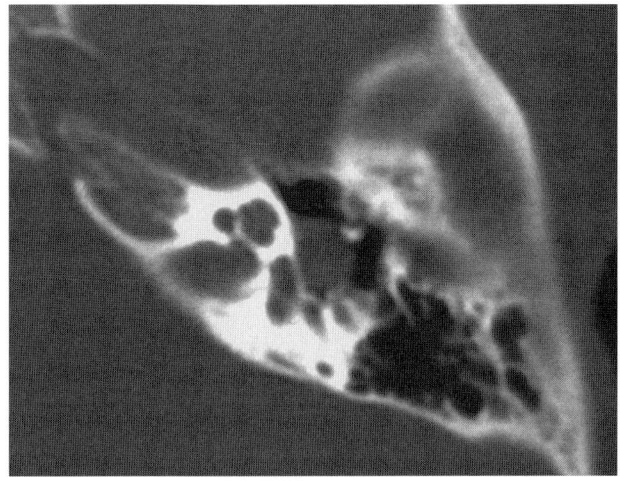

Figure 38B

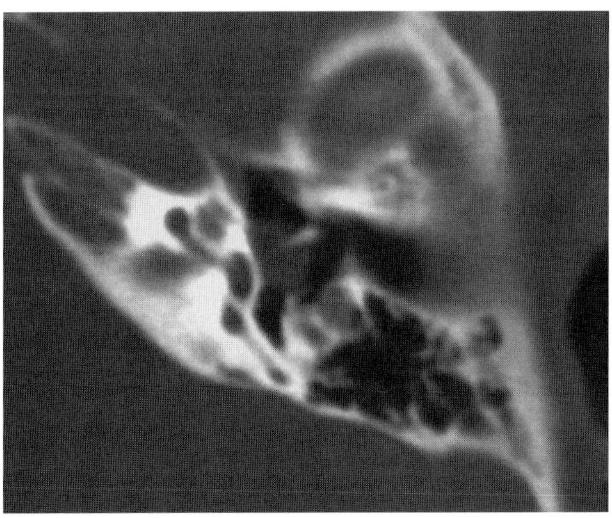

Figure 38C

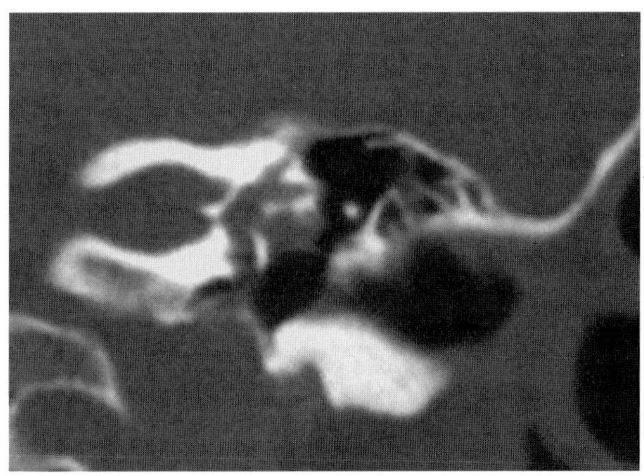

Figure 38D

1. Exactly where is the mass?
2. Is this a usual location for acquired cholesteatoma?
3. Given the history, physical findings, and computed tomography (CT) study, what is your diagnosis? List five other "non-cholesteatomatous" masses that can present in the middle ear behind an intact tympanic membrane.

Findings

An abnormal soft tissue between the body and long process of the incus and the incudomalleolar joint and the medial wall of the left middle ear cavity. The lesion fills the oval window niche. The stapes superstructure is at least demineralized and probably eroded. The mass is medial to the ossicles entirely and no evidence is seen of mastoid or other possible middle ear mucosal thickening.

Problem

A child with a middle ear mass behind an intact tympanic membrane.

Anatomy

A. Middle ear (tympanic) cavity
   1. Epitympanum
   2. Mesotympanum
   3. Hypotympanum
   4. Protympanum
B. Ossicles
   1. Malleus (manubrium)
   2. Incus (long and lentiform processes)
   3. Stapes (head and suprastructure)

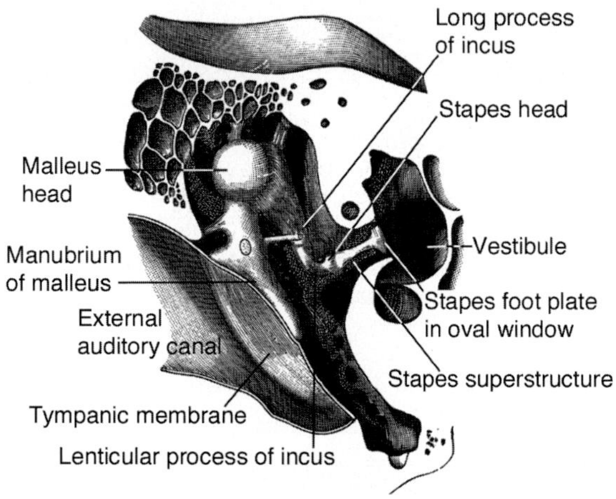

Figure 38E

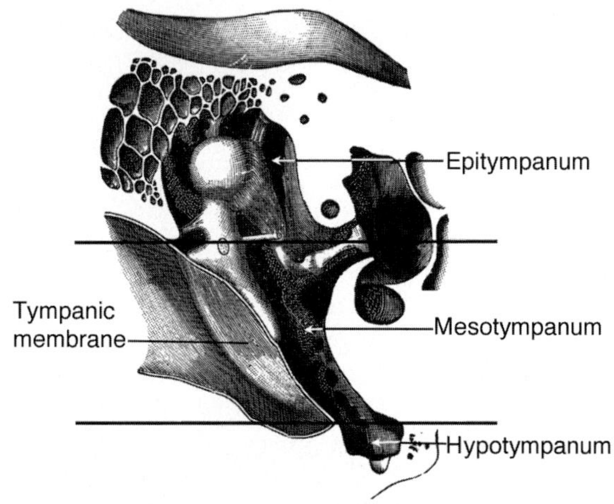

Figure 38F

Differential Diagnosis

Cholesteatoma (acquired or congenital); glomus tympanicum (rare in a child); adenoma or carcinoma (both are very rare), sarcoma (never present when the mass is this small), meningioma (usually middle ear extensions of intracranial lesions—rare in a child), aberrant carotid artery; high jugular bulb

Diagnosis

Congenital cholesteatoma

Diagnostic Imaging Approach

A. Is the middle ear mass discrete or present in addition to or as part of a more generalized process?
B. Is there bone erosion (e.g., of ossicles, scutum, tegmen)?
C. Is there displacement of the ossicles?
D. Is the mass originating outside the middle ear (e.g., ectopic carotid, meningoencephalocele)?
E. Does the mass extend beyond the middle ear (e.g., into middle ear, along facial canal)?

Clinical Points Of Importance And Supplemental Information

A. *Congenital*:
   1. Cholesteatomas are usually medial to the ossicles; the tympanic membrane will be intact.
B. *Acquired*:
   1. Cholesteatomas will be lateral to the ossicles in 70% to 80% of cases.
C. Either type of cholesteatoma can dissect along air cell tracts to involve the petrous portion of the temporal bone; these can be extensive.

Answers To Questions

1. Medial to the ossicles over the oval window region
2. No. But it is frequently for a congenital one.
3. Congenital cholesteatoma. Encephalocele, vascular, glomus tumor, meningioma, adenoma, schwannoma

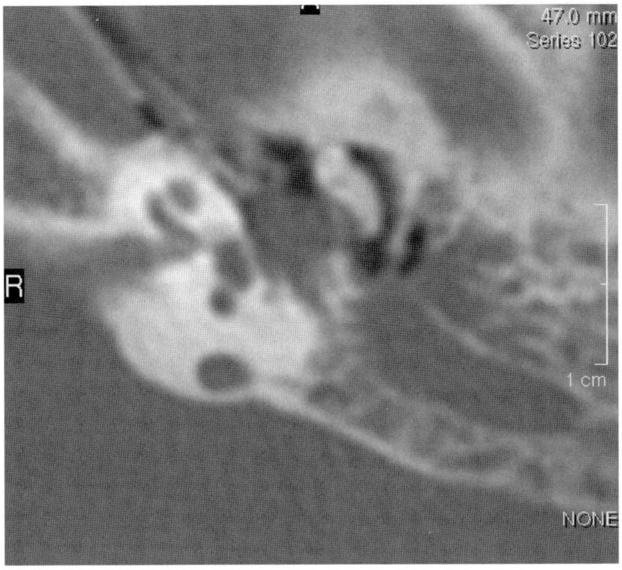

Figure 38G. Patient 1 with congenital cholesteatoma, showing mucosal thickening medial to body and short process of the incus, possibly growing along the tympanic segment of the facial canal. Axial computed tomography image.

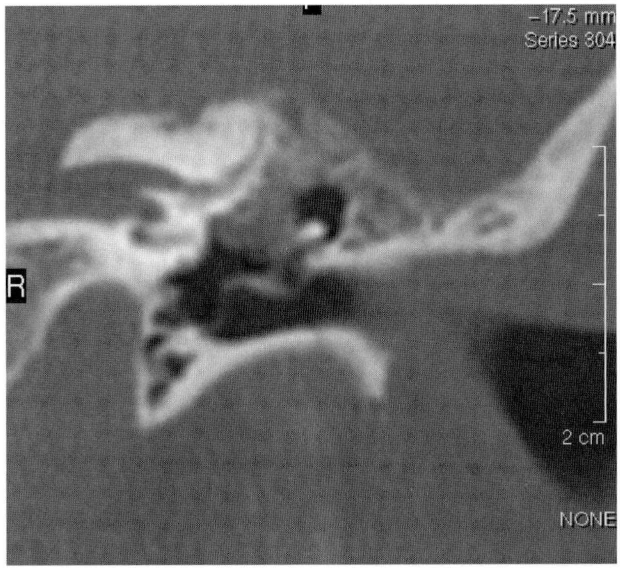

Figure 38H. Patient 1 with congenital cholesteatoma, showing focal mucosal thickening medial to body and long process of the incus, extending into the oval window niche and surrounding the tympanic segment of the facial canal. Coronal computed tomography image.

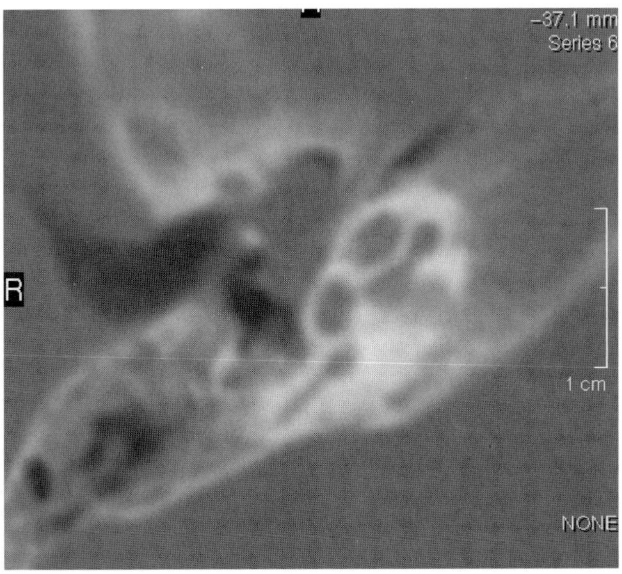

Figure 38I. Patient 2 with congenital cholesteatoma, also showing mucosal thickening medial to the ossicles (manubrium of the malleus and long process of the incus). The stapes superstructure is eroded. The cholesteatoma extends into protympanum and sinus tympani. Axial computed tomography image.

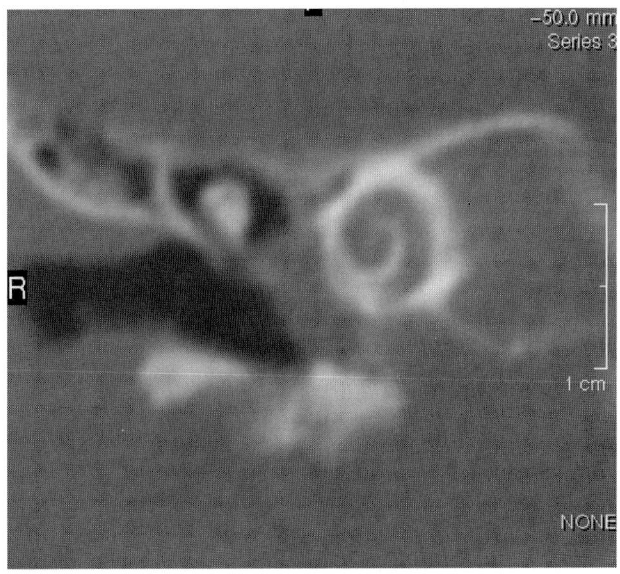

Figure 38J. Patient 2 with congenital cholesteatoma. Coronal computed tomography image, again showing disease medial to the ossicles, with demineralization of the manubrium of the malleus and the bone over the carotid canal.

CASE 39

Clinical History: A 35-year-old man presents with pulse synchronous tinnitus and a mass in the middle ear.

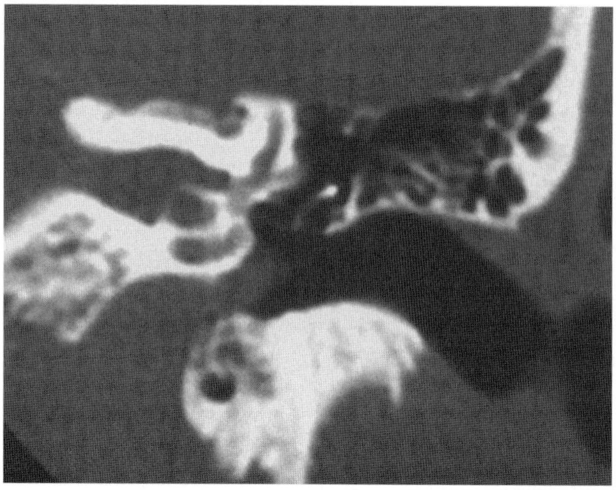

Figure 39A

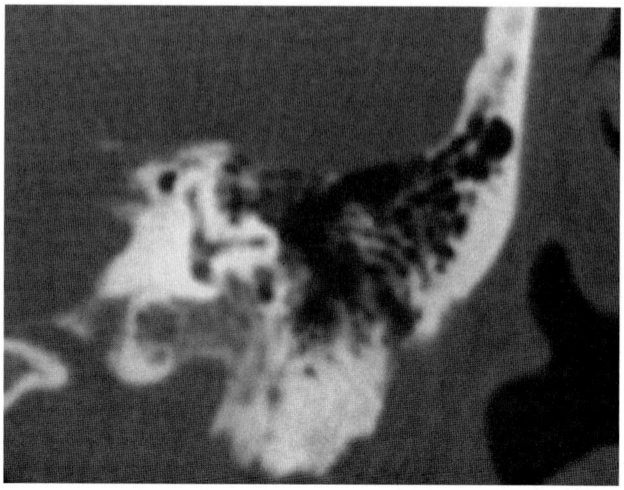

Figure 39B

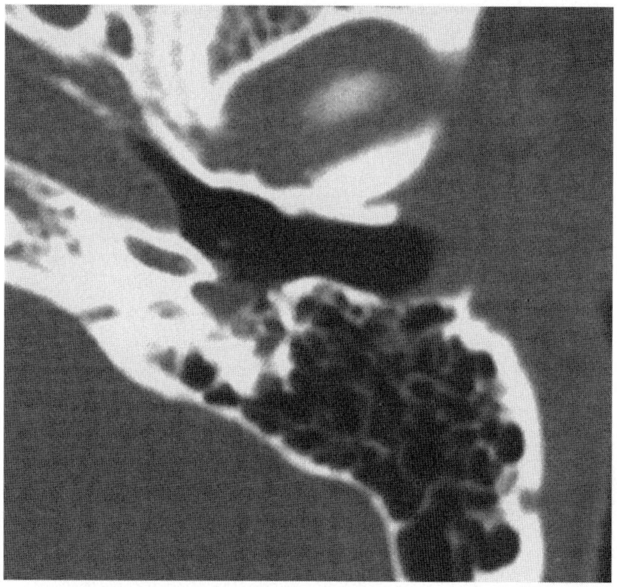

Figure 39C

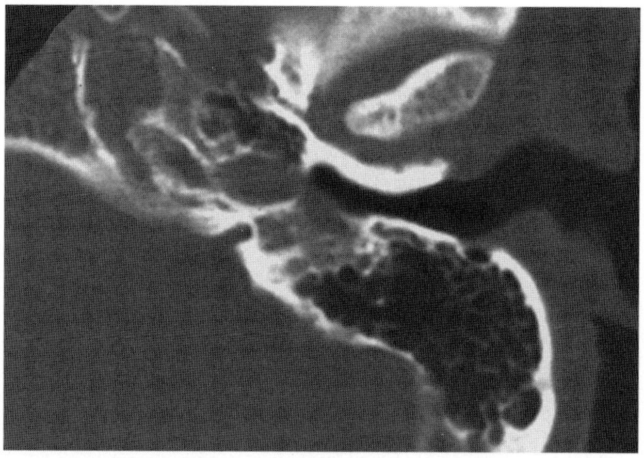

Figure 39D

1. Can the mass be safely removed by transcanal excision via a tympanotomy?
2. Is angiography necessary?
3. Name four varieties of paragangliomas. Are they commonly (> 40% of the time) multiple?
4. How might one screen for multiple tumors?

Findings

A soft tissue mass in the hypotympanum of left middle ear cavity. The lesion erodes a bony wall over the left jugular fossa; the inferior tympanic canaliculus and/or the caroticotympanic canal is the focus of this lesion.

Problem

Pulse synchronous tinnitus and a middle ear mass in an adult

Anatomy

A. Middle ear
   1. Promontory
   2. Hypotympanum (see 38F)
B. Carotid canal and jugular fossa
C. Inferior tympanic and caroticotympanic canaliculi

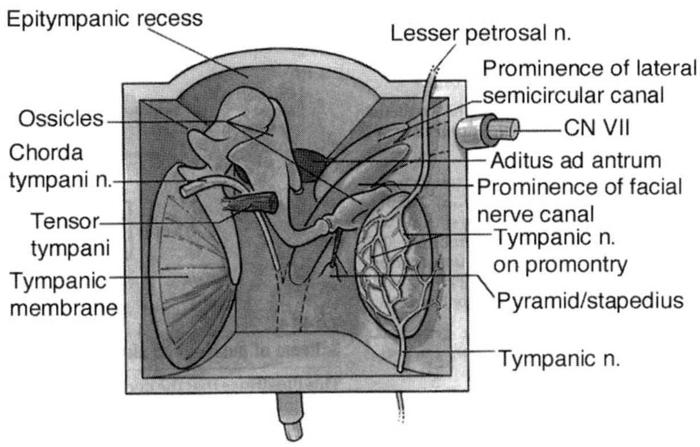

Figure 39E

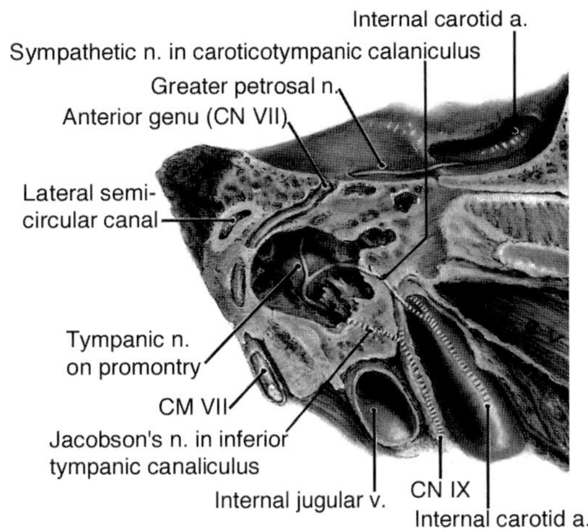

Figure 39F

Differential Diagnosis

Glomus tympanicum, upward extension of glomus jugulare, ectopic carotid artery, high jugular bulb—others are rare

Diagnosis

Glomus tympanicum type of paraganglioma extending to the top of the jugular fossa, probably via the inferior tympanic canaliculus

Diagnostic Imaging Approach

A. The evaluation of this specific problem is possible with axial noncontrast computed tomography (CT) done with contiguous 1- to 1.5-mm sections.
B. Exclude ectopic carotid artery or high jugular bulb as causing the signs and symptoms.
C. Establish the presence of a middle ear mass and evaluate its full extent, especially inferiorly.
D. Realize that a glomus tumor can mechanically obstruct the eustachian tube so that the middle ear may show complete opacification rather than a discrete mass . This is a difficult diagnostic situation and the middle ear might need to be explored and drained or an angiography performed to establish the diagnosis.

Clinical Points Of Importance And Supplemental Information

A. It is *absolutely essential* to establish that an apparent glomus tympanicum is restricted to the middle ear cavity. Recognizing downward extension along the inferior tympanic canaliculus or that the tumor is actually an upward extension of a glomus jugulare helps ensure complete removal of the mass without excessive blood loss.
B. Paraganglioma types include glomus tympanicum, jugulare, vagale, and carotid body tumors. Screening for multiple lesions can be done with CT (for lesions >15 mm), but it is more definitive with conventional angiography.

Answers To Questions

1. No!
2. Not unless the clinician insists
3. Tympanicum, jugulare, vagale, carotid body tumor. No.
4. CT or angiography; magnetic resonance imaging, if you wish

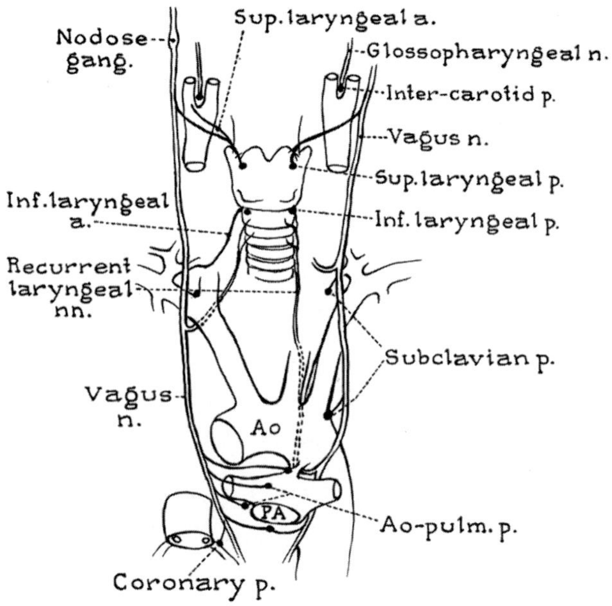

Figure 39G. Location of brachimetric and intravagal paraganglia with their anatomic relationship.

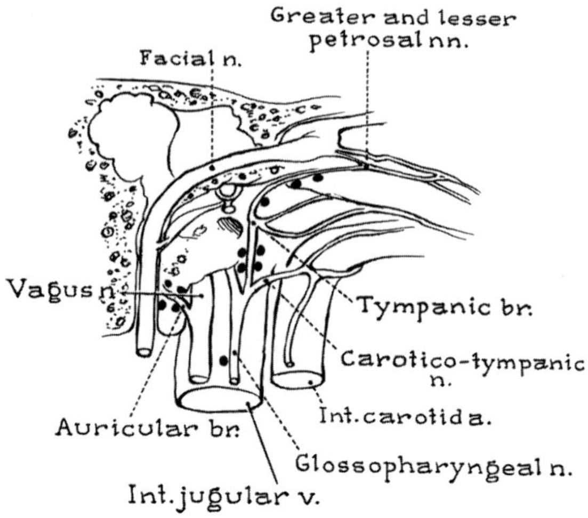

Figure 39H. Location of paraganglia within the temporal bone.

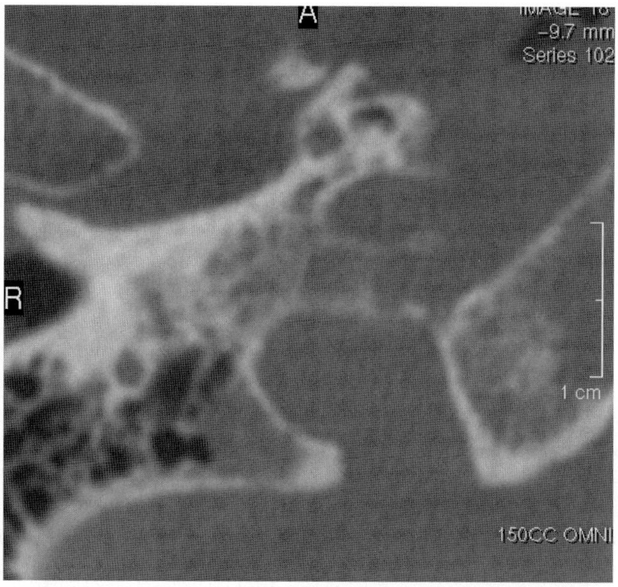

Figure 39I. Patient 1 with a jugulotympanic paraganglioma, showing extensive permeative bony change around the jugular fossa but only a very tiny middle ear component. It is extremely important to the surgeon that this situation is recognized in patients believed to have paraganglioma limited to the middle ear (isolated "glomus tympanicum"). Axial computed tomography image at bone window setting.

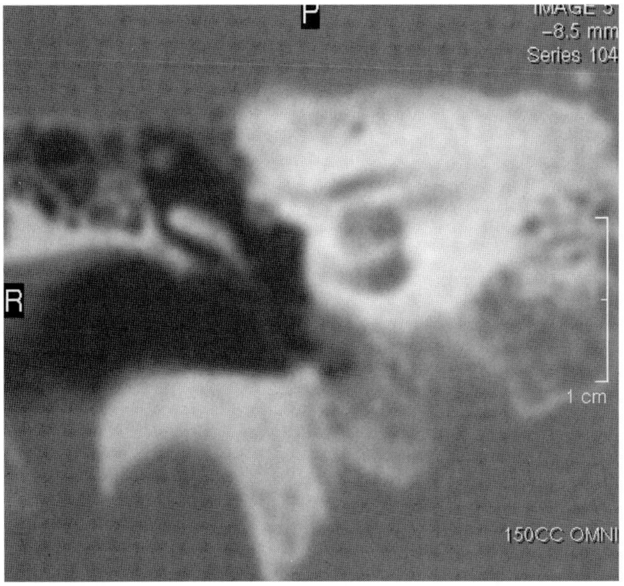

Figure 39J. Patient 1 with jugulotympanic paraganglioma. Coronal computed tomography image at bone window setting showing soft tissue mass adjacent to the lower portion of the promontory with abnormal bony change around the jugular fossa.

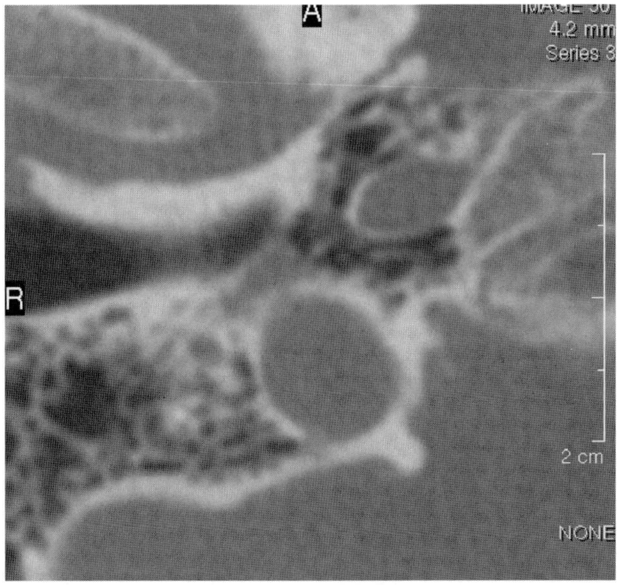

Figure 39K. Patient 2 with jugulotympanic paraganglioma, showing soft tissue mass in the posterolateral aspect of the hypotympanum with localized permeative change of adjacent bone between the mass and jugular fossa. Axial computed tomography image at bone window setting.

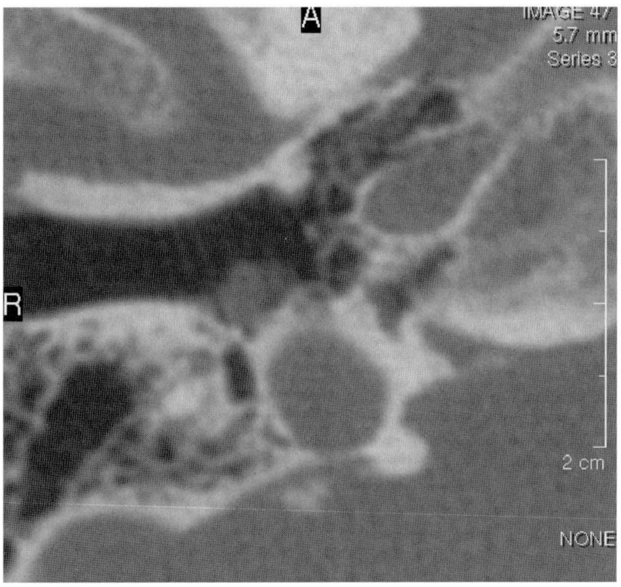

Figure 39L. Patient 2 with jugulotympanic paraganglioma. Axial computed tomography image cephalad to 39K, showing soft tissue mass just medial to the tympanic membrane.

CASE 40

Clinical History: An 18-year-old man presents with fevers, earache, headache, and papilledema.

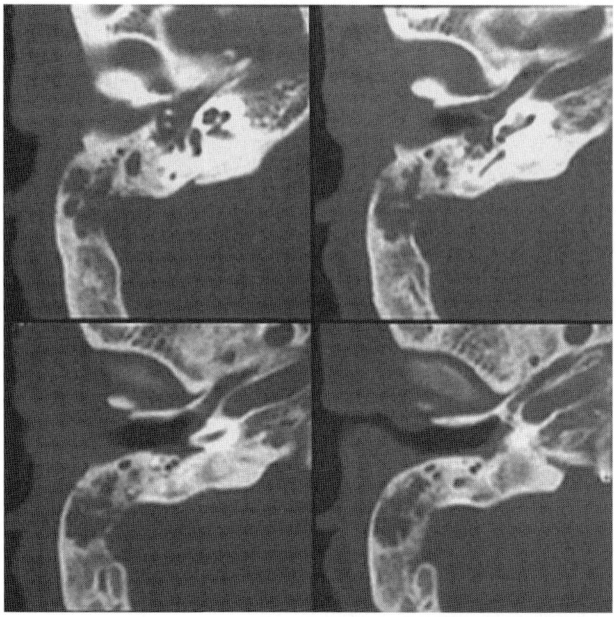

Figure 40A

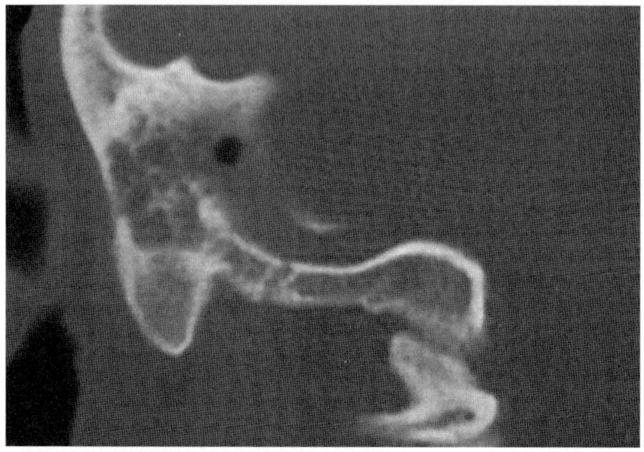

Figure 40B

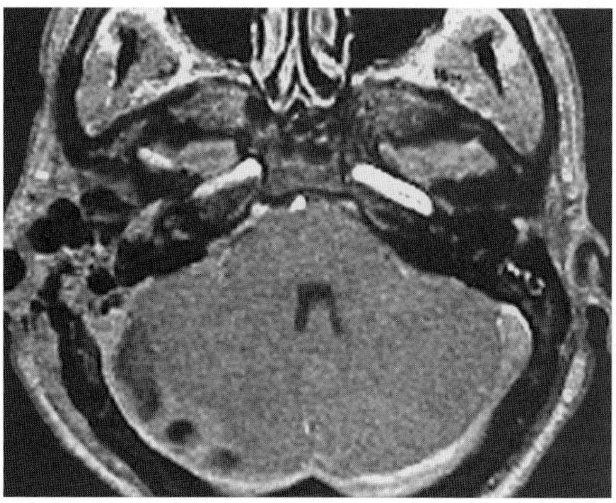

Figure 40C

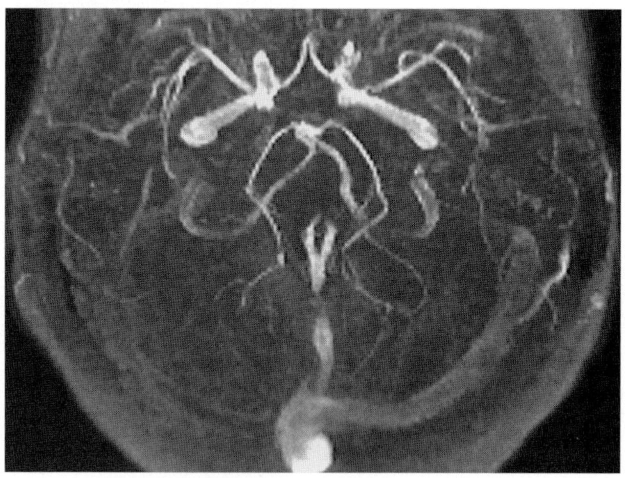

Figure 40D

1. What is the fundamental disease process?
2. List three complications of this disease demonstrated in this patient, and two others that can occur.
3. List three possible causes for the papilledema.

Findings

Abnormal soft tissue density in the middle ear and the mastoid on the right. Bone destruction is noted in the mastoid portion of the temporal bone, with erosion of cortical bone along the sigmoid plate. Coronal computed tomography (CT) image shows intracranial air in the sigmoid sinus.

The right sigmoid and transverse sinuses are occluded, as seen on both source and maximal intensity projection magnetic resonance imaging (MRI).

Problem

Otomastoiditis with intracranial complications

Anatomy

A. Mastoid
   1. Antrum, central mastoid canal
   2. Sigmoid plate
B. Transverse, sigmoid and petrosal venous sinuses

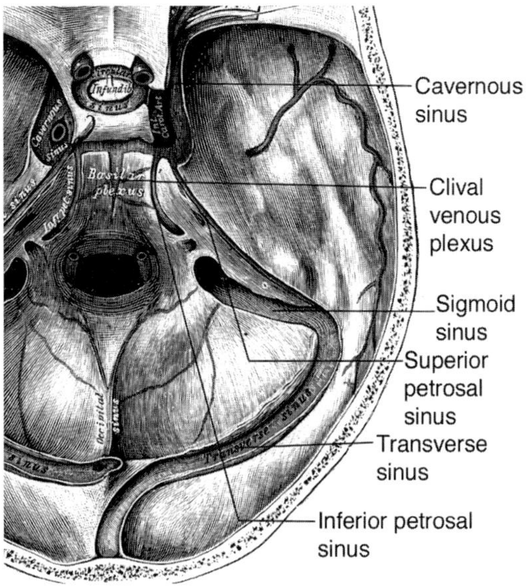

Figure 40E

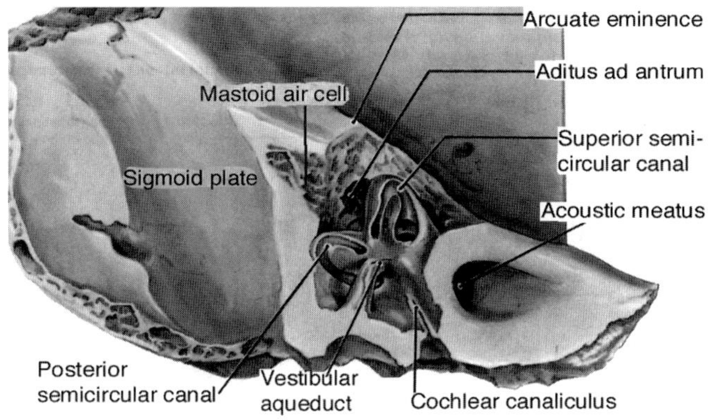

Figure 40F

Differential Diagnosis

Not applicable

Diagnosis

Coalescent (probably suppurative) otomastoiditis, with osteomyelitis and epidural empyema; secondary dural sinus thrombosis—probably septic

Diagnostic Imaging Approach

A. Determine whether the disease in the mastoid is aggressive.
   1. Air cell walls destroyed or demineralized:
      a. Coalescent mastoiditis
      b. Ossicles demineralized or eroded
   2. Cortical bone destruction: osteomyelitis
   3. Subperiosteal abscess
B. Has disease spread beyond the temporal bone intracranially?
   1. Epidural or subdural empyema
   2. Dural sinus or cortical venous thrombosis (bland or suppurative)
   3. Cerebritis or brain abscess
   4. Meningitis
   5. Other intracranial complications including "otitic" hydrocephalus, generalized brain edema or herniation
C. Has disease spread elsewhere (e.g., deep neck abscess, jugular thrombophlebitis)?

Clinical Points Of Importance And Supplemental Information

Most patients with acute otomastoiditis are treated successfully without imaging. The minority of patients who have complications of this disease require highly detailed, contrast-enhanced CT and sometimes MRI studies to assure prompt intervention before advanced, life-threatening disease develops.

Answers To Questions

1. Acute, pyogenic otomastoiditis
2. Osteitis, epidural abscess, dural sinus thrombosis, subdural empyema, brain abscess
3. Hydrocephalus, arachnoiditis, cerebral edema

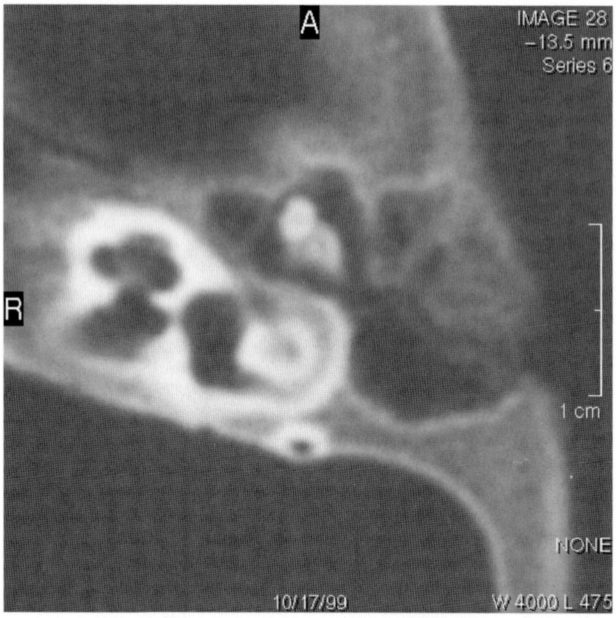

Figure 40G. Patient 1 with coalescent mastoiditis, showing extensive mucosal thickening throughout the middle ear and mastoid, with disruption of the outer cortex of the mastoid bone. Axial computed tomography image at bone window setting.

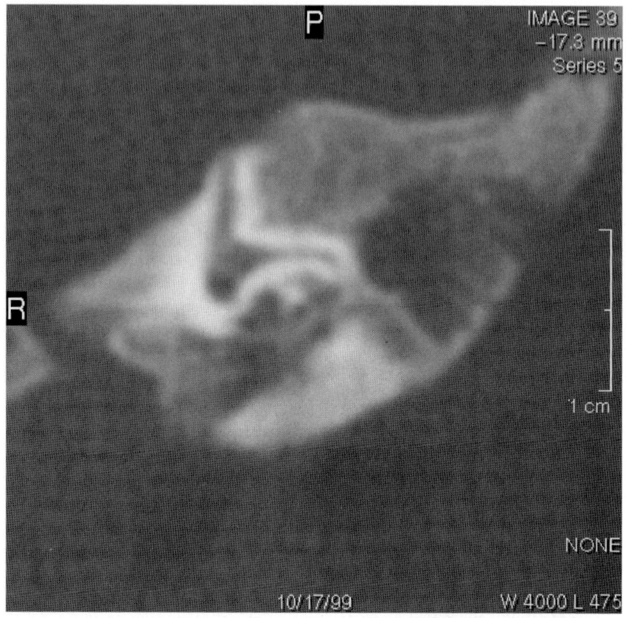

Figure 40H. Patient 1 with coalescent mastoiditis. Coronal computed tomography image, also showing mucosal thickening in the mastoid, with disruption of the outer cortex of the mastoid bone.

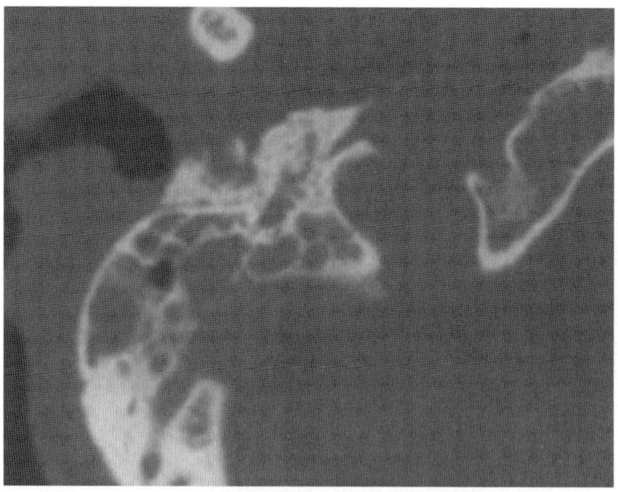

Figure 40I. Patient 2 with coalescent mastoiditis, showing mucosal thickening of the mastoid, with more extensive dehiscence of the adjacent sigmoid plate than seen in the 18-year-old in the case history presented. Axial computed tomography image at bone window setting.

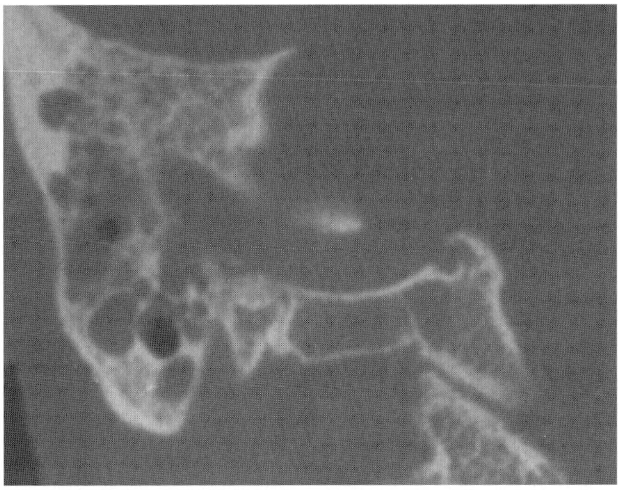

Figure 40J. Patient 2 with coalescent mastoiditis. Coronal computed tomography image at bone window setting showing erosive change of the sigmoid plate and septa of the mastoid air cells.

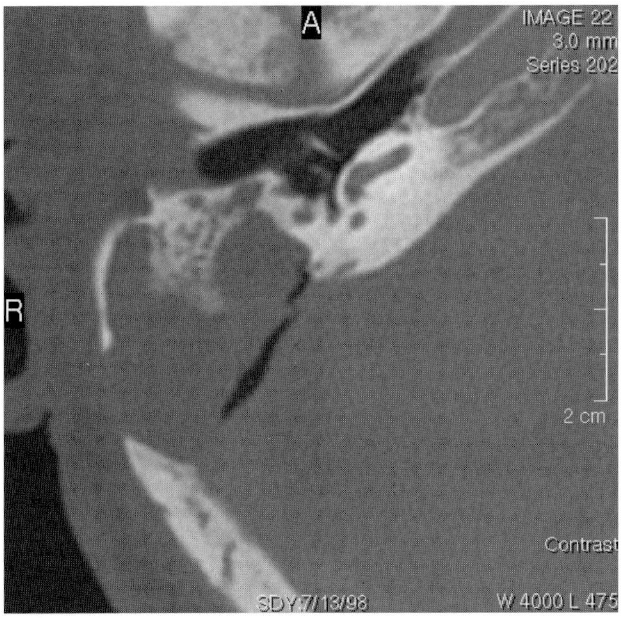

Figure 40K. Patient 3 with acquired cholesteatoma. Axial computed tomography image at bone window setting showing mastoid disease with erosion of the outer cortex and sigmoid plate, nearly resulting in automastoidectomy, as contrasted with the erosive changes seen in more acute disease in other cases presented in this section.

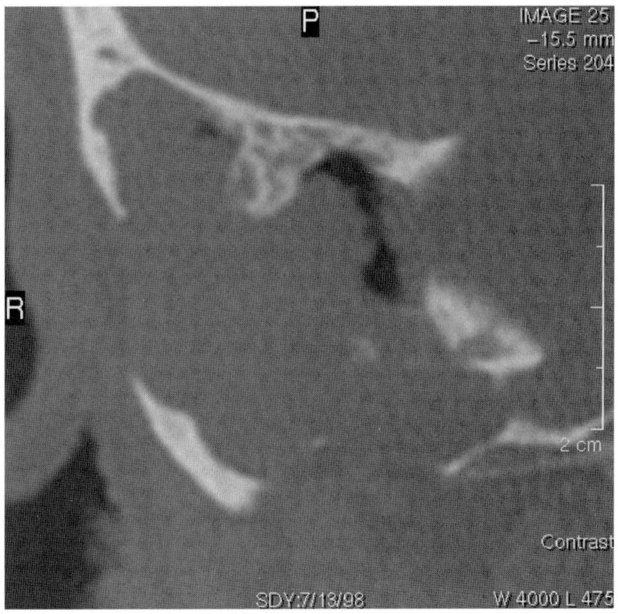

Figure 40L. Patient 3 with acquired cholesteatoma. Coronal computed tomography image at bone windows.

CASE 41

Clinical History: A 5-year-old girl presents for possible cochlear implantation.

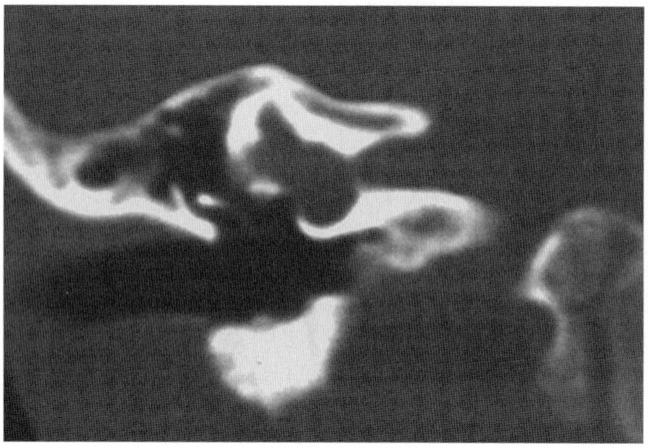

Figure 41A

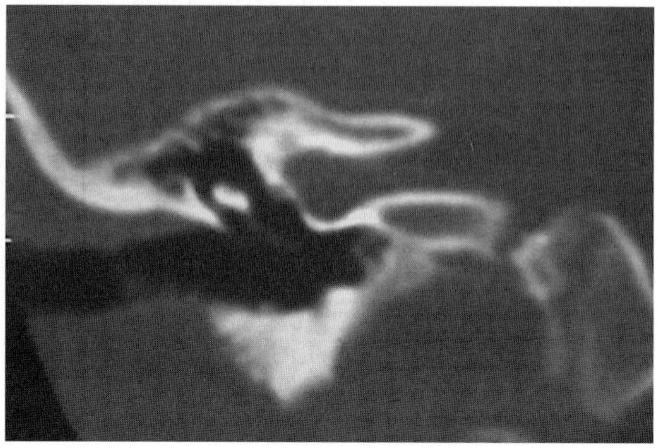

Figure 41B

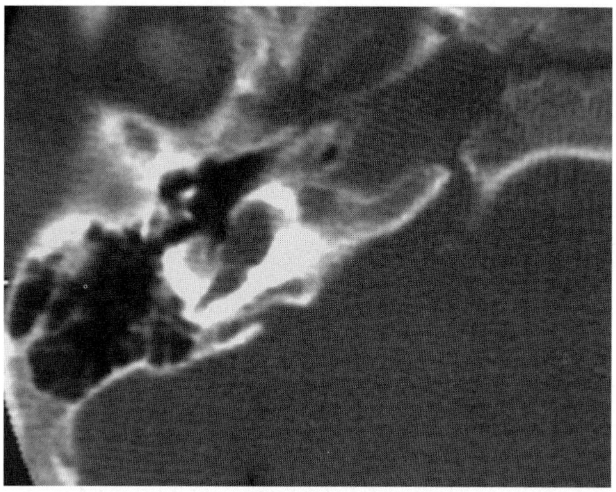

Figure 41C

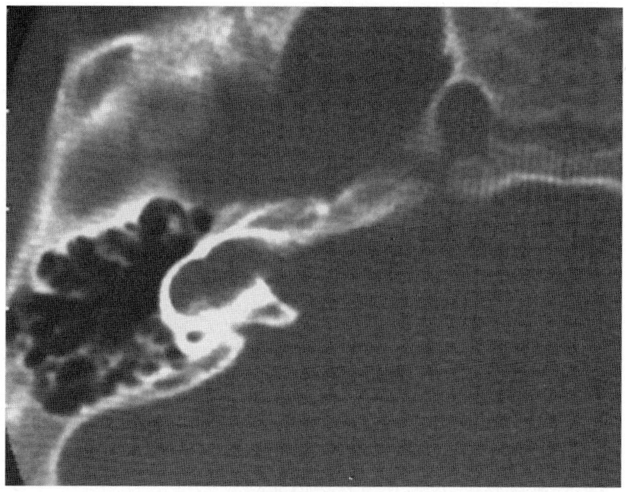

Figure 41D

1. What is the cause of the deafness?
2. The right ear is not suitable for safe implantation. Why?

Findings

Markedly dilated cochlea and vestibule communicate with the fundus of the internal auditory canal. The number of cochlear turns is reduced. The oval window is larger than normal. The ossicles, middle ear cavity, and mastoid air cells have developed normally. The vestibular aqueduct is enlarged.

Problem

A child with deafness caused by severe inner ear anomalies presents for cochlear implantation.

Anatomy

A. Inner ear
   1. Cochlea, vestibule, semicircular canals
   2. Modiolus
B. Internal auditory canal and how the VIIIth cranial nerve divisions reach their end organs
C. Facial recess

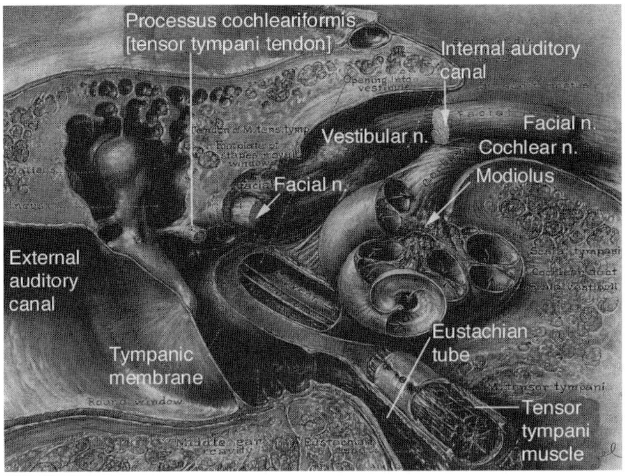

Figure 41E

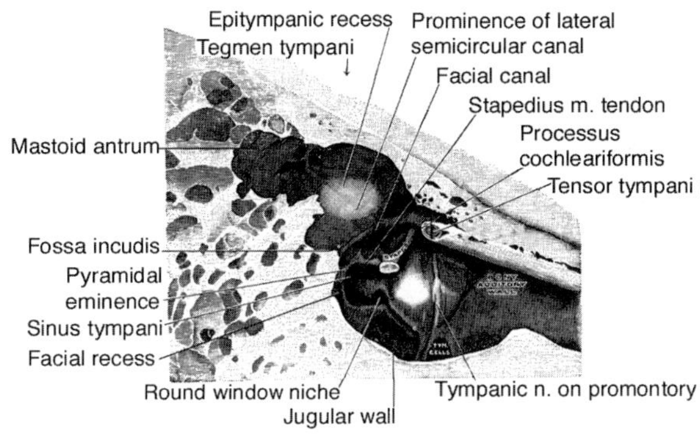

Figure 41F

Differential Diagnosis

Not applicable

Diagnosis

Severe, bilateral (only one side shown) inner ear anomalies, with broad opening between the internal auditory canal and deformed cochlea and vestibule

Diagnostic Imaging Approach

A. Evaluate the bone of the otic capsule.
B. Evaluate the cochlea:
   1. Number of turns, bony margins, round window, modiolus
C. Evaluate the vestibule and semicircular canals:
   1. Presence and size of oval window
D. Look for evidence of middle ear disease.
E. Establish that the anatomy of the facial recess and descending facial canal is normal.

Clinical Points Of Importance And Supplemental Information

A. A wide-opened communication between the internal auditory canal and inner ear as well as the large oval window seen in this patient indicates a high probability for perilymphatic "gusher" during round window manipulation; this can result in a dead ear. This is the only radiographic finding with a clear and consistent predictive value for the risk of perilymphatic fistula; an abnormal stapes footplate and a large cochlear aqueduct also can have some predictive value for the risk of a perilymphatic "gusher".
B. Computed tomography (CT) imaging is mandatory in the evaluation of cochlear implant patients. CT findings are one of several major factors used in determining the suitability of implantation. Other factors include a range of considerations from whether the deafness is prelingual to the results of psychological testing.

Answers To Questions

1. Congenital malformation of the inner ear
2. Because the wide communication between the cochlea and internal auditory canal (at the maculae cribrosae) might lead to "gusher" and a dead inner ear.

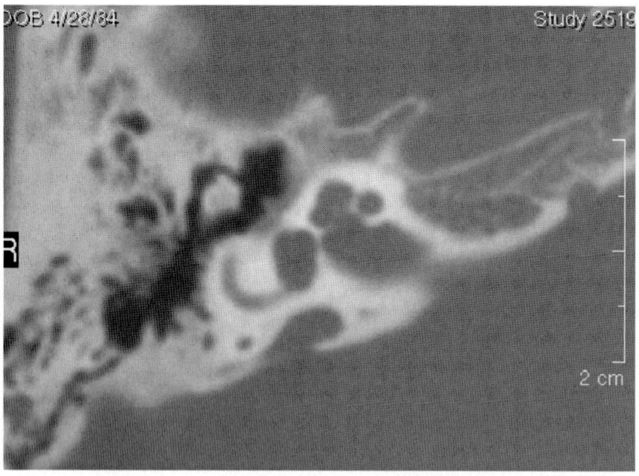

Figure 41G. Patient 1 with inner ear anomaly. Axial computed tomography image of the right temporal bone showing enlargement of the vestibular aqueduct and a relatively normal appearing modiolus—the modiolus is deficient in well over 80% of cases when the vestibular aqueduct is enlarged.

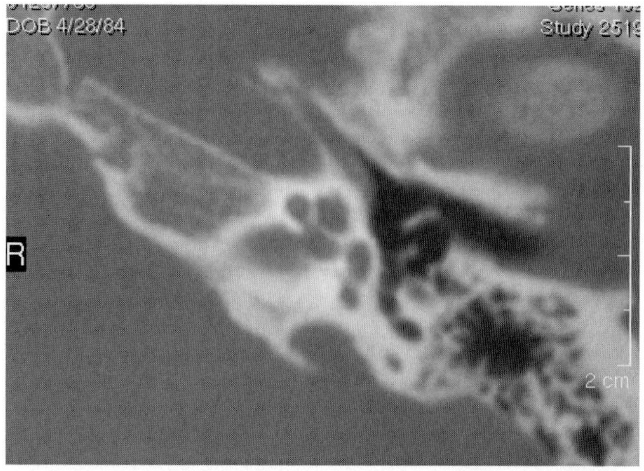

Figure 41H. Patient 1 with inner ear anomaly. Axial computed tomography image of the left temporal bone showing exactly the same finding as the opposite side (see 41G).

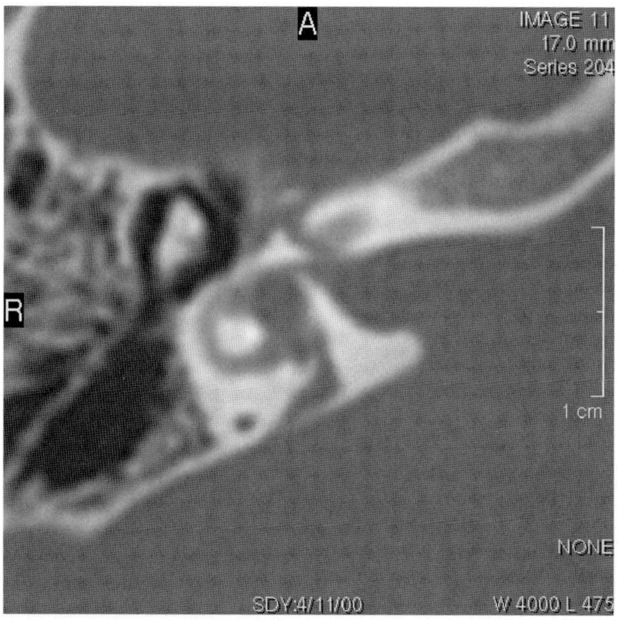

Figure 41I. Patient 2 with inner ear anomaly. Axial computed tomography at bone window setting showing an enlarged vestibular aqueduct.

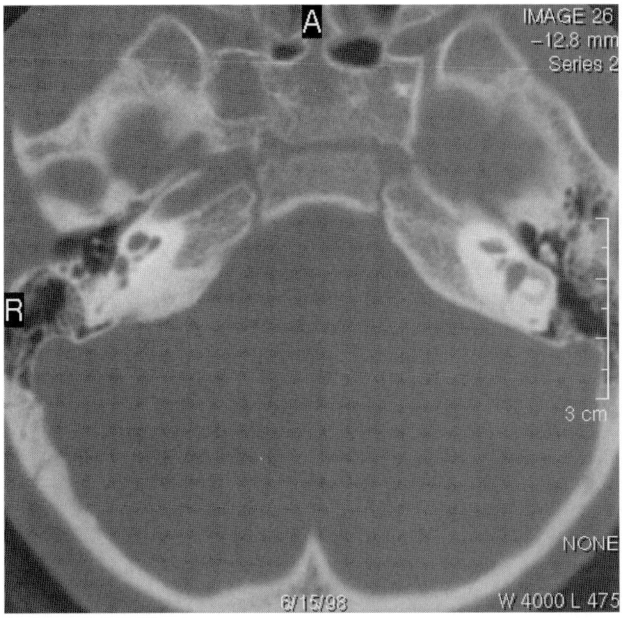

Figure 41J. Patient 3 with sensorineural hearing loss, showing lack of both internal auditory canals. Axial computed tomography image at bone window setting.

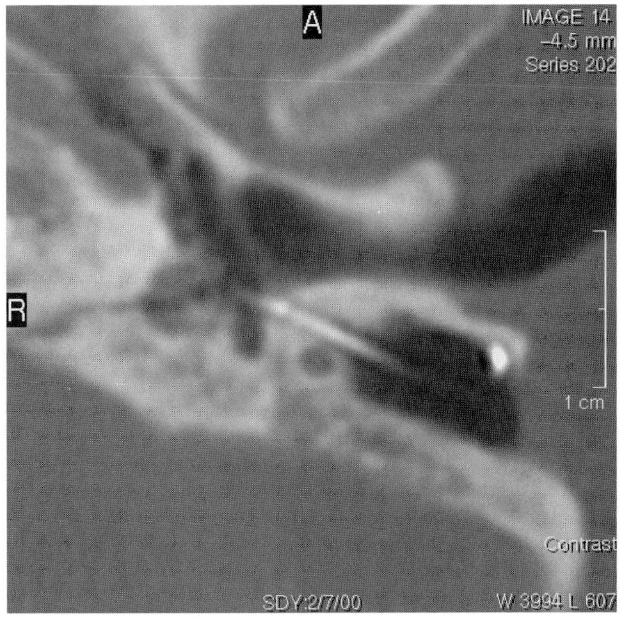

Figure 41K. Patient 4, status after cochlear implant. Axial computed tomography image at bone window setting showing electrode of the cochlear implant entering from the mastoid bowl into the middle ear cavity through an opened facial recess.

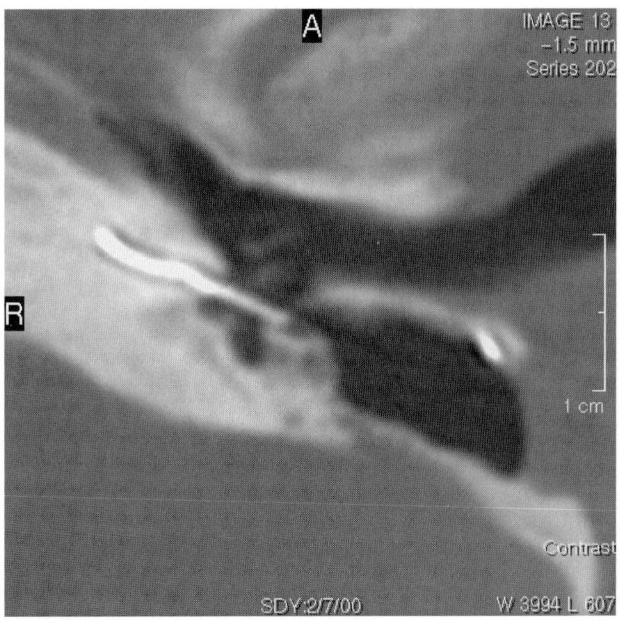

Figure 41L. Patient 4, status after cochlear implant. Axial computed tomography image cephalad to 41K showing the electrode inserted into the basal turn of the cochlea through the round window.

CASE 42

Clinical History: A 35-year-old man presents for possible cochlear implantation.

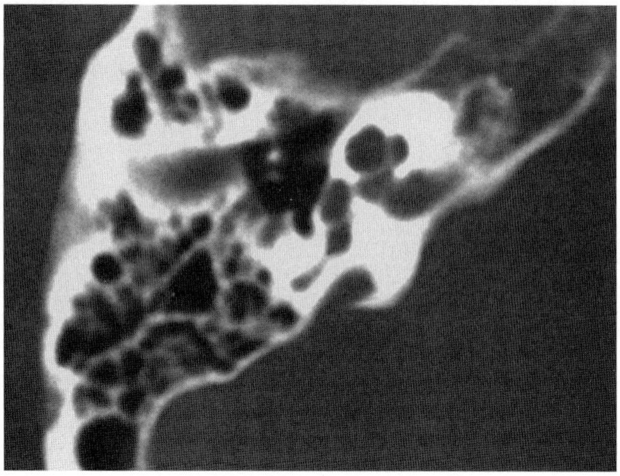

Figure 42A

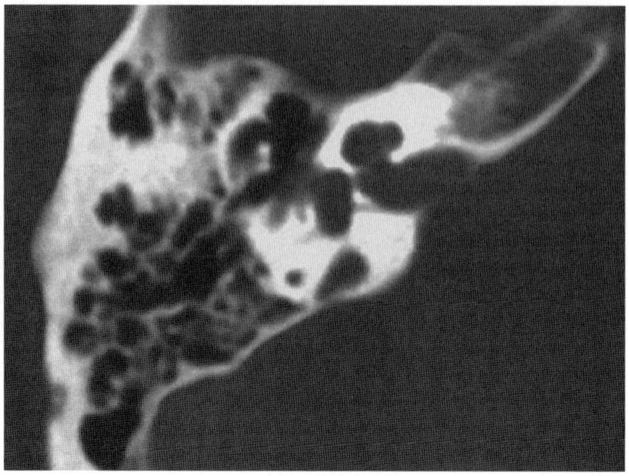

Figure 42B

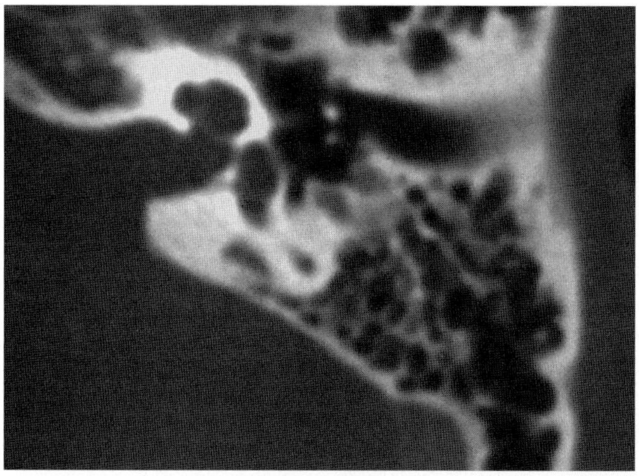

Figure 42C

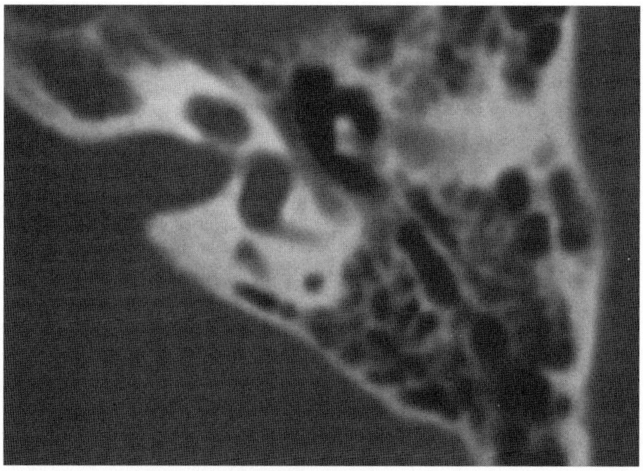

Figure 42D

1. Describe, precisely, one major and one minor abnormality.
2. What is the cause of the deafness?
3. Can the patient safely receive a cochlear implant?

Findings

An enlargement of the vestibular aqueduct on both sides, with the finding more pronounced on the right. The modiolus is deficient bilaterally. The cochlear turns are not fully developed on either side.

Problem

An adult candidate for cochlear implantation with bilaterally enlarged vestibular aqueducts

Anatomy

A. Cochlea
   1. Apical, basal, and middle turns
   2. Modiolus
B. Otic capsule (see Fig. 36D)
C. Vestibular and cochlear aqueducts
D. Descending facial canal, facial recess, and posterior external auditory canal wall

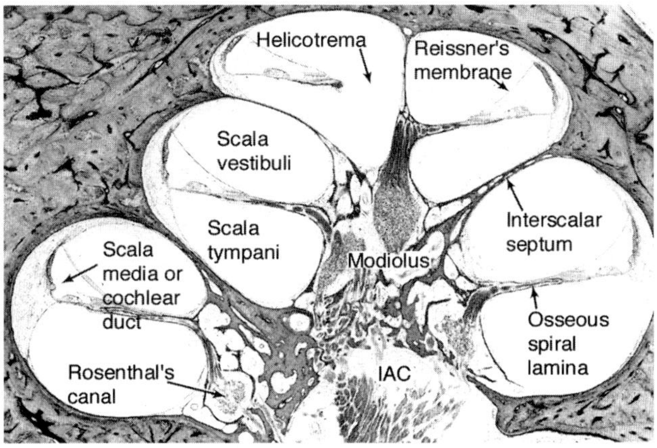

Figure 42E

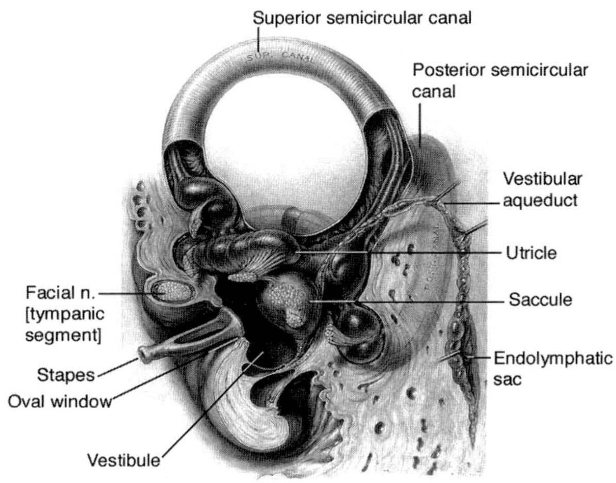

Figure 42F

Differential Diagnosis

Not applicable

Diagnosis

Anomalous inner ears bilaterally manifested by enlarged vestibular aqueducts and minor cochlear anomalies (poorly defined apical and middle turns and modiolus)

Diagnostic Imaging Approach

A. Evaluate the otic capsule, cochlea, vestibule, and semicircular canals.
B. Evaluate the vestibular and cochlear aqueducts: presence, size, position.
C. Ensure patency of round window.
D. Ensure normal anatomy of descending facial canal and facial recess and normal mastoid and middle ear.

Clinical Points Of Importance And Supplemental Information

A. Large vestibular aqueducts indicate that the hearing loss is related to inner ear maldevelopment (a normal vestibular aqueduct measured at its midpoint should be $\leq$1.5 mm) even with no other obvious abnormality of the bony labyrinth.
B. Cochlear implants are usually placed into the round window via a canal wall-up mastoidectomy and facial recess approach to the middle ear; the anatomic suitability of this pathway and the lack of inflammatory middle ear disease are two adjunctive pieces of data available from computed tomography imaging.

Answers To Questions

1. Enlarged vestibular aqueducts and a deficient modiolus on both sides
2. Cochlear dysplasia
3. Yes

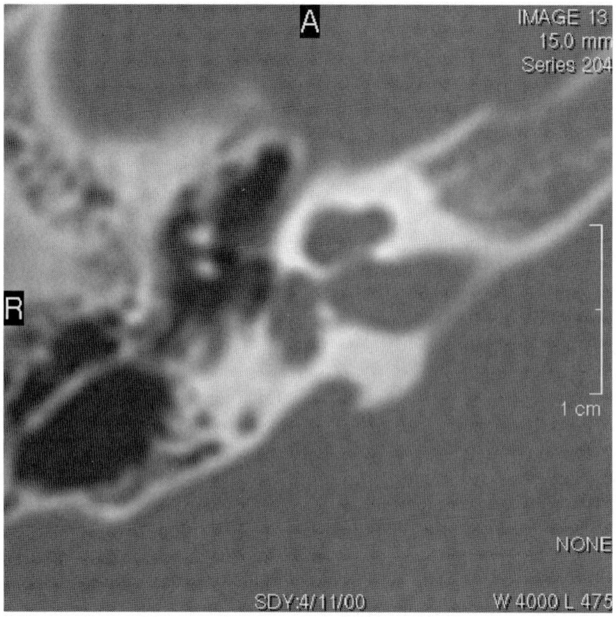

Figure 42G. Patient 1 with inner ear anomaly, showing enlarged vestibular aqueduct at its junction with the endolymphatic sac. Axial computed tomography image at bone window setting.

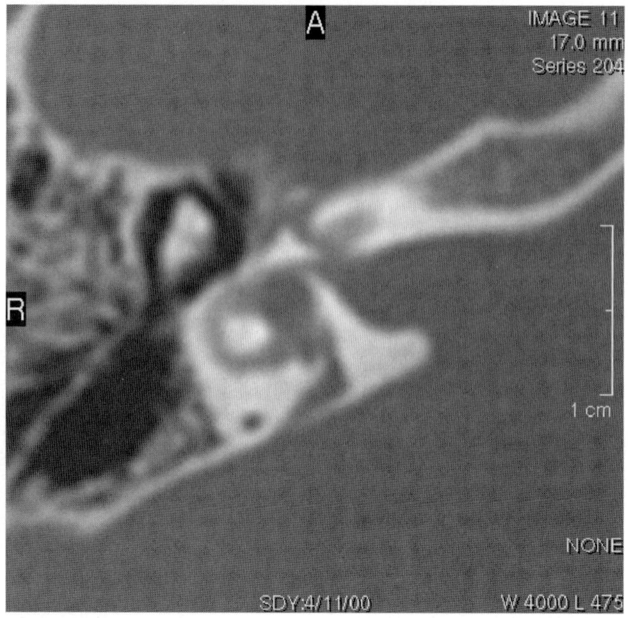

Figure 42H. Patient 1 with inner ear anomaly. Axial computed tomography image cephalad to 42G showing enlarged vestibular aqueduct.

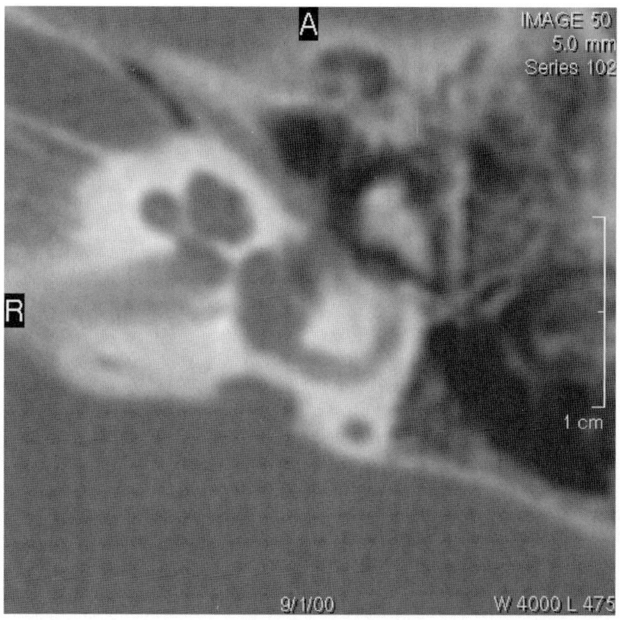

Figure 42I. Patient 2 with mild maldevelopment of the cochlea, showing mildly deformed second and apical turn of the cochlea and an enlarged vestibular aqueduct. Axial computed tomography image.

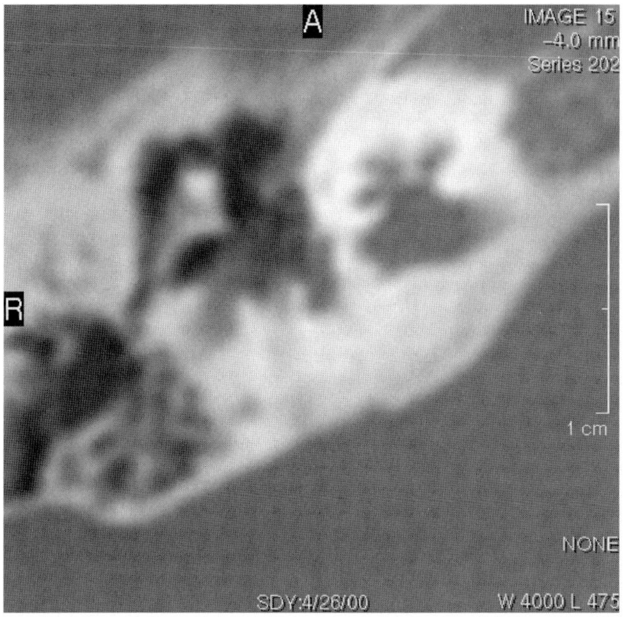

Figure 42J. Patient 3 with labyrinthitis ossificans. Axial computed tomography image at bone window setting showing obliteration of normal lucent areas of membranous labyrinth by bone density.

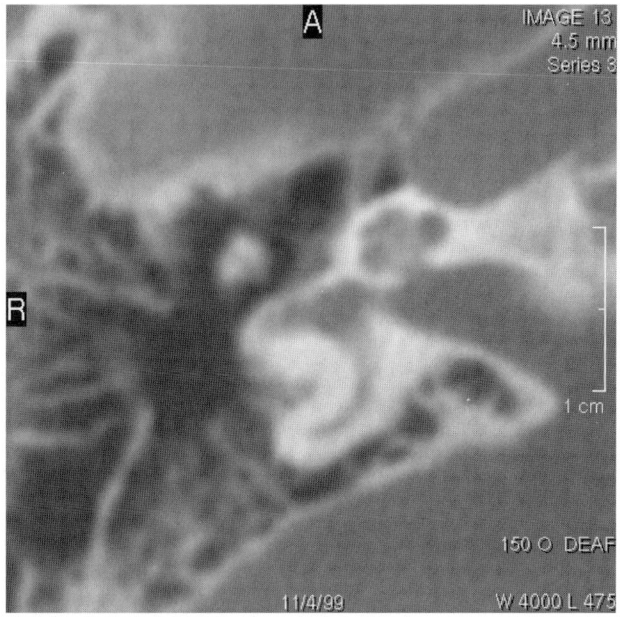

Figure 42K. Patient 4 with labyrinthitis ossificans. Axial computed tomography of the right temporal bone showing bone productive changes centered on the modiolus and interscalar septa (compare with 42L)

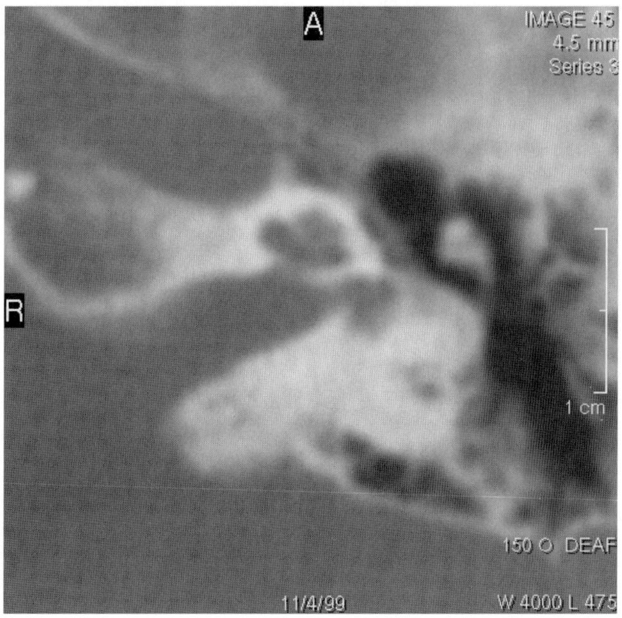

Figure 42L. Patient 4 with labyrinthitis ossificans. Axial computed tomography of the left temporal bone showing subtle obliteration of the apical and middle turn of the cochlea and vestibular involvement.

CASE 43

Clinical History: A 70-year-old man presents with bilateral hearing loss. The hearing loss is most severe on the side shown. Cochlear implantation is contemplated.

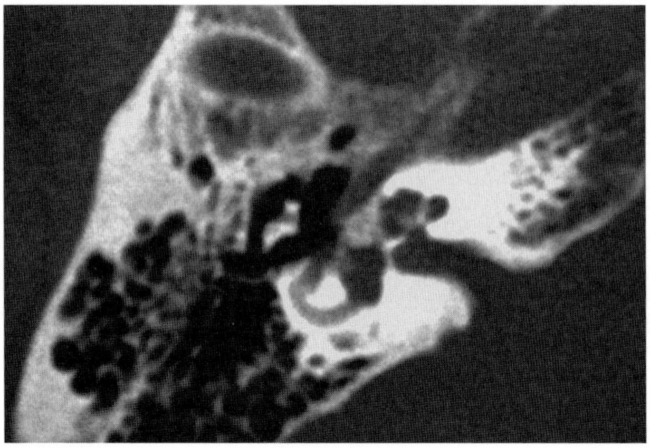

Figure 43A

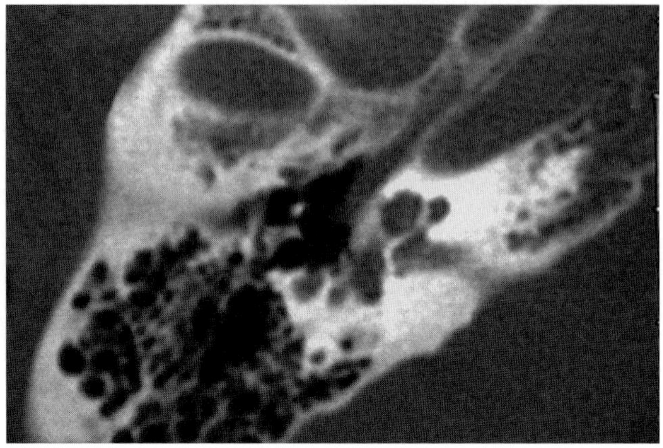

Figure 43B

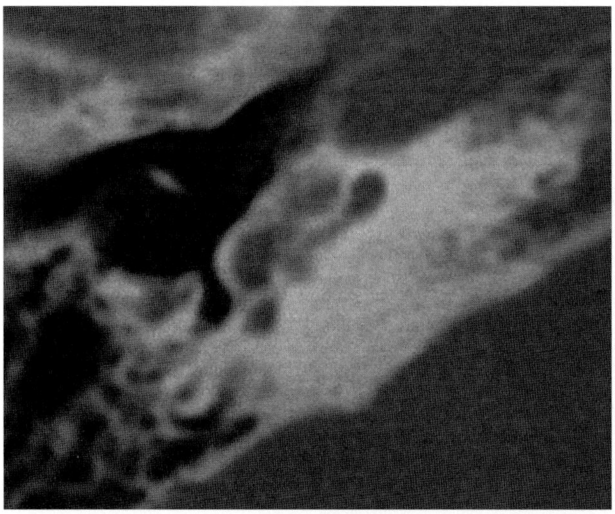

Figure 43C

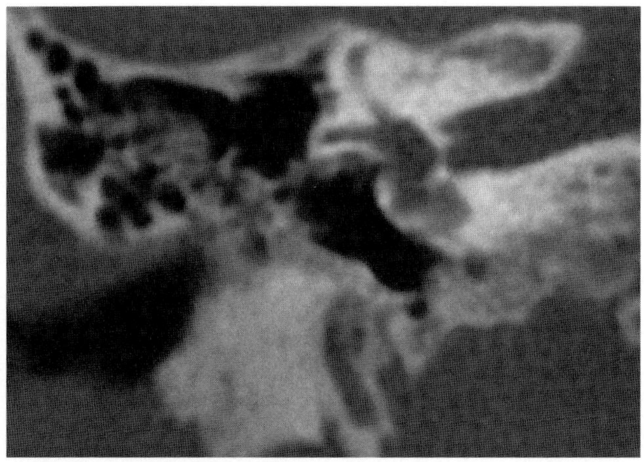

Figure 43D

1. Describe precisely, at least three different locations involved by the abnormalities present.
2. Name the two general categories of this disease.
3. What disease elsewhere in the body shows similar histologic changes?

Findings

A focal area of demineralization at the fissula antefenestram, with involvement of the oval window (see Fig. 43A) that encroaches on the oval window (see Fig. 43B); more inferior involvement with the round window (see Fig. 43D).

Problem

A hearing impaired adult candidate for cochlear implantation with abnormal appearing cochlea and otic capsule

Anatomy

A. Cochlea and round window (see Fig. 41F)
B. Vestibule, oval window, fissula antefenestram
C. Stapes: suprastructure (head and crura), footplate

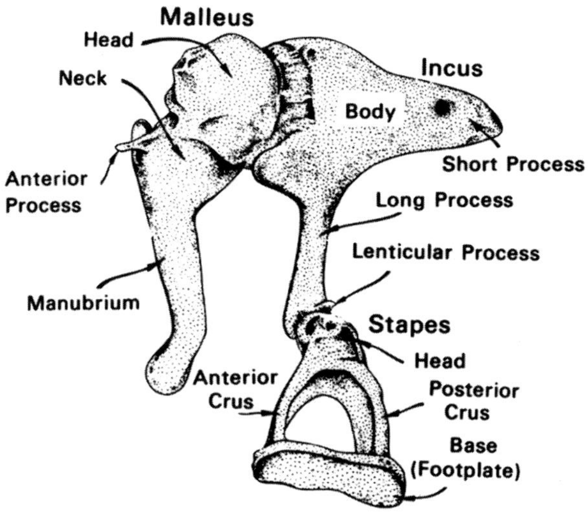

Figure 43E

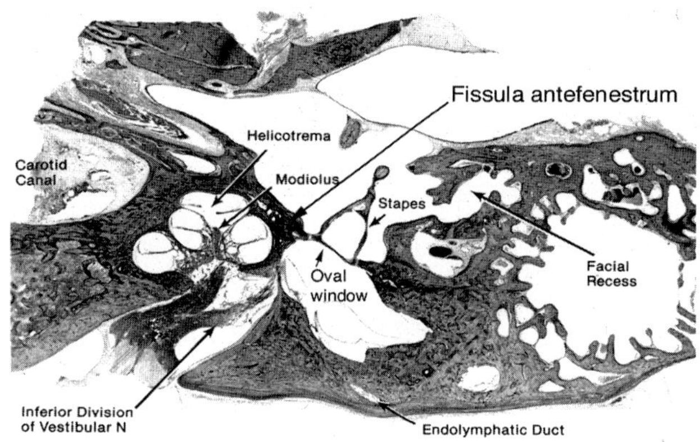

Figure 43F

Differential Diagnosis

Not applicable

Diagnosis

Otosclerosis

Diagnostic Imaging Approach

A. Establish a probable cause for hearing loss.
   1. Evaluate otic capsule, cochlea, vestibule, semicircular canals.
   2. Evaluate vestibular and cochlear aqueducts.
   3. If abnormality is present, determine if it primarily affects the otic capsule or inner ear.
   4. Which side is more severely affected?
B. Anticipate possible difficulties with surgery:
   1. Status of round window
   2. Middle ear inflammatory disease
   3. Anatomy of facial recess and tympanic and descending portions of the facial canal
   4. High jugular bulb

Clinical Points Of Importance And Supplemental Information

A. Otosclerosis has been divided into predominantly fenestral (round and oval window involvement) and predominantly cochlear varieties. In reality, it is a multifocal disease that can affect the entire otic capsule as well as the cochlea, vestibule, and stapes. Early involvement may first appear at the fissula antefenestram. Histopathologically, otosclerosis resembles Paget's disease.
B. It is important to identify complete round window obliteration in patients with otosclerosis patients, because stapedectomy will not restore hearing in these patients. Such information is also helpful to the cochlear implant surgeon.

Answers To Questions

1. Fissula antefenestram, oval window, stapes footplate
2. Fenestral and cochlear
3. Paget's disease

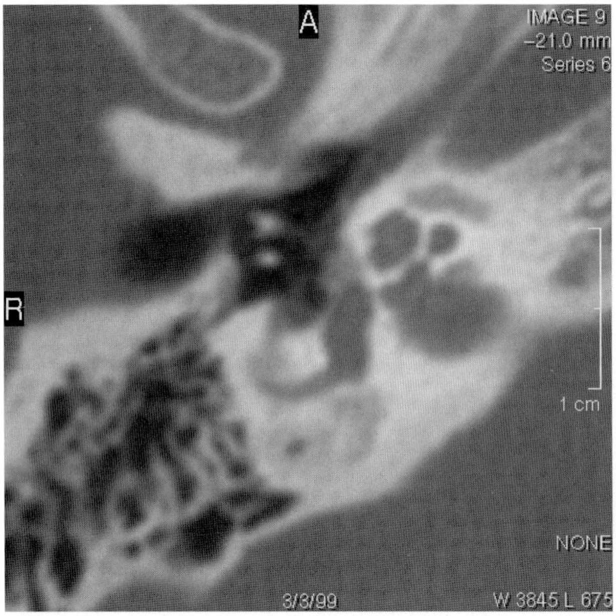

Figure 43G. Patient 1 with otosclerosis. Axial computed tomography image of the right temporal bone showing areas of abnormal demineralization and bony productive changes in the fissula antefenestram and around cochlea and semicircular canals.

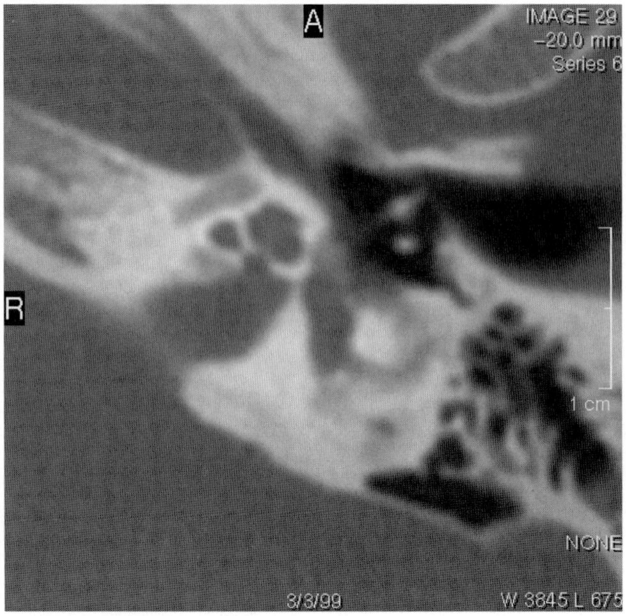

Figure 43H. Patient 1 with otosclerosis. Axial computed tomography of the left temporal bone also showing similar change with the opposite side (see 43G).

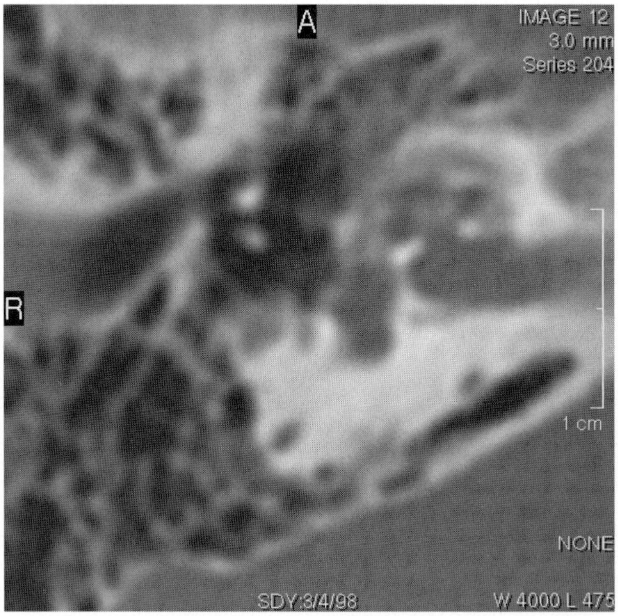

Figure 43I. Patient 2 with otosclerosis. Axial computed tomography image showing advanced osteolytic phase areas surrounding the cochlea representing double cochlear sign, which also involves the region of the fissula antefenestram.

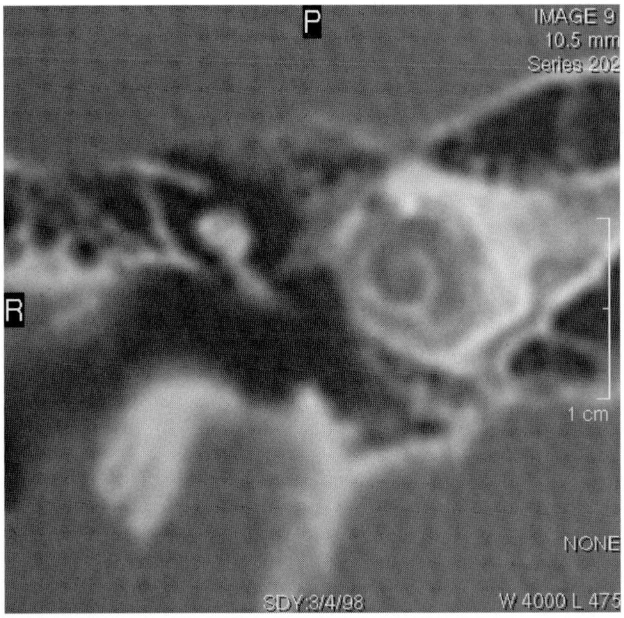

Figure 43J. Patient 2 with otosclerosis. Coronal computed tomography image showing abnormal demineralization around the cochlea.

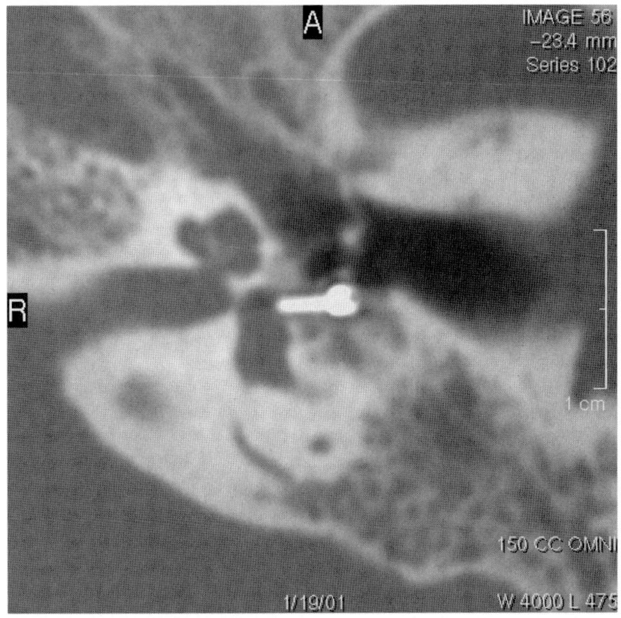

Figure 43K. Patient 3 with otosclerosis. Axial computed tomography image showing area of demineralization at the fissula antefenestram. Metallic prosthesis within the "heaped up" bone in the oval window niche, the tip of which is slightly more medial and anterior because of the regrowth of otosclerotic bone.

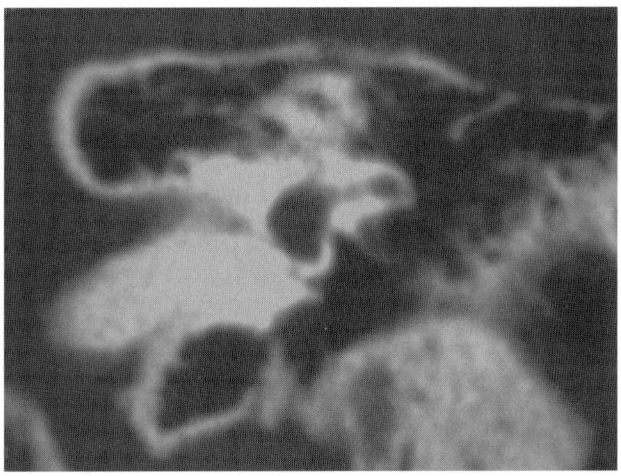

Figure 43L. Patient 4 with otosclerosis. Coronal computed tomography image at bone window showing bony obliteration of the round window.

CASE 44

Clinical History: A 43-year-old man presents with sensorineural hearing loss and balance difficulties.

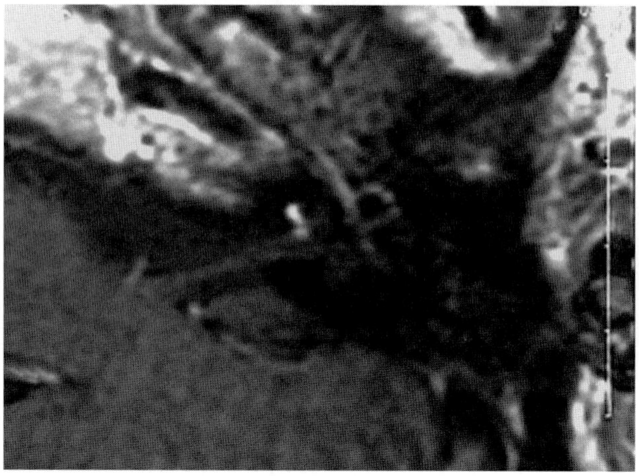

Figure 44A

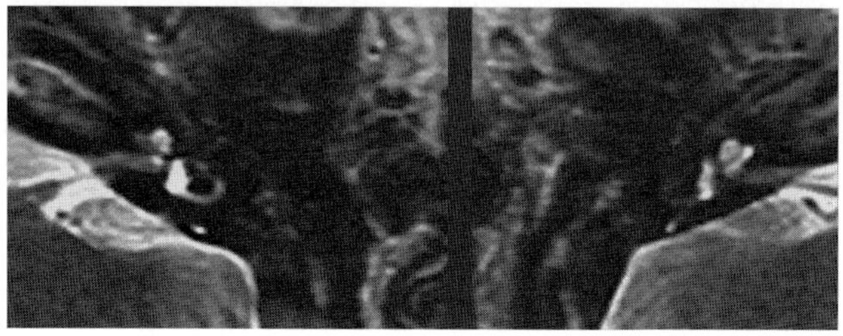

Figure 44B

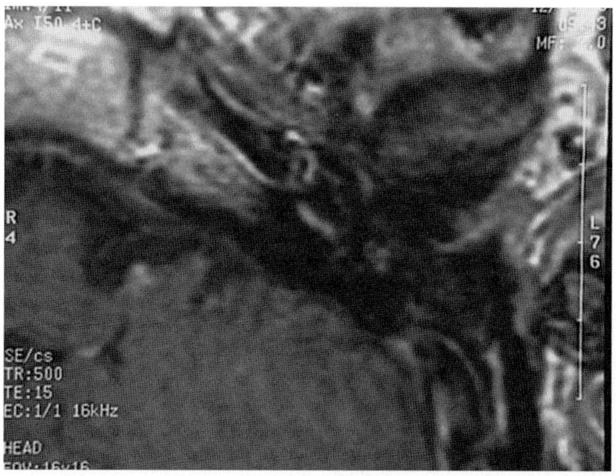

Figure 44C

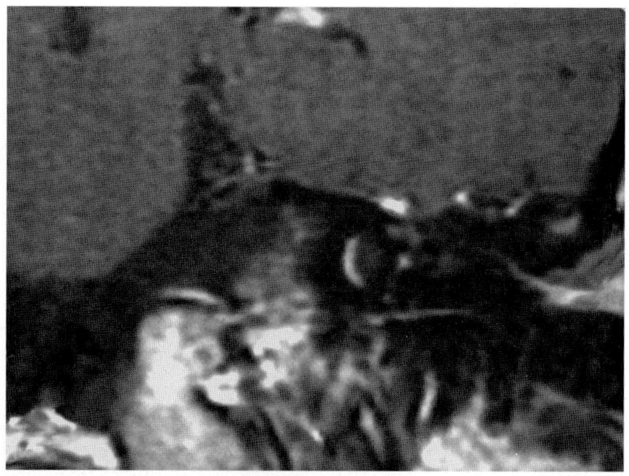

Figure 44D

1. What are the findings?
2. List two general categories of disease that might produce such findings.
3. If the findings are unchanged at 1-year follow up, what is the most likely diagnosis? What is the diagnosis if they resolve within 3 months?

Findings

Abnormal enhancement of the membranous labyrinth in a basal turn of the cochlea on the left. Signal intensity of a basal turn of the left cochlea is somewhat low on T2-weighted image.

Problem

An adult with cochlear and vestibular symptoms and focal contrast enhancement within the cochlea

Anatomy

Cochlea and vestibule as seen on high resolution T1- and T2-weighted magnetic resonance images (MRI)

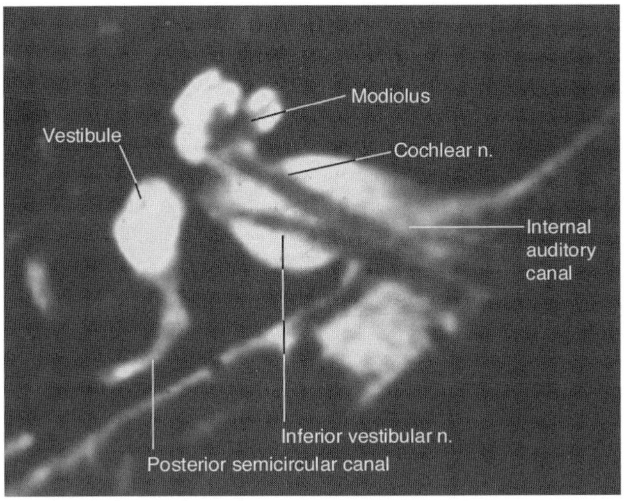

Figure 44E

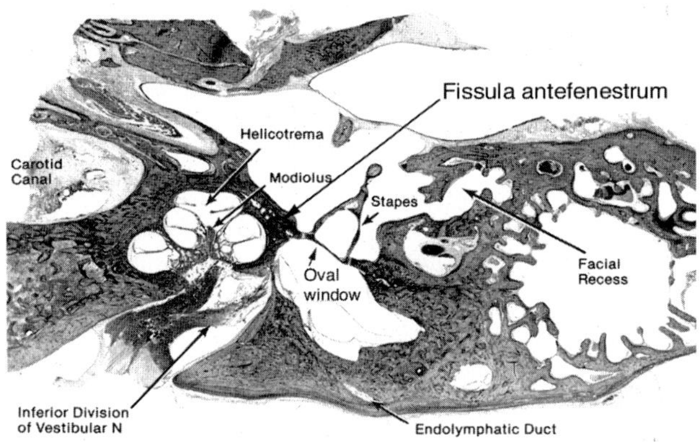

Figure 44F

Differential Diagnosis

Cochlear schwannoma or neurofibroma vs. labyrinthitis (e.g., viral, syphilitic, autoimmune, Wegener's, sarcoidosis)

Diagnosis

Cochlear schwannoma (presumptive)

Diagnostic Imaging Approach

A. Evaluate the entire cochleovestibular pathway in the brainstem.
B. Trace major divisions of the VIIIth cranial nerve (cisternal segment and canalicular segment) from their root entry zones to cochlea and vestibule.
C. Look for abnormal enhancement or loss of cerebrospinal fluid (CSF) signal (T2-weighted image) within the inner ear.
D. Identify abnormal meningeal or subarachnoid space enhancement.

Clinical Points Of Importance And Supplemental Information

A. Subtle enhancement (<10 mm foci) of the VIIIth cranial nerve or within the inner ear should be considered inflammatory until proved otherwise.
B. High-resolution MRI should be repeated 3 months after the initial study and, if appropriate, clinical testing (e.g., sedimentation rate, antineutrophil cytoplasmic antibodies [ANCA], CSF for syphilis) can be done during this interval. Most inflammatory conditions will show a decreased or no enhancement in 3 months if treated appropriately.
C. The average VIIIth cranial nerve schwannoma grows less than1 mm/year.

Answers To Questions

1. Focal, nodular enhancement of membranous labyrinth in the cochlea
2. Inflammatory and neoplastic
3. Schwannoma. Neuritis.

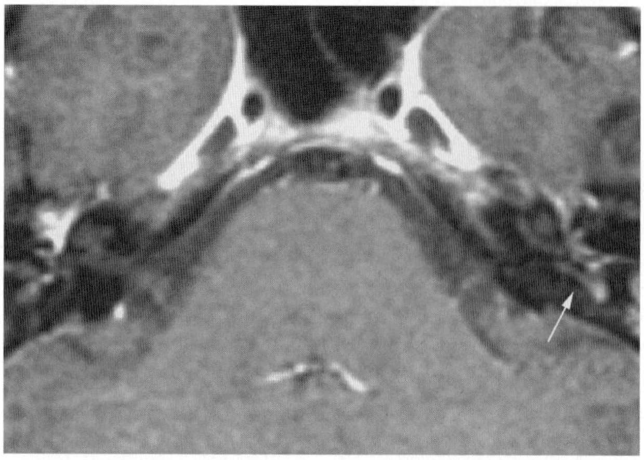

Figure 44G. Patient 1 with presumed viral labyrinthitis. T1-weighted axial image with contrast showing abnormal enhancement of the left posterior semicircular canal.

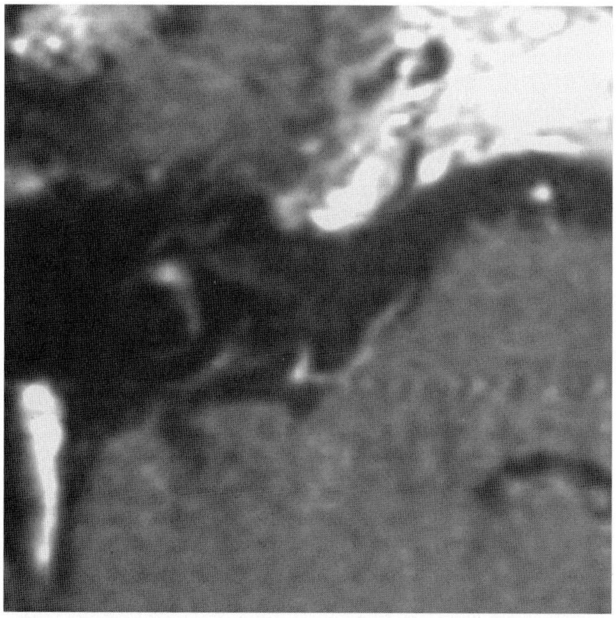

Figure 44H. Patient 2 with presumed viral labyrinthitis. T1-weighted axial image with contrast showing abnormal enhancement of the vestibule and posterior and lateral semicircular canals.

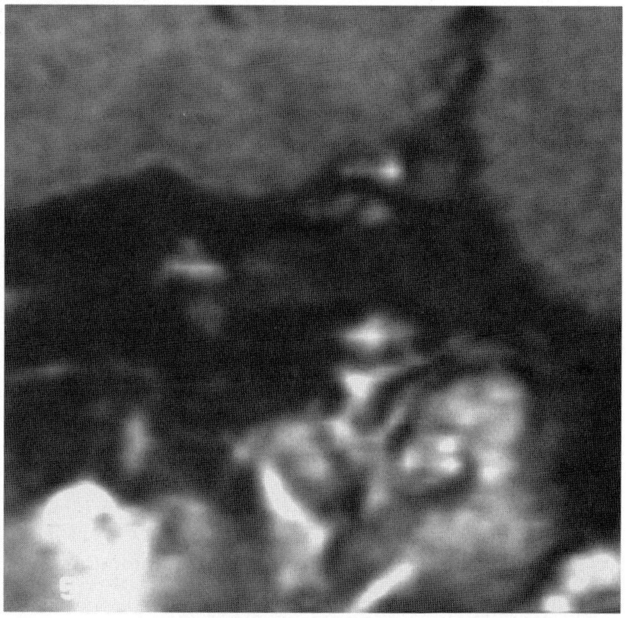

Figure 44I. Patient 2 with presumed viral labyrinthitis. T1-weighted coronal image with contrast also showing abnormal enhancement of the vestibular system.

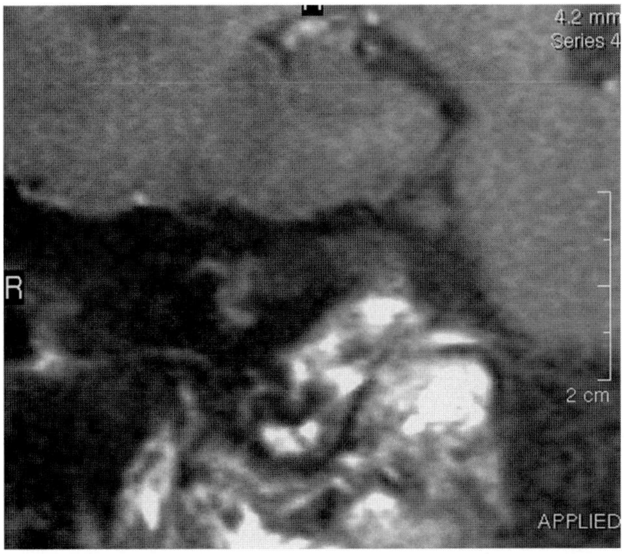

Figure 44J. Patient 3 with sensorineural hearing loss with presumptive viral labyrinthitis, showing abnormal enhancement of membranous labyrinth. T1-weighted coronal image with contrast.

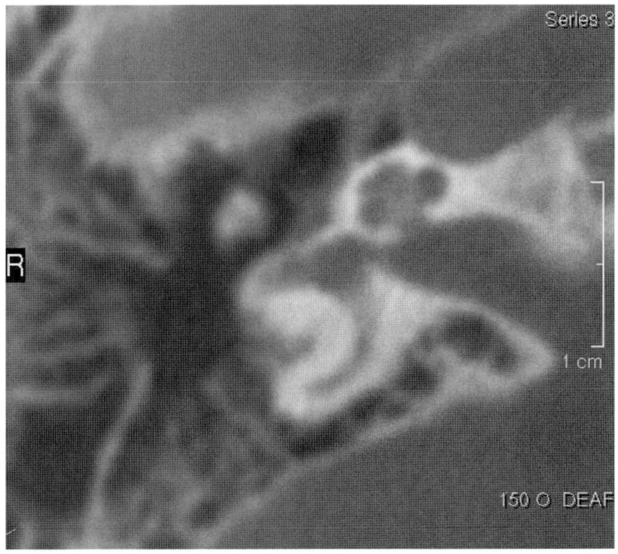

Figure 44K. Patient 4 with labyrinthitis ossificans. Axial computed tomography image of the right temporal bone showing bone productive changes centered on the modiolus and interscalar septa.

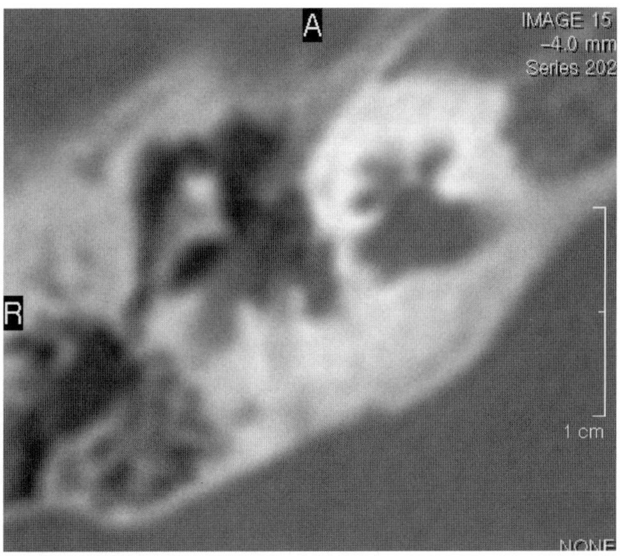

Figure 44L. Patient 5 with labyrinthitis ossificans (end stage of bacterial labyrinthitis). Axial computed tomography image at bone window setting showing obliteration of normal lucent areas of membranous labyrinth by bone density.

CASE 45

Clinical History: A 32-year-old man presents with left vocal cord paralysis and difficulty swallowing.

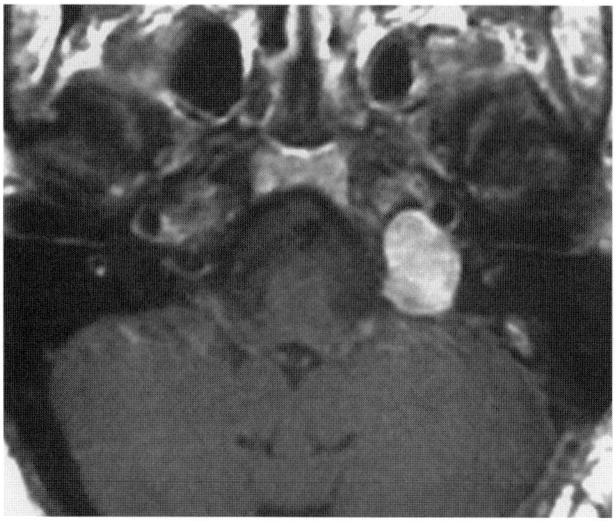

Figure 45A

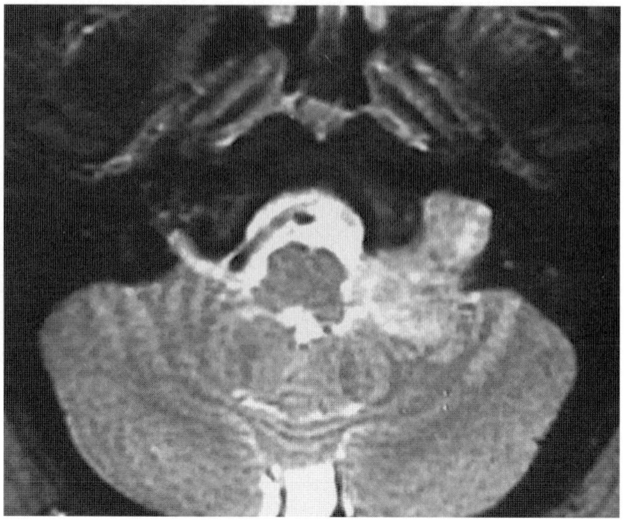

Figure 45B

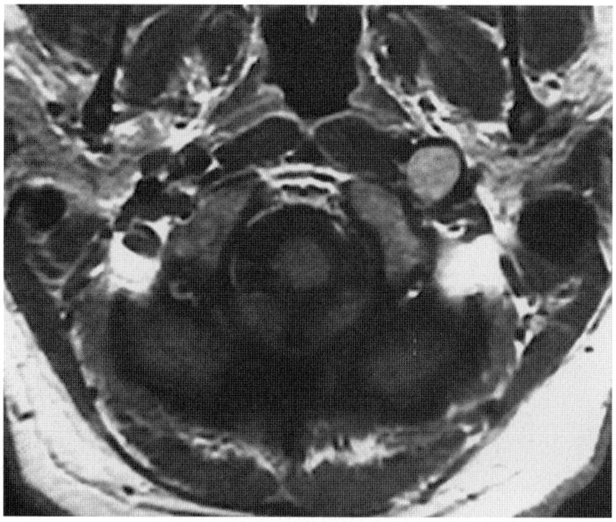

Figure 45C

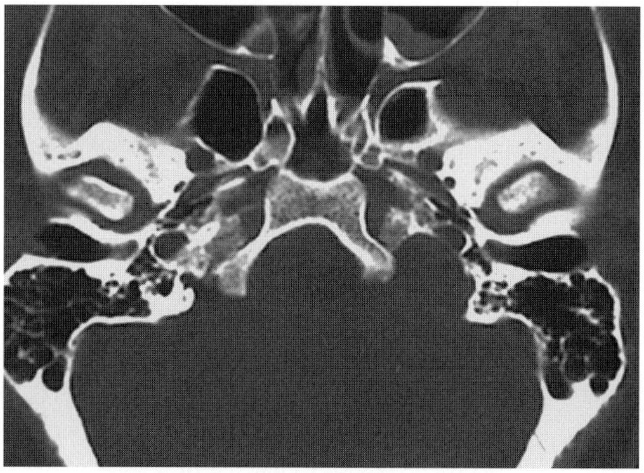

Figure 45D

1. Where is the lesion centered?
2. What is the most likely diagnosis?
3. What is the most helpful imaging feature for the differential diagnosis?

Findings

An enhancing mass in the left-sided posterior fossa extending into retrostyloid compartment of the parapharyngeal space via the enlarged left jugular foramen. The bony margins of the jugular fossa are smoothly remodeled and well corticated. The lesion intervenes between the internal carotid artery and the internal jugular vein just below the skull base.

Problem

An adult with vagal neuropathy and a mass centered in the jugular fossa

Anatomy

A. Brain stem: nuclei related to the vagus nerve
B. Jugular fossa: pars nervosa, pars venosum
C. Poststyloid parapharyngeal space

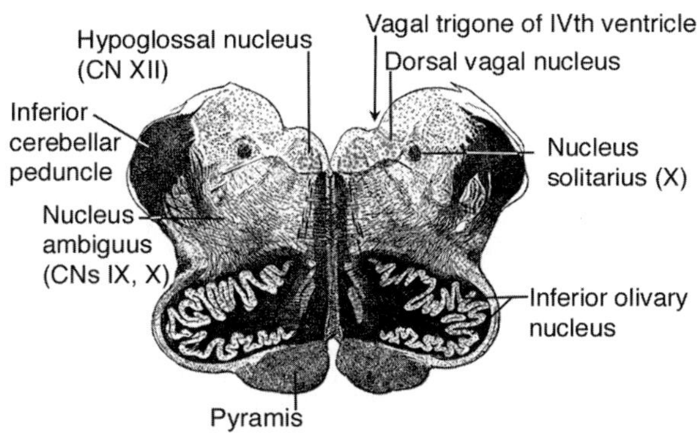

Figure 45E

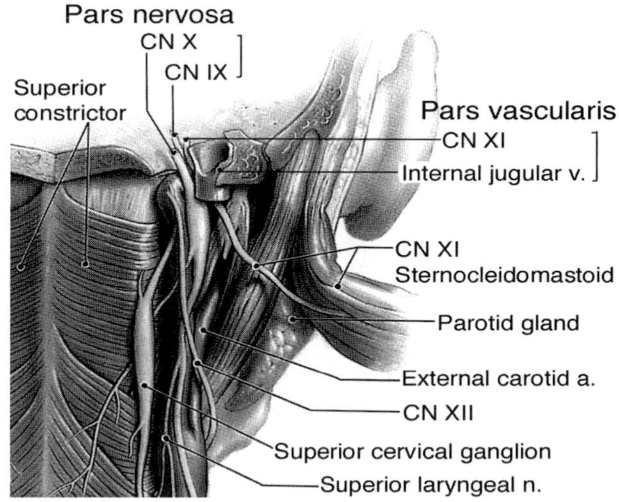

Figure 45F

Differential Diagnosis

Schwannoma or neurofibroma, paraganglioma (glomus vagale), meningioma, hemangiopericytoma, metastasis (rare)

Diagnosis

Schwannoma, most likely arising from the vagus nerve

Diagnostic Imaging Approach

A. Evaluate the vagus nerve from its nuclei of origin in the brainstem to end organs, including:
   1. Cisternal segment
   2. Jugular fossa
   3. Poststyloid parapharyngeal space
   4. Carotid sheath
   5. Recurrent laryngeal nerves
B. Consider specific deficits (end organ and other cranial neuropathy) when determining most likely level of vagal nerve involvement.
C. For a mass in the jugular fossa, evaluate:
   1. Enhancement
   2. Flow voids
   3. T1- or T2-morphology
   4. Calcifications
D. If differential diagnosis between paraganglioma and schwannoma is not certain, perform a noncontrast computed tomography (CT) study to look at bony margins of jugular fossa; aggressive erosion is almost always paraganglioma (never schwannoma).
E. Conventional angiography if differential diagnosis is still in question.

Clinical Points Of Importance And Supplemental Information

A. Accurate differential diagnosis is essential for management.
B. Schwannomas of this sort will usually be treated by a neurootologic or neurosurgical team, either with a combined or staged intracranial and extracranial approach.
C. Stereotactic radiosurgery is sometimes used as adjunctive therapy for control of residual tumor, for patients who refuse or are not candidates for surgery, or if more extensive surgery would require sacrifice of additional, functioning nerves.

Answers To Questions

1. Jugular fossa
2. Lower cranial nerve schwannoma
3. Smooth bony margins of the jugular fossa

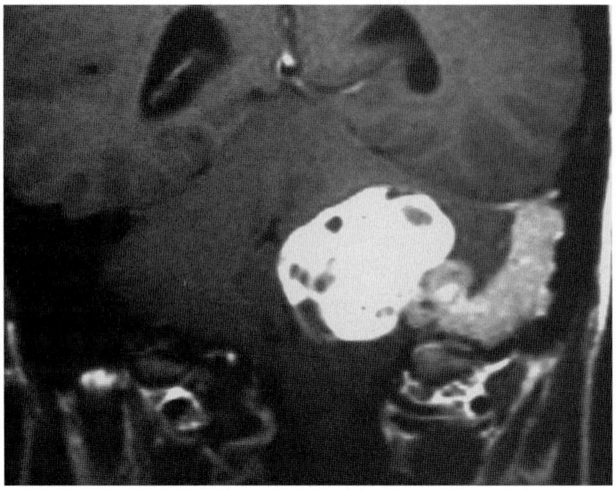

Figure 45G. Patient 1 with hemangiopericytoma, showing enhancing mass with several cystic components in the left cerebellar hemisphere contiguously extending into the sigmoid sinus. T1-weghted coronal image with contrast.

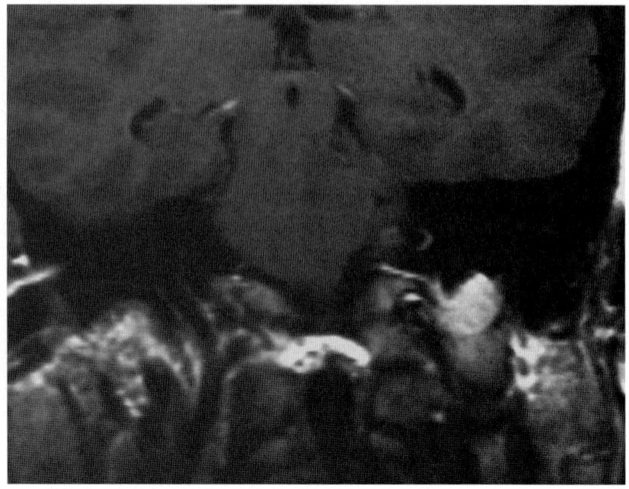

Figure 45H. Patient 1 with hemangiopericytoma. T1-weighted coronal image with contrast anterior to 45G showing extension of the enhancing mass within the jugular fossa.

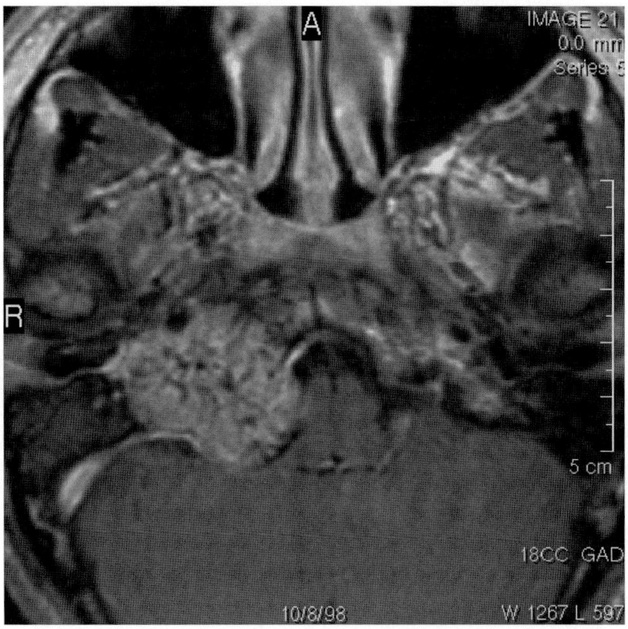

Figure 45I. Patient 2 with glomus jugulare type paraganglioma, showing intensely enhancing mass containing tumor vessels seen as areas of signal void, centered in the right jugular fossa. Nonaggressive mastoid disease resulting from mechanical dysfunction of eustachian tube. T1-weighted axial image with contrast.

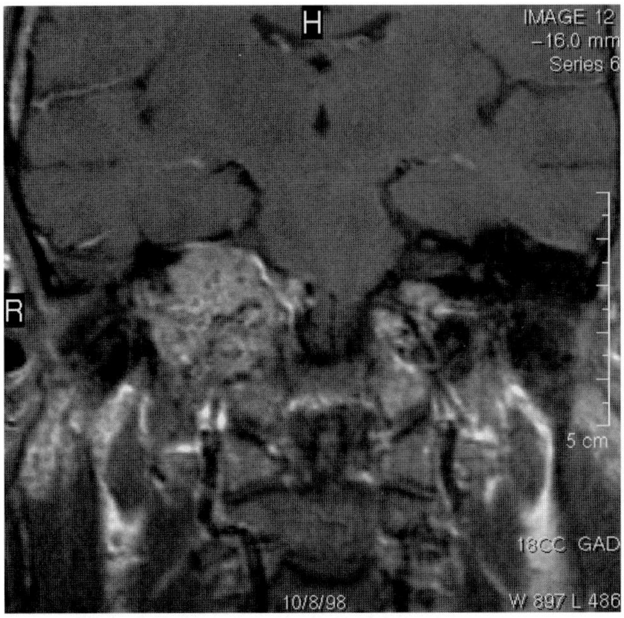

Figure 45J. Patient 2 with glomus jugulare type paraganglioma. T1-weighted coronal image with contrast.

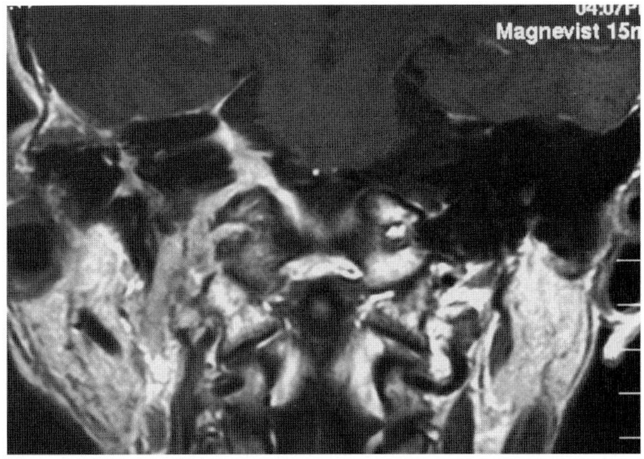

Figure 45K. Patient 3 with transcranial meningioma, showing *en plaque* meningioma extending extracranially through the jugular foramen.

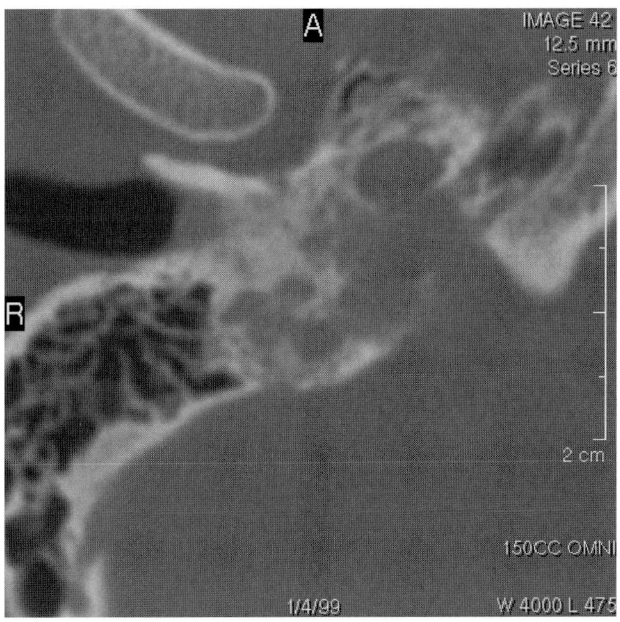

Figure 45L. Patient 4 with jugulotympanic paraganglioma, showing irregular bone destruction of the wall of the jugular foramen with permeative bony change around it. Axial computed tomography image at bone window setting.

CASE 46

Clinical History: A 43-year-old woman presents with left vocal cord paralysis and difficulty swallowing.

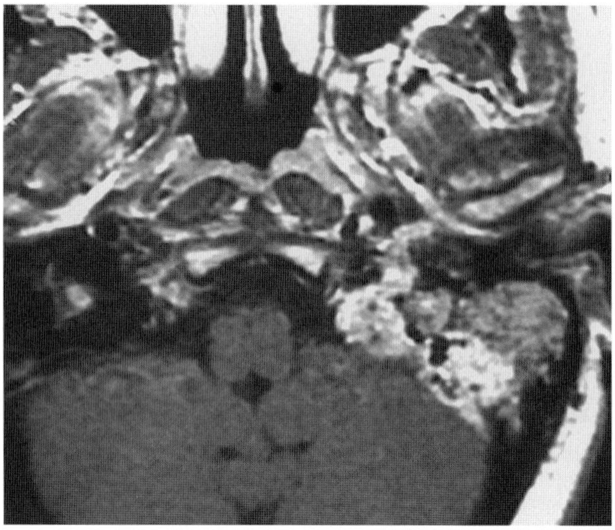

Figure 46A

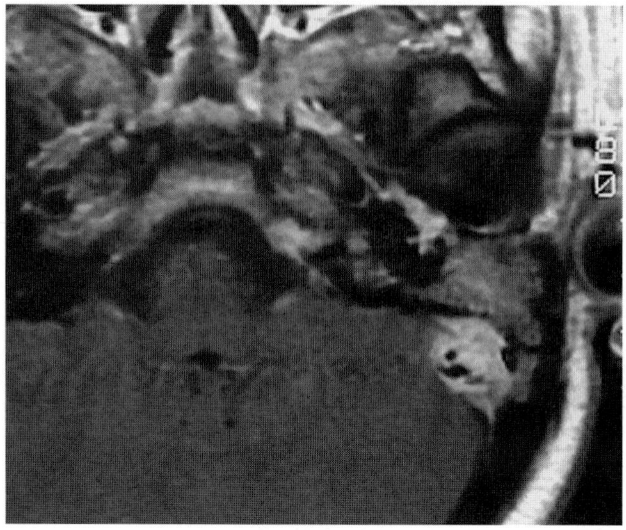

Figure 46B

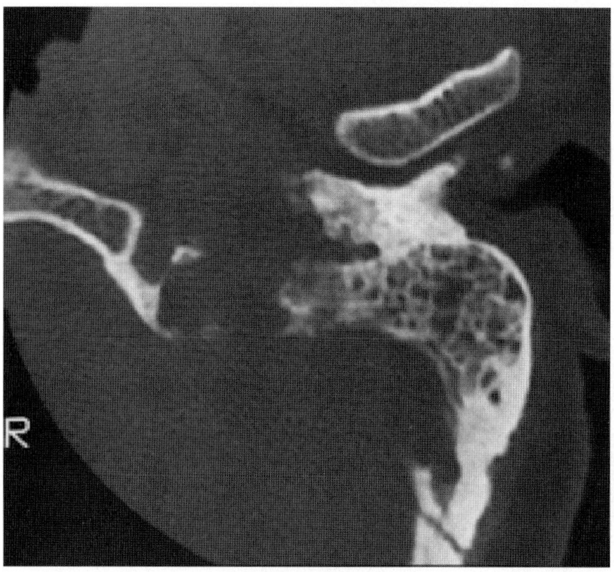

Figure 46C

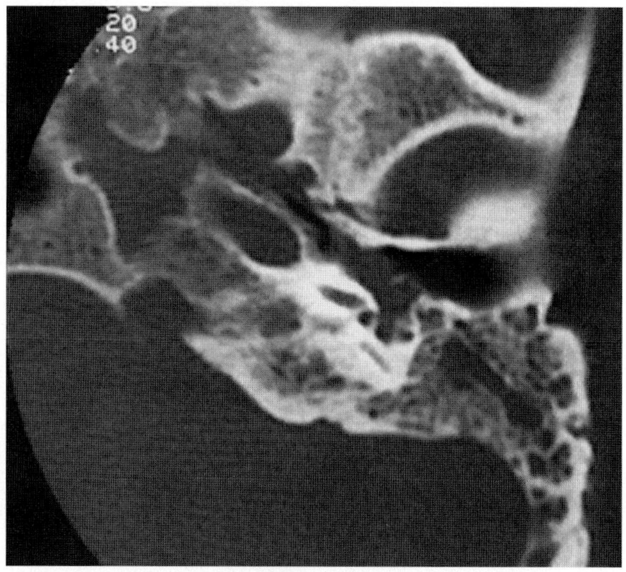

Figure 46D

1. Where is the lesion centered?
2. List the two most helpful differentiating features (one from the computed tomography (CT) study and one from the magnetic resonance imaging (MRI) study.
3. What is the most medial extent of this lesion? (Extra credit for a precise answer.)

Findings

An irregularly shaped mass containing flow voids centered in the left jugular fossa, the margins of which are aggressively eroded. The lesion enhances intensely on postcontrast images and contiguously involves the posterior aspect of the petrous bone, the sigmoid sinus, and the inferior petrosal sinus. The mucosa of the mastoid and middle ear is enhancing because of obstructive, inflammatory otomastoiditis

Problem

An adult with probable vagal neuropathy and a mass centered in the jugular fossa

Anatomy

A. Jugular fossa
B. Dural venous sinuses: superior and inferior petrosal, sigmoid, and transverse

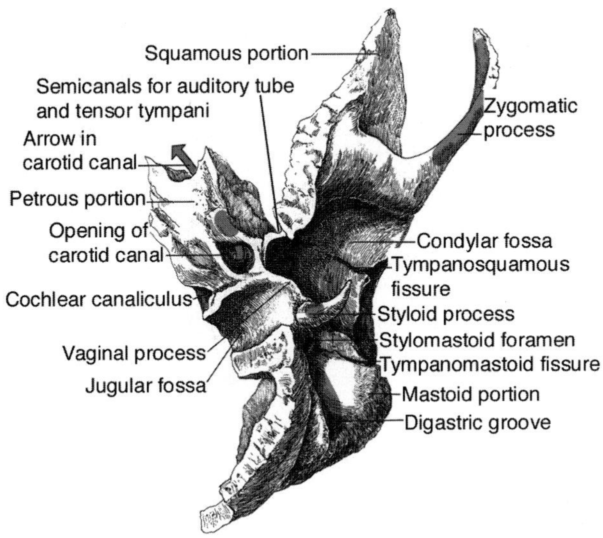

Figure 46E

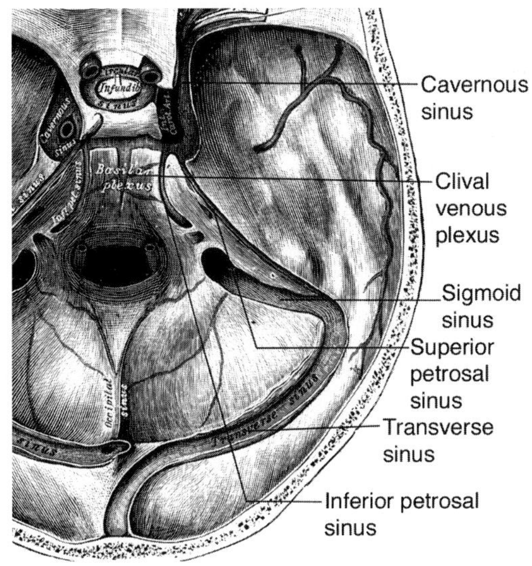

Figure 46F

Differential Diagnosis

Paraganglioma, schwannoma or neurofibroma, meningioma, hemangiopericytoma, metastasis (rarely centered in the jugular fossa)

Diagnosis

Paraganglioma (glomus jugulare type) with intracranial extension and invasion of the sigmoid and inferior petrosal sinuses

Diagnostic Imaging Approach

A. Locate the likely epicenter of the mass.
B. Evaluate enhancement, flow voids, T1- or T2-morphology, calcifications, adjacent bony margins.
C. Determine extent of the lesion:
   1. Middle ear
   2. Jugular fossa
   3. Poststyloid parapharyngeal space (within or outside the jugular vein)
   4. Facial nerve canal
   5. Hypoglossal canal
   6. Intracranial (intra- or extradural)
   7. Invasion of dural venous sinuses; spread to petrous apex, internal auditory canal, brain
D. Perform conventional angiography for confirmation of diagnosis and possible adjunctive endovascular therapy.

Clinical Points Of Importance And Supplemental Information

A. Accurate differential diagnosis is essential for management. Paragangliomas are frequently managed with radiotherapy.
B. CT, MRI and conventional angiography (followed by endovascular therapy) are all frequently necessary in the planning and treatment of lesions arising in the jugular fossa.

Answers To Questions

1. Jugular fossa
2. CT: aggressive bone erosion. MRI: flow voids.
3. Inferior petrosal sinus

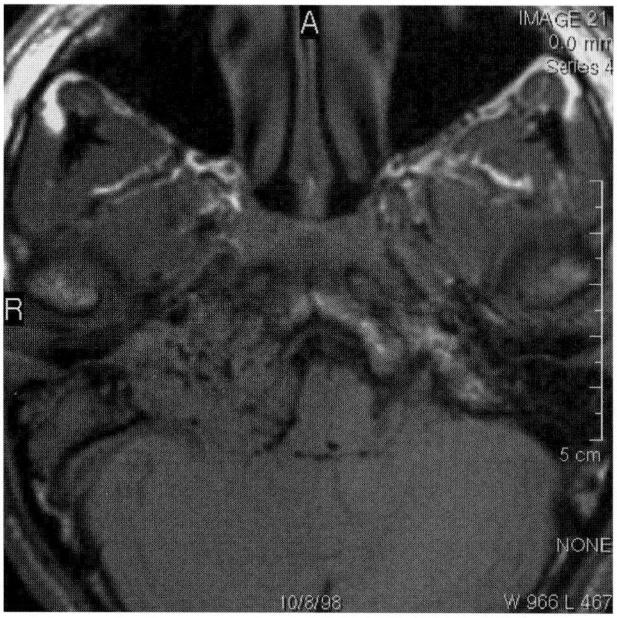

Figure 46G. Patient 1 with glomus jugulare type of paraganglioma, showing a mass centered in the right jugular fossa containing multiple areas of signal void and distorting adjacent pons and cerebellum, intracranially. Nonaggressive right mastoid disease. T1-weighted axial image without contrast.

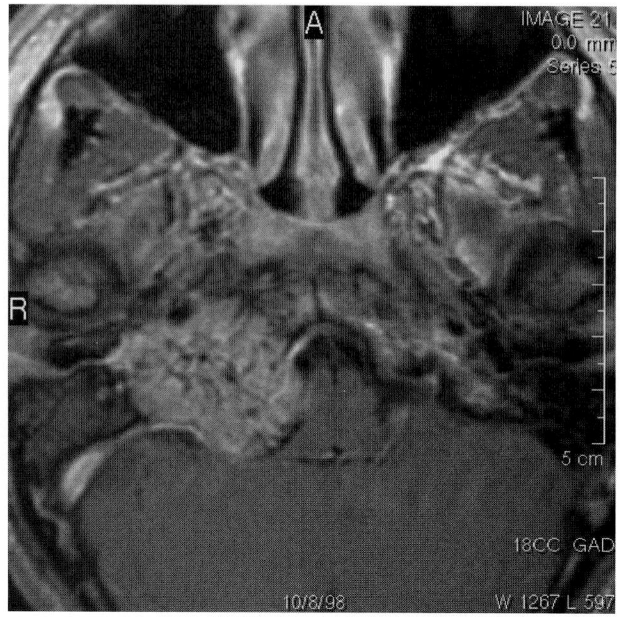

Figure 46H. Patient 1 with glomus jugulare type of paraganglioma. T1-weighted axial image with contrast showing intense enhancement of the mass.

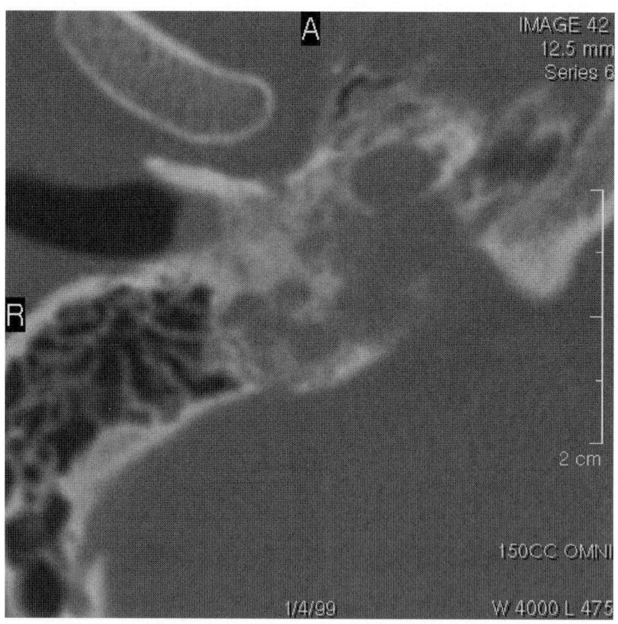

Figure 46I. Patient 2 with glomus jugulotympanicum type of paraganglioma, showing extensive, permeative bony change around the jugular fossa. Axial computed tomography image at bone window setting.

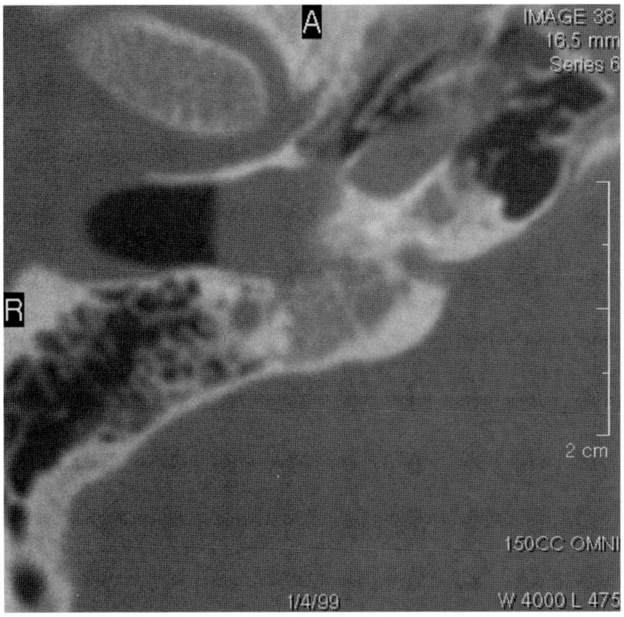

Figure 46J. Patient 2 with glomus jugulotympanicum type of paraganglioma. Axial computed tomography image cephalad to 46I showing the same bony change and mass filling the low middle ear cavity and protruding into proximal external auditory canal.

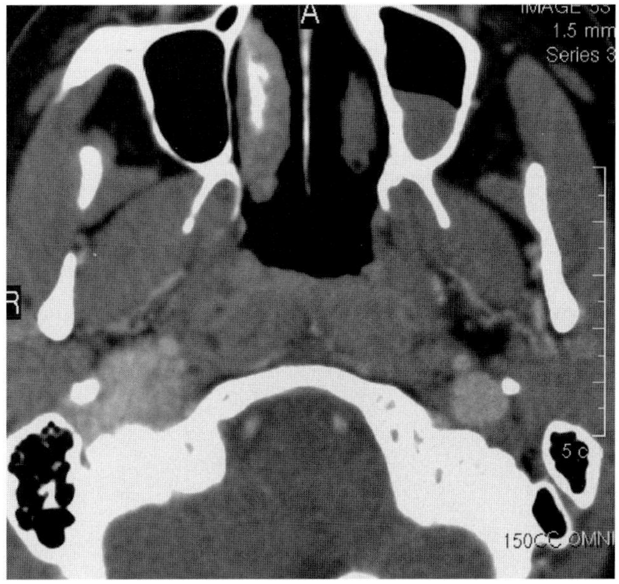

Figure 46K. Patient 2 with glomus jugulotympanicum type of paraganglioma. Axial computed tomography image with contrast at soft tissue window setting showing homogeneously enhancing mass involving retrostyloid parapharyngeal space just below the skull base.

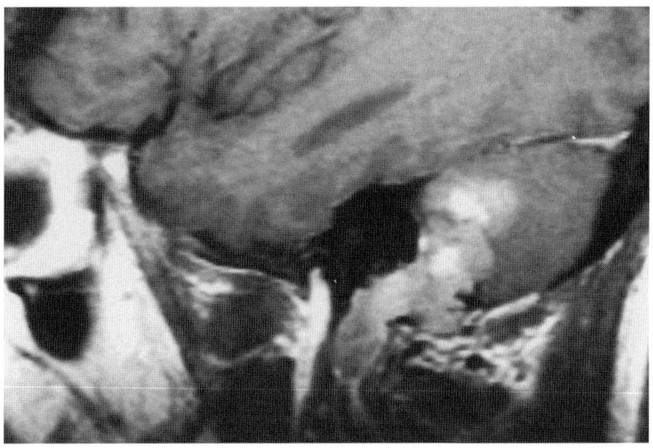

Figure 46L. Patient 3 with hemangiopericytoma. T1-weighted sagittal image with contrast showing enhancing tumor filling the sigmoid sinus and extending into the proximal internal jugular vein through the jugular foramen.

CASE 47

Clinical History: A 47-year-old man presents with left-sided tongue weakness and atrophy.

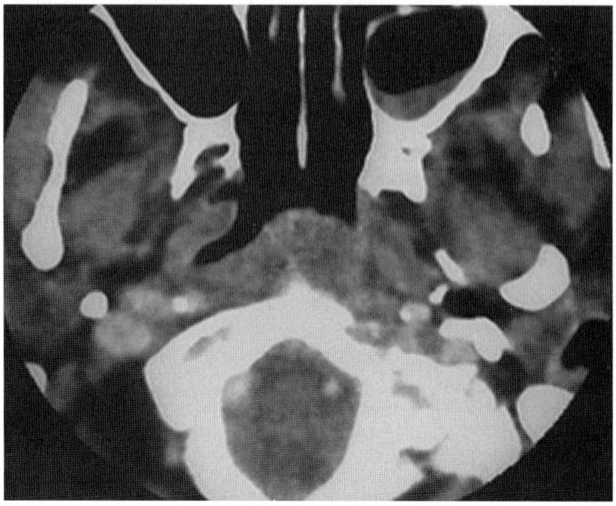

Figure 47A

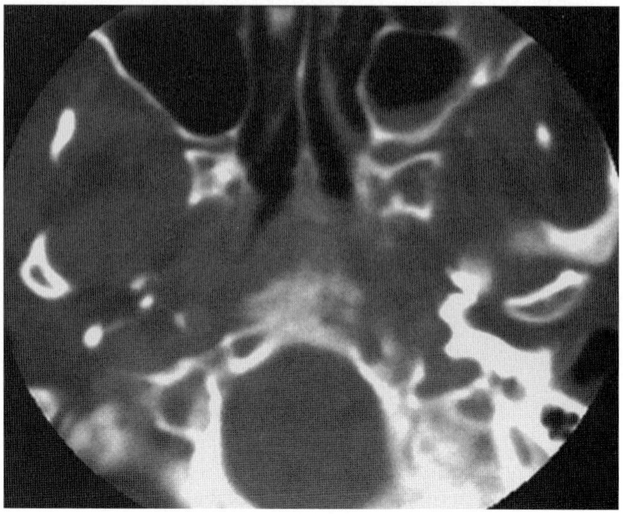

Figure 47B

1. Where is the pathology centered?
2. Is the hypoglossal canal involved?
3. What is the most likely diagnosis?

Findings

Permeative bone destruction in left basiocciput. The lesion involves the left hypoglossal canal and forms small extraosseous soft tissue mass extracranially.

Problem

An adult with hypoglossal neuropathy, a destructive skull base lesion and infiltration of surrounding soft tissues

Anatomy

A. Skull base: basisphenoid, basiocciput, hypoglossal canal, jugular fossa, condylar canal
B. Hypoglossal (XIIth) cranial nerve: nucleus, root entry zone, cisternal segment, hypoglossal canal, poststyloid parapharyngeal space, suprahyoid course of the nerve to the tongue as it runs lateral to hyoglossus muscle

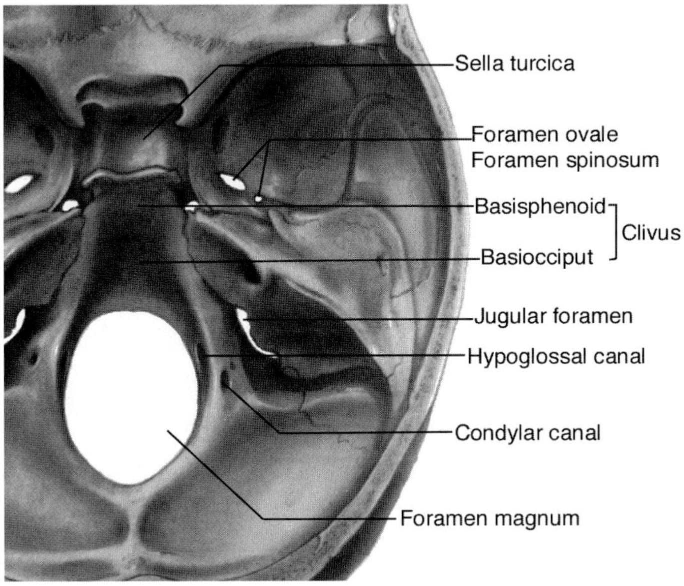

Figure 47C

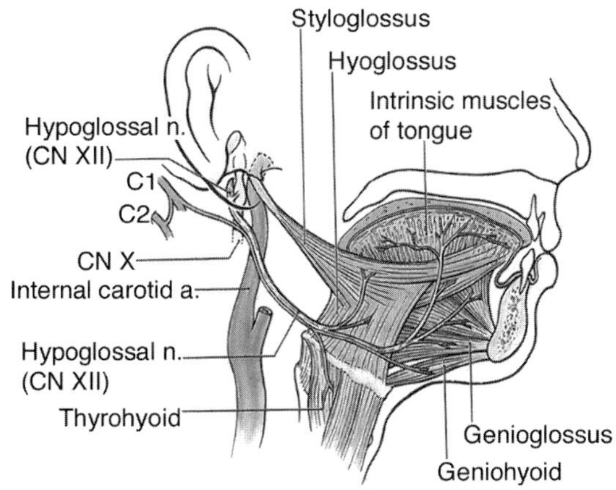

Figure 47D

Differential Diagnosis

Metastasis, myeloma, lymphoma (everything else unusual to rare); granulomatous process (e.g., actinomycosis or blastomycosis); neurogenic sarcoma, hemangiopericytoma

Diagnosis

Carcinoma of the lung with a metastasis to the basiocciput involving the hypoglossal canal and nerve

Diagnostic Imaging Approach

A. Evaluate the hypoglossal nerve from nucleus to tongue.
B. Look for denervation atrophy of intrinsic tongue muscles to confirm motor deficit.
C. Identify epicenter of lesion precisely (e.g., basiocciput vs. jugular foramen).
D. Define morphology of mass: infiltrative, well-defined, pattern of bone destruction, enhancement, vascularity, calcifications.
E. Solitary, multifocal diffuse abnormality?

Clinical Points Of Importance And Supplemental Information

A. Aggressive lesions in this location are *frequently* mistaken as arising in the jugular fossa and, therefore, erroneously believed to be paragangliomas. A destructive lesion in this location is a metastasis until proved otherwise; if it is hypervascular, consider renal cell origin.
B. An adult with an isolated hypoglossal neuropathy will usually have a causative structural lesion and it will usually be a metastasis to the skull base.

Answers To Questions

1. Posterior central skull base to lower clivus
2. Yes
3. Metastasis

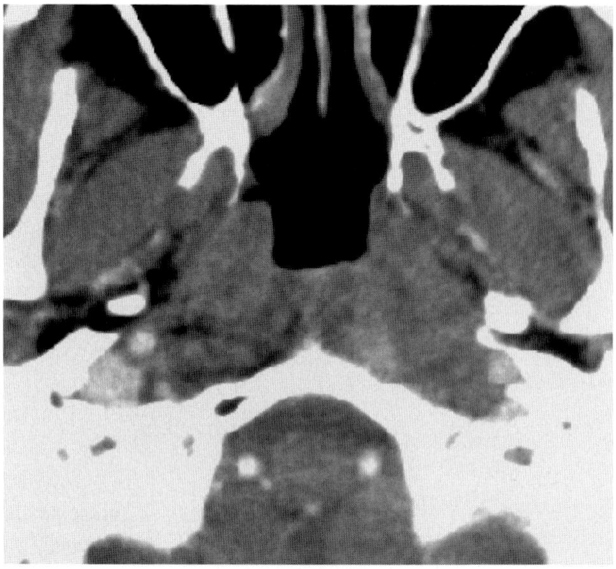

Figure 47E. Patient 1 with nasopharyngeal carcinoma, showing infiltrative mass centered in the left lateral pharyngeal recess (fossa of Rosenmüller's) with involvement of adjacent retrostyloid parapharyngeal space and prevertebral space. Sclerotic change of left-sided basiocciput is also identified. Contrast-enhanced computed tomography image at soft tissue window setting.

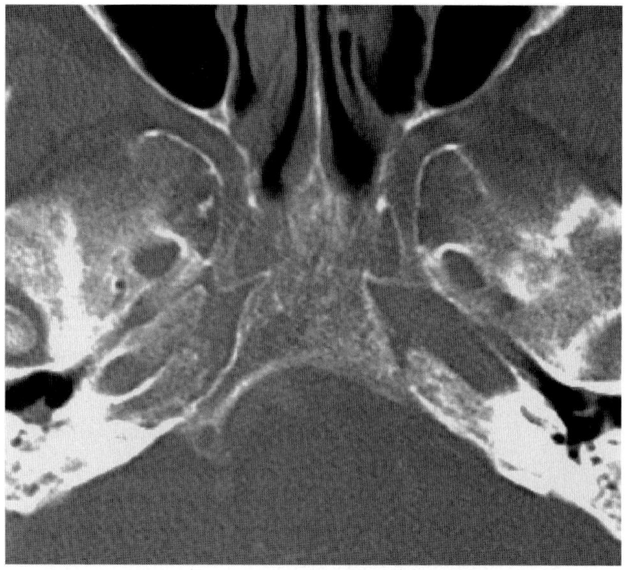

Figure 47F. Patient 1 with nasopharyngeal carcinoma, showing sclerotic change of left-sided body of the sphenoid bone and left petrous apex. Axial computed tomography image at bone window setting.

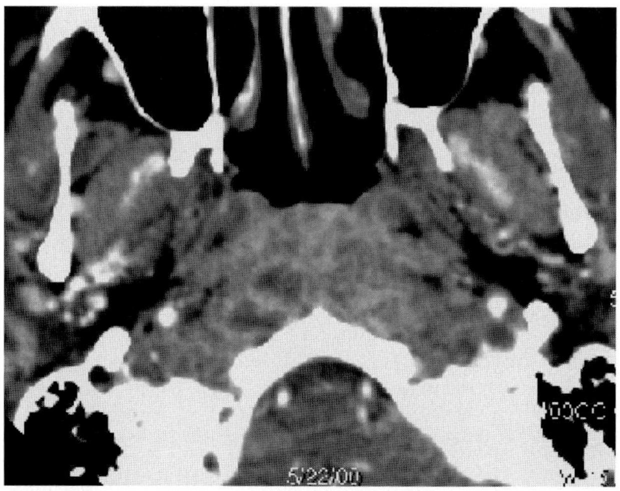

Figure 47G. Patient 2 with skull base osteomyelitis and XIIth cranial nerve deficit. Contrast-enhanced computed tomography image showing infiltrative process involving the prevertebral space and retrostyloid parapharyngeal space bilaterally, which contained several areas of fluid attenuation.

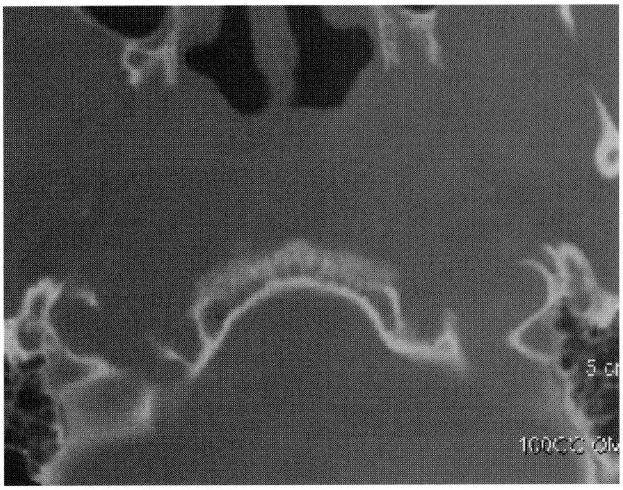

Figure 47H. Patient 2 with skull base osteomyelitis and XIIth cranial nerve deficit. Computed tomography image at bone window setting showing small area of air density within the marrow cavity of the right-sided basiocciput and soft tissue infiltration along the extracranial course of the XIIth cranial nerve where it exits the skull base.

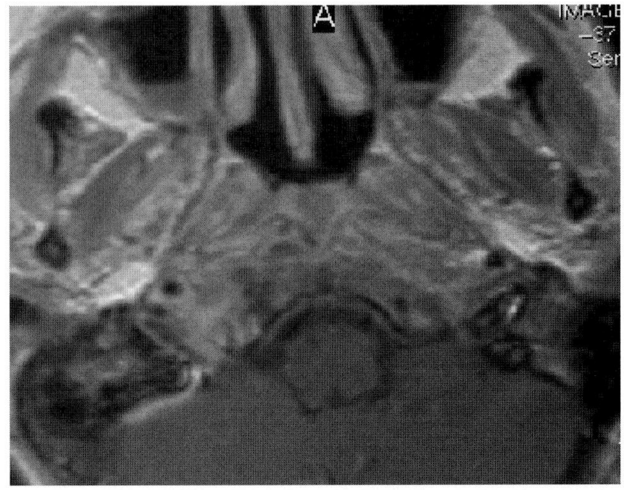

Figure 47I. Patient 2 with skull base osteomyelitis. T1-weighted axial image with contrast showing infiltrating process involving not only soft tissue of the prevertebral and retrostyloid parapharyngeal spaces but also the marrow cavity of the clivus in the region of the hypoglossal canal. The patient had XIIth nerve and multiple other lower cranial nerve deficits on both sides.

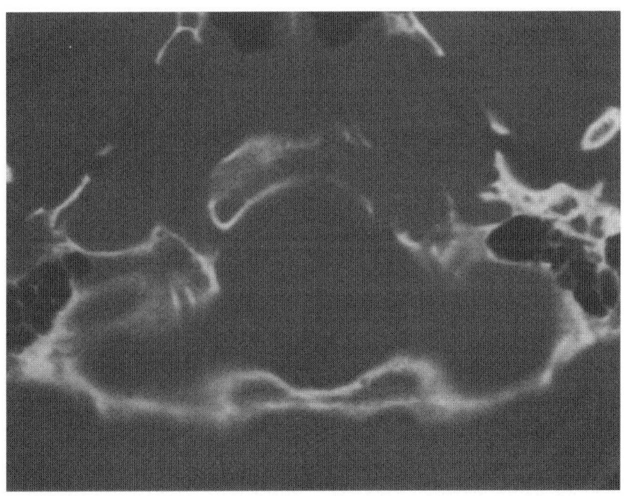

Figure 47J. Patient 3 with metastasis to the skull base from renal cell carcinoma, showing osteolytic lesion involving left-sided basiocciput around the hypoglossal canal with a somewhat expansile appearance. The patient presented with a XIIth cranial nerve deficit.

CASE 48

Clinical History: A 55-year-old man presents with multiple cranial nerve deficits. No lesion is visible in the nasopharynx.

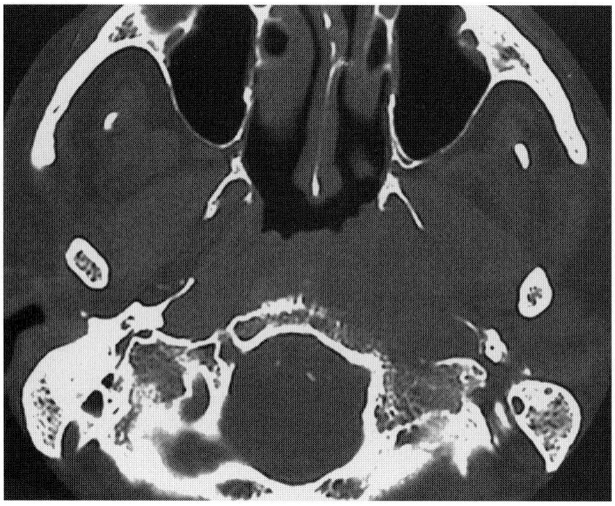

Figure 48A

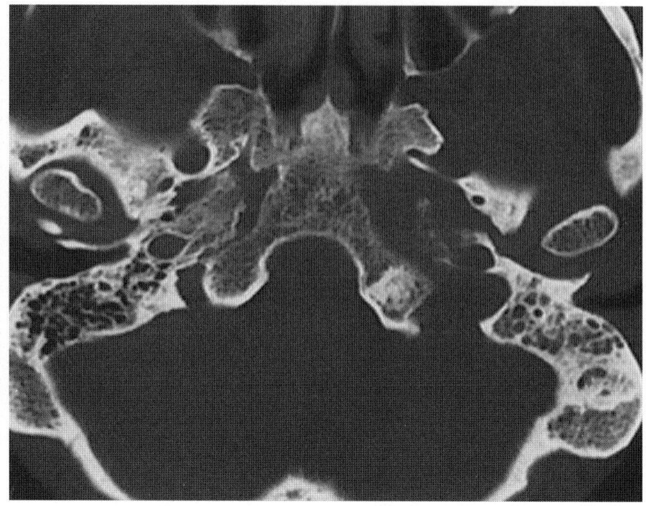

Figure 48B

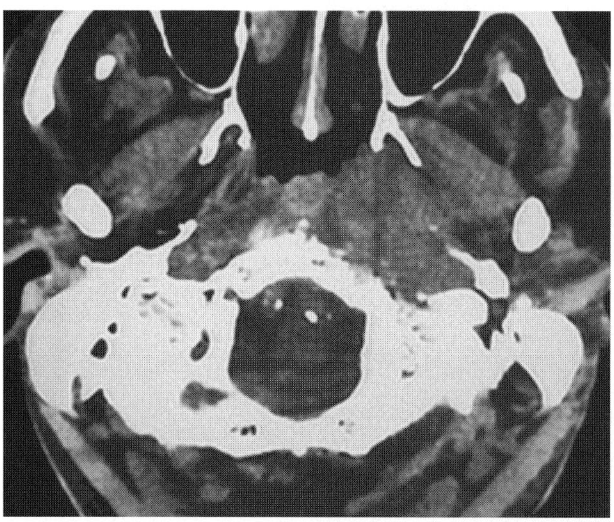

Figure 48C

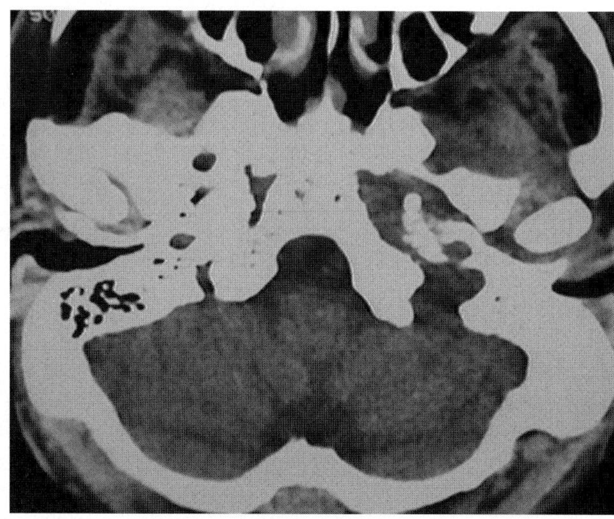

Figure 48D

1. Predict which nerves are abnormal.
2. Where is the pathology centered?
3. What are the two most likely diagnoses?

Findings

An infiltrative soft tissue mass centered in the left parapharyngeal space contiguously involves left retropharyngeal space and the prevertebral space. Aggressive bony erosion is seen of the adjacent skull base, including the left jugular fossa, petrous apex, and the hypoglossal canal. Left lateral pharyngeal recess is severely distorted by the lesion.

Problem

An adult with multiple cranial nerve deficits and an infiltrating, entirely submucosal, mass invading the skull base

Anatomy

A. Posterior skull base (see Fig. 21F)
B. Relationship of nasopharynx to skull base
C. Course of cranial nerves IX to XII, after passing through their exit foramina

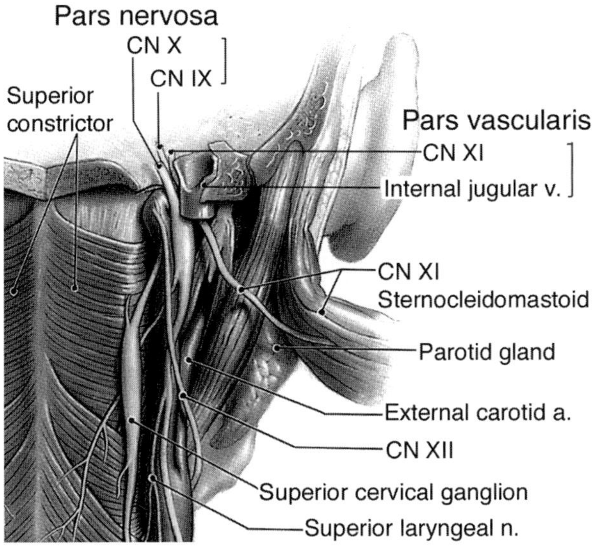

Figure 48E

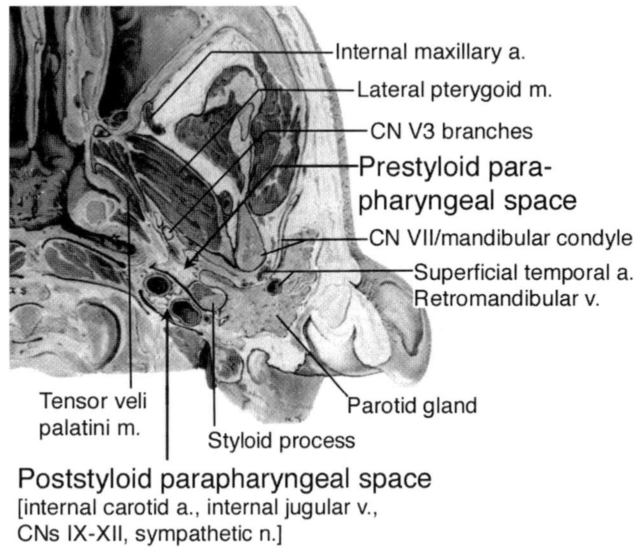

Figure 48F

Differential Diagnosis

Carcinoma, lymphoma, plasmacytoma (unusual) of the nasopharynx; rhabdomyosarcoma (child); Wegener's granulomatosis (unusual); metastatic disease (rare)

Diagnosis

Plasmacytoma of the nasopharynx with skull base invasion

Diagnostic Imaging Approach

A. Evaluate course of all cranial nerves in question, from the brainstem to "end organ."
B. If a mass lesion is present, establish its likely origin (epicenter).
C. Morphology of mass: infiltrative vs. well-circumscribed, T1- or T2-weighted appearance, enhancement, vascularity, calcifications.
D. Determine if focal, multifocal, or diffuse disease process.

Clinical Points Of Importance And Supplemental Information

A. "Submucosal" nasopharyngeal masses can truly arise beneath the mucosa (e.g., adenoidcystic carcinoma in minor salivary glands) or actually arise in the eustachian tube and spread deeply (e.g., carcinoma, Wegener's granulomatosis). The skull base can also be a *source* of a submucosal mass.
B. A "submucosal" nasopharyngeal mass must be biopsied once a vascular lesion (e.g., aneurysm, paraganglioma) has been excluded. If endoscopic biopsy is unsuccessful, computed tomography- or magnetic resonance image-directed sampling is indicated.

Answers To Questions

1. IXth to XIIth and the sympathetic nerves
2. Lower clivus central skull base and posterior nasopharynx
3. Nasopharyngeal cancer (squamous cell carcinoma or lymphoma), plasmacytoma, metastasis

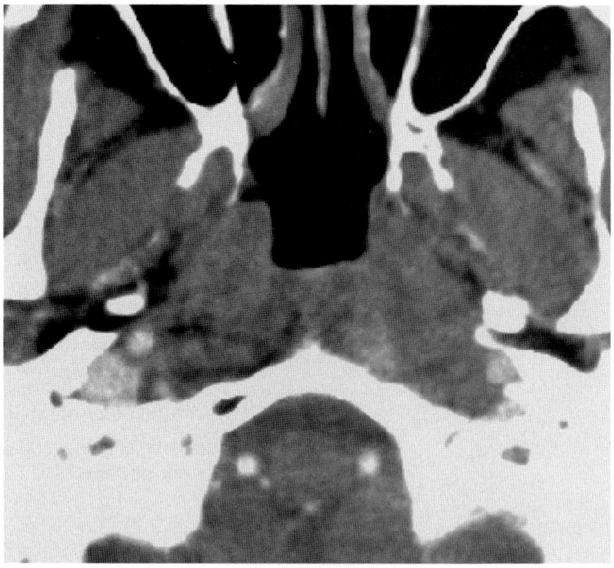

Figure 48G. Patient 1 with nasopharyngeal carcinoma, showing an infiltrative mass centered in left lateral pharyngeal recess (fossa of Rosenmüller) with involvement of adjacent retrostyloid parapharyngeal space and prevertebral space. Sclerotic change of left basiocciput is also identified, which could be a reactive change or be caused by early skull base invasion. Contrast-enhanced computed tomography image at soft tissue window setting.

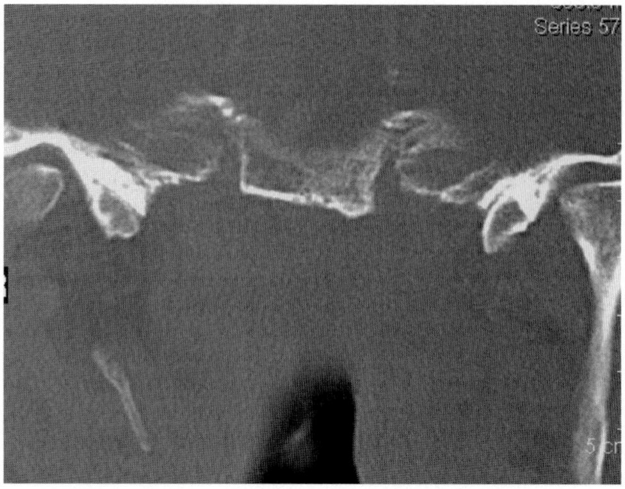

Figure 48H. Patient 1 with nasopharyngeal carcinoma. Coronal computed tomography image at bone window setting showing sclerotic change of the clivus on the left.

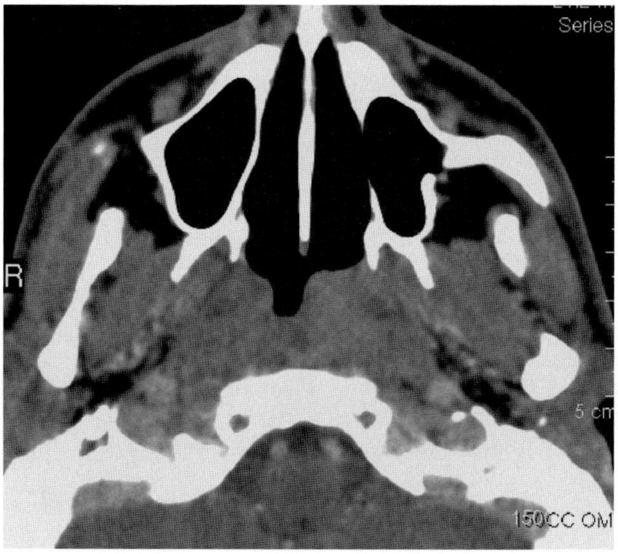

Figure 48I. Patient 2 with high-grade non-Hodgkin's lymphoma, showing infiltrative mass involving the nasopharynx, predominantly on the left.

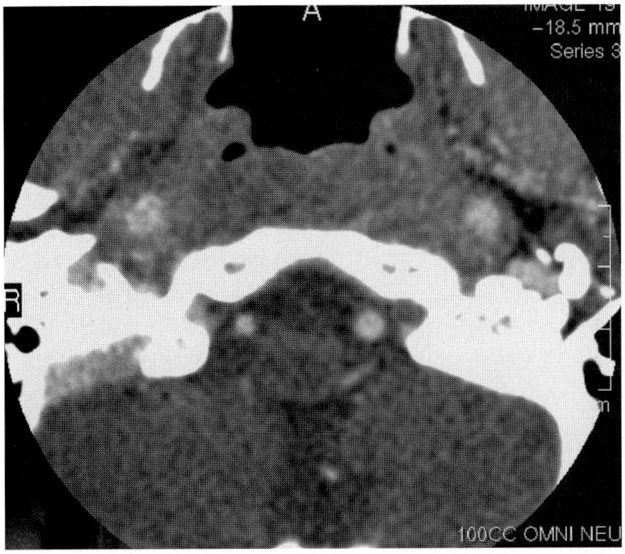

Figure 48J. Patient 3 with skull base osteomyelitis, showing a diffuse, infiltrative process involving soft tissue anterior to the clivus that encompasses both internal carotid arteries.

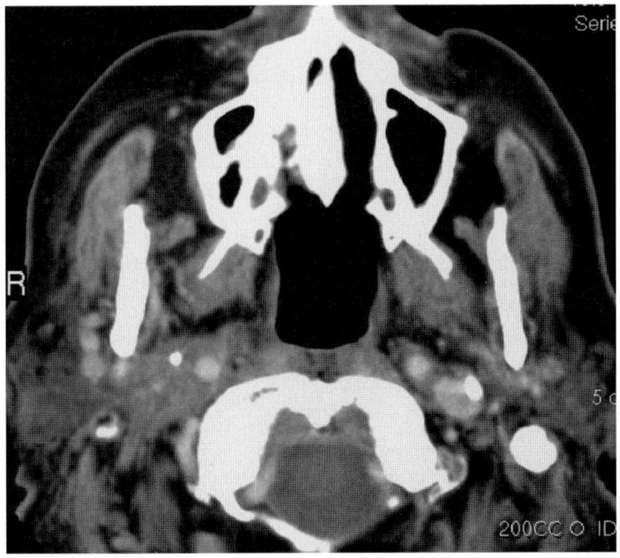

Figure 48K. Patient 4 with recurrent neuroendocrine carcinoma of the submandibular gland, now having lower cranial nerve symptoms. Contrast-enhanced computed tomography image showing an infiltrative process involving the poststyloid parapharyngeal space on the right.

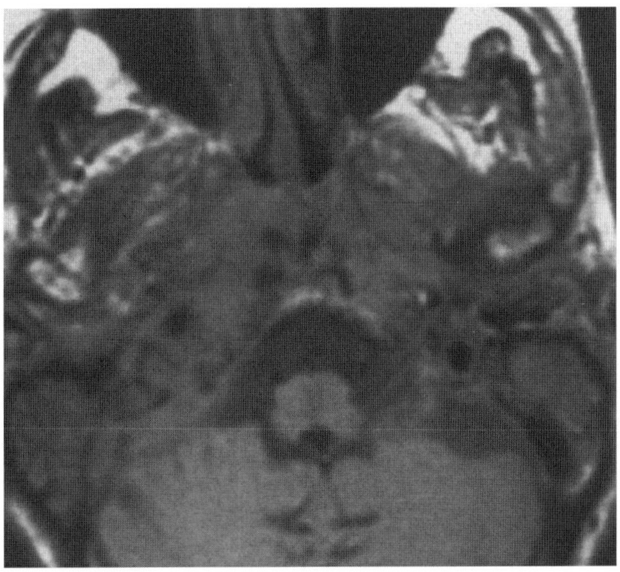

Figure 48L. Patient 5 with skull base invasion of actinomycosis. T1-weighted axial image showing an infiltrative process involving the clivus and adjacent soft tissue of the nasopharynx. The disease process also involves the right jugular fossa and extends intracranially. Fluid collection in the mastoid sinus on each side is caused by eustachian tube involvement.

CASE 49

Clinical History: A 10-year-old boy with three episodes of recurrent meningitis over a 9-month period. The patient had been struck in the head with a baseball bat 10 months earlier. Two prior computed tomography (CT) studies at other institutions showed no skull base or temporal bone fractures.

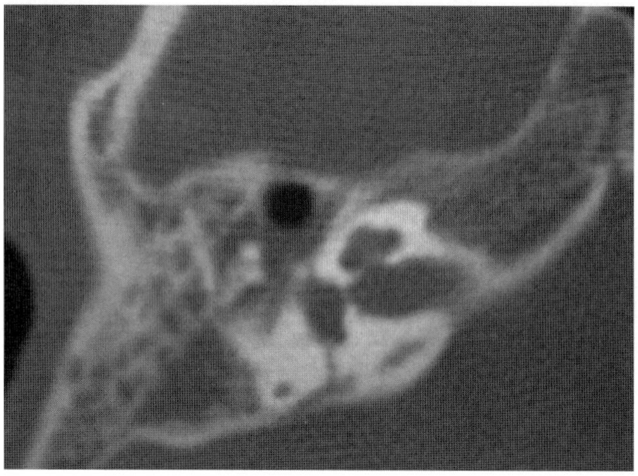

Figure 49A

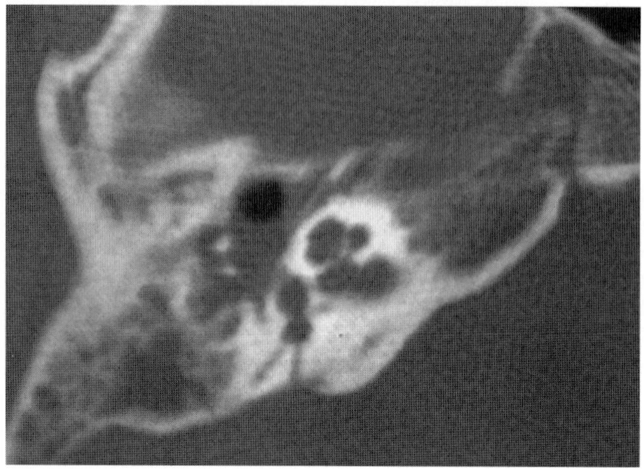

Figure 49B

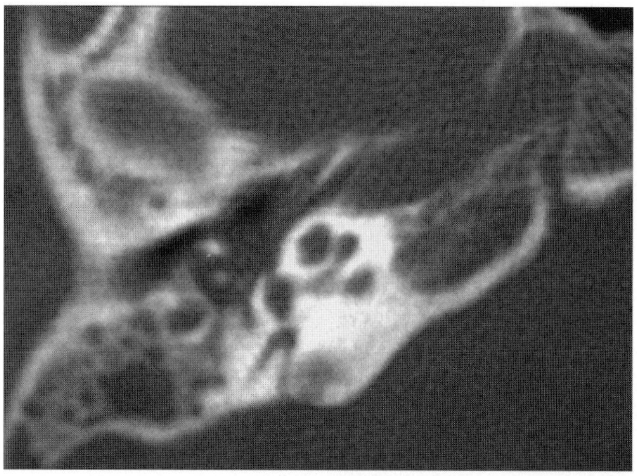

Figure 49C

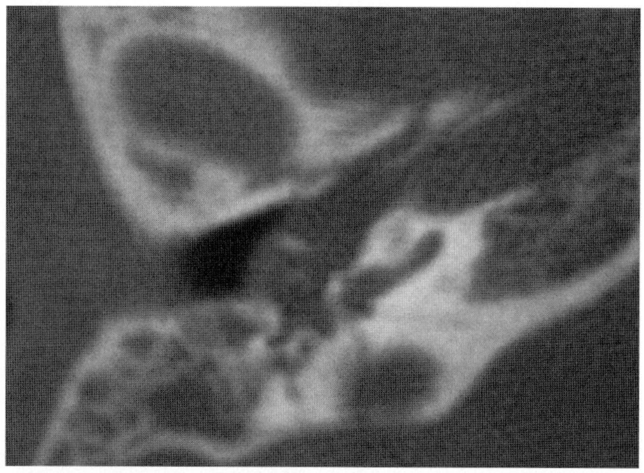

Figure 49D

1. Is there a temporal bone fracture?
2. Is there a finding that explains the recurrent meningitis?
3. List one acute and three chronic complications of temporal bone trauma that require diagnostic imaging evaluation by CT scan or magnetic resonance imaging (MRI). Match the complications to the imaging study(ies) required.

Findings

A fracture line partly traverses the right petrous bone across its long axis. The oval window and likely the stapes footplate are fractured. Some fluid or mucosal thickening is present the right middle ear cavity and mastoid air cells likely related to leakage of fluid from the membranous labyrinth.

Problem

A child with recurrent meningitis following head trauma with two prior negative CT examinations; a more current study shows a temporal bone fracture

Anatomy

A. Oval window, stapes (footplate and suprastructure)
B. Vestibule and posterior semicircular canal

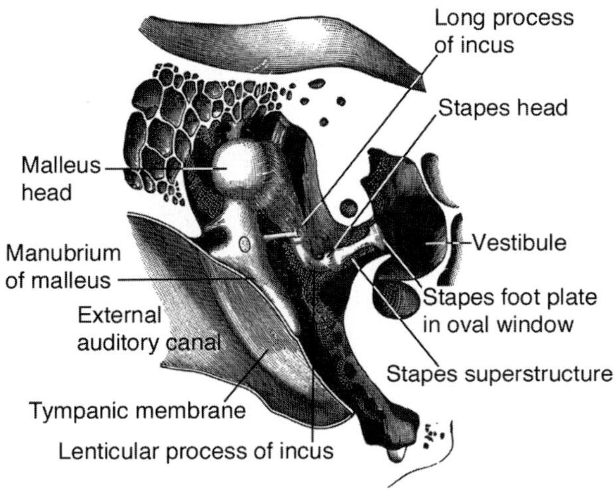

Figure 49E

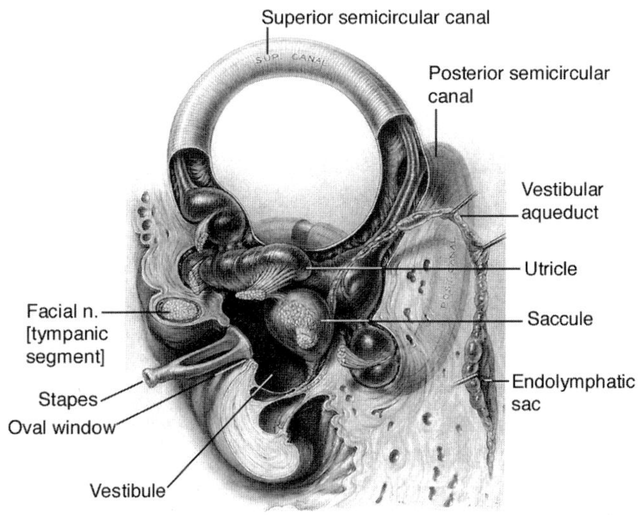

Figure 49F

Differential Diagnosis

Not applicable

Diagnosis

A. Transverse temporal bone fracture involving the oval window and stapes footplate
B. Opacification of the middle ear and mastoid caused by otomastoiditis or cerebrospinal fluid (CSF) otorrhea

Diagnostic Imaging Approach

A. Very high resolution CT required (1 mm sections, FOV 10 cm or smaller) with magnification of areas of interest
B. Identify source of recurrent meningitis; intrathecal contrast might be required to confirm CSF leak.
C. Differential diagnosis (of CSF otorrhea):
   1. Prior trauma: meningoencephalocele, sites of arachnoid granulations, tumors eroding to or from intracranial compartment
   2. Congenital lesions associated with a dermal sinus

Clinical Points Of Importance And Supplemental Information

A. Accurate diagnosis of temporal bone pathology requires very high spatial resolution.
B. CSF leakage into the temporal bone (middle ear) can present as rhinorrhea (via eustachian tube).

Answers To Questions

1. Yes
2. Oval window or stapes footplate fracture creates a path of infection from the middle ear to the CSF.
3. Acute: facial nerve palsy (CT). Chronic: CSF leak (CT); recurrent meningitis (CT); encephalocele (MRI)

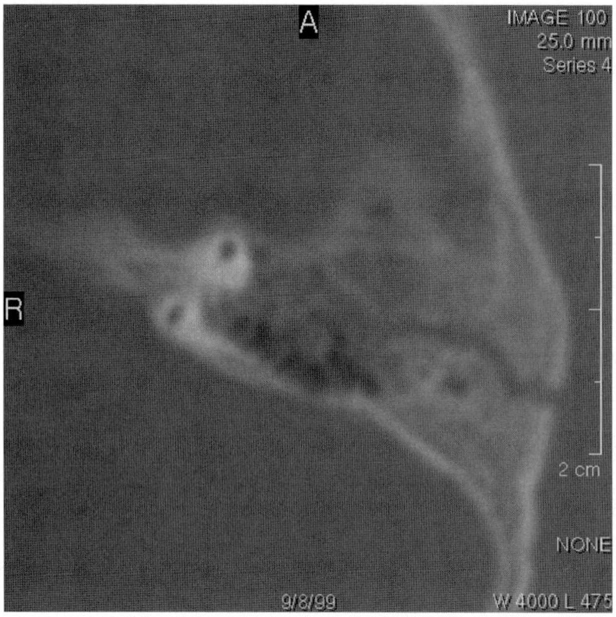

Figure 49G. Patient 1 with temporal bone fracture (longitudinal type). Axial computed tomography image at bone window setting showing fracture line parallel to the long axis of left petrous bone.

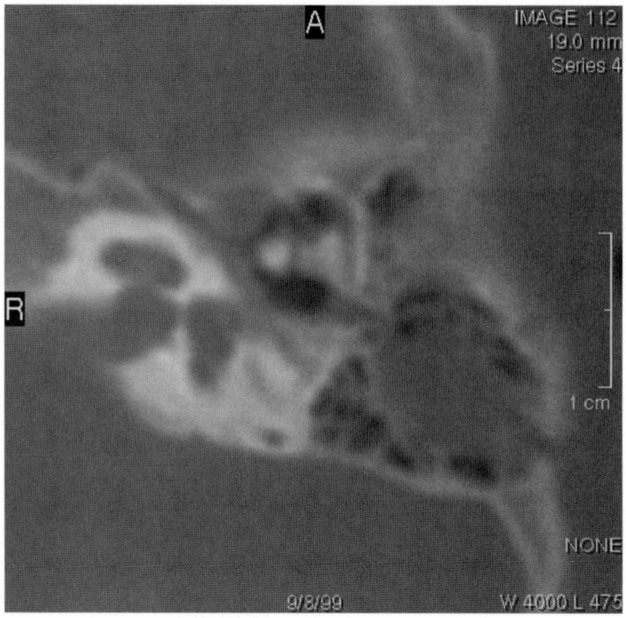

Figure 49H. Patient 1 with temporal bone fracture (longitudinal type). Axial computed tomography caudal to 49G also showing fracture line and abnormal arrangement of malleus head and incus body (dislocation of incudomalleal joint).

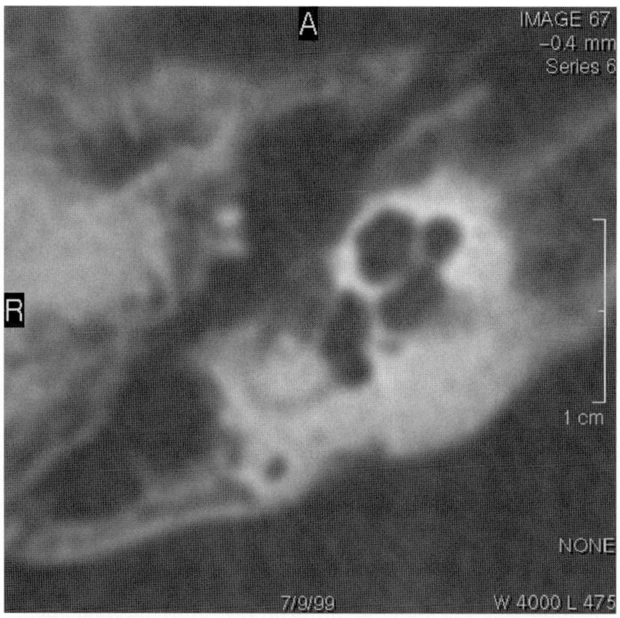

Figure 49I. Patient 2 with skull base fracture involving the temporal bone. Axial computed tomography image at bone window setting showing fracture line traversing mastoid and tympanic bones obliquely. Malleus and incus are laterally displaced in an opacified middle ear cavity, as manifest by their distance from the stapes superstructure.

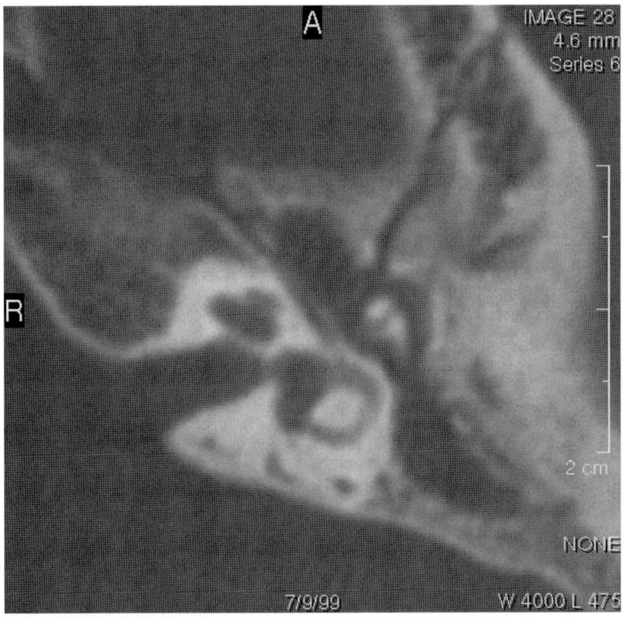

Figure 49J. Patient 3 with skull base fracture involving the temporal bone. Axial computed tomography image at bone window setting showing fracture line traversing the mastoid and tympanic membrane.

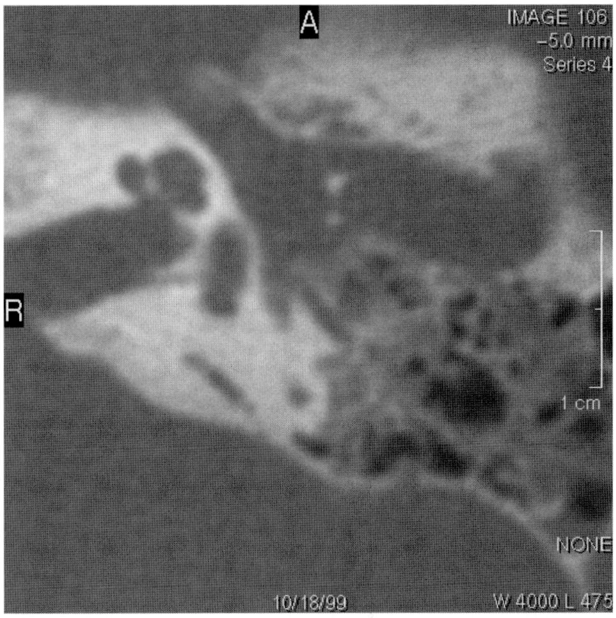

Figure 49K. Patient 3 with temporal bone fracture. Axial computed tomography image at bone window setting showing dislocation of the incudostapedial joint with lateral displacement of the long process of the incus.

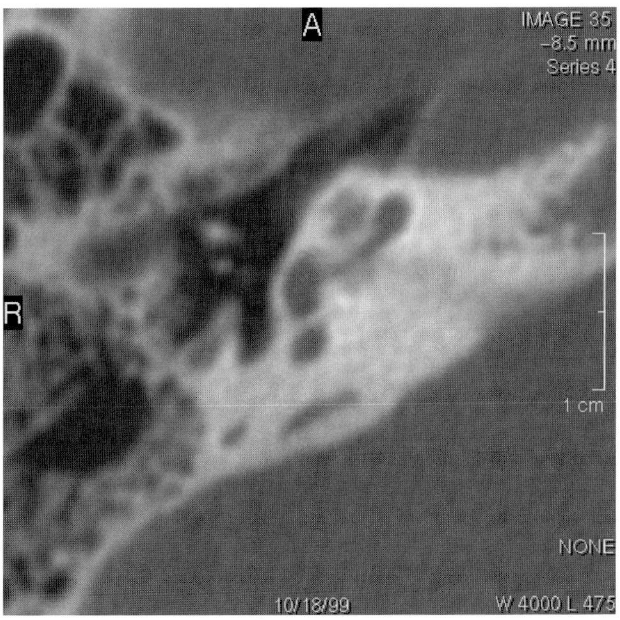

Figure 49L. Patient 3 with temporal bone fracture. Axial computed tomography image of the opposite side of the temporal bone showing normal alignment of the incudostapedial joint.

CHAPTER 4

SINONASAL REGION

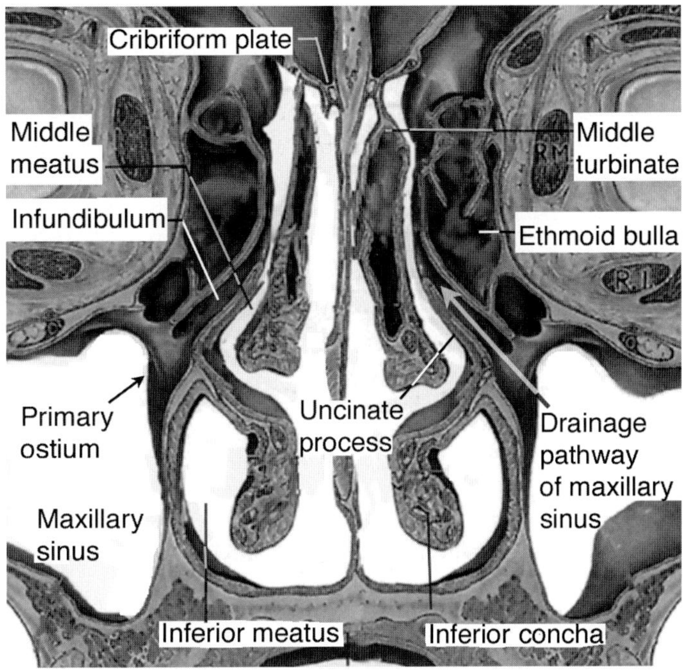

CASE 50

Clinical History: A 1-year-old boy presents with a probable nasal dermoid noted on physical examination.

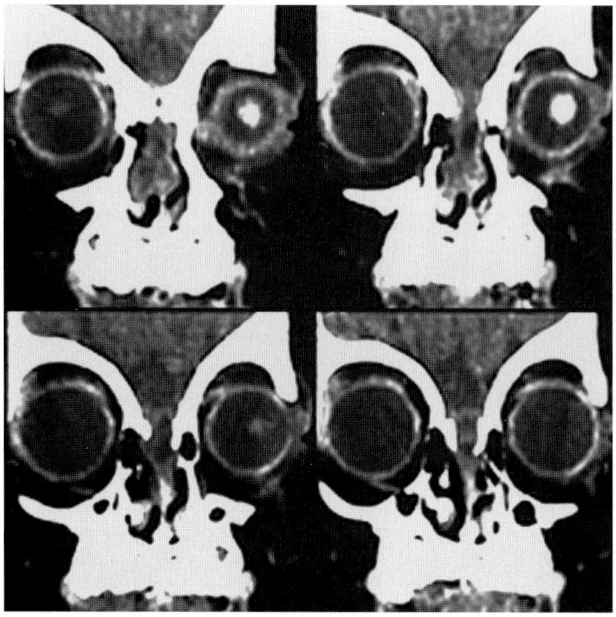

Figure 50A

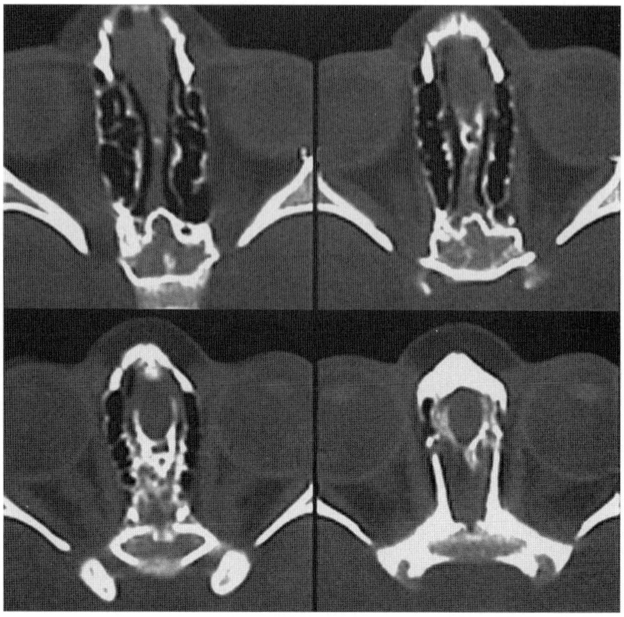

Figure 50B

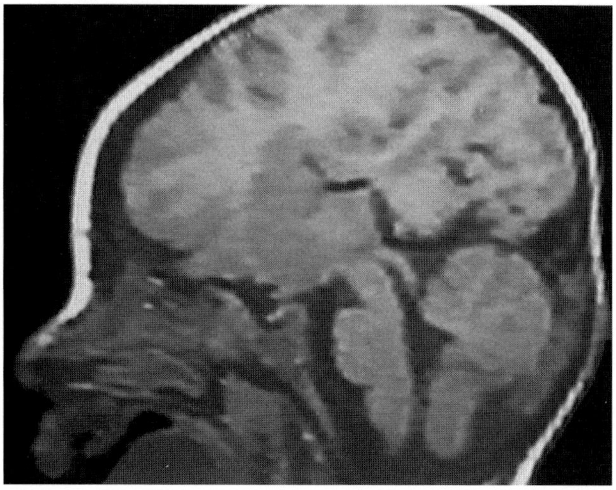

Figure 50C

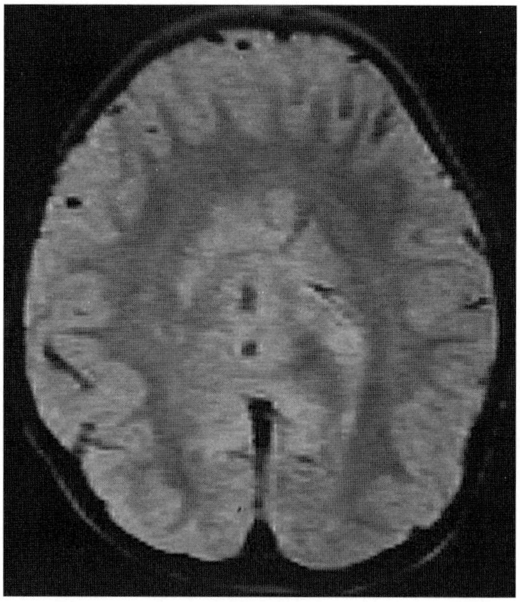

Figure 50D

1. Can the dermoid be removed by a strictly extracranial, transfacial approach?
2. What are the radiologist's responsibilities in evaluating congenital mass lesions of the facial and sinonasal region?

Findings

A mass in the superior and anterior aspect of the midline of the nasal cavity, at least partially within the nasal septum. Internal attenuation of the lesion is lower than cerebrospinal fluid, which is suggestive of a fatty or cystic component. The foramen cecum is enlarged but no connection to the brain is evident. A holoprosencephaly is present intracranially.

Problem

A child with a possible nasal dermoid and tract leading toward the brain noted on the computed tomography (CT) study

Anatomy

A. Nasal bone or frontal bone relationship
B. Foramen cecum, crista galli, skull base anterior to the anterior ethmoid artery

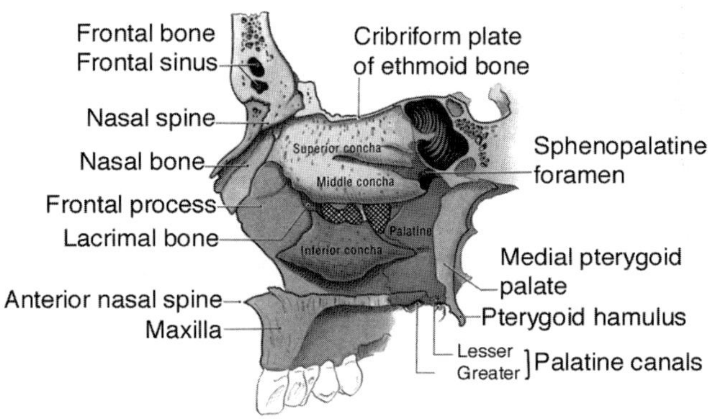

Figure 50E

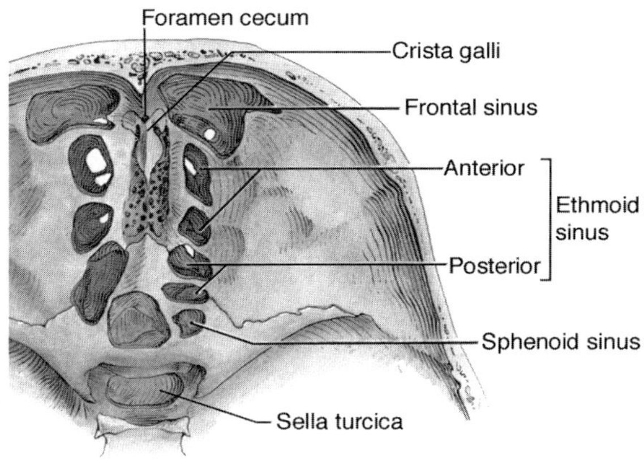

Figure 50F

Differential Diagnosis

Not applicable

Diagnosis

Nasal dermoid cyst with a sinus ending blindly at the foramen cecum

Diagnostic Imaging Approach

A. Establish local extent of dermoid (e.g., nose, nasal septum, bony).
B. Determine if a related tract extends intracranially and whether it is associated with an intracranial mass or is connected to the central nervous system (CNS) (e.g., meningocele, meningoencephalocele).
C. Evaluate for intracranial anomalies (e.g., of olfactory tracts, pituitary gland, brain).
D. Differential diagnosis: meningoencephalocele, ectopic brain?

Clinical Points Of Importance And Supplemental Information

A. Imaging studies must determine whether the mass can be safely removed by an entirely extracranial approach.
B. Study protocols must include detailed evaluation of the face as well as the intracranial structures.

Answers To Questions

1. Yes
2. Define any connection to the CNS, identify other intracranial anomalies, and anticipate altered anatomy that might affect the surgical approach.

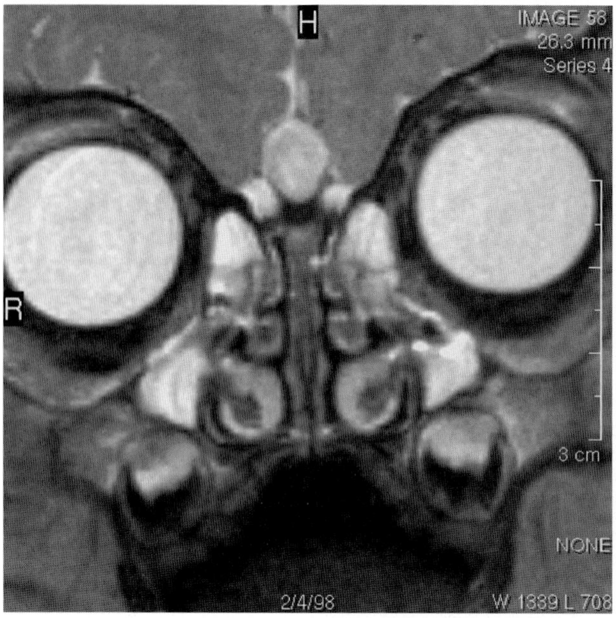

Figure 50G. Patient 1 with a pit in the dorsum of the nose. Coronal T2-weighted image showing elliptical high-intensity mass adjacent superior to the area of foramen cecum, splaying a bifid appearing crista galli, consistent with nasal dermoid.

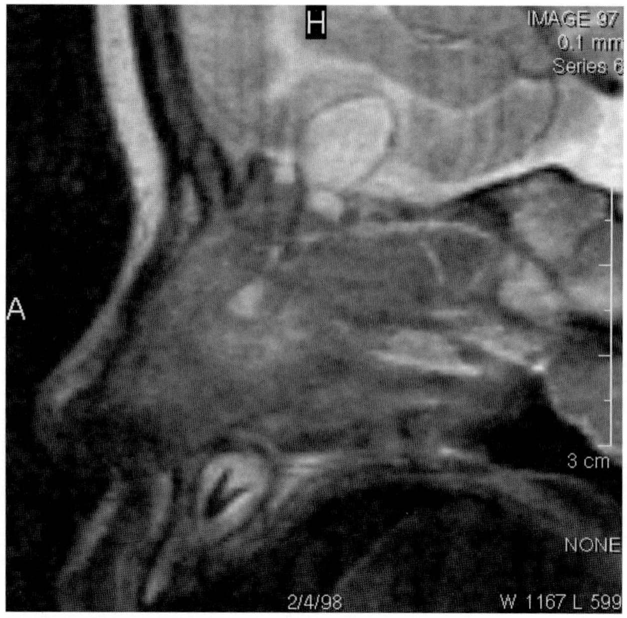

Figure 50H. Patient 1 with pit in dorsum of nose—T2- weighted midline sagittal image showing connection of the mass with the anterior skull base.

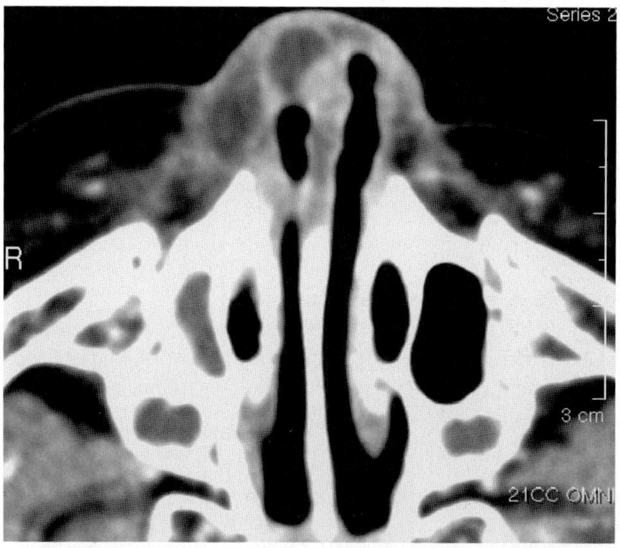

Figure 50I. Patient 2 with an infected nasal dermoid. Axial computed tomography image with contrast showing a thick-walled, cystic lesion in the dorsum of the nose partially indenting in the superior nasal cartilage.

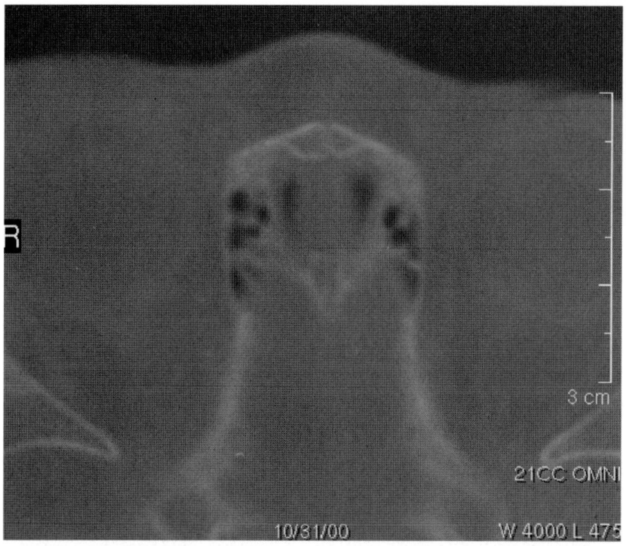

Figure 50J. Patient 2 with presumed infected nasal dermoid. Axial computed tomography image superior to 50I at bone window setting showing soft tissue and lack of mineralization anterior to the crista galli that could represent a superior extension of the mass or just be normal for age.

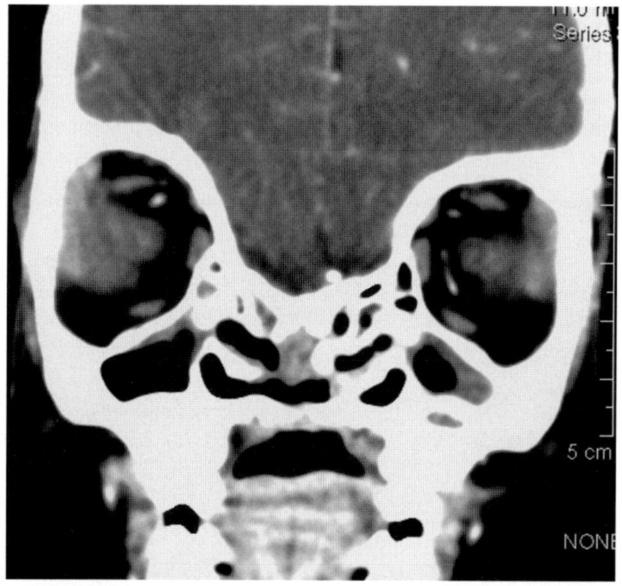

Figure 50K. Patient 3 with anterior meningoencephalocele, showing the frontal lobe protruding inferiorly between both orbits, with hypertelorism. Coronal computed tomography image at soft tissue window setting.

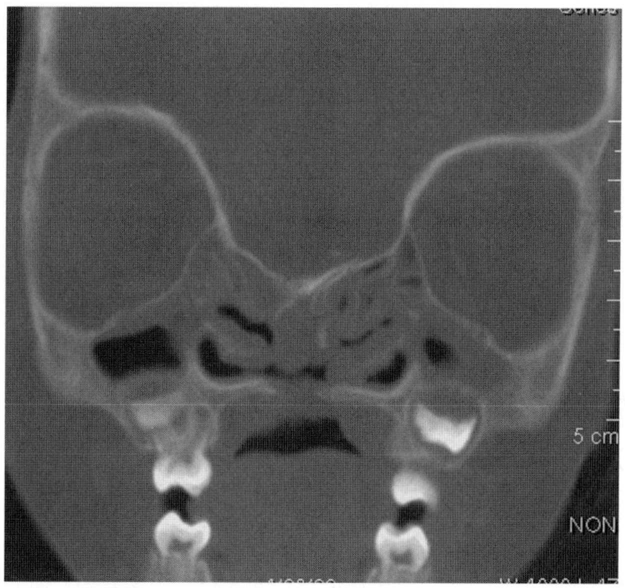

Figure 50L. Patient 3 with anterior meningoencephalocele. Coronal computed tomography image at bone window setting showing dysmorphism of the nasal septum and conchae and a cleft of the hard palate.

CASE 51

Clinical History: A 4-year-old boy presents with sinusitis and orbital cellulitis.

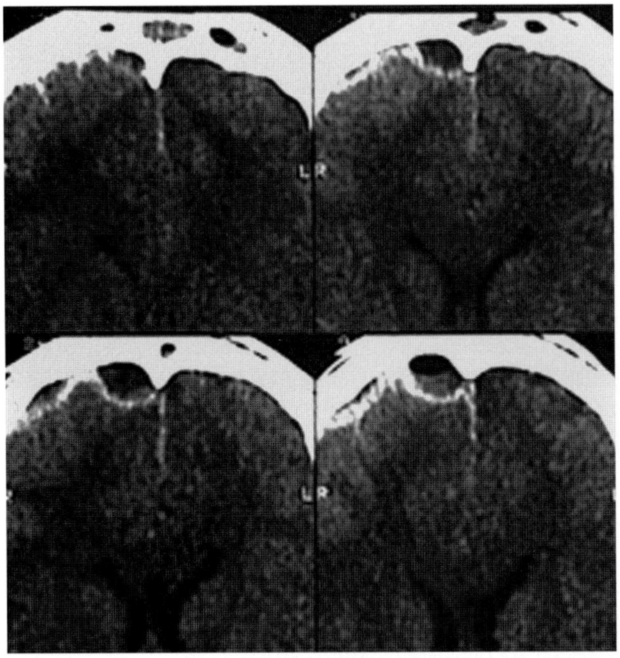

Figure 51A

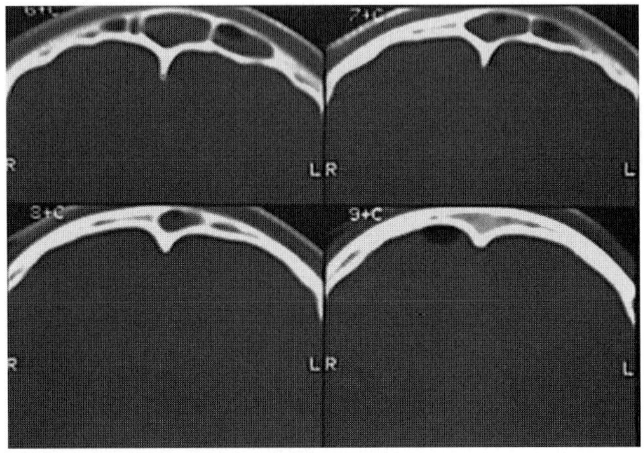

Figure 51B

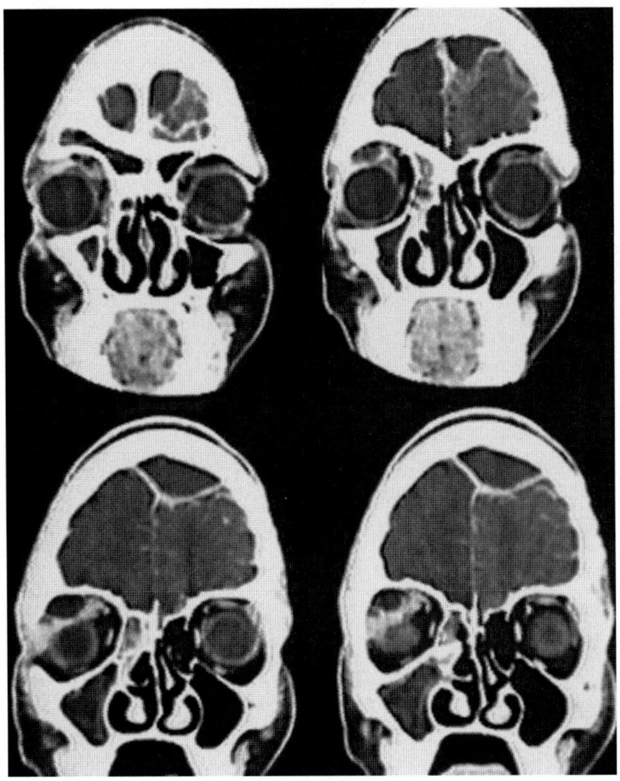

Figure 51C

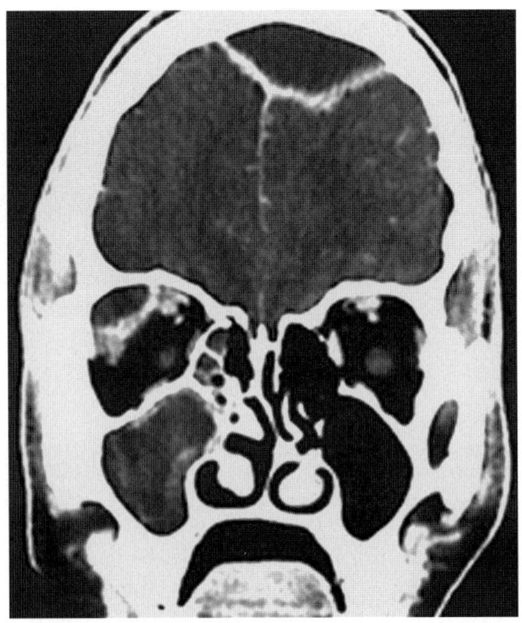

Figure 51D

1. Name three specific circumstances when the evaluation of rhinosinusitis requires a contrast-enhanced, two-plane computed tomography (CT) study.
2. Name three routes of spread for intracranial complications of pyogenic sinonasal infections.
3. Name six intracranial complications of pyogenic sinus infection.

Findings

Opacified frontal sinus and left maxillary and ethmoid sinuses with fluid and marked mucosal thickening; localized fluid collection with rim enhancement in the superolateral aspect of the right orbit; loculated fluid collections with thickening and enhancement of the adjacent dura mater in the epidural space in the frontal region. Air is seen within one fluid collection. No bone erosion is seen at any of the sites of these probable abscesses.

Problem

A child with acute, pyogenic sinusitis, orbital cellulitis, and possible intraorbital and intracranial complications of that disease

Anatomy

A. Frontal bone and sinus: inner or outer table
   1. Variants in sinus relationship to orbits
   2. Diploic vessels and their relationship to the dura mater and brain
B. Orbit: orbital periosteum (periorbita)

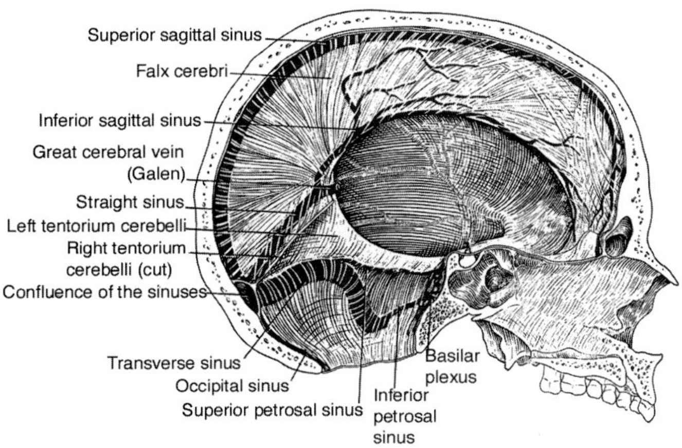

Figure 51E

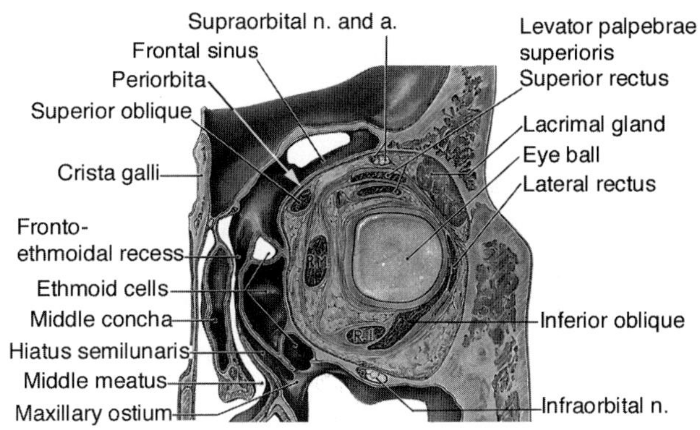

Figure 51F

Differential Diagnosis

Not applicable

Diagnosis

Sinusitis (probably pyogenic), with subperiosteal orbital abscess and subdural, epidural empyema, or both

Diagnostic Imaging Approach

A. With regard to the possible orbital complications, look for both postseptal and preseptal disease.
   1. Determine if postseptal disease is an abscess or phlegmon (cellulitic).
   2. Evaluate optic nerve–sheath complex for compression and involvement.
   3. Look for evidence of "tension orbit" and orbital venous thrombosis.
B. With regard to possible intracranial complications, evaluate for:
   1. Osteomyelitis of the frontal bone inner table.
   2. Subdural or epidural empyema.
   3. Meningitis.

4. Cerebritis or brain abscess.
5. Cavernous sinus, other dural sinus, or cortical venous thrombosis.

C. Precisely describe the position and likely mode of extension of any collection of pyogenic material (e.g., directly through sinus wall vs. thrombophlebitic spread).

Clinical Points of Importance and Supplemental Information

A. The presence of an abscess or empyema is frequently the result of thrombophlebitic spread of pyogenic material so that the collection may not be obviously in continuity with the sinus disease (i.e., through an osteomyelitic defect). The precise localization of orbital abscesses will aid greatly in planning drainage.

B. Findings indicative of subdural empyema may be subtle and occasionally manifest only by lucency in the interhemispheric region. High spatial resolution techniques and effective use of contrast are required for imaging of these patients. Magnetic resonance imaging (MRI) may help identify subtle interhemispheric subdural empyema or early brain complications.

Answers to Questions

1. Preseptal cellulitis, visual problems, altered mental status
2. Thrombophlebitis (valveless veins); directly through bone (osteomyelitis); through existing foramina
3. Osteomyelitis, subdural abcess, epidural abcess, meningitis, cerebritis, brain abcess.

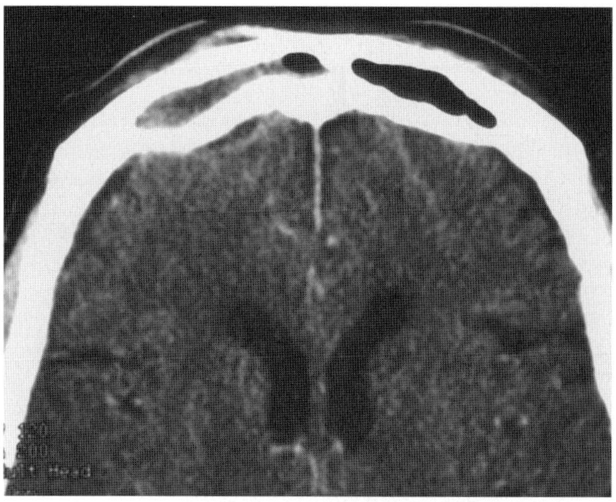

Figure 51G. Patient 1 with intracranial complication of frontal sinusitis, showing fluid collection or mucosal thickening of the right frontal sinus with a small subdural fluid collection adjacent to the inner table of the frontal sinus. Subperiosteal fluid collection along outer table is also seen. Axial computed tomography image.

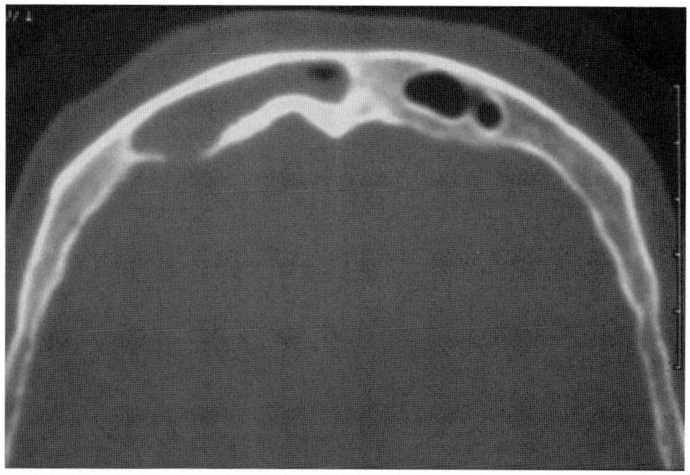

Figure 51H. Patient 1 with intracranial complication of frontal sinusitis. Computed tomography image at bone window setting showing erosion at the inner table of the opacified right frontal sinus.

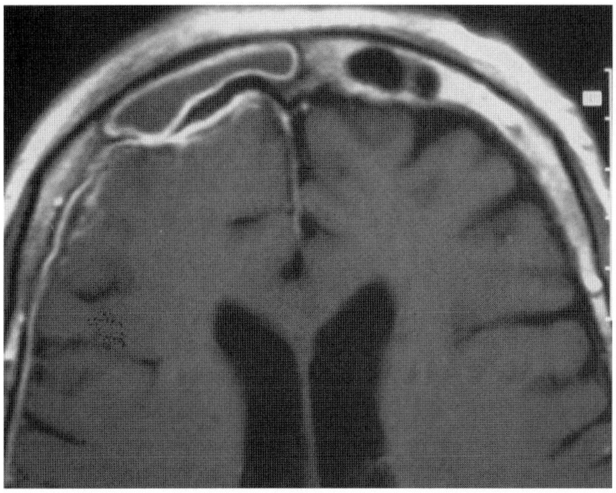

Figure 51I. Patient 1 with intracranial complication of frontal sinusitis. T1-weighted axial image with contrast showing enhancement of the thickened mucosa in the opacified right frontal sinus. Intracranial complication is manifested by leptomeningeal enhancement in the adjacent right frontal region; at surgery, no pus was found in the subdural space.

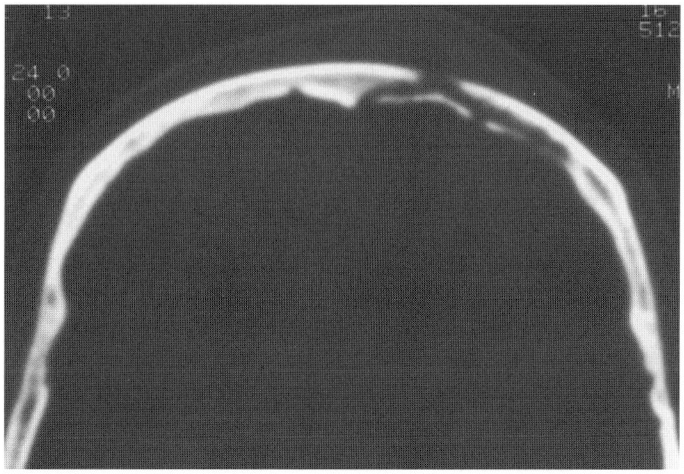

Figure 51J. Patient 2 with frontal osteomyelitis caused by to sinusitis, showing fragmentation of the left frontal bone with disruption in several areas of both outer and inner tables. Axial computed tomography image at bone window setting.

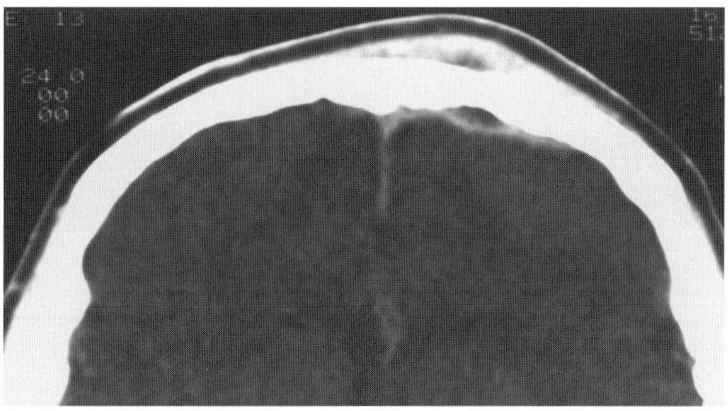

Figure 51K. Patient 2 with frontal osteomyelitis caused by sinusitis. Contrast-enhanced axial computed tomography image showing a small extraaxial fluid collection with enhancement of adjacent dura mater suggestive of subdural or epidural empyema. Small periosteal abscess present in an area of the adjacent forehead, formerly called "Pott's puffy tumor."

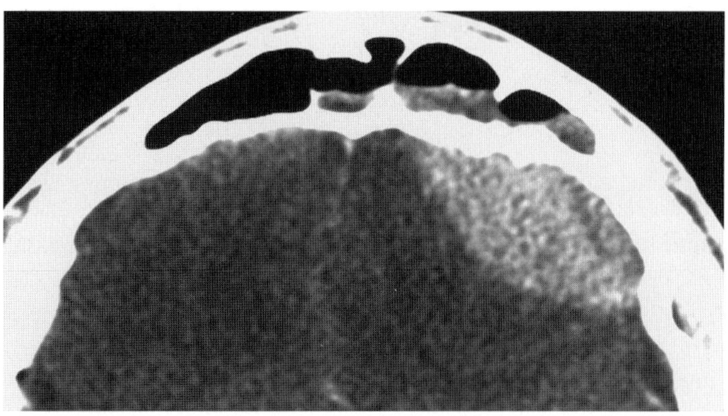

Figure 51L. Patient 3 with intracranial complication of frontal sinusitis, showing air–fluid levels in the frontal sinus with epidural hematoma presumably resulting from intracranial complication of acute frontal sinusitis; at surgery, pus was also found in the predominant hematoma.

CASE 52

Clinical History: A 28-year-old man presents with nasal stuffiness and a bulge in the right superior medial orbital region.

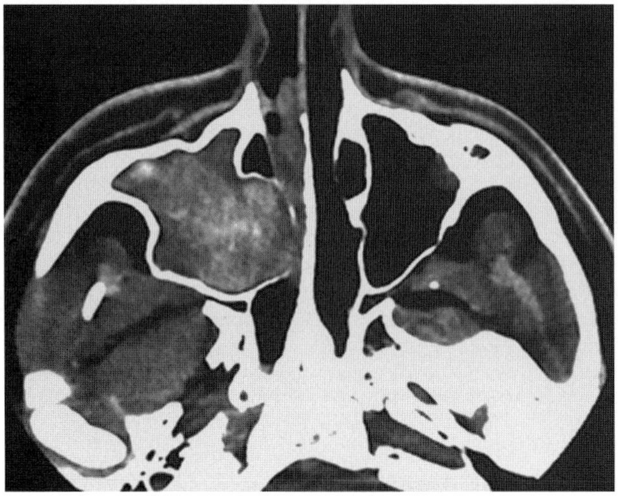

Figure 52A

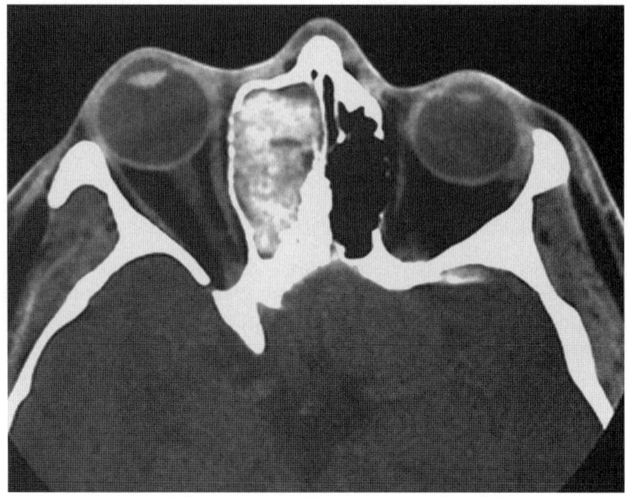

Figure 52B

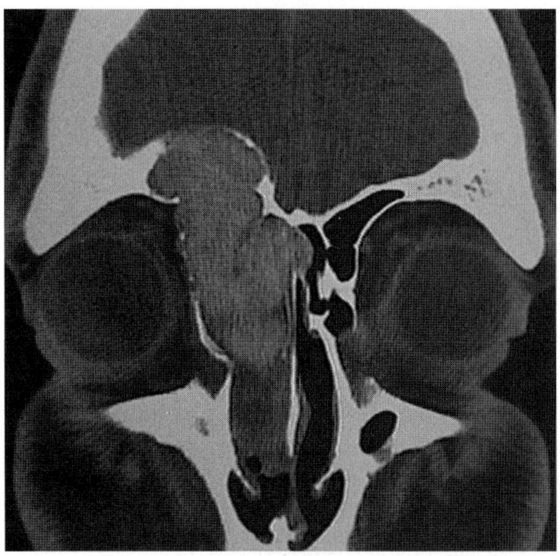

Figure 52C

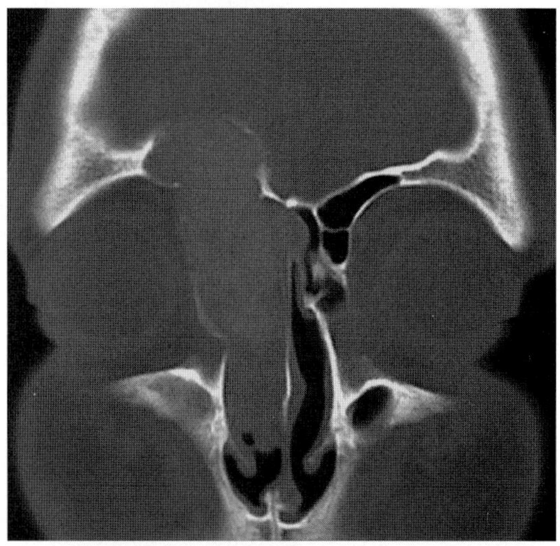

Figure 52D

1. Give a complete diagnosis.
2. Give two reasons for the increased attenuation of the sinus contents on this *non*-contrast-enhanced computed tomography (CT) image.
3. What might be the appearance of these sinus secretions on T2-weighted magnetic resonance images (MRI)?

Findings

An expansile sinonasal mass involving the right maxillary, ethmoid, and frontal sinuses, with remodeling of their walls. The lesion contains a diffuse, amorphous high-attenuation area. Lateral displacement of the medial wall of the right orbit results in exophthalmos.

Problem

An adult with unilateral, expansile-appearing ethmoid and maxillary sinuses filled with relatively high attenuation material

Anatomy

A. Maxillary sinus and its drainage pathway
B. Ethmoid sinuses and their drainage pathways

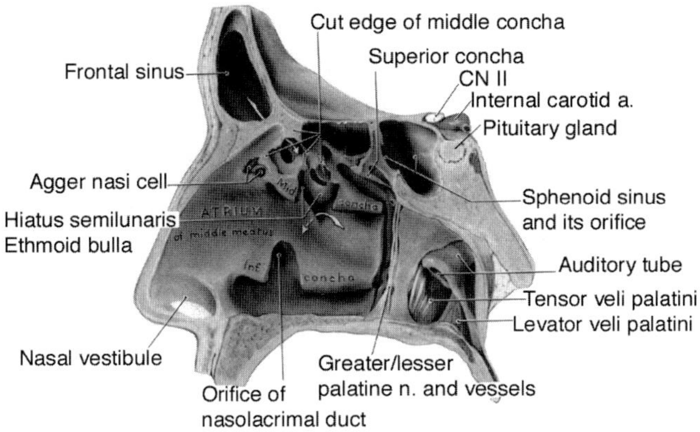

Figure 52E

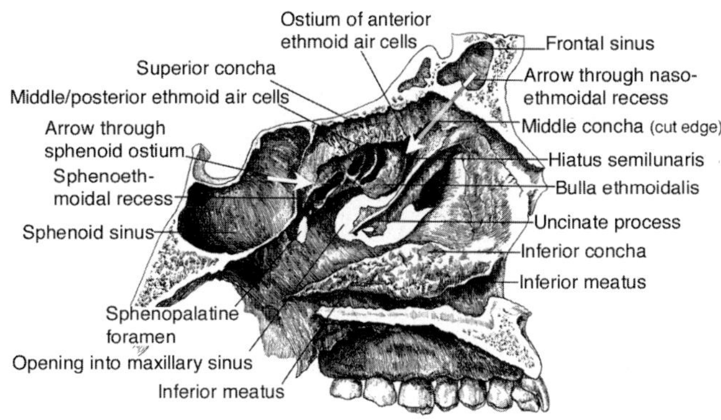

Figure 52F

Differential Diagnosis

None. However, such changes could mimic a localized fibroosseous lesion, and an inverting papilloma might cause (by obstruction) or resemble this disease process.

Diagnosis

Unilateral maxilloethmoid mucocele containing desiccated secretions with probable fungal colonization of the sinus contents. Rule out a causative obstructing mass

Diagnostic Imaging Approach

A. Is the disease process arising primarily in the sinus(es), nasal cavity, or elsewhere (e.g., from bone)?
B. Is the affected sinus(es) airless? Does it appear expanded?
C. Any bone destruction?
D. Is the disease bilateral or unilateral?
E. An obstructing mass present?

Clinical Points of Importance and Supplemental Information

A. It must be emphasized in diagnostic reports that this fungal disease is likely *colonization, not* invasive fungal disease.
B. Patients with these changes frequently have chronic allergic polypoid rhinosinusitis.

Answers to Questions

1. Maxilloethmoidal mucocele with desiccated secretions, possibly colonized with fungi
2. Desiccation and fungal colonization of secretions
3. Darker than muscle—almost appearing as a signal void

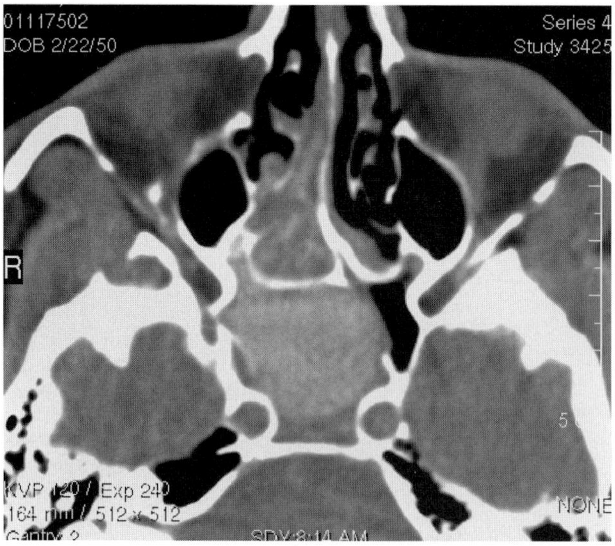

Figure 52G. Patient 1 with sphenoethmoidal mucocele and fungal colonization. Axial computed tomography image showing relatively high attenuation, and complete opacification of the sphenoid sinus with somewhat expansile change.

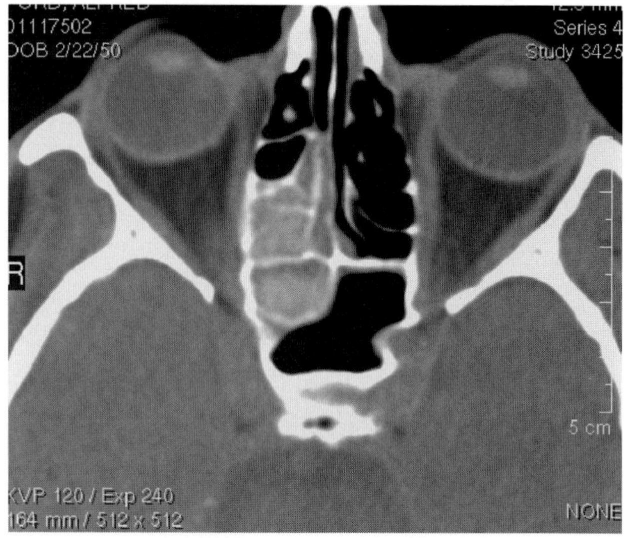

Figure 52H. Patient 1 with sphenoethmoidal mucocele and fungal colonization. Axial computed tomography image cephalad to Fig. 52G showing complete opacification of the posterior ethmoidal air cells with slightly expansile change.

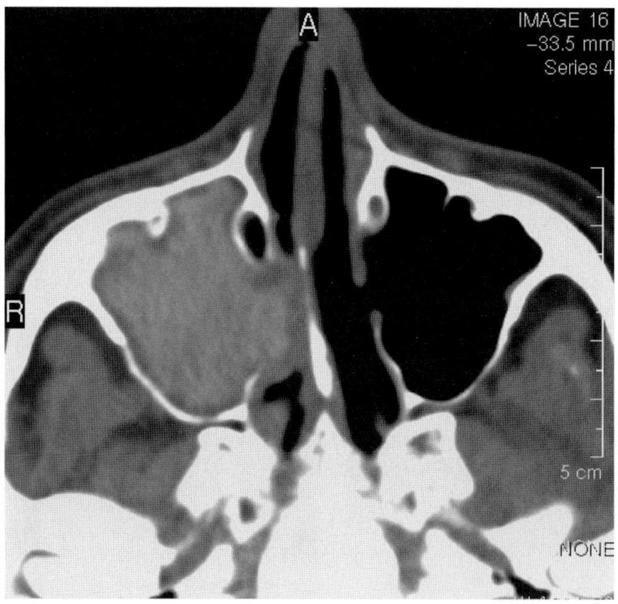

Figure 52I. Patient 2 with maxillary mucocele. Axial computed tomography image at soft tissue window setting showing complete opacification of the right maxillary antrum by relatively high attenuation with expansile appearance; in this situation, an obstructing nasal cavity mass must always be excluded by careful nasal endoscopy.

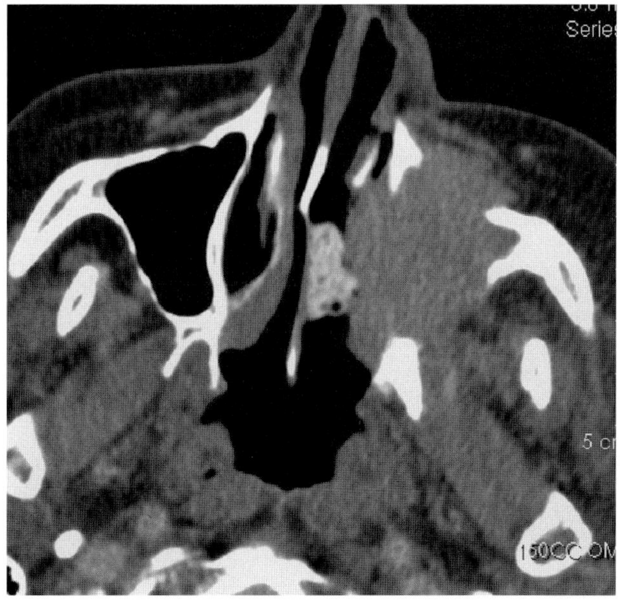

Figure 52J. Patient 3 with maxillary sinus carcinoma. Axial computed tomography image at soft tissue window setting showing a soft tissue density mass filling the left maxillary sinus, extending into the middle meatus medially; soft tissue in the cheek anteriorly and the buccal fat pad posterolaterally, with destruction of the sinus walls—for comparison with other benign cases.

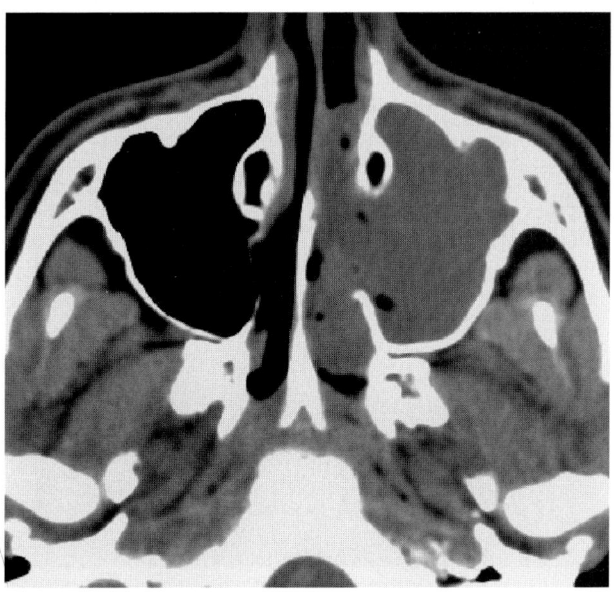

Figure 52K. Patient 4 with antrochoanal polyp, showing polypoid mass occupying the left maxillary antrum, with extension into the left nasal cavity through the secondary ostium.

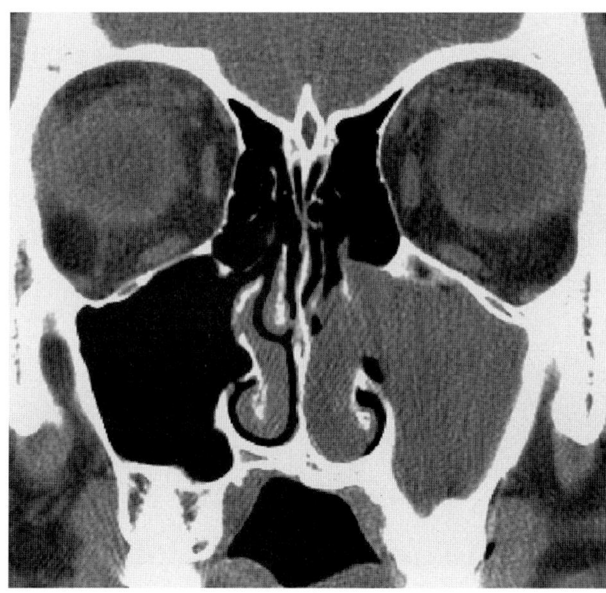

Figure 52L. Patient 4 with antrochoanal polyp. Coronal computed tomography image showing a relatively low density mass filling the left maxillary antrum, with extension into the left middle meatus through the secondary ostium.

CASE 53

Clinical History: A 29-year-old woman presents with midface pain and extensive "crusting" in the nasal cavity. Some minor restriction of ocular motility on the left was also noted. She had no history of sinonasal surgery or cocaine abuse.

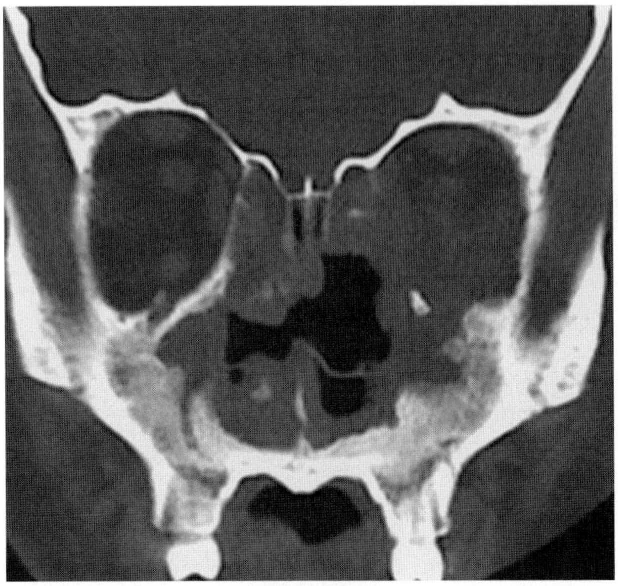

Figure 53A

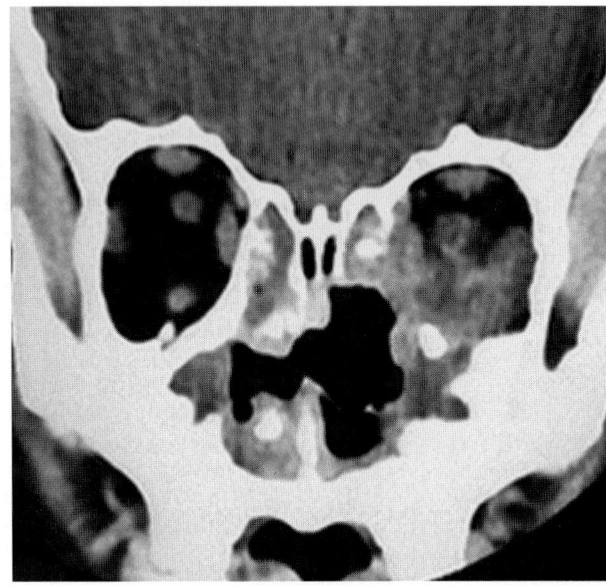

Figure 53B

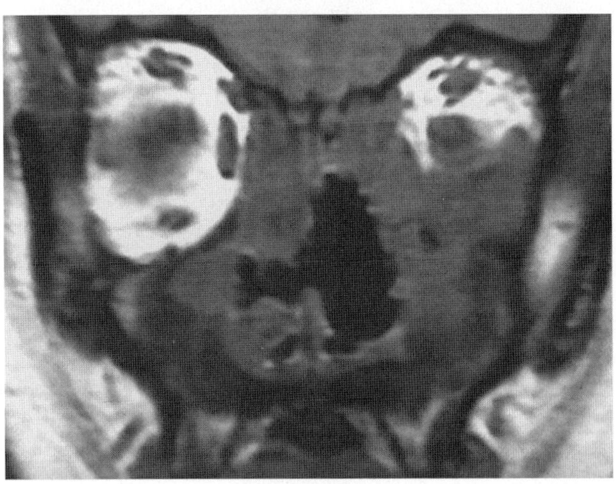

Figure 53C

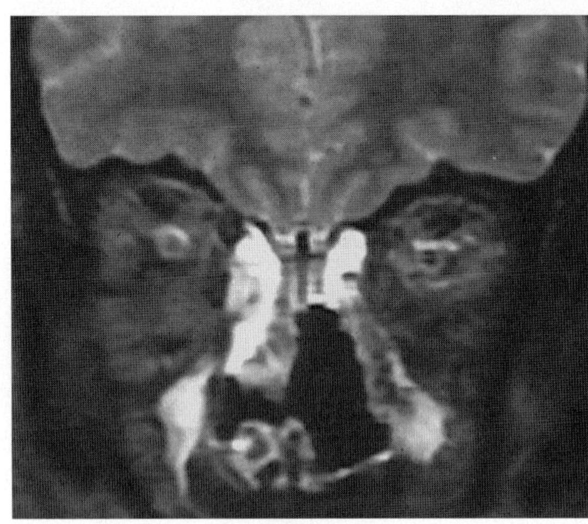

Figure 53D

1. Name two varieties of the disease process that is producing these computed tomography (CT) findings.
2. Name three types of noninfectious inflammatory lesions that commonly involve the sinonasal region.

Findings

Extensive bony destruction of the nasal septum, nasal conchae, medial wall of both maxillary antra, and inferomedial wall of the left orbit. Extensive soft tissue thickening of mixed intensity on STIR image in these area, which enhances on the CT images. The process involves the left orbit.

Problem

A young adult with diffuse, aggressive sinonasal disease destroying the nasal septum and turbinates

Anatomy

A. Nasal cavity: nasal septum (three parts); turbinates (origin and attachments)
B. Maxilla and medial wall of maxillary sinus: contributions from maxilla and palatine bones

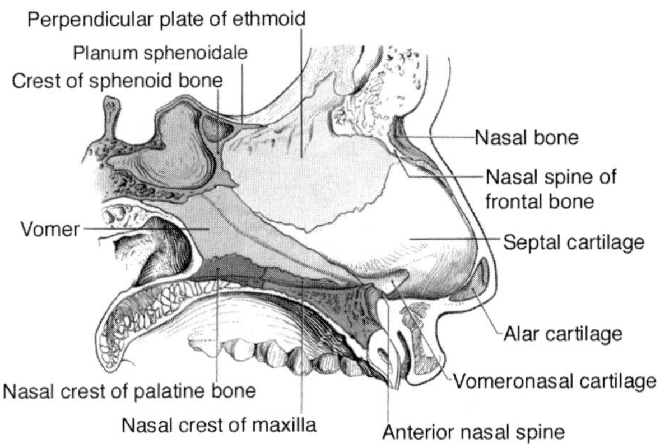

Figure 53E

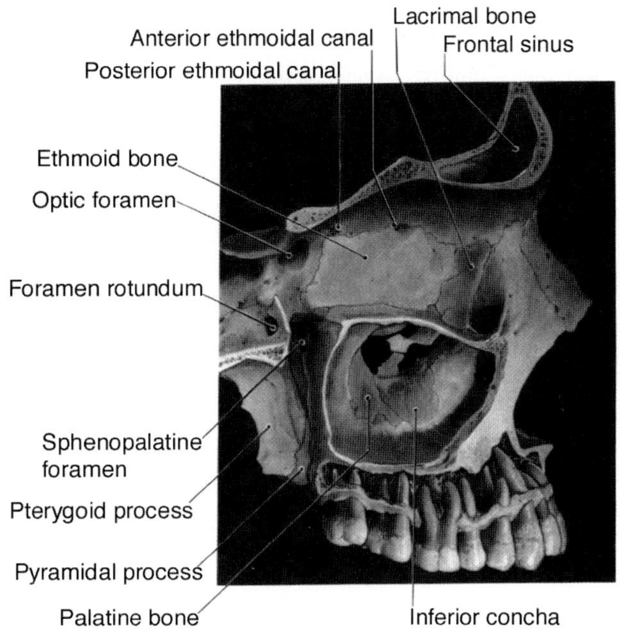

Figure 53F

Differential Diagnosis

Granulomatoses (sarcoidosis, Wegener's granulomatosis, midline granuloma, lymphomatoid granulomatosis), lymphoma, Langerhan's cell histiocytosis (child), plasmacytoma, cocaine abuse

Diagnosis

Wegener's granulomatosis

Diagnostic Imaging Approach

A. Is the disease originating from the nasal cavity or a sinus(es)?
B. Focal, multifocal or diffuse disease?
C. Is the process infiltrative or well defined? Analyze T1- and T2-weighted signal, enhancement, vascularity.
D. Is there bone destruction?
E. If the disease involves the nasal cavity, is the nasal septum destroyed?
F. Are any surrounding areas involved, including orbits, intracranial sites, nasopharynx?

Clinical Points of Importance and Supplemental Information

A. The diagnosis of Wegener's granulomatosis or midline granuloma can be strongly suggested when this or a similar pattern of sinonasal disease is observed. The clinician should be alerted to order an antineutrophil cytoplasmic antibodies (ANCA) test; cyclophosphamide therapy needs to begin promptly in this disease to preserve renal and pulmonary function.
B. Wegener's granulomatosis is probably at the most benign (inflammatory) end of a disease spectrum that includes the progressively more severe midline granuloma, lymphomatoid granulomatosis, and lymphoma. Midline granuloma may actually be more easy to control than Wegener's granulomatosis because of its lack of systemic involvement (i.e., it can be controlled with radiotherapy).

Answers to Questions

1. Midline granuloma; Wegener's granulomatosis
2. Sarcoidosis, Wegener's granulomatosis, histiocytosis

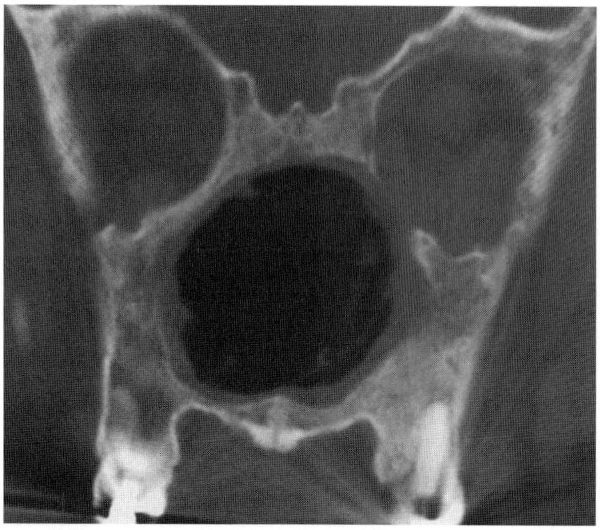

Figure 53G. Patient 1 with endstage Wegener's granulomatosis. Coronal computed tomography image at bone window setting showing destruction of the nasal septum and conchae, with chronic inflammatory change of the bone. (This is the same patient as presented in the 53A–D, several years later.)

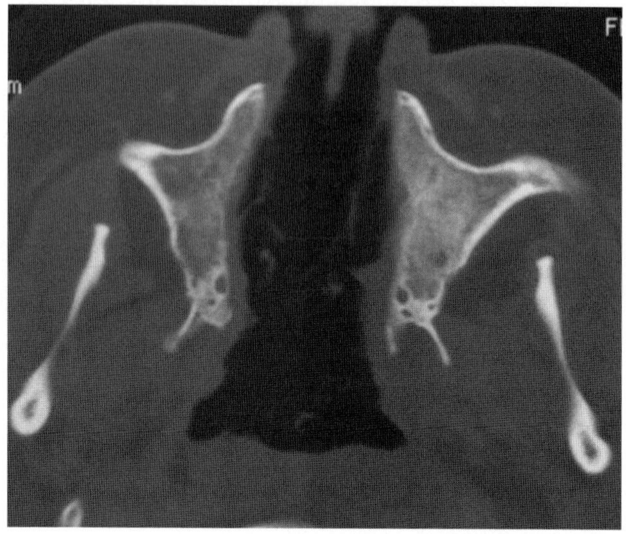

Figure 53H. Patient 1 with Wegener's granulomatosis. Axial computed tomography image at bone window setting showing destruction of the bony portion of the nasal septum and conchae. Sinus obliteration with reactive bone also seen.

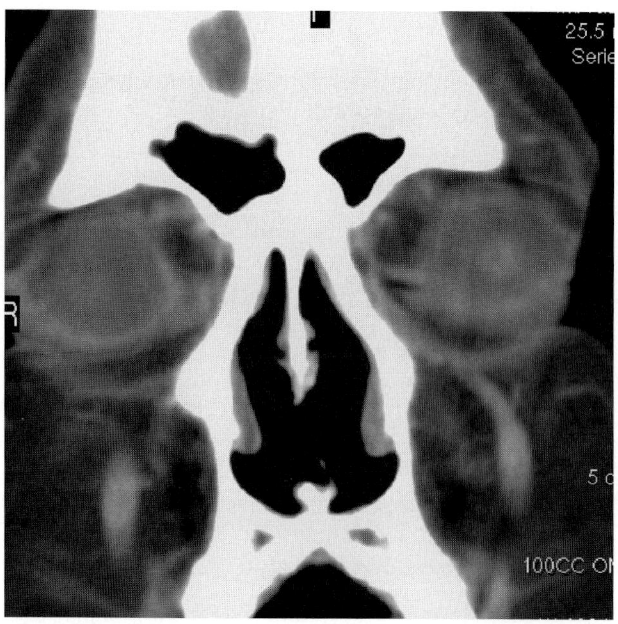

Figure 53I. Patient 2 with invasive fungal sinusitis. Coronal computed tomography image at soft tissue window setting showing a large septal perforation.

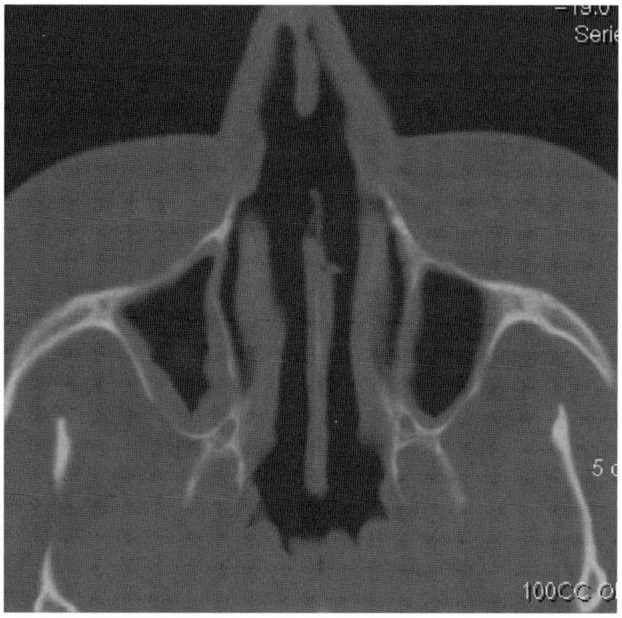

Figure 53J. Patient 2 with invasive fungal sinusitis. Axial computed tomography image at bone window setting.

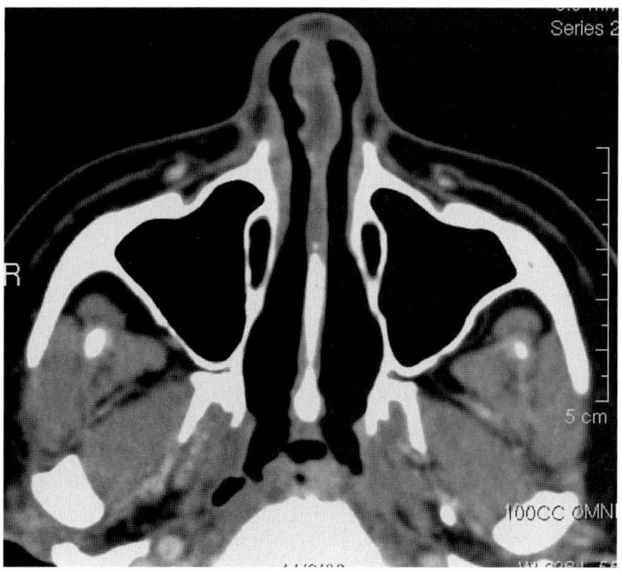

Figure 53K. Patient 3 with acute myeloid leukemia, showing soft tissue swelling in the cartilaginous portion of the nasal septum caused by invasive fungal disease. Axial computed tomography image at soft tissue window setting.

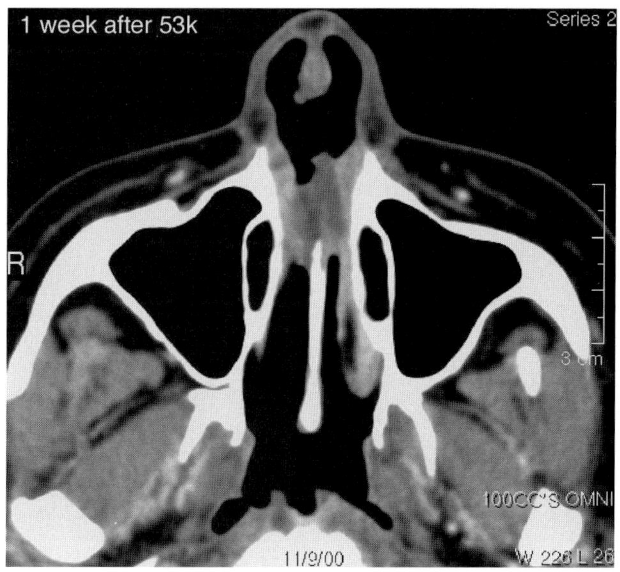

Figure 53L. Patient 3 with acute myeloid leukemia. Axial computed tomography image, 1 week after Fig. 53K, showing necrosis and perforation of the nasal septum.

CASE 54

Clinical History: A 55-year-old man presents with retroorbital headaches radiating to the vertex and occiput.

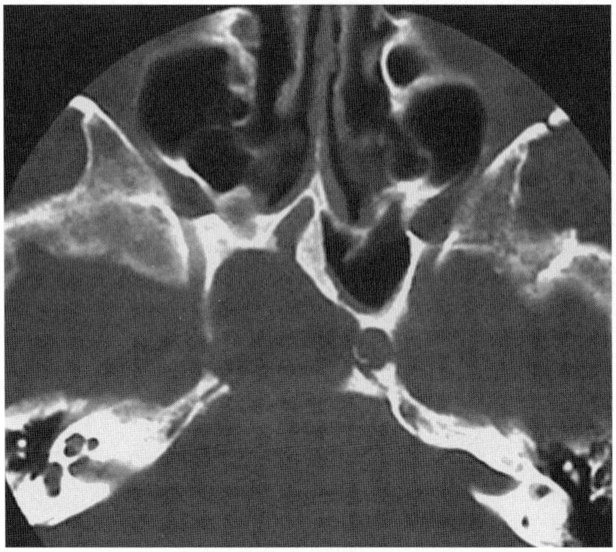

Figure 54A

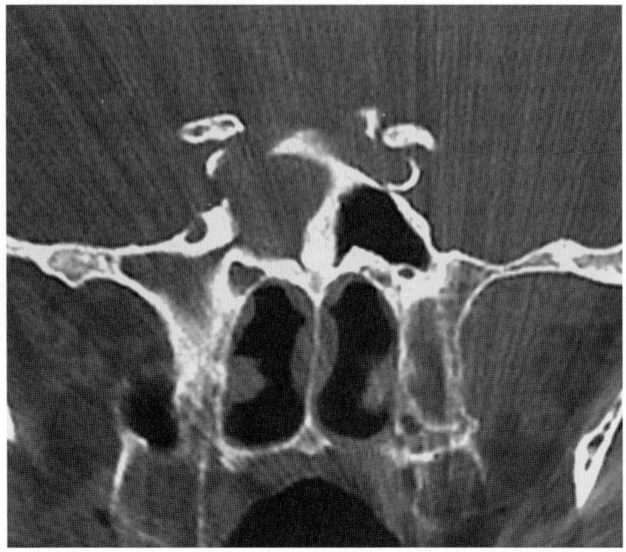

Figure 54B

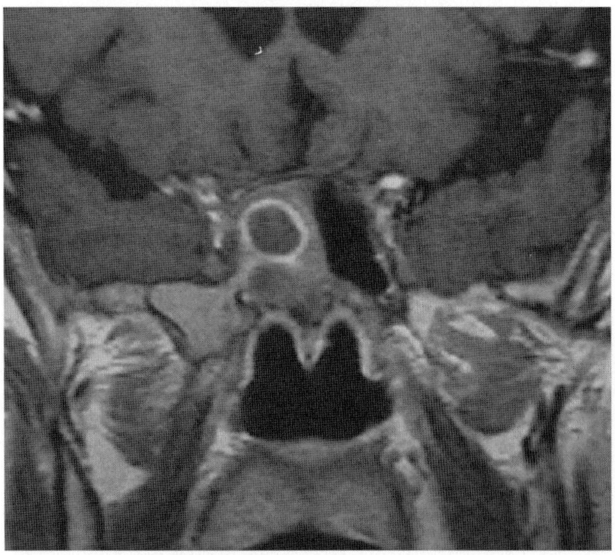

Figure 54C

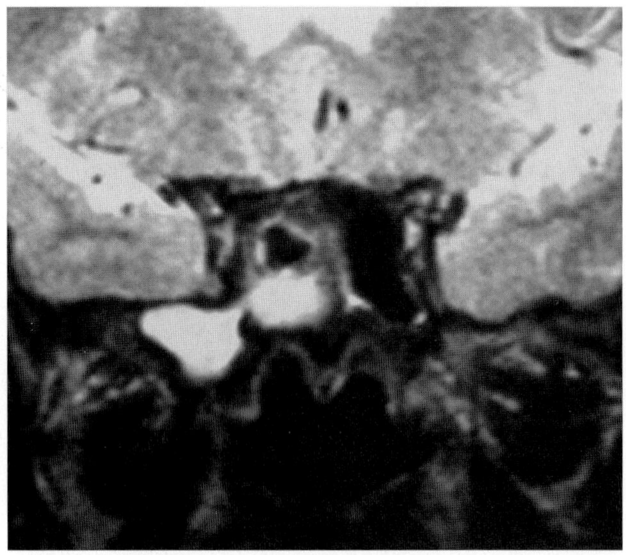

Figure 54D

1. What accounts for the dark central focus on the T2-weighted magnetic resonance image?
2. Give the most likely complete diagnosis.
3. When unilateral or isolated sinus disease is present, especially in an adult, what are the three prime obligations of the radiologist?

Findings

An abnormal soft tissue density in the expansile-appearing sphenoid sinus. The lesion is generally of high intensity after contrast-enhanced T1-weighted images with a rim-enhancing low intensity area within it. T2-weighted image shows the central area of opacification actually of low signal intensity, which contiguously involves the right lateral extension of the sphenoid sinus. Coronal computed tomography image at bone window setting shows concentric enlargement of the right Vidian canal.

Problem

An adult with vertex headaches and pathology centered in the sphenoid sinus

Anatomy

A. Sphenoid sinus: relationship to dura mater of sella, clivus, and cavernous sinus, and to carotid arteries and orbits
B. Nasal cavity: sphenoid sinus ostia, sphenoethmoidal recess, superior meatus, posterior ethmoidal arteries

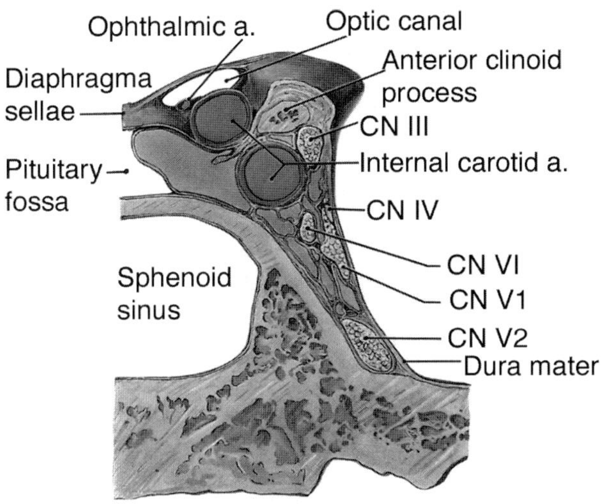

Figure 54E

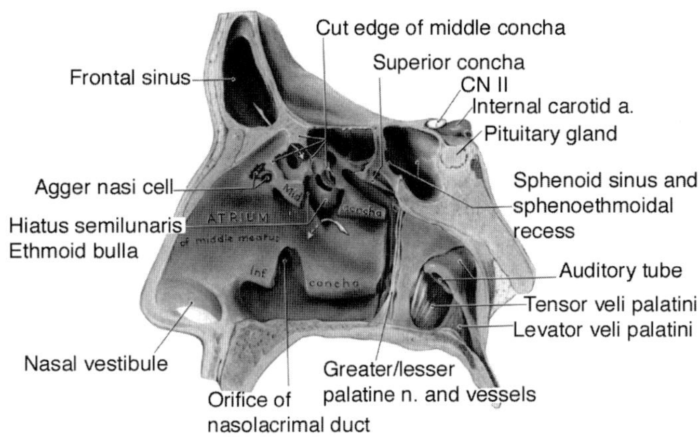

Figure 54F

Differential Diagnosis

Not applicable

Diagnosis

Sphenoid sinus mucocele with secondary fungal colonization

Diagnostic Imaging Approach

A. Is the disease originating from the nasal cavity or a sinus(es)?
B. If it is related to a sinus, is the sinus:
   1. Completely opacified?
   2. Expanded?
   3. Walls eroded?
C. Is there extension to surrounding structures (e.g., cavernous sinus, orbit, meninges, brain, pituitary, skull base, cranial nerves)?
D. Evaluate morphology of sinus contents: is the pattern suggestive of mucosal disease with trapped secretions (e.g., mucocele pattern) or a mass?
E. Is an obstructing mass in the nasal cavity (especially if one sinus or one side is involved)?

Clinical Points of Importance and Supplemental Information

A. Vertex headaches strongly suggest sphenoid sinus or central skull base pathology.
B. The low signal intensity of the sinus concretions is probably caused by desiccation (decrease in free water) of sinus secretions and fungal colonization (heavy metals within the fungal elements).

Answers to Questions

1. Fungal colonization
2. Sphenoid sinus mucocele colonized with fungi
3. Exclude an obstructing mass lesion, identify bone destruction, and anticipate critical complications (e.g., optic neuropathy or cavernous sinus involvement)

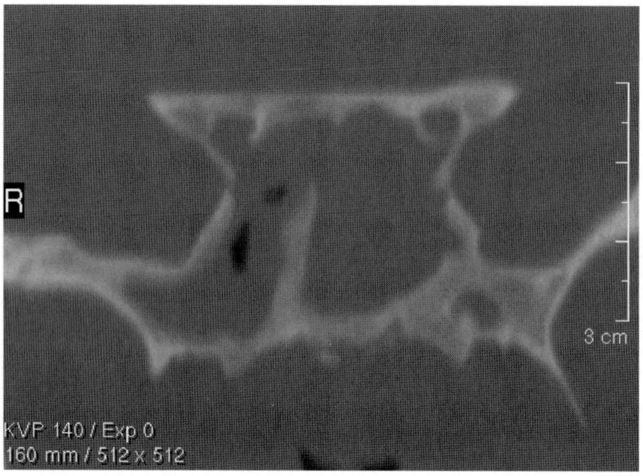

Figure 54G. Patient 1 with sphenoid sinusitis, showing mucosal thickening of the sphenoid sinus, with diffuse bony wall thickening suggestive of chronic inflammation. Bone dehiscence is seen over the right optic canal; this is an important surgical consideration. Coronal computed tomography image at bone window setting.

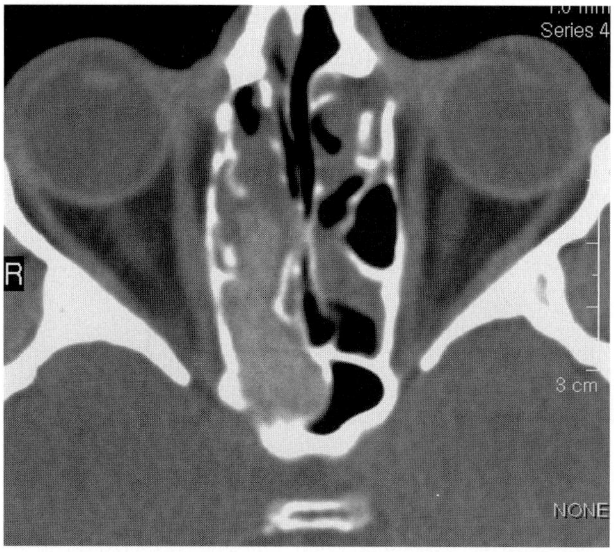

Figure 54H. Patient 2 with sphenoethmoidal mucocele. Axial computed tomography image showing complete opacification of the right sphenoid and posterior ethmoid sinuses, with expansile change. Bone dehiscence over the optic canal is identified on the right, which is an important surgical consideration.

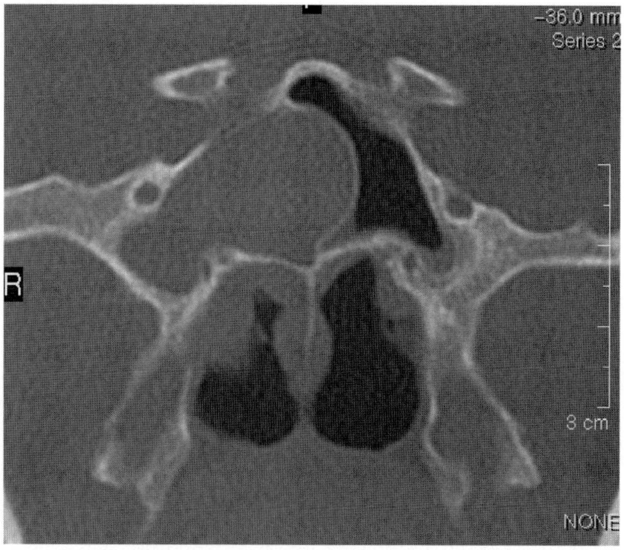

Figure 54I. Patient 2 with sphenoethmoidal mucocele. Coronal computed tomography image at bone window setting showing complete opacification of right sphenoid sinus, with expansile change.

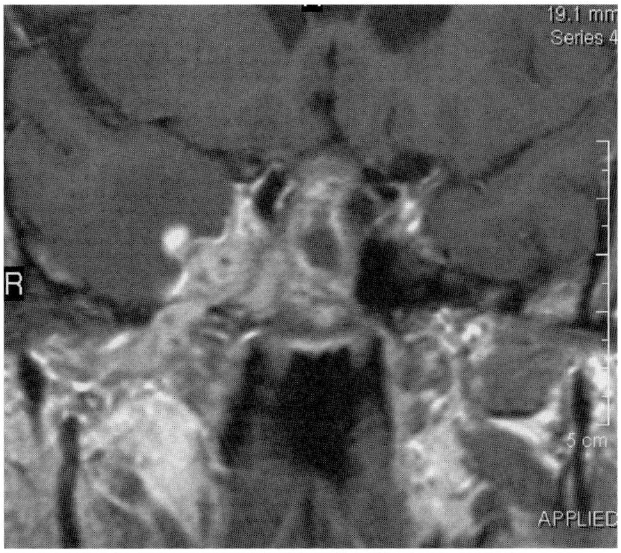

Figure 54J. Patient 3 with intracranial complication of invasive fungal sinusitis. T1-weighted coronal image with contrast showing enhancing tissue in the sphenoid sinus, with direct invasion of adjacent right cavernous sinus and brain parenchyma in the medial aspect of the right temporal lobe.

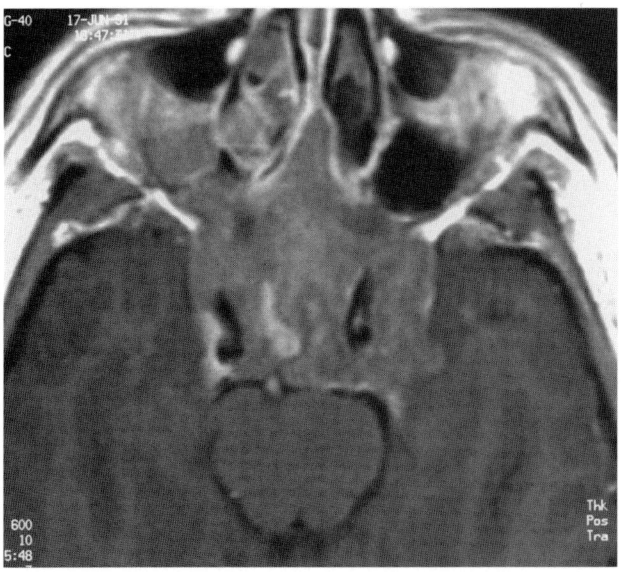

Figure 54K. Patient 4 with invasive pituitary adenoma, showing infiltrative, inhomogeneously enhancing mass involving the pituitary fossa and cavernous sinus on both sides and encasing the internal carotid artery. T1-weighted axial image with contrast.

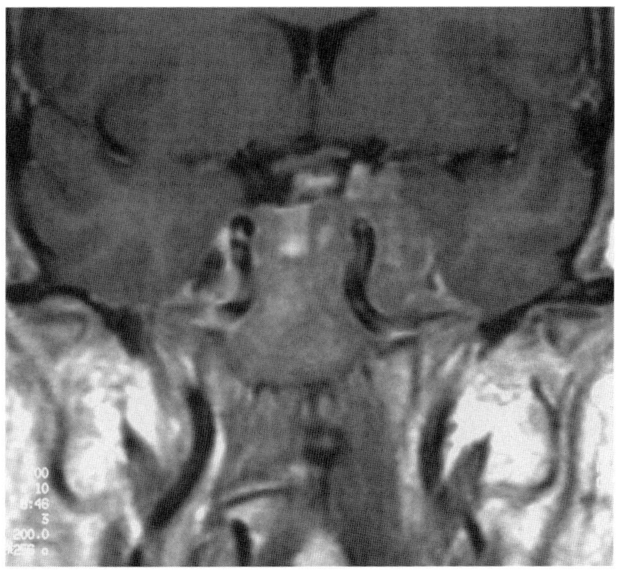

Figure 54L. Patient 4 with invasive pituitary adenoma. T1-weighted coronal image with contrast.

CASE 55

Clinical History: A 46-year-old man who presents with chronic polypoid rhinosinusitis had this study as part of an evaluation for possible endoscopic sinus surgery.

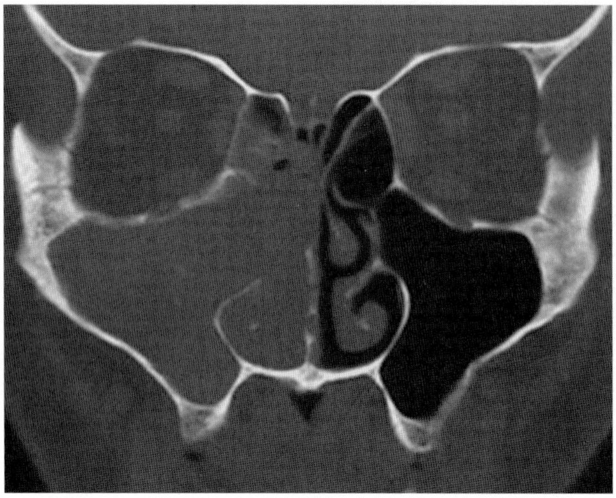

Figure 55A

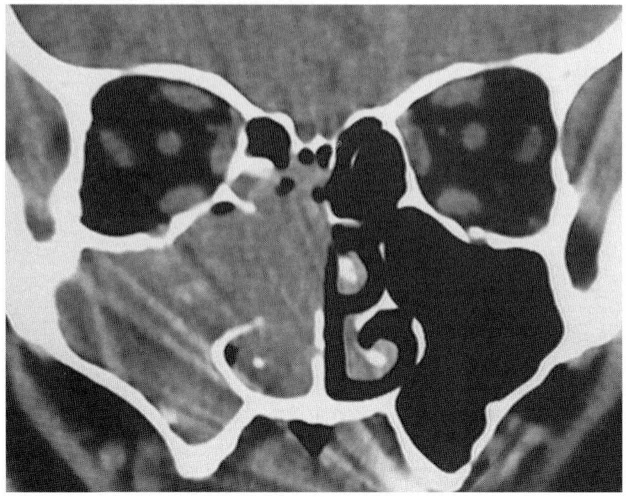

Figure 55B

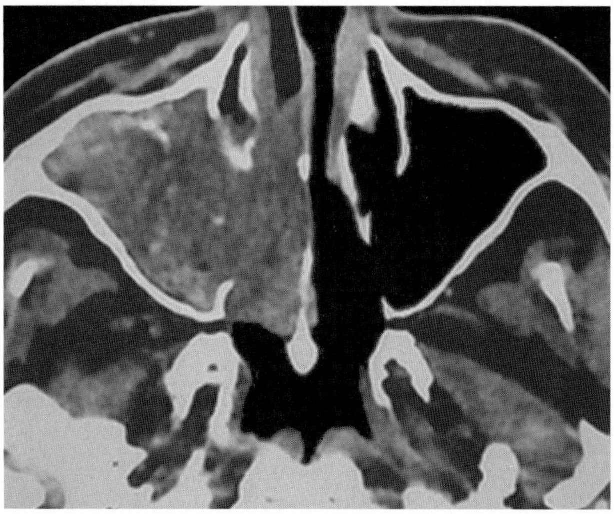

Figure 55C

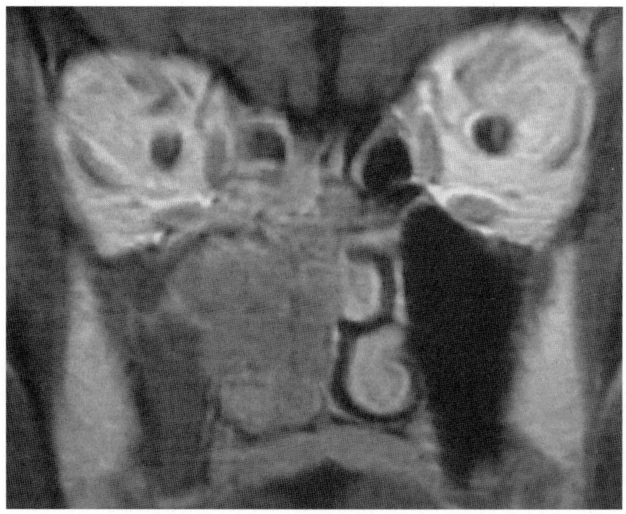

Figure 55D

1. Are all the changes present attributable to chronic "allergic" polyposis?
2. Why does a large portion of the normal maxillary sinus medial wall frequently appear non-ossified?
3. Are the densities within the sinus contents (axial view) helpful in the differential diagnosis?

Findings

Computed tomography (CT) shows an abnormal soft tissue density opacifying the right maxillary antrum and right nasal fossa, with destruction of the medial wall of the antrum and part of the middle and inferior nasal conchae. Spotty calcific densities are seen in it. Internal density of the lesion is inhomogeneous on soft tissue setting CT image. Anterior and posterolateral walls of the involved right maxillary antrum are thicker than the opposite. Contrast-enhanced T1-weighted image discloses inhomogeneously enhancing tissue centered in the medial aspect of the right maxillary antrum and nasal fossa, with obstructive sinusitis of more peripheral maxillary antrum.

Problem

An adult with a sinonasal mass that appears to be eroding bone

Anatomy

A. Maxillary sinus: primary ostium, secondary ostium, "fibrous" portion ("fontanelle") of medial wall (see Fig. 52F)
B. Nasal cavity: infundibulum, uncinate process, hiatus semilunaris, ethmoidal bulla, middle turbinate (vertical and horizontal attachments); middle meatus

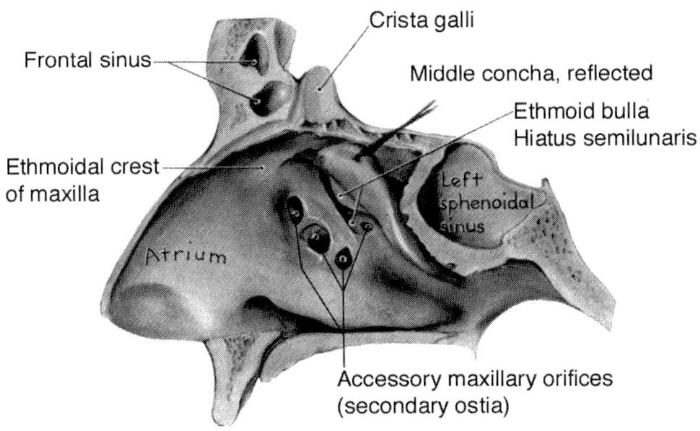

Figure 55E

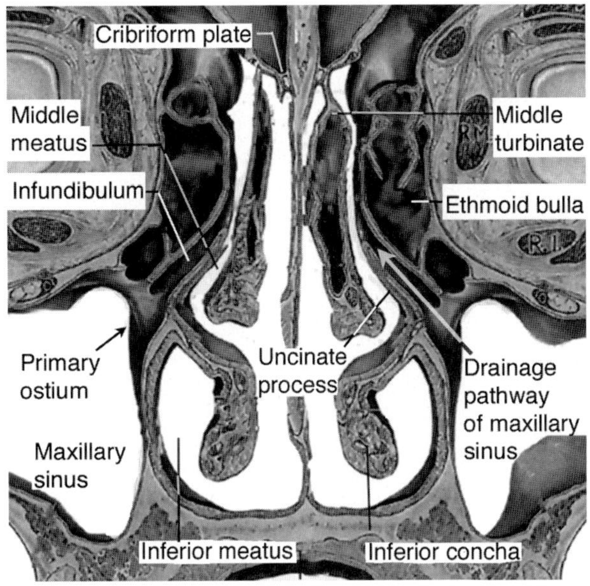

Figure 55F

Differential Diagnosis

Inverted papilloma, antrochoanal polyp, carcinoma, olfactory neuroblastoma, lymphoma, plasmacytoma, melanoma, extracranial meningioma, hemangiopericytoma, rhabdomyosarcoma (child), other sarcoma, metastases

Diagnosis

Inverted papilloma containing foci of squamous cell carcinoma

Diagnostic Approach

A. Is the disease originating from the nasal cavity or a sinus(es)?
B. If nasal cavity origin, is it from the lateral wall, turbinates, or septum? Is the septum destroyed?
C. Focal, multifocal, or diffuse disease?
D. Well-circumscribed or infiltrative disease?
E. Is there bone destruction? Sclerosis?
F. If there is a mass, analyze morphology: T1- or T2-weighted signal, enhancement, vascularity, calcified matrix, other calcifications (or focal density).
G. Is there extension to adjacent structures: other sinuses, intracranial, nasopharynx, orbits, hard palate, perineural?

Clinical Points of Importance and Supplemental Information

A. Inverted papilloma will contain foci of squamous cell carcinoma in about 10% to 15% of cases. They must be resected with clear margins, even if this requires craniofacial resection.
B. The medial wall of the maxillary sinus has a "fontanelle" or "fibrous" portion between the contributions of the palatine bone and maxilla to the medial wall; it is here that the sinus will bulge most easily and where bone erosion may be misdiagnosed.

Answers to Questions

1. No
2. A gap (fontanelle) exists between the contribution of the maxillary sinus medial wall and the palatine bone contributions to the lateral nasal wall
3. Yes, suggestive of inverted papilloma but also suggest fungal colonization

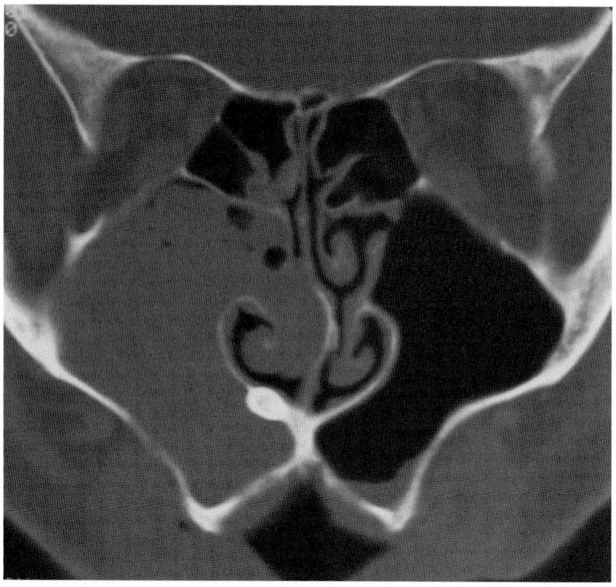

Figure 55G. Patient 1 with inverted papilloma, showing a soft tissue mass filling the right maxillary sinus, with destruction of the medial wall of the sinus and a direct extension into the middle meatus. Coronal computed tomography image at bone window setting.

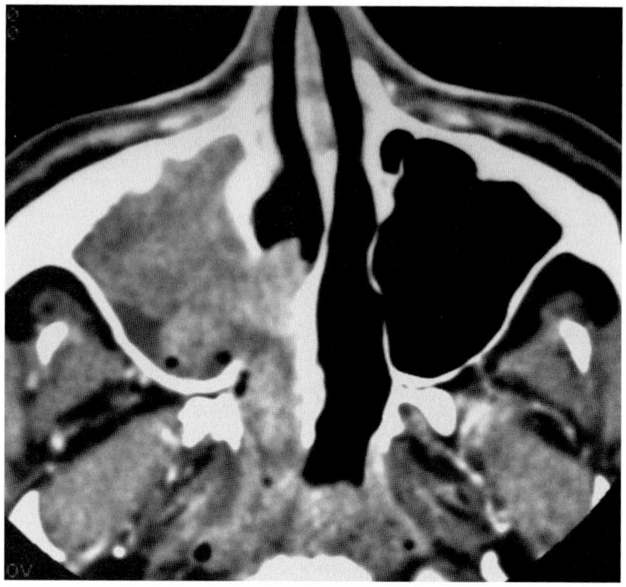

Figure 55H. Patient 1 with inverted papilloma. Contrast-enhanced axial computed tomography image showing a solid enhancing mass involving the right maxillary sinus, with direct extension into the right nasal cavity.

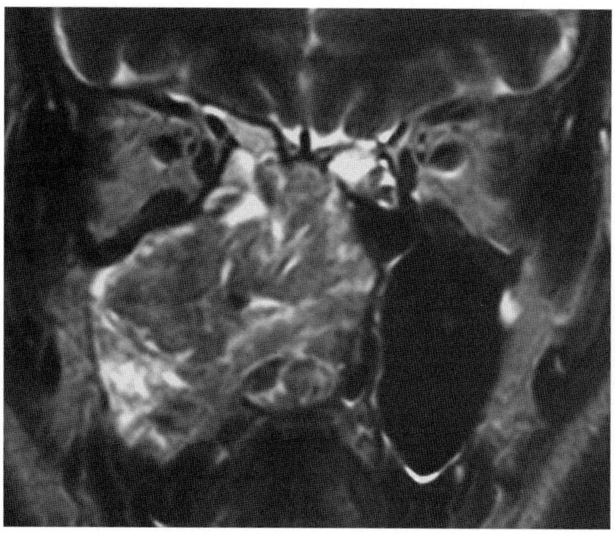

Figure 55I. Patient 2 with inverted papilloma, showing a solid mass of convoluted cerebriform pattern involving the right maxillary sinus and nasal cavity. T2-weighted coronal image.

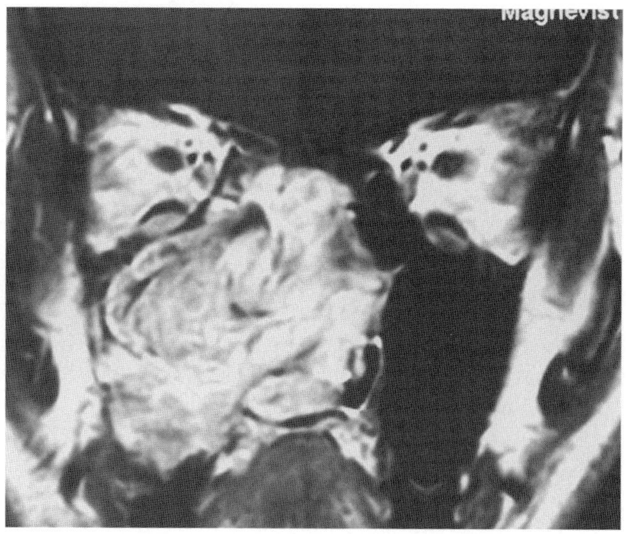

Figure 55J. Patient 2 with inverted papilloma. T1-weighted coronal image with contrast showing enhancement of the mass, with convoluted cerebriform pattern.

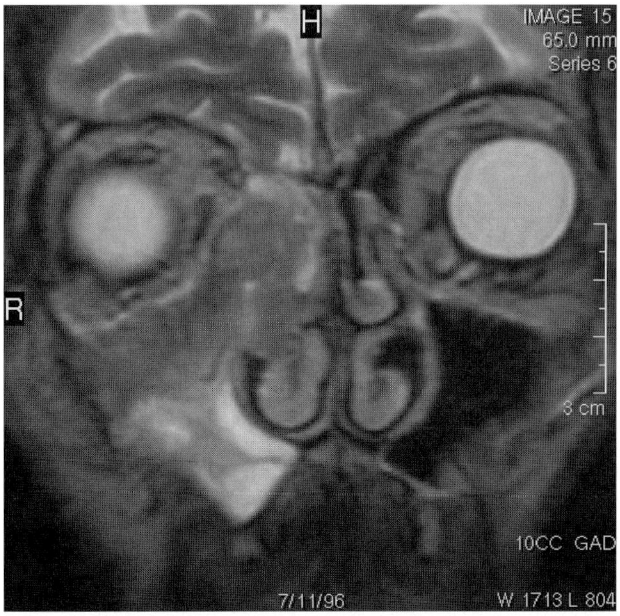

Figure 55K. Patient 3 with maxillary sinus carcinoma. T2-weighted coronal image showing relatively low-intensity mass extending into the right ethmoid and middle meatus from the right maxillary sinus through the enlarged primary ostium. Inflammatory mucosal thickening in the lower maxillary sinus reveals much higher intensity than the mass.

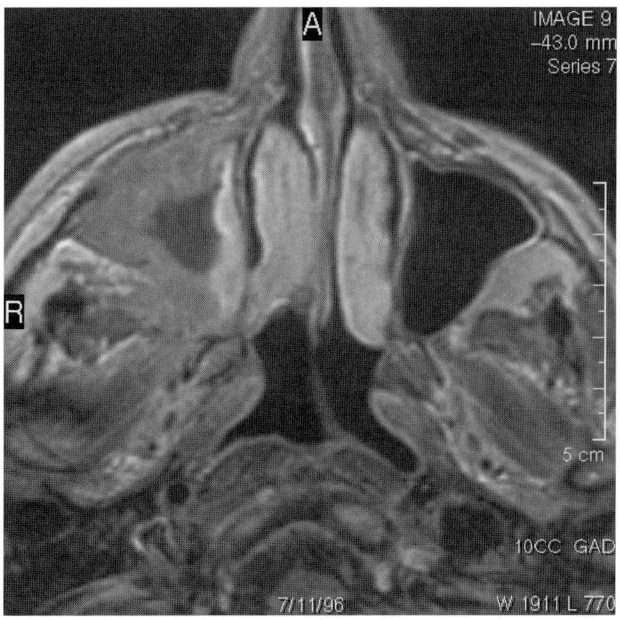

Figure 55L. Patient 3 with maxillary sinus carcinoma, showing an enhancing mass mainly involving the anterior and posterolateral aspect of the right maxillary sinus with extension into the retroantral fat pad and soft tissue under the superficial musculoaponeurotic system in the cheek. Inflammatory mucosal thickening enhances more intensely than the mass.

CASE 56

Clinical History: A 69-year-old woman presents with nasal stuffiness.

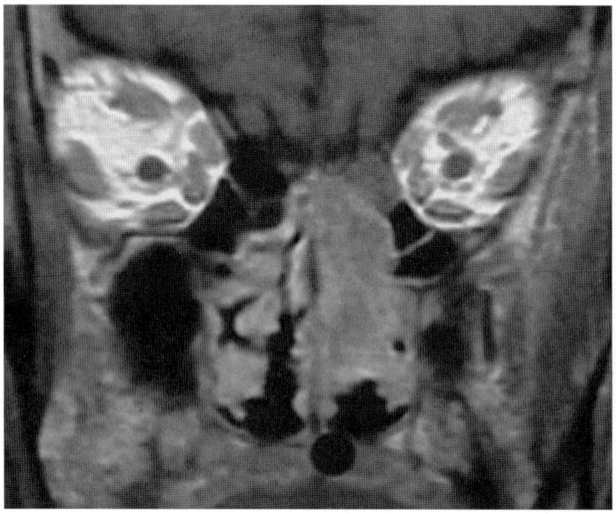

Figure 56A

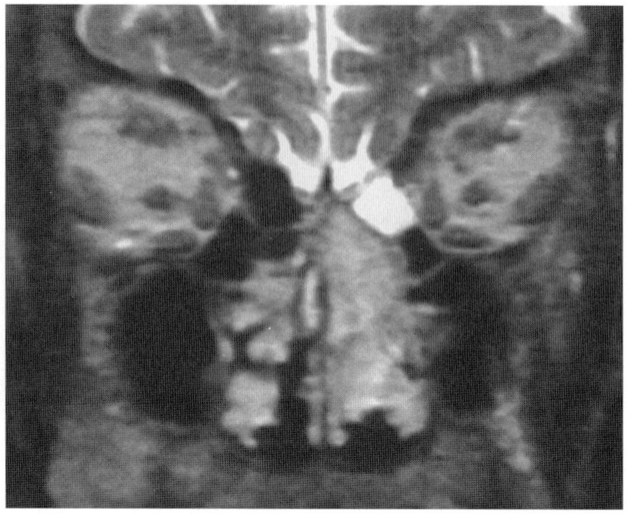

Figure 56B

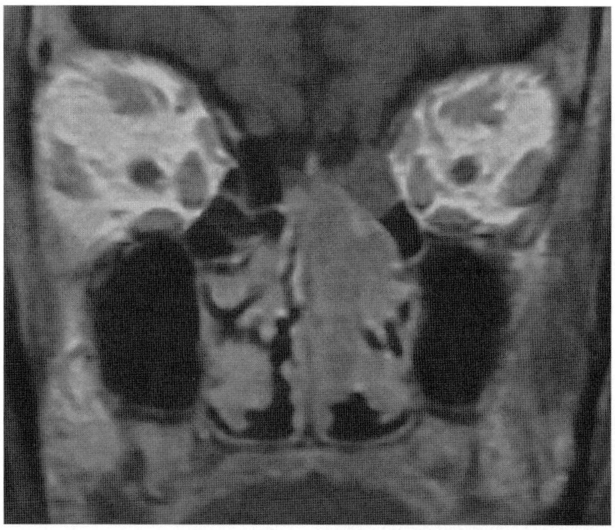

Figure 56C

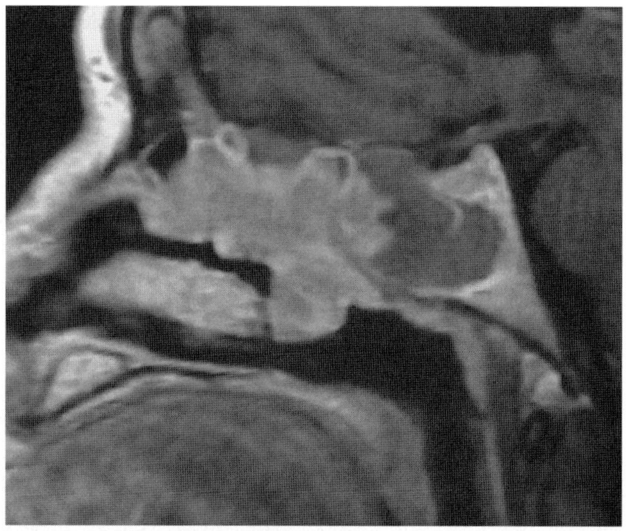

Figure 56D

1. Precisely, from where is the mass arising?
2. Does the mass cross the cribriform plate on the images shown? If the answer is "yes," the patient will require a craniofacial resection.
3. How do you identify the position of the anterior ethmoid artery on coronal computed tomography (CT) or magnetic resonance imaging (MRI)? Would such knowledge be required in this case?

Findings

An inhomogeneously enhancing mass in the left ethmoid sinus and the nasal cavity. The lesion abuts the cribriform plate, with small intracranial extension seen on the coronal MRI minimally displacing the left olfactory bulb and tract. The lesion contiguously involves the anterior part of the sphenoid sinus via sphenoethmoidal recess and results in obstructive sphenoid sinusitis. Secondary fluid collection is also identified in left ethmoid bulla.

Problem

An elderly woman with a mass arising in the superior portion of the nasal cavity

Anatomy

A. Middle meatus (see Fig. 55F)
B. Nasal septum: vertical plate of the ethmoid, vomer and cartilaginous portions (see Fig. 53E)
C. Cribriform plate (see Fig. 55F)
D. Anterior ethmoid canal and nasal slit
E. Planum sphenoidale

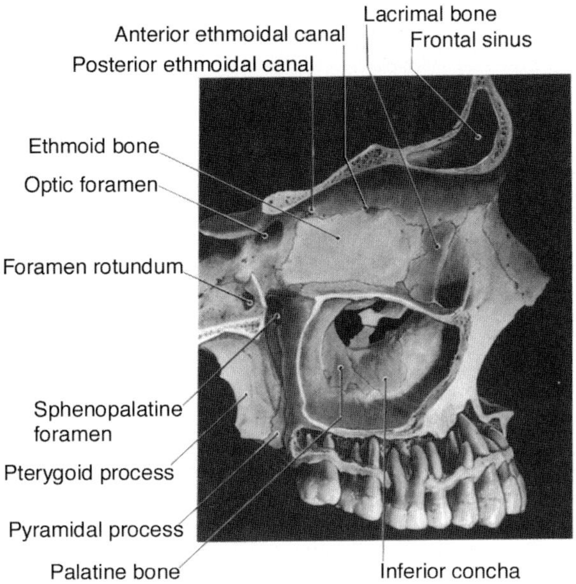

Figure 56E

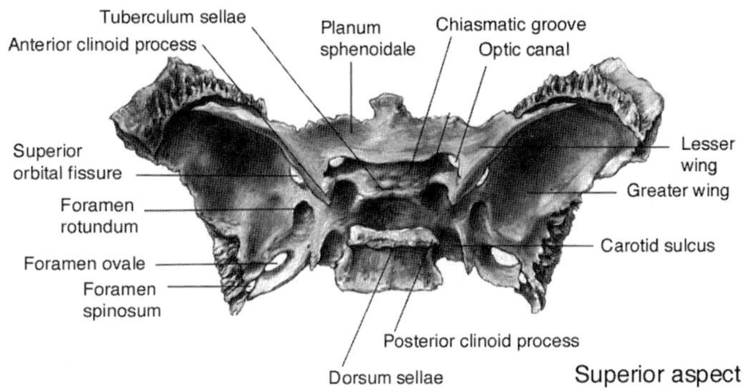

Figure 56F

Differential Diagnosis

Carcinoma, lymphoma, melanoma, sarcoma, metastasis, meningioma

Diagnosis

Olfactory neuroblastoma (esthesioneuroblastoma), with early intracranial spread across the cribriform plate

Diagnostic Imaging Approach

A. Determine whether the mass *arises* in the nasal cavity, paranasal sinus(es), orbit, or intracranially.
B. Look for bone destruction and, if present, determine whether it suggests a rapid growth rate (weeks to months, e.g., aggressive inflammation or cancer) or slower growth rate (months to years, e.g., benign lesion or slowly growing malignancy).
C. Determine extent:
   1. Local spread to nasal septum or to adjacent sinus(es)?
   2. Orbit?
   3. Intracranial (extradural, dural, pia-arachnoid or subarachnoid space, brain involvement)?
   4. Perineural spread?
   5. Retropharyngeal or other adenopathy?
D. Determine precise relationship of tumor to the anterior skull base (anterior and posterior ethmoid arteries, planum sphenoidale).

Clinical Points of Importance and Supplemental Information

Olfactory neuroblastoma can grow intracranially via the olfactory neuroepithelium and related nerves *without* CT or MRI evidence of intracranial spread. Tumor abutting the cribriform plate should be presumed to have spread intracranially, at least microscopically.

Answers to Questions

1. Nasal cavity, mainly anteriorly and superiorly
2. Yes
3. Find the anterior ethmoid canal at the down slope of the crista galli. Yes.

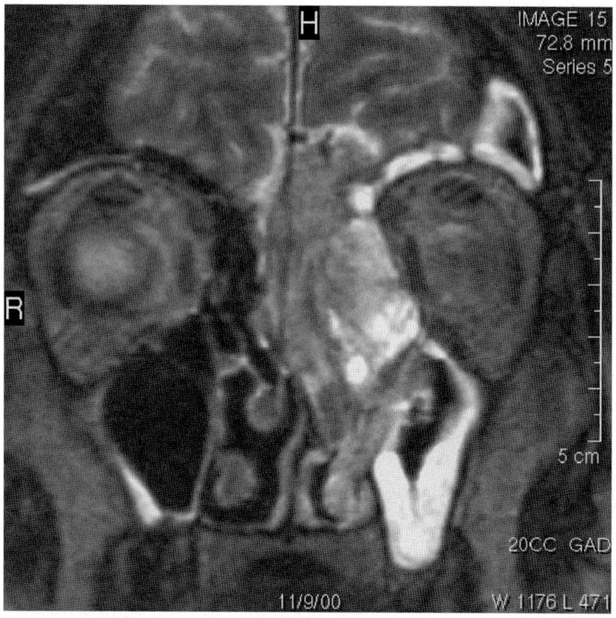

Figure 56G. Patient 1 with olfactory neuroblastoma, showing a mass involving the left ethmoid sinus and nasal cavity that stays centered in the expected position of the left olfactory groove. The mass extends intracranially, with destruction of the cribriform plate. The signal intensity of the mass is lower than inflammatory mucosa. T2-weighted coronal image.

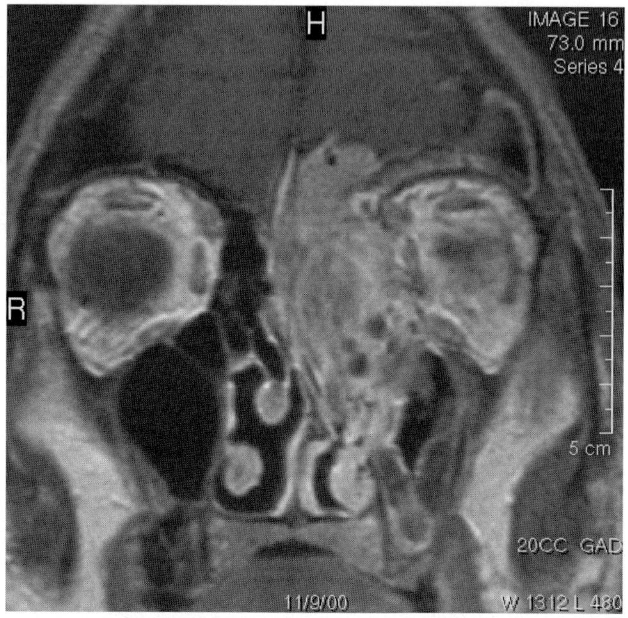

Figure 56H. Patient 1 with olfactory neuroblastoma. T1-weighted coronal image with contrast showing inhomogeneous enhancement of the mass, which is much more than that of inflammatory mucosa. Pial enhancement adjacent to the intracranial component of the mass is seen in the base of the left frontal lobe.

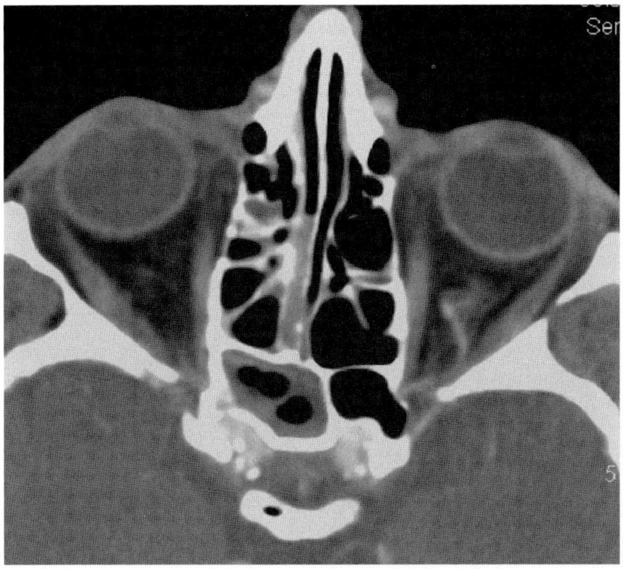

Figure 56I. Patient 2 with olfactory neuroblastoma. Axial computed tomography showing solid, enhancing mass within the right posterior olfactory groove, which is impossible to differentiate from more “routine” mucosal disease on these images.

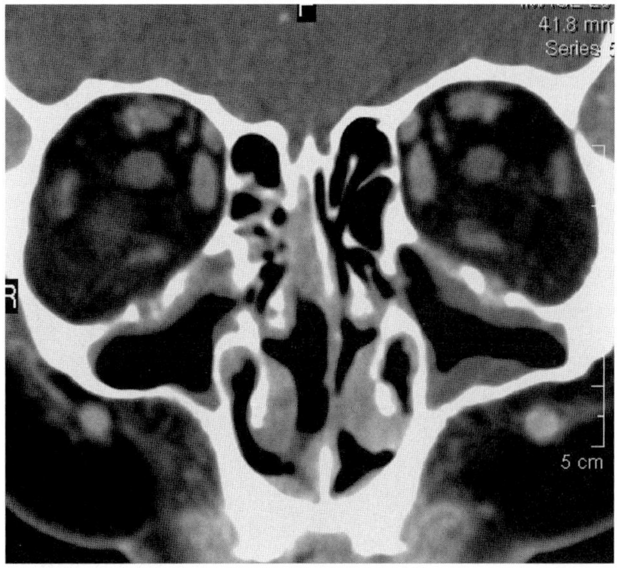

Figure 56J. Patient 2 with olfactory neuroblastoma. Coronal computed tomography image also showing enhancing mass in the right olfactory groove.

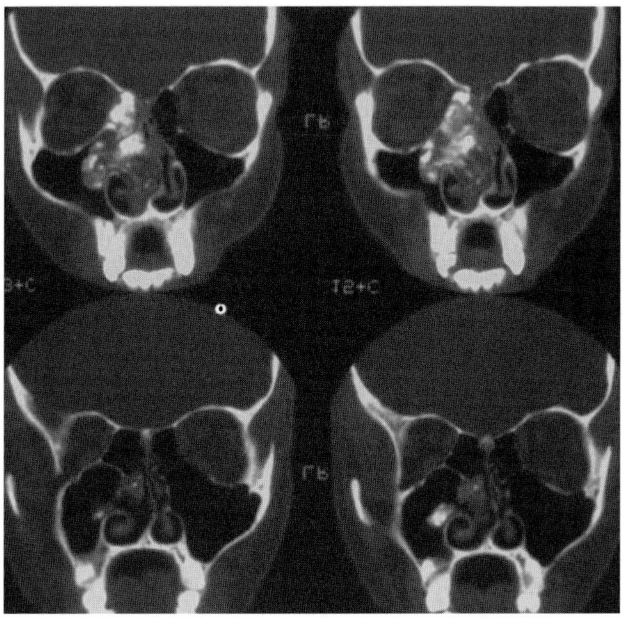

Figure 56K. Patient 3 with calcifying olfactory neuroblastoma. Coronal computed tomography images at bone window setting showing soft tissue mass, with calcification involving the ethmoidal and maxillary sinuses and superior nasal cavity, including the area of the olfactory groove.

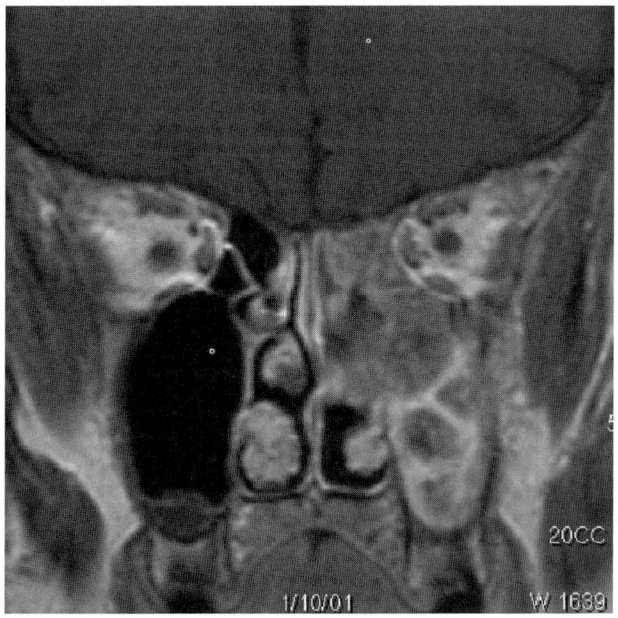

Figure 56L. Patient 4 with moderately differentiated squamous cell carcinoma of the sinonasal cavity. T1-weighted coronal image with contrast showing inhomogeneously enhancing mass involving the left upper nasal cavity and adjacent ethmoid and superomedial aspect of the maxillary sinus, although apparently sparing the olfactory groove.

CASE 57

Clinical History: A 69-year-old woman presents with facial pain.

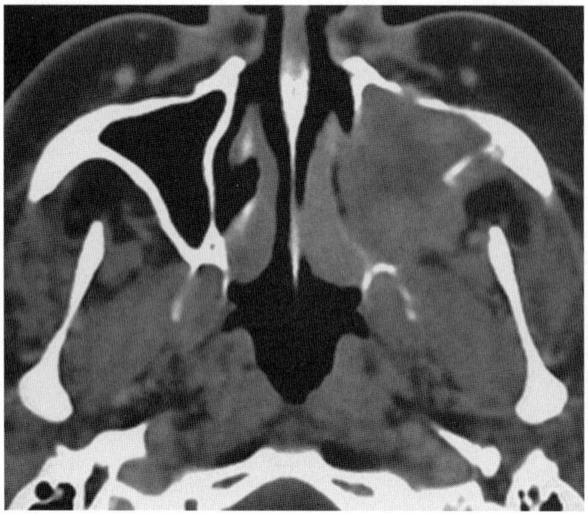

Figure 57A

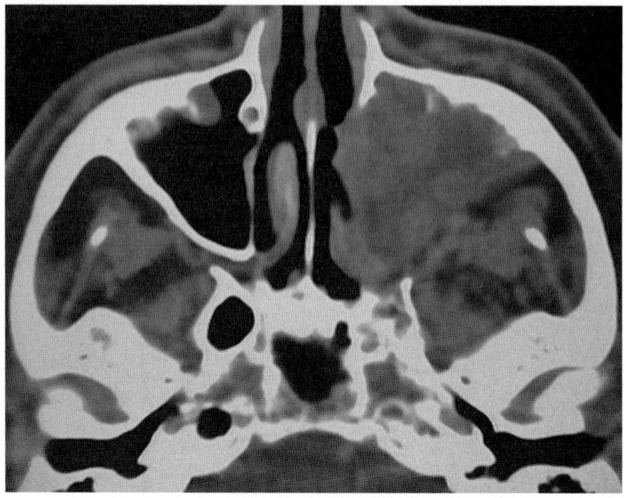

Figure 57B

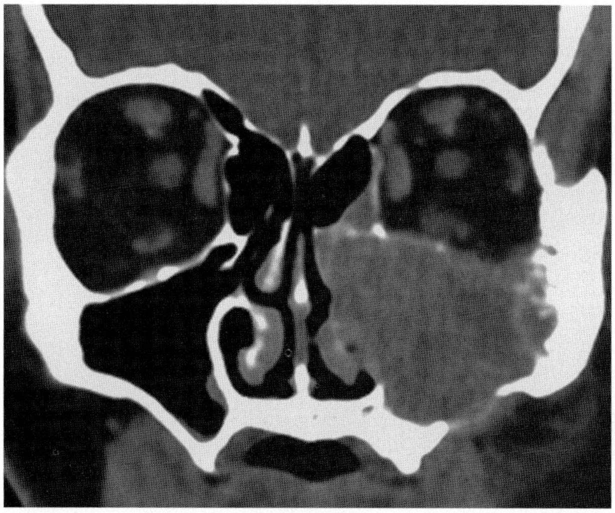

Figure 57C

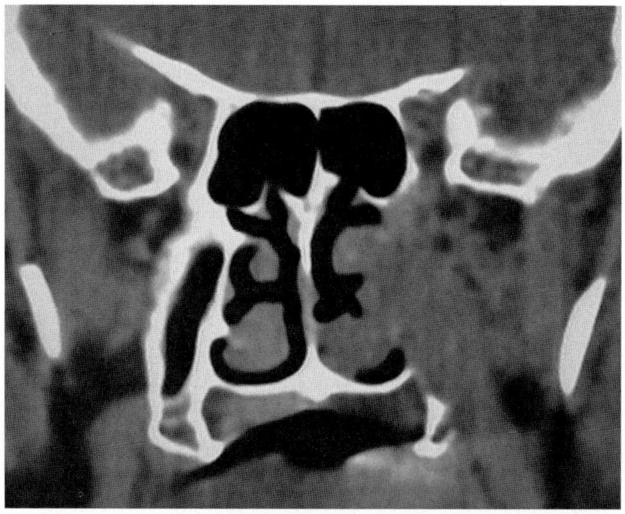

Figure 57D

1. Is the lesion more likely inflammatory or neoplastic?
2. What is the hallmark of aggressive sinonasal pathology?
3. In sinonasal cancer, what four prime areas of involvement will influence the choice of therapy? Prognosis?

Findings

Soft tissue density fills the left maxillary antrum and contiguously involves the infratemporal fossa (buccal space), including pterygopalatine fossa posteriorly, lateral nasal cavity medially, left orbit superiorly, alveolar process inferiorly, and soft tissue of the cheek anteriorly (presumably through the inferior orbital foramen), with extensive bony destruction. An area of greater palatine foramen is imbedded in the lesion. The left inferior orbital fissure is partly involved by the lesion.

Problem

An elderly woman with facial pain caused by an aggressive mass centered in the left maxillary sinus

Anatomy

A. Maxillary sinus: maxillary, zygomatic, and palatine bone portions
B. Ostiomeatal unit: middle meatus, uncinate process, ethmoid bulla, primary ostium of maxillary sinus and infundibulum, hiatus semilunaris (see Fig. 55F)
C. Infraorbital canal, greater and lesser palatine canals and foramina, pterygopalatine fossa (see Fig. 54F)
D. Infratemporal fossa

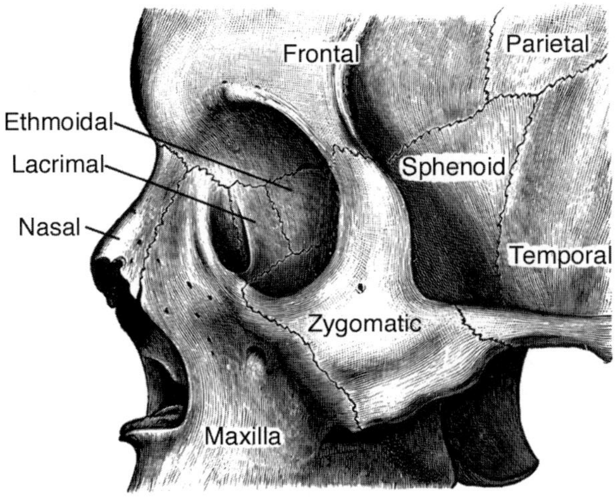

Figure 57E

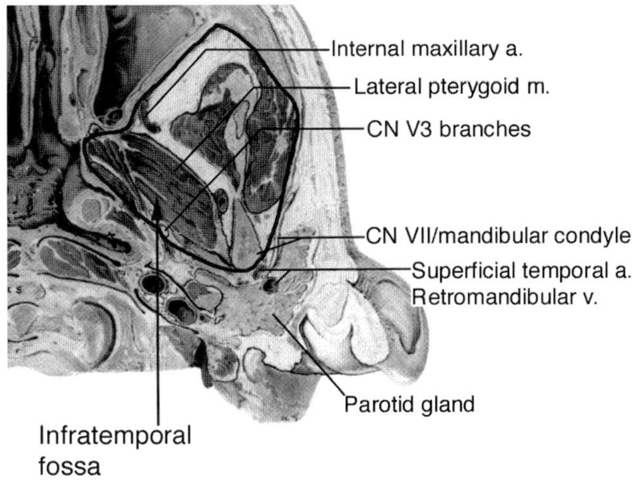

Figure 57F

Differential Diagnosis

Carcinoma, lymphoma, melanoma, sarcoma, granulocytic sarcoma, invasive fungal disease (diabetic), histiocytoses, granulomatoses (rare)

Diagnosis

Plasmacytoma of the maxillary sinus, with spread to the orbit, nasal cavity, face, and infratemporal fossa

Diagnostic Imaging Approach

A. Where is the mass centered?
B. Is there bone destruction? Other bony changes (sclerosis)? What do the bony abnormalities *suggest* about the degree of aggressiveness (growth rate) of this lesion?
C. Evaluate enhancement, vascularity, density, T1- or T2-weighted signal intensity, calcifications, matrix.
D. Evaluate extent of abnormalities: local, orbital, intracranial, infratemporal fossa, pterygopalatine fossa, nasopharynx, face, perineural, nodes.

Clinical Points of Importance and Supplemental Information

A. It is sometimes difficult, even with high precision imaging, to determine whether a tumor is involving or displacing dura mater or orbital periosteum.
B. Demonstrating perineural spread or retropharyngeal adenopathy in sinonasal cancer drastically alters therapy and prognosis.

Answers to Questions

1. Neoplastic–no evidence of "edema"
2. Bone destruction or invasion of surrounding soft tissues
3. Orbit, intracranial, infratemporal fossa, nasopharynx, perineural

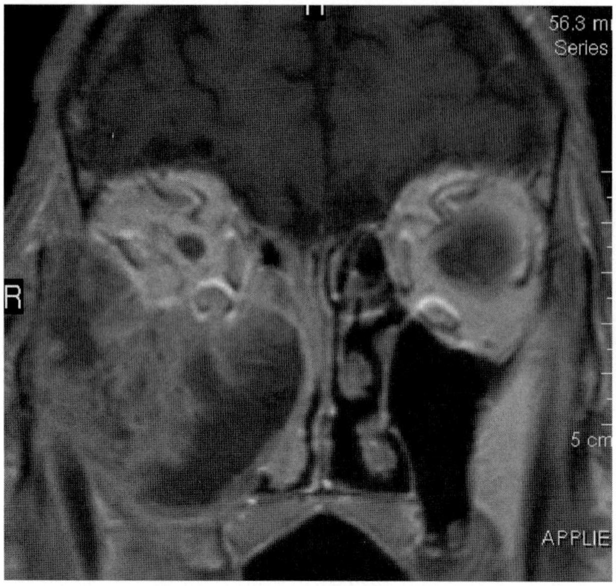

Figure 57G. Patient 1 with maxillary sinus carcinoma, showing inhomogeneously enhancing mass involving the right maxillary sinus with direct invasion of the orbit and soft tissue in the cheek. T1-weighted coronal image with contrast.

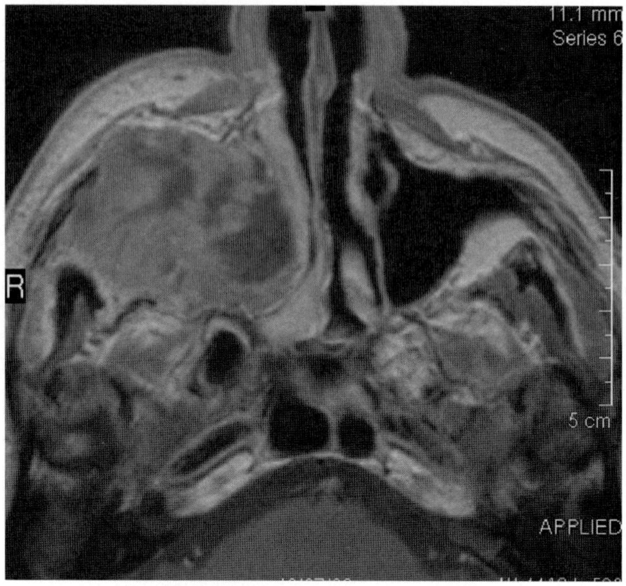

Figure 57H. Patient 1 with maxillary sinus carcinoma. T1-weighted axial image with contrast showing involvement of the pterygopalatine fossa and buccal fat pad posteriorly and soft tissue in the cheek anteriorly.

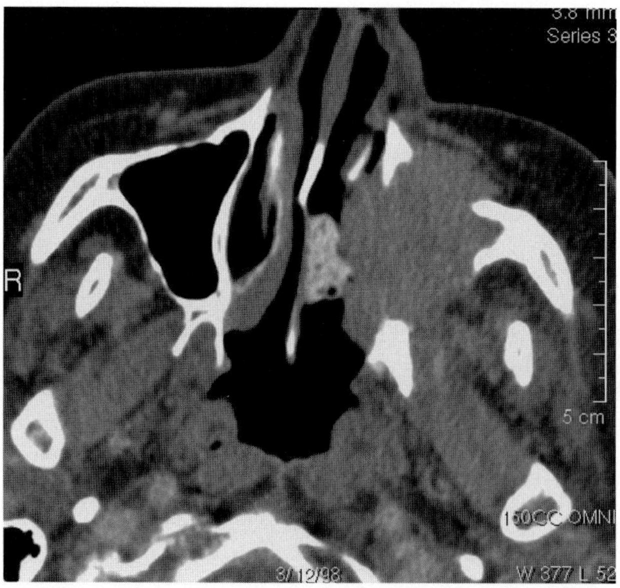

Figure 57I. Patient 2 with maxillary sinus carcinoma, showing soft tissue mass involving the left maxillary sinus, with destruction of the anterior, medial, and posterolateral walls of the sinus and extension into soft tissue of the cheek and retroantral fat pad.

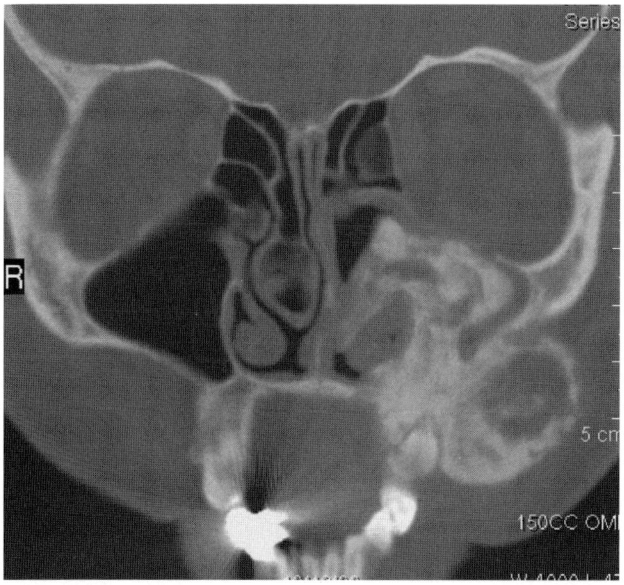

Figure 57J. Patient 3 with atypical appearing Ewing's sarcoma of the maxilla, showing a mass involving the maxilla, with marked matrix mineralization pretreatment, which partially presents as a maxillary sinus mass. Coronal computed tomography image at bone window setting.

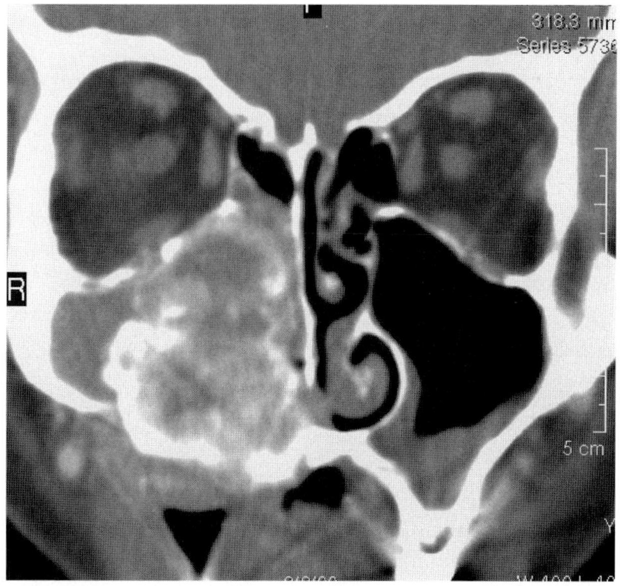

Figure 57K. Patient 4 with osteosarcoma of the maxilla. Coronal computed tomography image showing soft tissue mass involving the right maxillary antrum and nasal cavity, which contains mineralization.

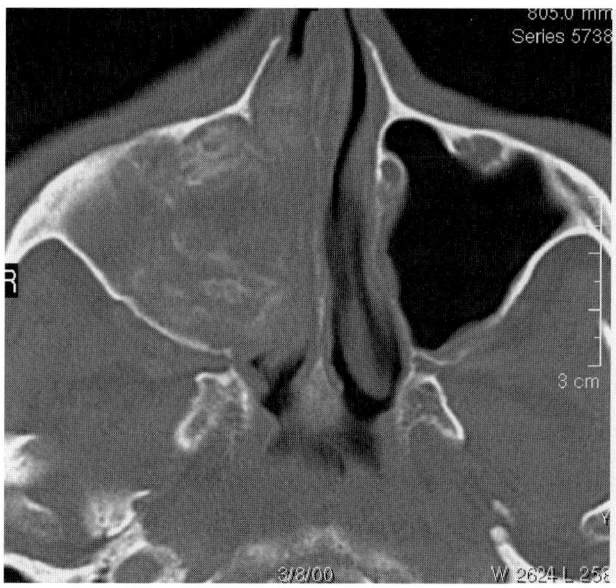

Figure 57L. Patient 4 with osteosarcoma of the maxilla. Axial computed tomography image at bone window setting showing detail of the mineralization in the mass, suggestive of osteoblastic type of sarcoma.

CASE 58

Clinical History: A 39-year-old woman who had a magnetic resonance imaging (MRI) study for headaches presents with no localizing symptoms.

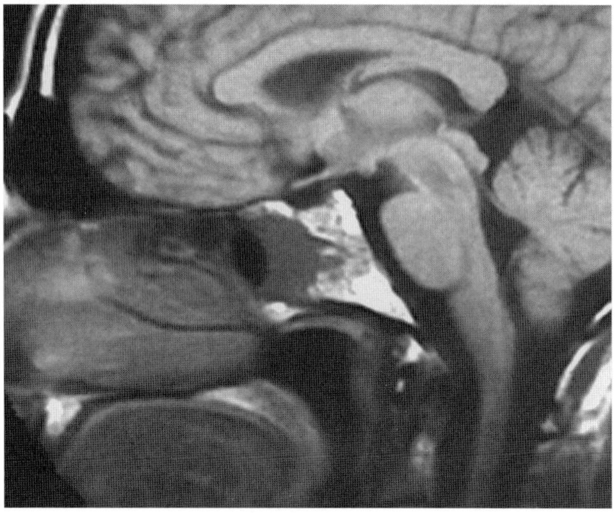

Figure 58A

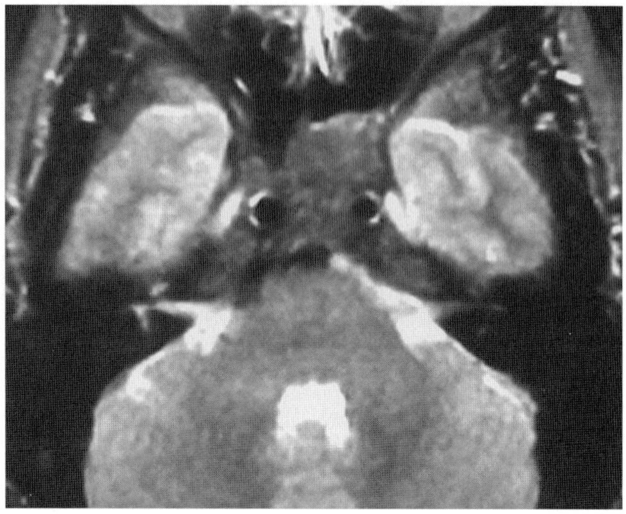

Figure 58B

1. Is the appearance of the clivus normal or abnormal?
2. What is the diagnosis?

Findings

An intermediate signal intensity lesion arises from sphenoid body partly protruding into the sphenoid sinus on T1-weighted image. The lesion might appear to be in the left cavernous sinus and the left orbital apex. Integrity of the left trigeminal cistern is maintained.

Problem

A woman with headaches and an abnormal appearance of the clivus on MRI

Anatomy

A. Sphenoid bone: body, basisphenoid, spheno-occipital synchondrosis, greater wing, lesser wing, pterygoid process, and plates
B. Sphenoid sinus: relationship to optic canals (nerves), cavernous sinus, carotid artery (see 54E)

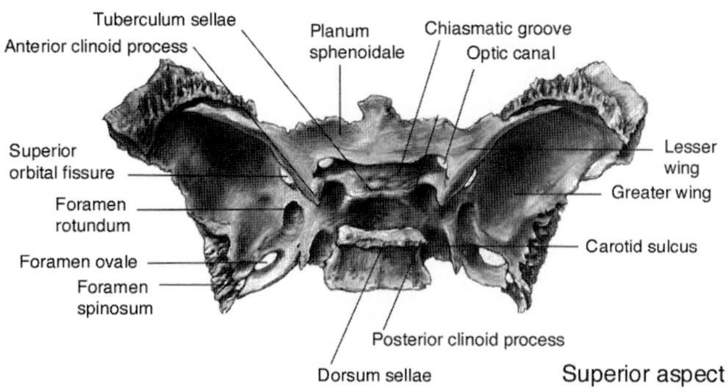

Figure 58C

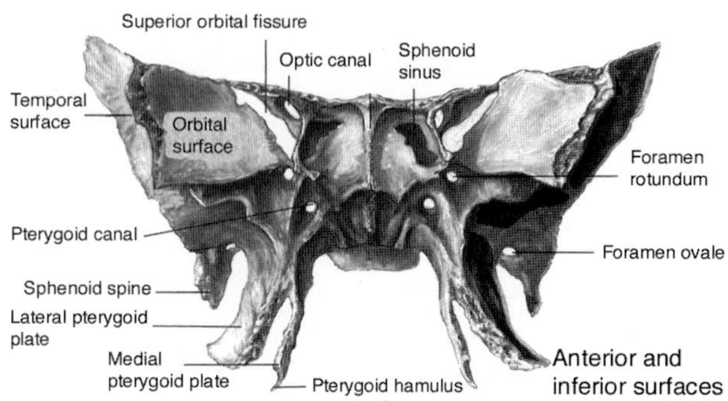

Figure 58D

Differential Diagnosis

Intraosseous meningioma (or reaction to adjacent meningioma) and metastasis are sometimes reasonable considerations.

Diagnosis

Fibrous dysplasia of the sphenoid bone

Diagnostic Imaging Approach

A. Are the findings a normal variation or pathologic?
B. If pathologic, is the disease process centered in the sinus, bone, nasal cavity, or nasopharynx?
C. Does the pattern of bone involvement suggest an indolent or aggressive process?
D. Evaluate morphologic features other than bone: T1- or T2-weighted signal intensity, density, enhancement, vascularity, matrix.
E. If calcified matrix is present, is it more likely osteoid, chondroid, or fibrous?
F. Are further studies necessary: computed tomography (CT), MRI, radionuclide, angiography?

Clinical Points of Importance and Supplemental Information

A. Fibrous dysplasia can display a wide range of morphology on MRI and CT. Some of this variability in sinonasal fibrous dysplasia is caused by trapped mucosa and secretions.
B. Prime clinical considerations are usually cosmetic or functional (e.g., proper occlusion); possible cranial nerve dysfunction; and possible secondary mucoceles.

Answers to Questions

1. Abnormal
2. Fibrous dysplasia

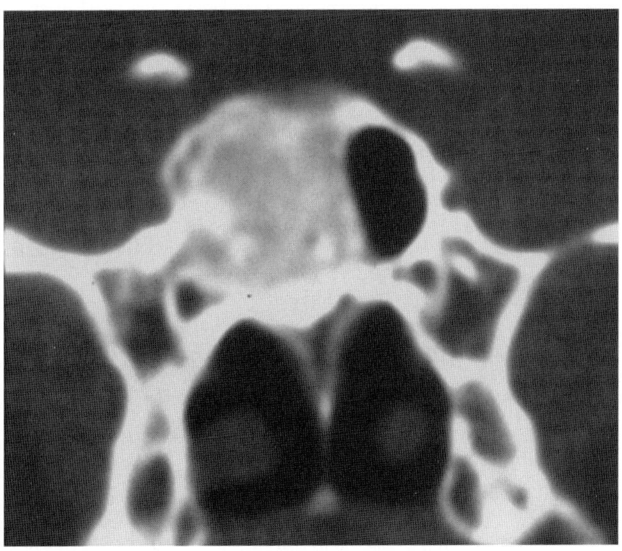

Figure 58E. Patient 1 with fibrous dysplasia of the sphenoid bone, showing a ground-glass pattern involving the body of the sphenoid bone with expansile appearance (This is the same patient as presented in the 58 A and B.)

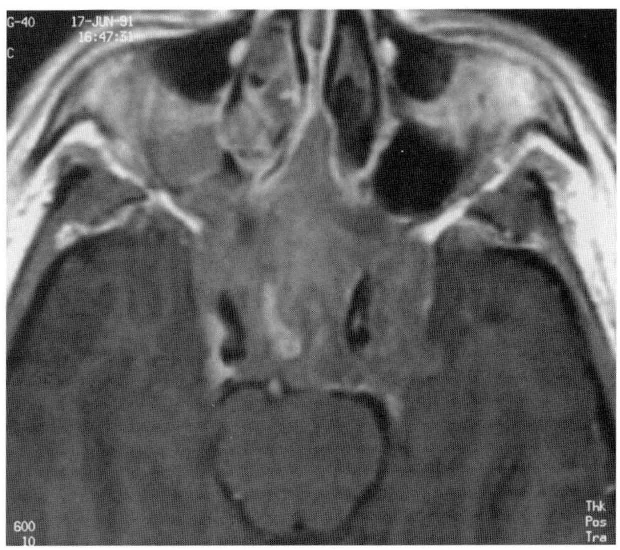

Figure 58F. Patient 2 with invasive pituitary adenoma, showing an infiltrative mass centered in the pituitary fossa with direct invasion of the cavernous sinus, posterior nasal cavity, and clivus, in which both carotid arteries are imbedded. T1-weighted axial image with contrast.

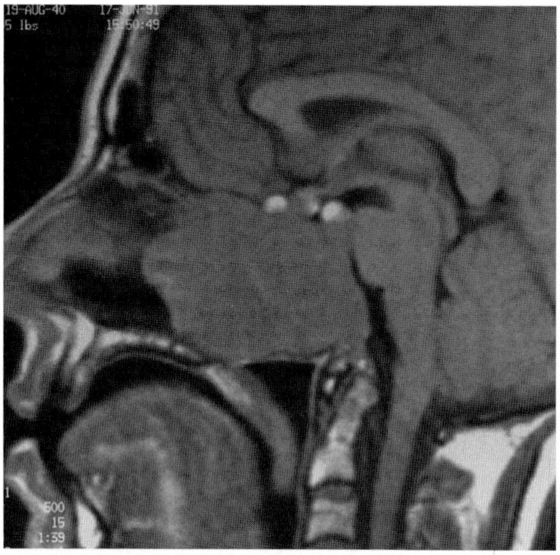

Figure 58G. Patient 2 with invasive pituitary adenoma. T1-weighted sagittal image without contrast showing a mass centered in the clivus involving the entire body of the sphenoid bone.

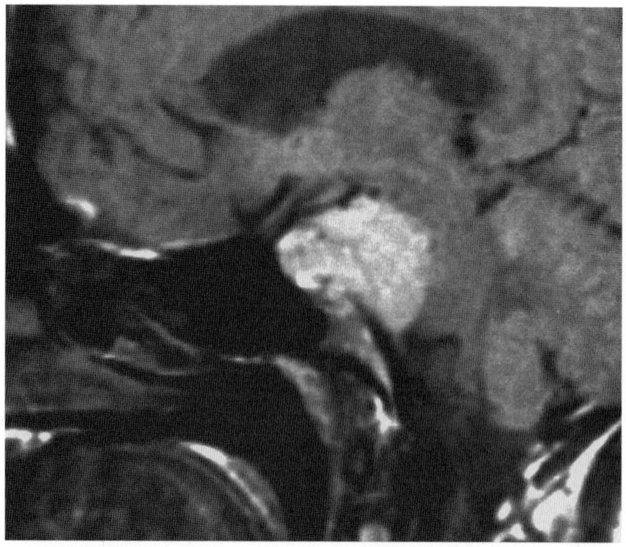

Figure 58H. Patient 3 with meningioma, showing a homogeneously enhancing extraaxial mass centered in the pituitary fossa, extending along the posterior aspect of the upper clivus, with erosion of the dorsum sella. The sphenoid sinus is intact. T1-weighted sagittal image with contrast.

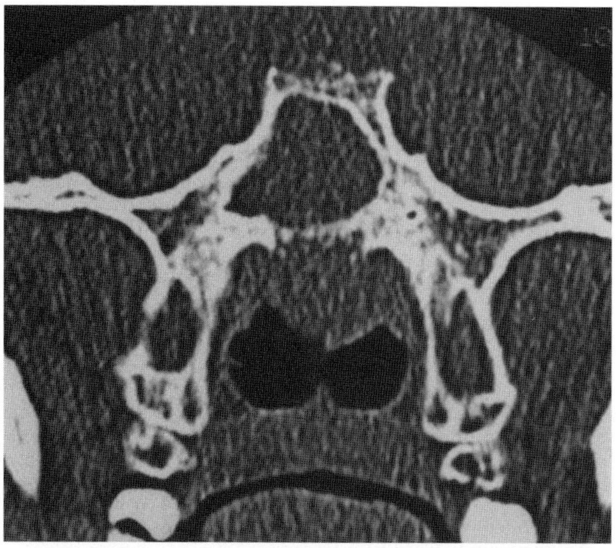

Figure 58I. Patient 4 with undifferentiated nasopharyngeal carcinoma with sphenoid sinus invasion. Coronal computed tomography image at bone window setting showing somewhat prominent soft tissue in the nasopharynx and soft tissue obliteration of the sphenoid sinus, with permeative change of the sinus floor.

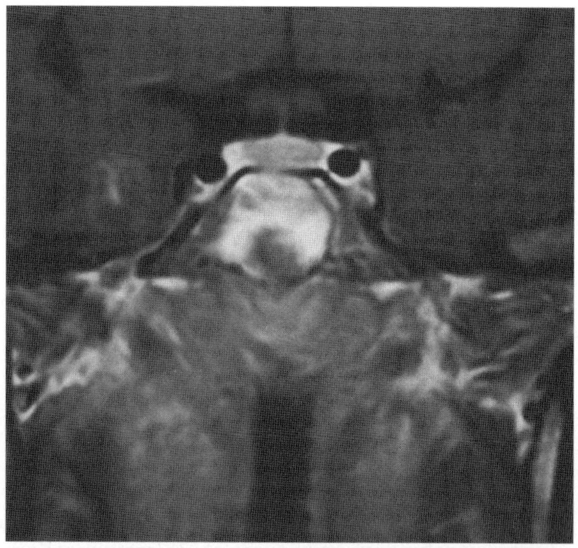

Figure 58J. Patient 4 with undifferentiated nasopharyngeal carcinoma with sphenoid sinus invasion, showing an inhomogeneously enhancing mass filling the sphenoid sinus, with disruption of low intensity cortical bone in both floor and roof of the sphenoid sinus. T1-weighted coronal image with contrast.

CASE 59

Clinical History: A 61-year-old woman presents with spontaneous cerebrospinal fluid (CSF) rhinorrhea confirmed by radionuclide studies. Two prior computed tomography (CT) studies (at other institutions) of the cribriform plate region were reportedly negative. She has no history of prior trauma.

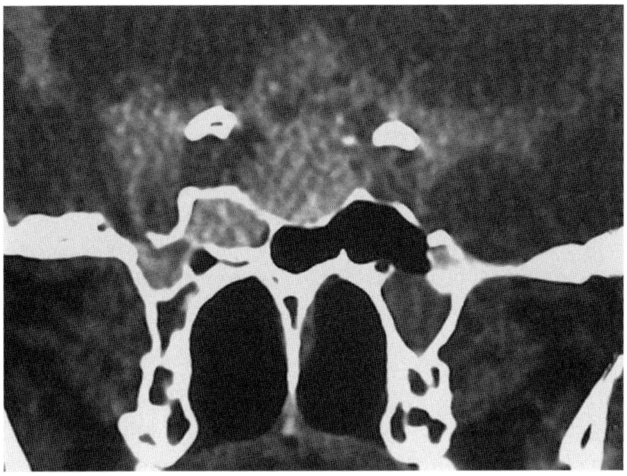

Figure 59A

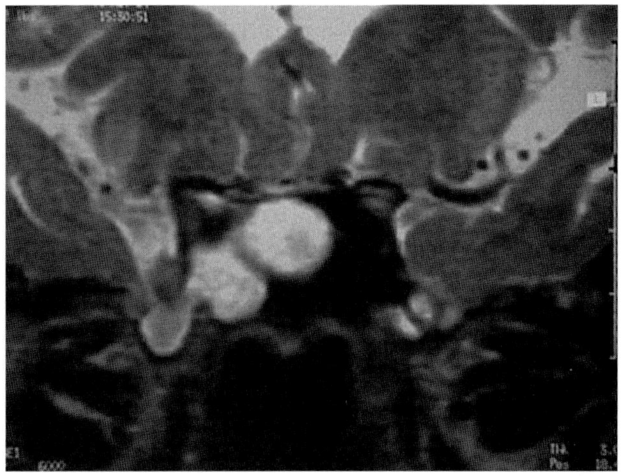

Figure 59B

1. Is contrast in the subarachnoid space required to detect the site of CSF leakage?
2. Give a complete diagnosis for the right- and left-sided abnormalities.
3. Why were the findings missed on the two prior studies?

Findings

Computed tomography cisternography shows an extravasation of contrast material into the sphenoid sinus through bony dehiscence. T2-weighted coronal image reveals herniation of the medial aspect of the right temporal lobe through the dehiscent and into the sphenoid sinus.

Problem

An adult with spontaneous CSF rhinorrhea and two prior CT studies showing no site of leakage

Anatomy

A. Sphenoid bone: body, basisphenoid, greater wing, lesser wing, pterygoid process, and plates
B. Foramen rotundum and course of V2 (maxillary division of the trigeminal nerve) (see Fig. 4F)

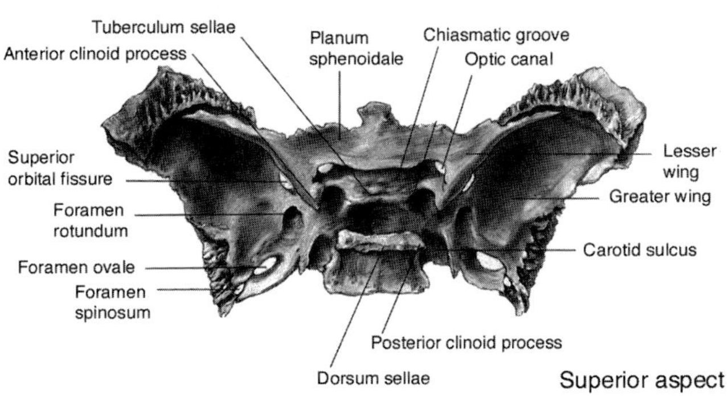

Figure 59C

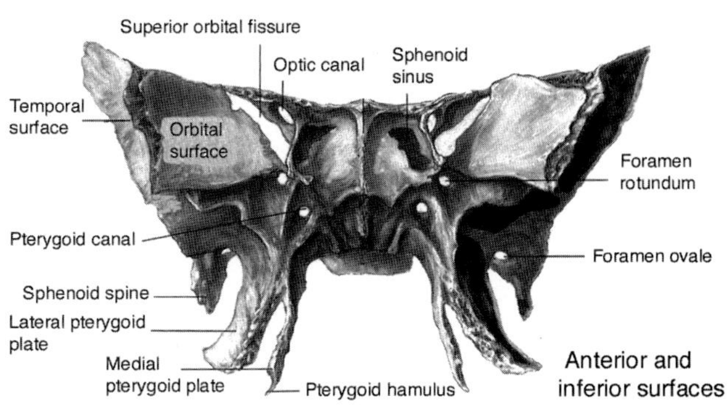

Figure 59D

Differential Diagnosis

Occasionally, a central, congenital meningocele or meningoencephalocele will produce a CSF leak; look for an associated mass lesion or hydrocephalus, which sometimes causes previously quiescent defects to begin leaking

Diagnosis

Dehiscence of the lateral extensions of the sphenoid sinus within the central skull base (right larger than left) causing CSF rhinorrhea, with a secondary meningoencephalocele on the right and a probable small meningocele on the left

Diagnostic Imaging Approach

A. Confirm CSF leakage: clinically (testing fluid for glucose); radionuclides (pledgets).
B. Noncontrast CT with 1- to 2-mm thick sections a 1- to 2-mm increment from the frontal bone to the dorsum sella (or further posterior for temporal bones) in the coronal plane.
C. Consider temporal bone as a source (via eustachian tube) and include in study as clinically appropriate.
D. Almost all defects can be found *without* the use of intrathecal contrast; if intrathecal contrast is used, do prone coronal scans of sinonasal and temporal bones; prone axial scans of the temporal bone may also be necessary; intrathecal contrast occasionally confirms leakage, but is not required to identify bony defects responsible for leak.

Clinical Points of Importance and Supplemental Information

A. The three most common errors in detection of CSF leaks are using thick (3- to 5-mm sections), not extending the study posterior enough, and not considering the temporal bone as a source of rhinorrhea or the sinonasal region as a source of otorrhea.
B. Repeated episodes of meningitis caused by sinonasal flora may require a similar search.

Answers to Questions

1. No
2. Bilateral meningoencephaloceles into lateral recesses of the sphenoid sinus
3. The studies were incomplete.

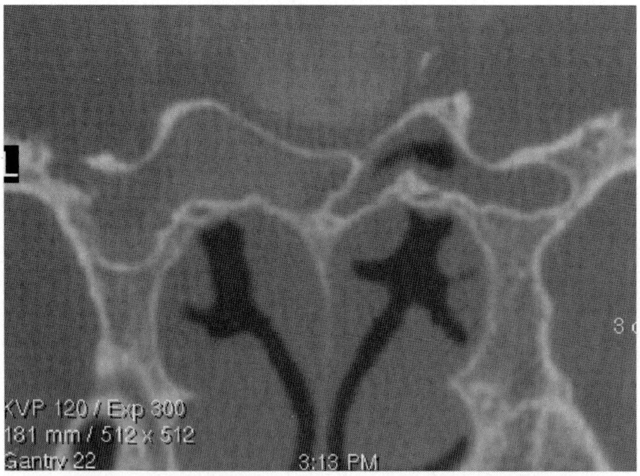

Figure 59E. Patient 1 with CSF rhinorrhea. Coronal computed tomography (CT) image (of CT cisternography) at bone window setting showing bony defect at the roof of the left sphenoid sinus, which is obliterated.

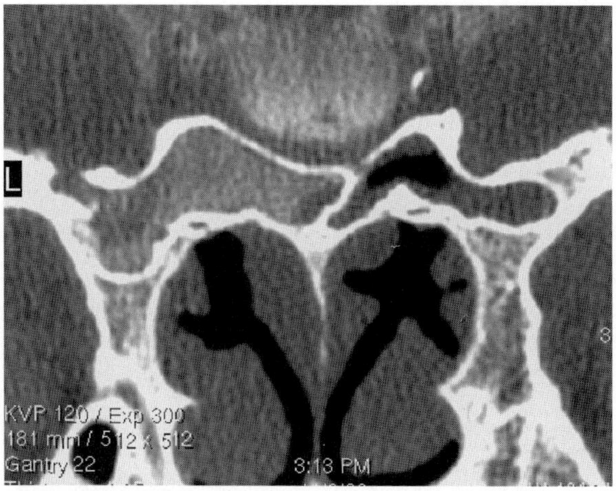

Figure 59F. Patient 1 with cerebrospinal fluid rhinorrhea. Computed tomography cisternograpy showing leakage of intrathecally injected contrast into the left sphenoid sinus through the bone defect. Less-enhancing area in the sphenoid sinus adjacent to the bony defect might represent encephalocele.

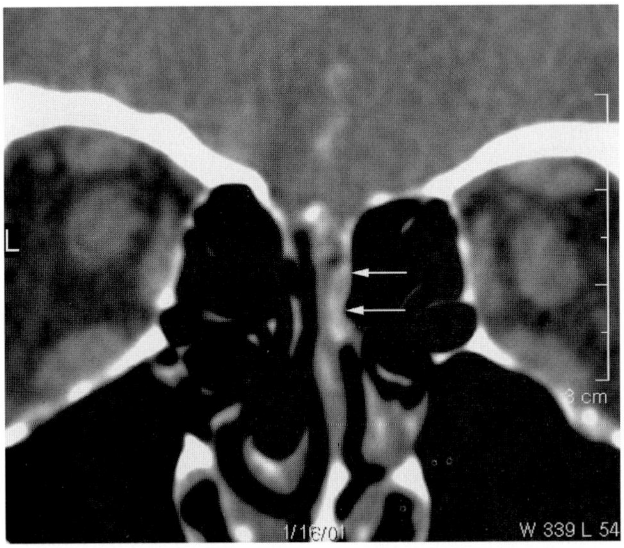

Figure 59G. Patient 2 with cerebrospinal fluid rhinorrhea. Computed tomography cisternography showing leakage of contrast into left olfactory groove.

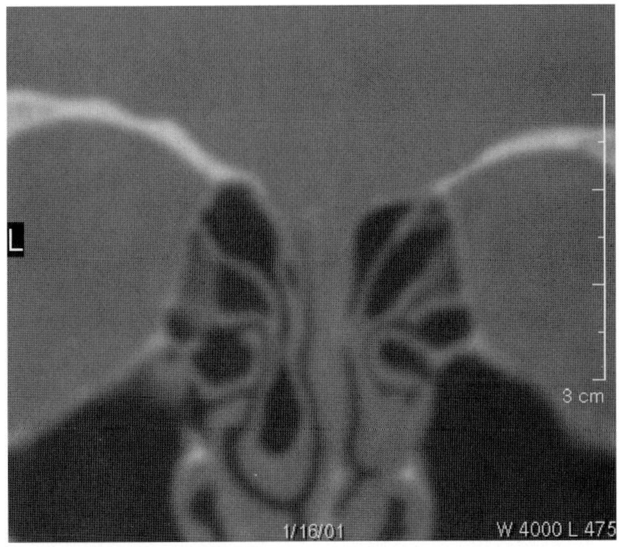

Figure 59H. Patient 2 with cerebrospinal fluid rhinorrhea. Coronal computed tomography image at bone window setting showing less mineralization of the cribriform plate in the adult than usual.

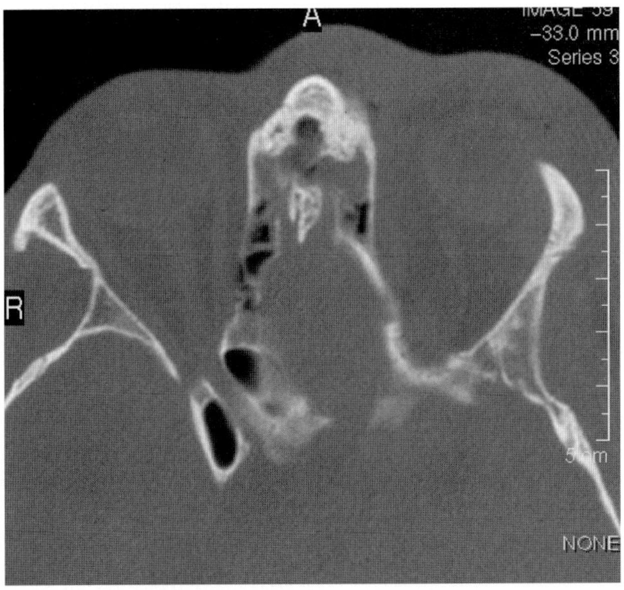

Figure 59I. Patient 3 with posttraumatic encephalocele. Axial computed tomography image showing expansile soft tissue mass, with bone remodeling superimposing upon the posterior ethmoid and sphenoid sinuses.

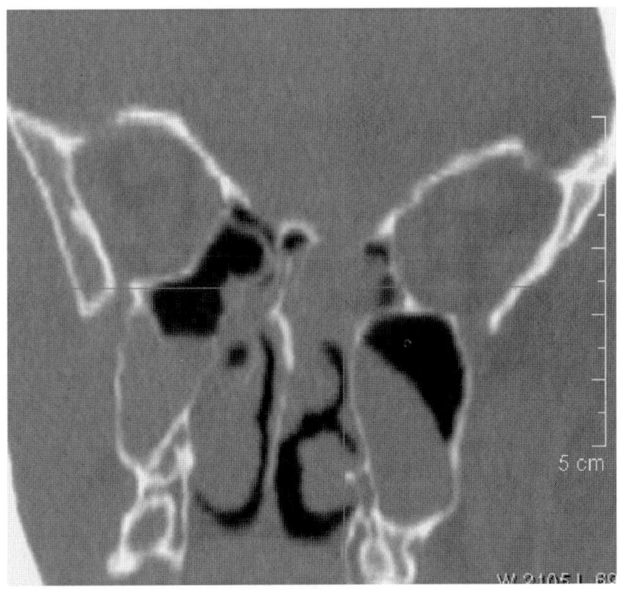

Figure 59J. Patient 3 with posttraumatic encephalocele. Reformatted coronal computed tomography image showing soft tissue mass in the left superior nasal cavity and ethmoid sinus subjacent to bone defect in the fovea ethmoidalis.

CHAPTER 5

MANDIBLE AND MAXILLA

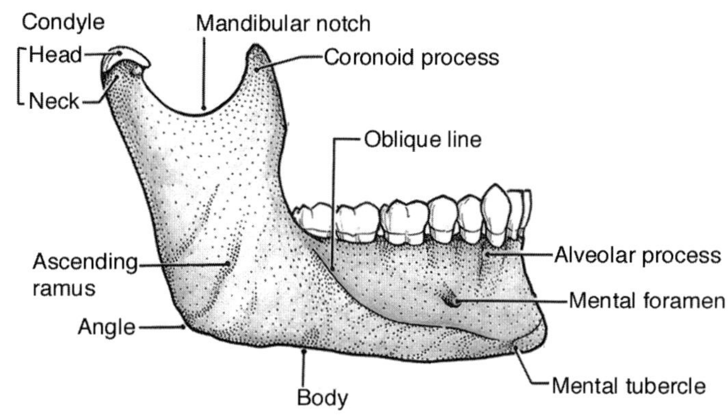

CASE 60

Clinical History: A 30-year-old woman presents with a lower jaw mass.

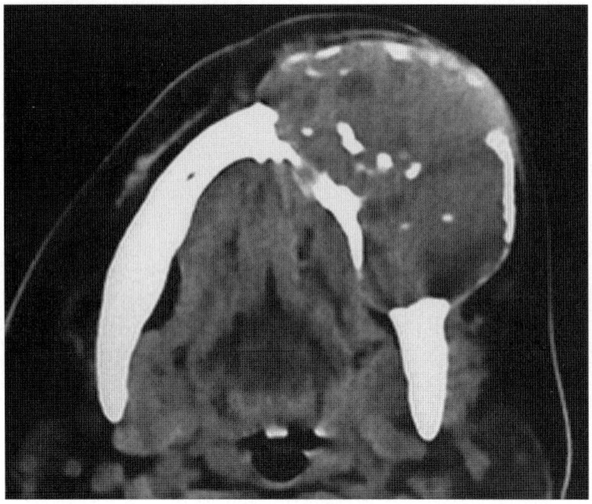

Figure 60A

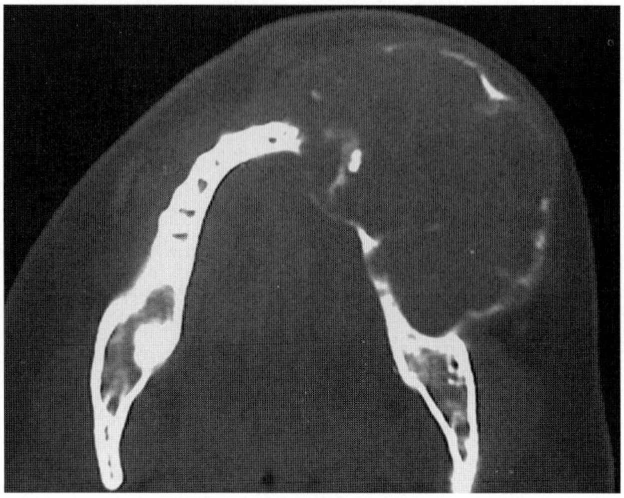

Figure 60B

1. Name the three most common odontogenic masses that can cause a large (>3 cm), expansile-appearing mandibular mass. Give the most likely diagnosis for this lesion.
2. List four prime responsibilities of the radiologist in evaluating such mandibular masses.

Findings

An expansile mass that is encompassed by a shell-like periosteal reaction arises from the left body of the mandible. Multiple septations are seen in the mass, with no obvious invasiveness of the lesion at the margins. Solid enhancement is identified in the lesion. These images do not definitively show an associated unerupted tooth.

Problem

An adult woman with an "expansile-appearing" mass of the mandible

Anatomy

A. Mandible: body, ascending ramus, retromolar trigone, inferior alveolar canal, mental foramen
B. Floor of the mouth and mylohyoid muscle

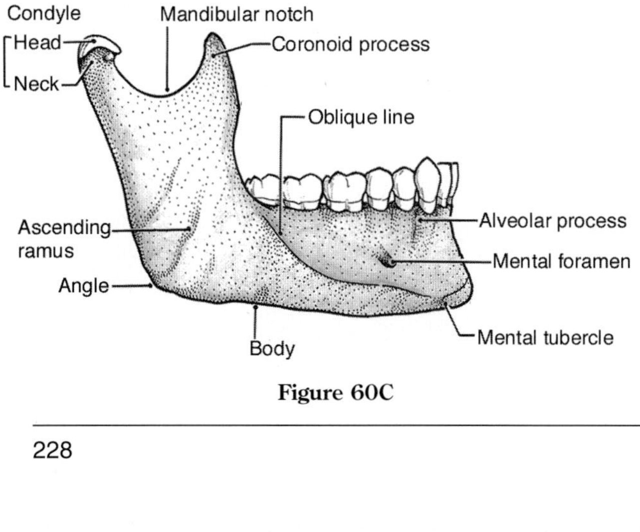

Figure 60C

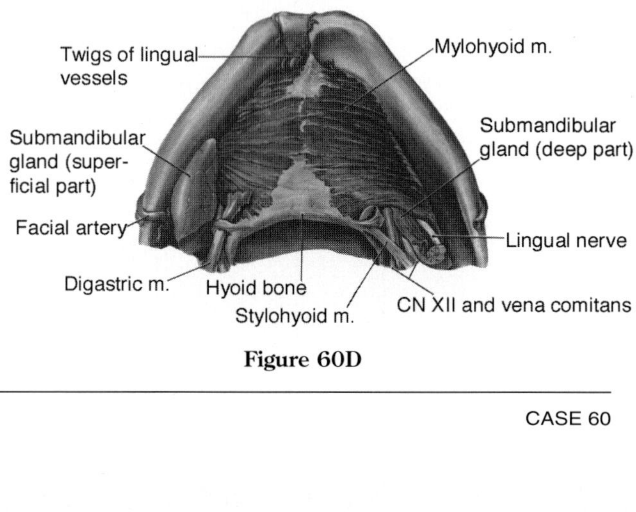

Figure 60D

Differential Diagnosis

1. If more cystic appearing, odontogenic keratocyst, dentigerous cyst
2. Osteo-, chondro-, or other sarcoma
3. Lymphoma or other round cell lesions, metastases (unlikely)

Diagnosis

Ameloblastoma of the mandible

Diagnostic Imaging Approach

A. Dental radiography is usually available or required for complete evaluation.
B. Is the mass arising within the mandible? If so, in what portion?
C. Is an associated unerupted tooth present?
D. Does the pattern of bone involvement suggest an aggressive or relatively indolent process? Is it multi- or unilocular?
E. Evaluate the internal morphology: solid vs. cystic, T1- or T2-weighted signal intensity, vascularity, enhancement, calcification, matrix.
F. Are the surrounding soft tissues involved?
G. What is the relationship of the lesion to the inferior alveolar nerve and more proximal portions of the mandibular nerve?

Clinical Points Of Importance And Supplemental Information

A. It is important to establish whether mandibular lesions are hypervascular (e.g., hemangioma) before biopsy.
B. The maxillofacial surgeon will always be interested in the proximity of the lesion to the inferior alveolar nerve and the extent of spread to surrounding soft tissues.

Answers To Questions

1. Dentigerous cyst, ameloblastoma, odontogenic keratocyst. Ameloblastoma—solid-appearing.
2. The prime diagnostic responsibilities are to establish the differential diagnosis, relationship to the inferior alveolar nerve, degree of vascularity, and soft tissue extent.

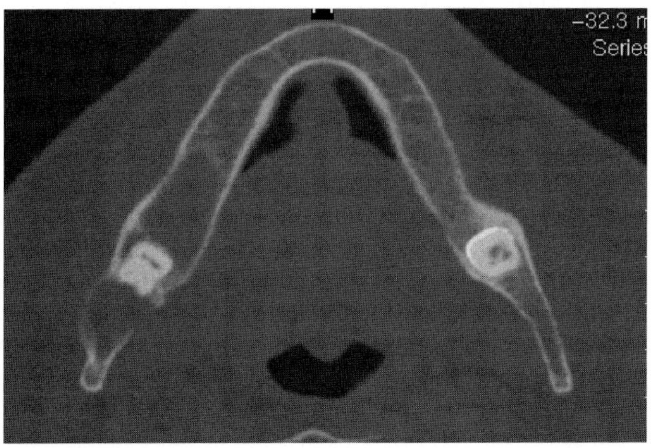

Figure 60E. Patient 1 with dentigerous cyst, showing expansile, unilocular lesion centered in the posterior body and ascending ramus of the mandible on the right, which contains an unerupted third molar. Defect of the cortical bone is seen in the lingual aspect.

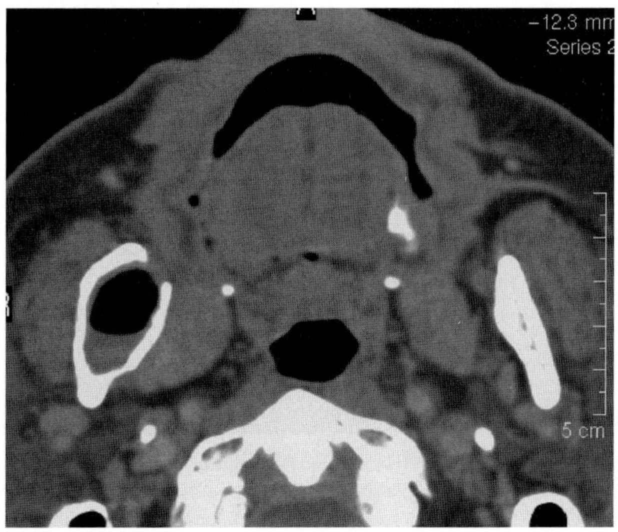

Figure 60F. Patient 1 with dentigerous cyst (status after curettage). Axial computed tomography image showing air–fluid level in the expansile mass in the right ascending ramus of the mandible.

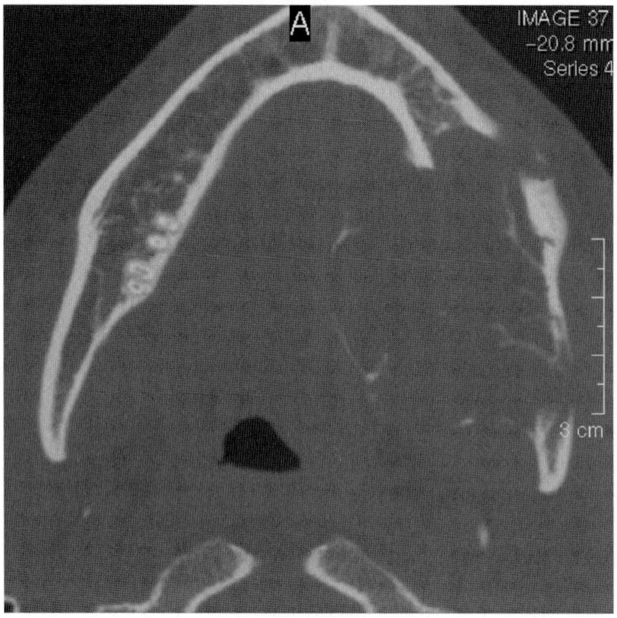

Figure 60G. Patient 2 with ameloblastoma, showing multilocular cystic mass involving the mid and posterior bodies of the mandible on the left, with bone remodeling and cortical interruption in several areas. Axial computed tomography image at bone window setting.

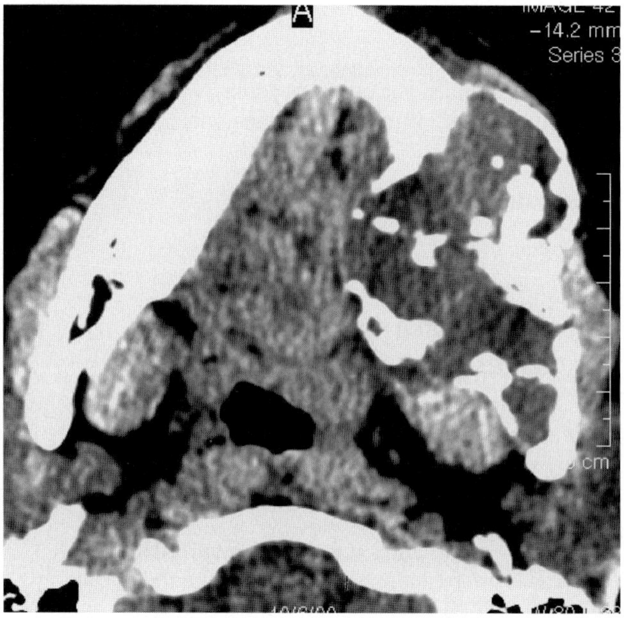

Figure 60H. Patient 2 with ameloblastoma. Axial computed tomography image with contrast showing the mass containing several enhancing components.

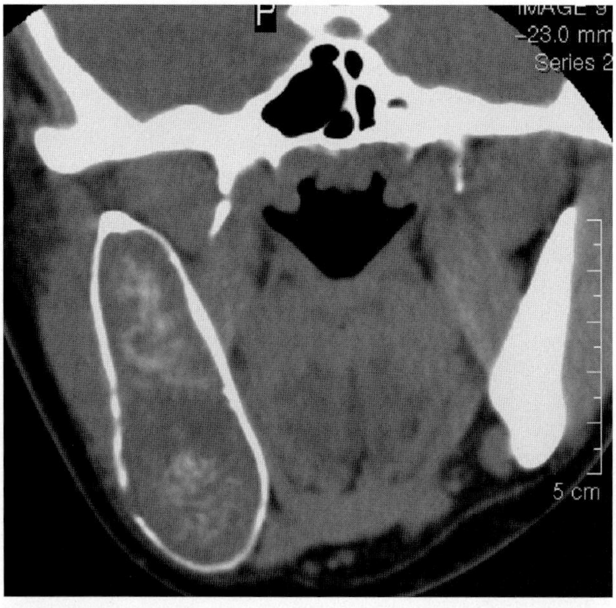

Figure 60I. Patient 3 with surgically proved odontogenic keratocyst, showing a unilocular, expansile lesion involving the ascending ramus of the mandible on the right, which contains speckled areas of high attenuation, which is a very atypical feature of these usually near-fluid attenuation contents. No obvious soft tissue involvement is seen, despite the bone defect in the outer cortex. Coronal computed tomography image.

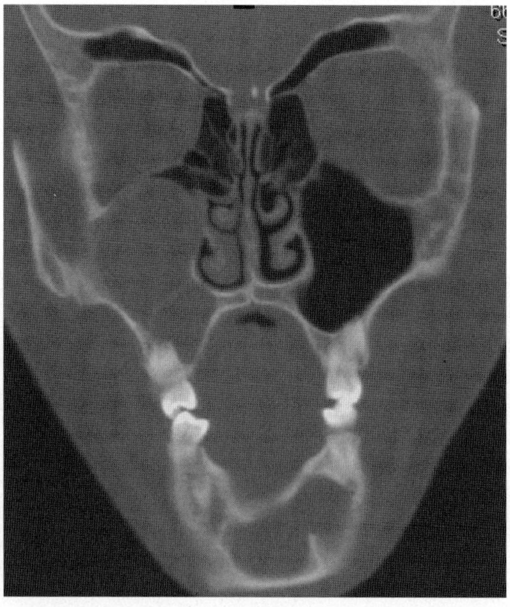

Figure 60J. Patient 4 with basal cell nevus syndrome, showing multiple unilocular expansile lesions involving both maxilla and mandible.

CASE 61

Clinical History: A 17-year-old boy presents with a "parotid" mass.

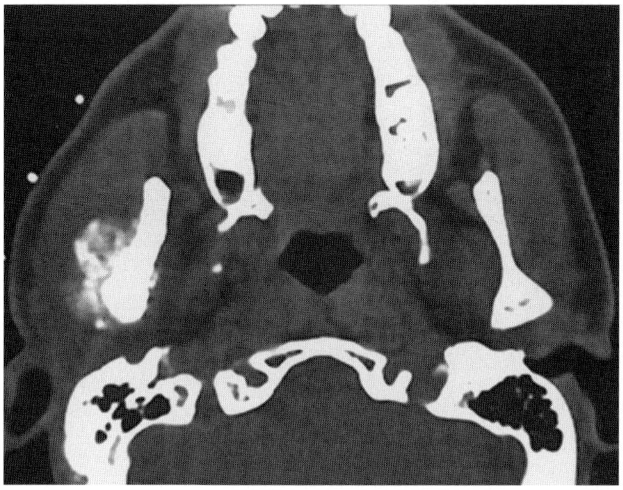

Figure 61A

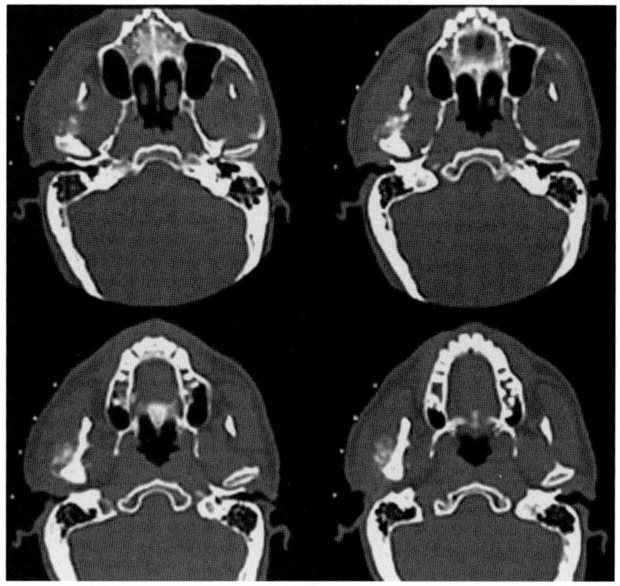

Figure 61B

1. What is the true origin of the mass?
2. What is the most likely diagnosis?
3. If the patient were 60 years of age, what would be your first choice for the diagnosis? Second choice?
4. Can you offer any further assistance in diagnosis?

Findings

A soft tissue mass that produces a bony matrix represented by spotty and amorphous calcific densities around the ascending ramus and the condylar process of the mandible on the right. The cortices are irregular and associated with some spiculation.

Problem

An older teenager with a parotid region mass on clinical examination shown to actually arise from the mandible

Anatomy

A. Mandible: condyle, ascending ramus, coronoid process
B. Masticator space and its relationship to the parotid gland
C. Parotidomasseteric fascia

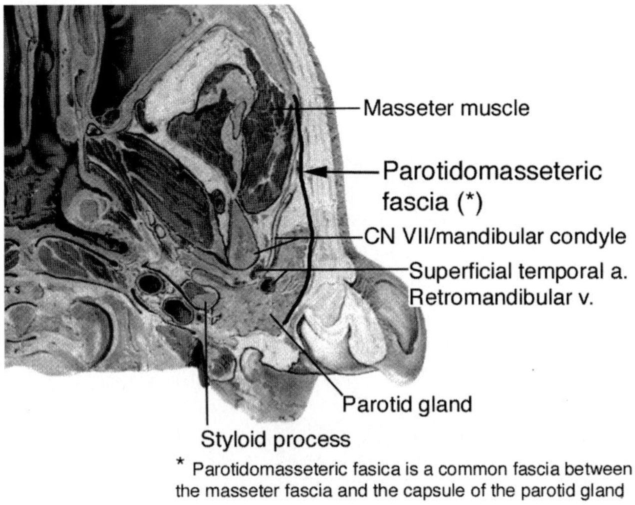

Figure 61C

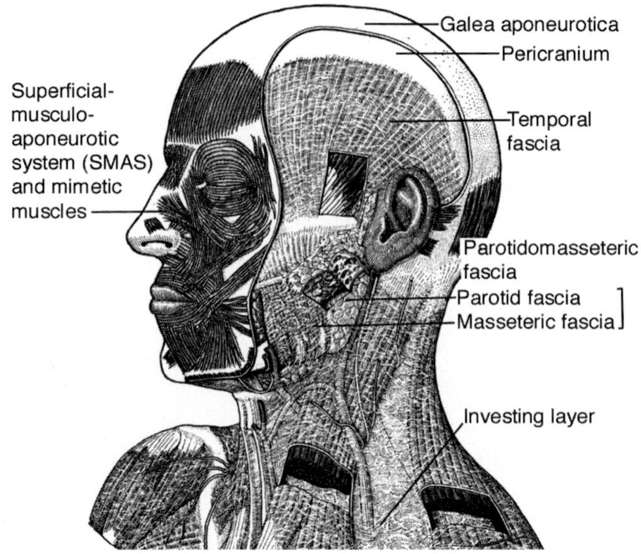

Figure 61D

Differential Diagnosis

Osteogenic sarcoma, metastasis, posttraumatic reaction (myositis ossificans)

Diagnosis

Osteosarcoma of the condyle and ascending ramus of the mandible

Diagnostic Imaging Approach

A. Is the mass intrinsic or extrinsic to the parotid gland (consider this only because of the clinical impression)?
B. Where is the mass centered?
C. Is the mandibular involvement localized, multifocal, or diffuse?
D. Does the pattern of bone involvement suggest an aggressive or relatively indolent process?
E. Evaluate the internal morphology for density, T1- or T2-weighted signal intensity, vascularity, enhancement, calcification, matrix.
F. Is there spread beyond the mandible? Perineural? Nodal?
G. Should additional tests (e.g., dental films, magnetic resonance imaging, radionuclide, angiography) be done?
H. Is the lesion suitable for imaging directed biopsy?

Clinical Points Of Importance And Supplemental Information

A. Masses believed to be parotid in origin on the basis of the physical examination frequently arise from periparotid sources.
B. Although some clinicians do not share this concept, needle biopsies of any potential malignancy are generally safe and do not have a significant risk of needle tract seeding. Imaging-guided biopsy should be done only after careful consideration of the likely histology and compatibility of the biopsy pathway (compartment resection) and method (fine needle aspiration vs. core needle aspiration) with the treatment plan.

Answers To Questions

1. Mandible—not the parotid
2. Osteosarcoma
3. Osteosarcoma. Metastasis.
4. Imaging-guided biopsy

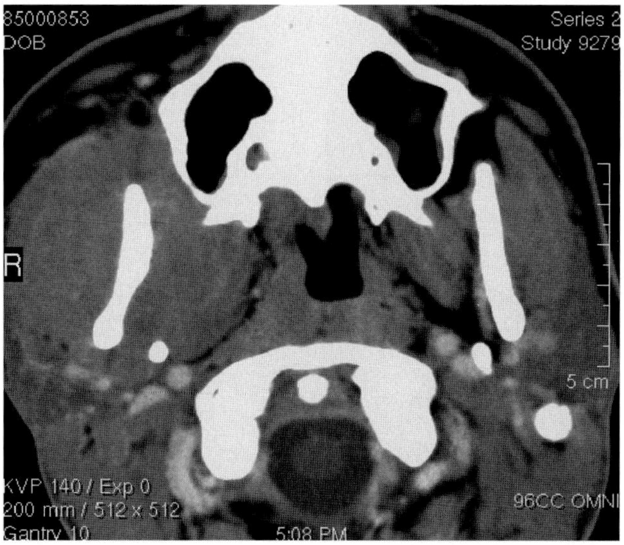

Figure 61E. Patient 1 with extranodal involvement of non-Hodgkin's lymphoma, showing an infiltrating mass surrounding the ascending ramus of the mandible on the right, with involvement of the adjacent masseter and pterygoid muscles. Parotid tail is displaced posterolaterally by the mass. Axial computed tomography image with contrast.

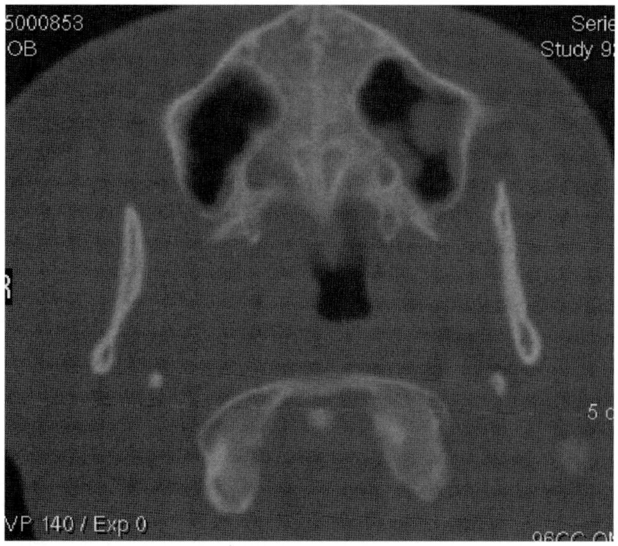

Figure 61F. Patient 1 with extranodal involvement of non-Hodgkin's lymphoma. Axial computed tomography image at bone window setting showing some remodeling of the ascending ramus of the mandible without destructive change.

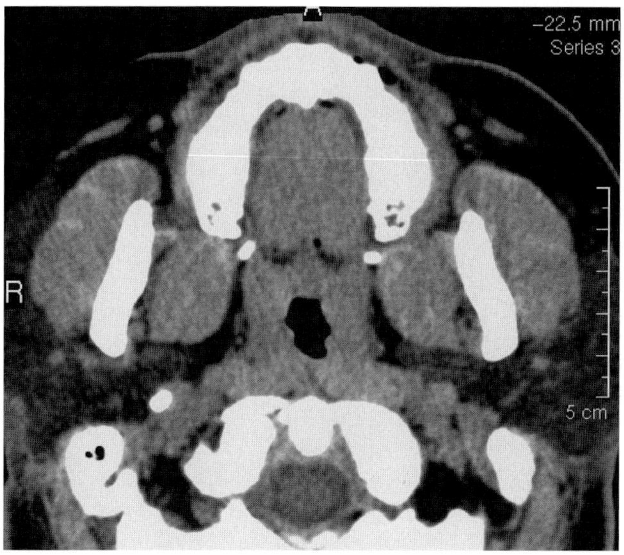

Figure 61G. Patient 2 with suspicious bilateral parotid swelling, showing hypertrophy of the masseter and pterygoid muscles bilaterally. Axial computed tomography image.

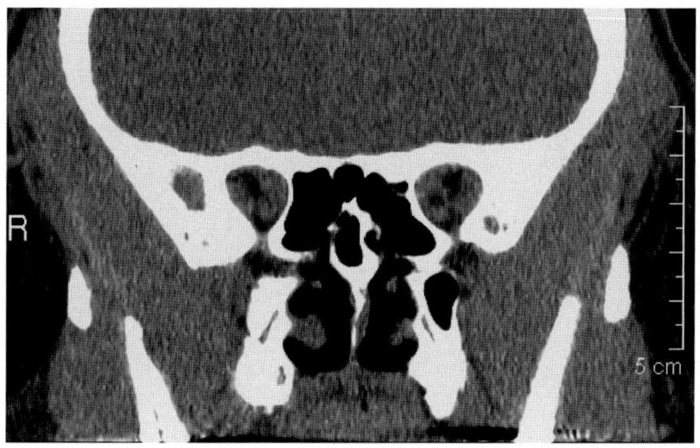

Figure 61H. Patient 2 with suspicious bilateral parotid swelling. Coronal computed tomography image showing hypertrophy of the masseter and temporalis muscles bilaterally.

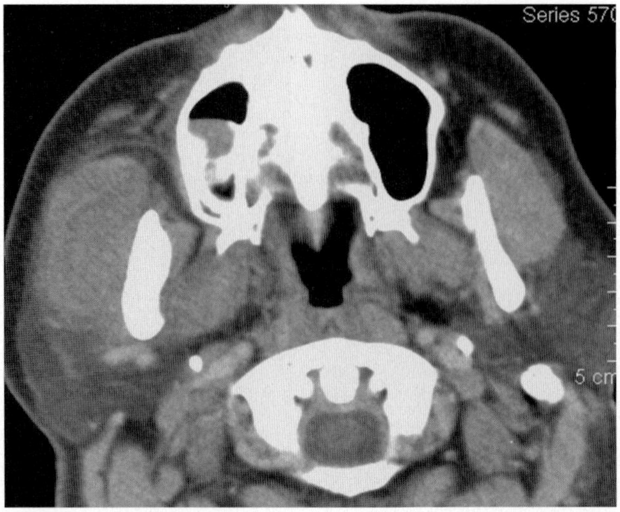

Figure 61I. Patient 3 with sclerosing osteomyelitis of the mandible, showing soft tissue swelling around the ascending ramus of the mandible on the right, especially of the masseter muscle. Axial computed tomography image at soft tissue window setting.

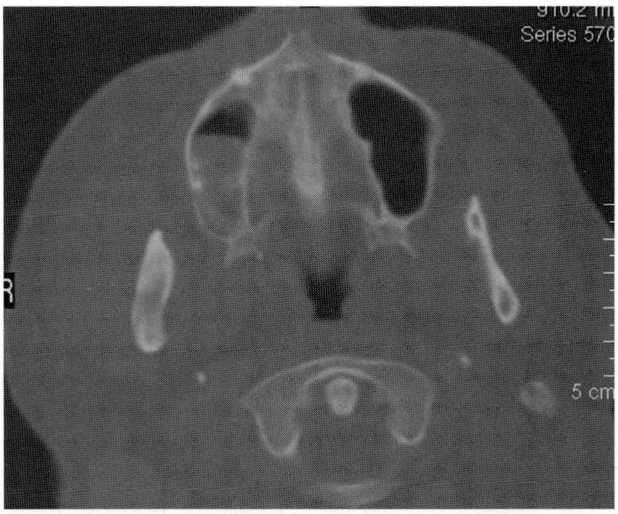

Figure 61J. Patient 3 with sclerosing osteomyelitis of the mandible. Axial computed tomography image at bone window setting showing sclerotic change of the ascending ramus of the mandible on the right.

CASE 62

Clinical History: A 7-year-old boy presents with a cheek mass.

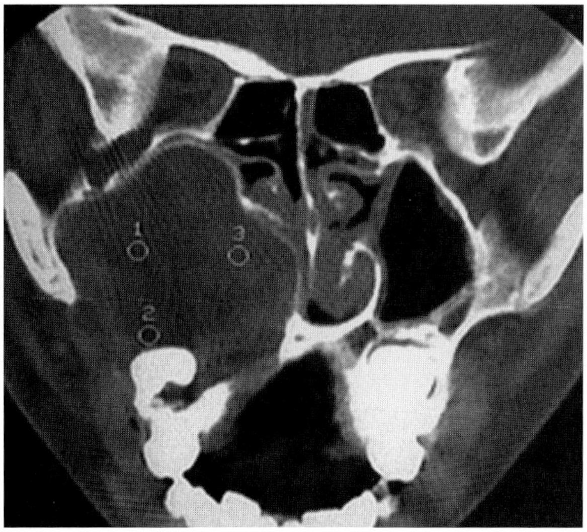

Figure 62A

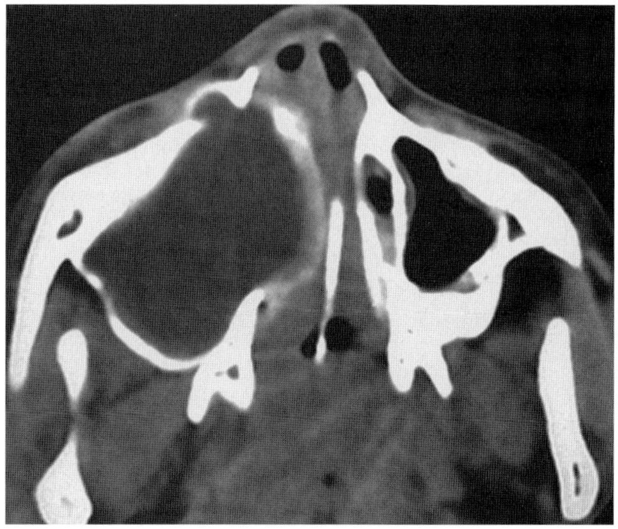

Figure 62B

1. What is the origin of the mass?
2. What is the most likely specific diagnosis?

Findings

An expansile fluid attenuation mass arises from the right upper molar region of the maxillary alveolar ridge, protruding superiorly into the maxillary antrum. The lesion contains an unerupted molar.

Problem

A 7-year-old with a cheek mass involving the maxilla

Anatomy

A. Maxilla: maxillary alveolar ridge and related teeth, maxillary tuberosity
B. Zygomatic and palatine bone contributions to maxillary sinus

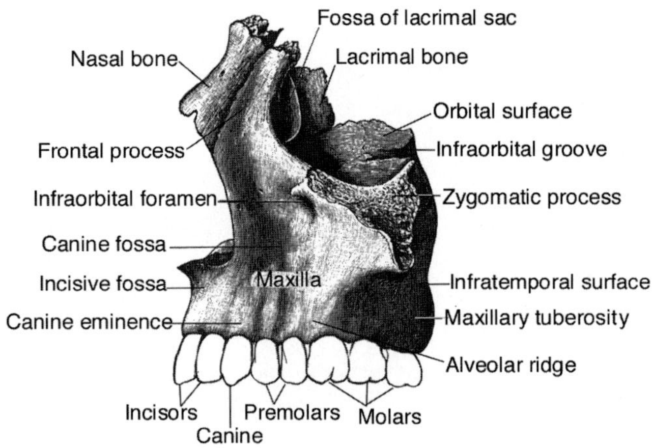

Figure 62C

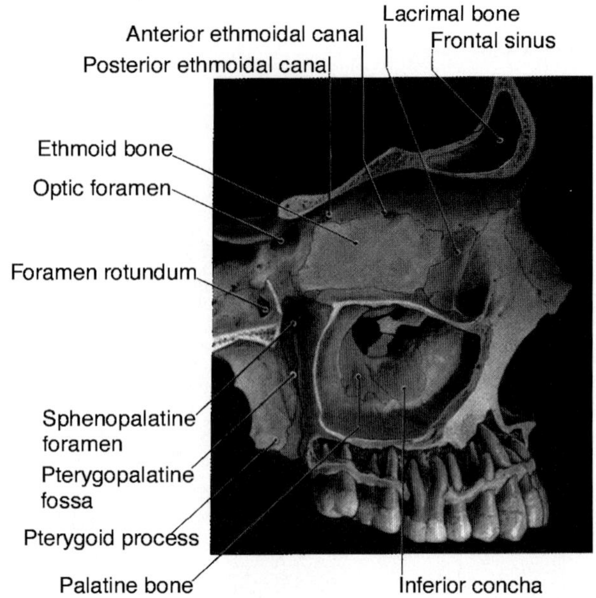

Figure 62D

Differential Diagnosis

Odontogenic cyst, keratocyst, mucocele of maxillary antrum (until double wall is recognized)

Diagnosis

Dentigerous cyst of the maxilla

Diagnostic Imaging Approach

A. Is the mass arising in the maxillary sinus or the alveolar ridge? Look for a double bony margin along the roof of the antrum (floor of the orbit).
B. If it possibly arises outside of the sinus, could it be odontogenic? Look for associated unerupted tooth; dental radiographs (orthopantomographs or intraoral views are usually necessary).
C. Does the pattern of bone involvement suggest a rapid or relatively indolent rate of "growth"?
D. Evaluate the internal morphology for density, T1- or T2-weighted signal intensity, vascularity, enhancement, calcification, matrix.
E. Focal, multifocal or diffuse disease?

Clinical Points Of Importance And Supplemental Information

When an isolated, expansile-appearing mass of the maxilla is present, always consider an odontogenic origin; these dental lesions are often mistaken for maxillary sinus mucoceles.

Answers To Questions

1. Odontogenic—"double" superior wall
2. Odontogenic cyst

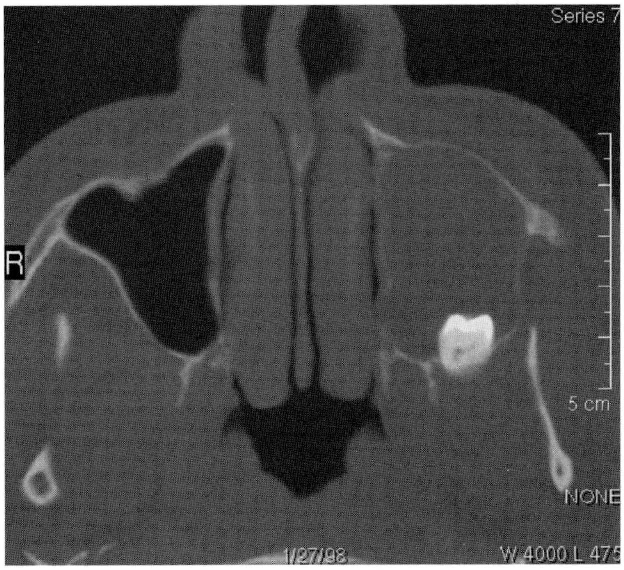

Figure 62E. Patient 1 with dentigerous cyst, showing expansile lesion protruding into the left maxillary sinus, which contains an unerupted molar. Axial computed tomography image at bone window setting.

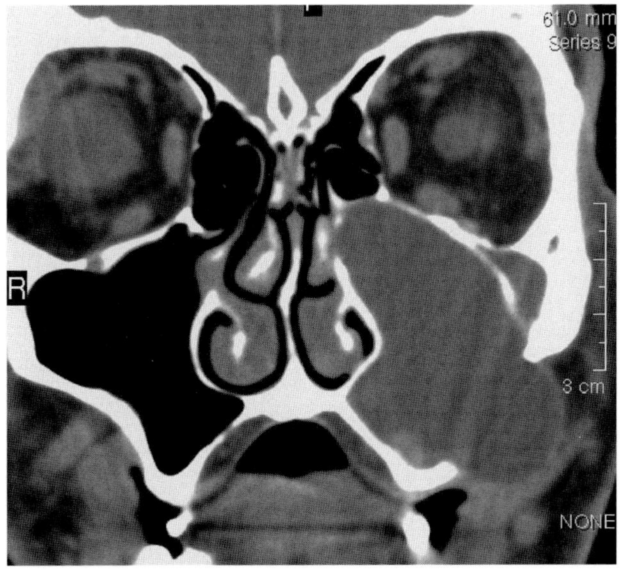

Figure 62F. Patient 1 with dentigerous cyst. Coronal computed tomography image showing an expansile lesion centered in the left maxillary sinus, bulging into the soft tissue of the cheek. The superior aspect of the mass has its own bony wall, distinct from the orbital floor, suggestive of odontogenic lesion.

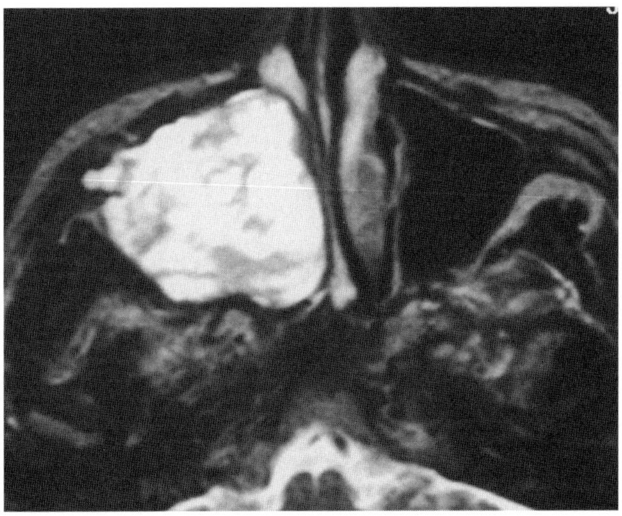

Figure 62G. Patient 2 with ameloblastoma, showing a multiloculated, high-intensity mass involving the right maxillary sinus. T2-weighted axial image.

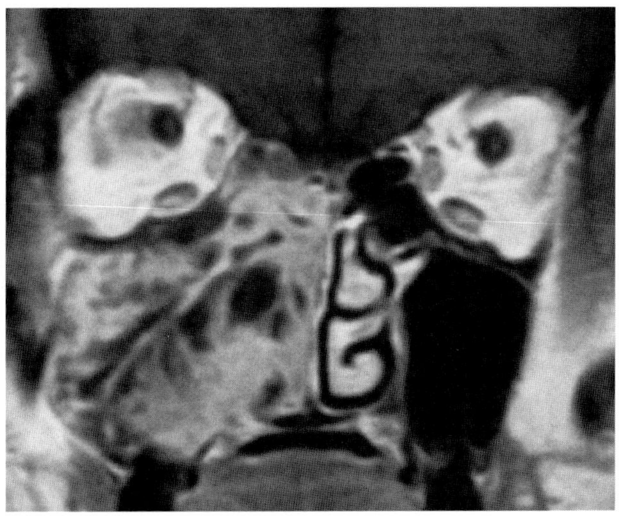

Figure 62H. Patient 2 with ameloblastoma, showing an enhancing mass with multiple cystic components involving the right maxillary sinus and nasal cavity. T1-weighted image with contrast.

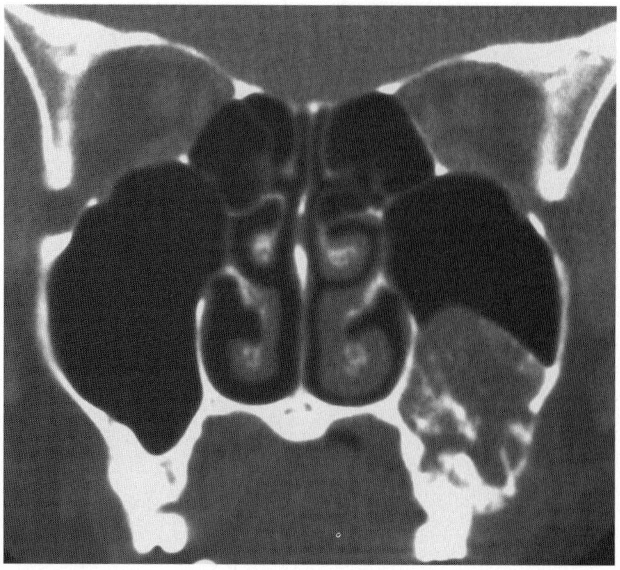

Figure 62I. Patient 3 with odontogenic fibromyxoma, showing a soft tissue mass, with lacelike calcification in the left maxillary sinus and involvement of subjacent alveolar process.

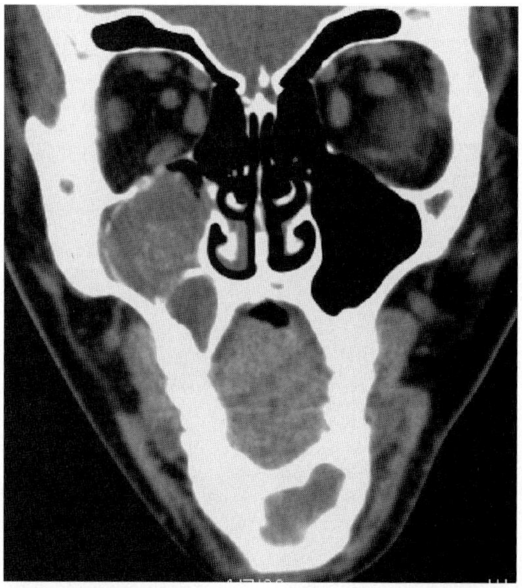

Figure 62J. Patient 4 with basal cell nevus syndrome, showing an expansile mass in the right maxillary sinus, with the appearance of "double wall," and another lesion in the body of the mandible.

CHAPTER 6

PAROTID AND SUBMANDIBULAR GLANDS

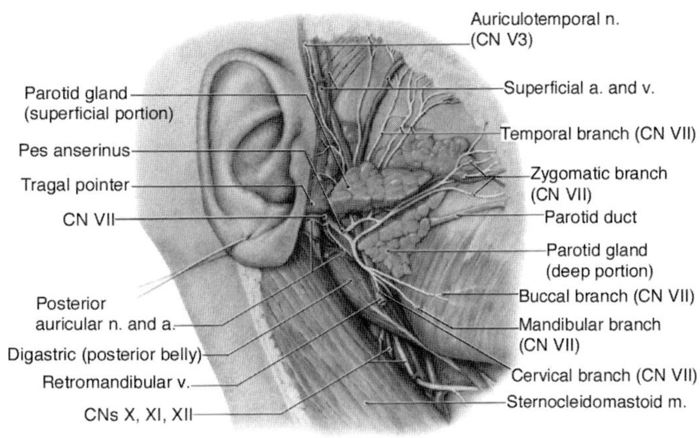

CASE 63

Clinical History: A 35-year-old man presents with a parotid mass and a slowly progressive, peripheral facial nerve deficit.

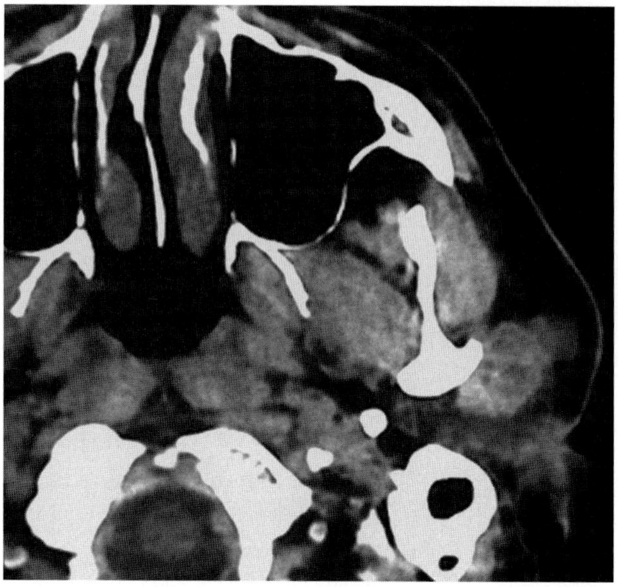

Figure 63A

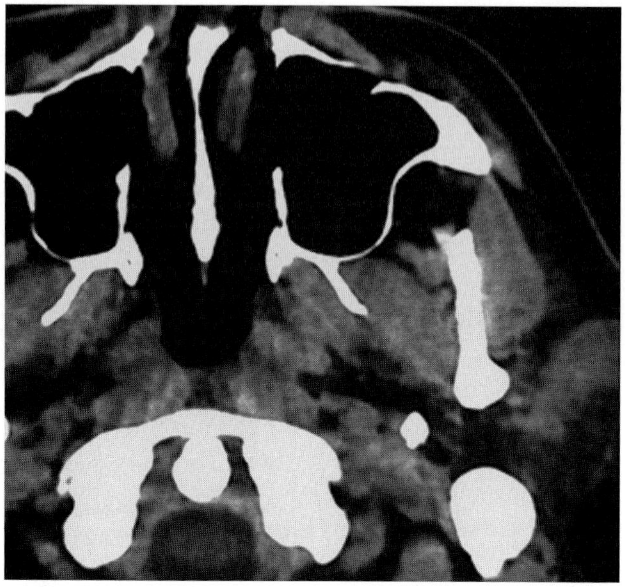

Figure 63B

1. Is the mass intrinsic or extrinsic to the parotid gland?
2. If it is intrinsic, what is its relationship to the facial nerve?
3. Is its gross morphology more suggestive of an aggressive or nonaggressive tumor?
4. What is the most likely diagnosis? What is the most likely explanation for the facial nerve deficit?

Findings

A lobulated mass with indistinct margins in the left parotid gland, mainly in the superficial portion of the gland. The lesion travels partly along the expected position of the main trunk of the facial nerve.

Problem

An adult with a solitary parotid mass and facial nerve dysfunction

Anatomy

A. Parotid gland: deep and superficial portions
B. Facial nerve landmarks: fat pad below the stylomastoid foramen, digastric groove and muscle, tragal pointer, retromandibular vein
C. Facial nerve: main trunk, pes anserinus, major divisions and their positions within the gland and more distally
D. Auriculotemporal nerve

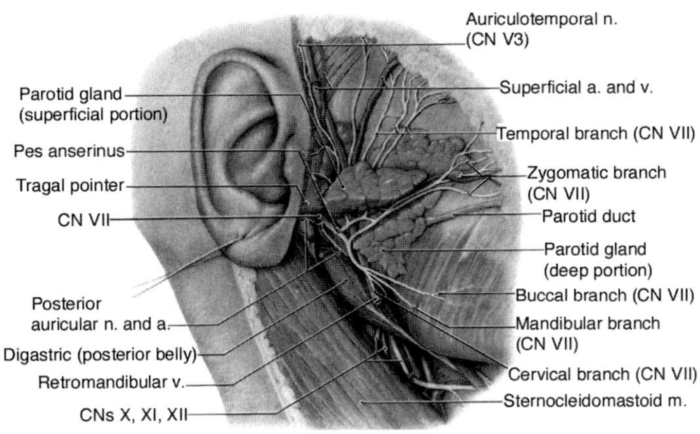

Figure 63C

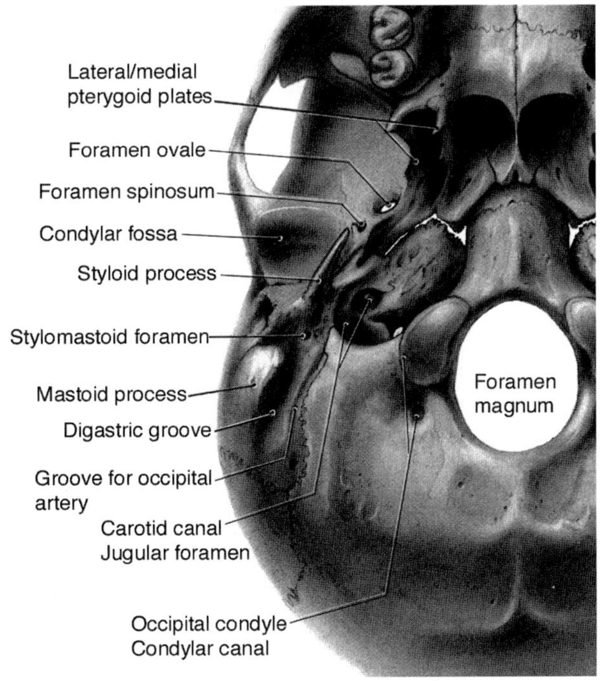

Figure 63D

Differential Diagnosis

Epithelial lesions of glandular origin, both benign and malignant, including benign mixed tumor (pleomorphic adenoma), Warthin's tumor, monomorphic adenoma, oncocytoma, adenoidcystic carcinoma, mucoepidermoid carcinoma, acinic cell carcinoma; metastatic (to parotid node) carcinoma—usually from skin cancer; nodal pathology of another cause (e.g., lymphoma, reactive)

Diagnosis

Adenocystic carcinoma of the parotid gland, with gross extension along the main trunk of the facial nerve

Diagnostic Imaging Approach

A. Is the parotid *region* mass intrinsic or extrinsic to the parotid *gland*?
B. If intrinsic, what is the relationship to the facial nerve?
C. Any sign that the mass is aggressive? Infiltrative margins? Perineural spread? Metastatic nodes?
D. Is the mass(es) solitary, multiple, or bilateral?
E. Evaluate the internal morphology for density, T1- or T2-weighted signal intensity, vascularity, enhancement, calcification.
F. Is there spread beyond the parotid gland?

Clinical Points Of Importance And Supplemental Information

Any patient with a gradual or "stuttering" onset of a peripheral facial nerve deficit *must* have the course of the facial nerve studied from the brainstem nucleus of origin to its peripheral sites of innervation (facial musculature for facial nerve). This *must* include a detailed evaluation of the entire parotid gland.

Answers To Questions

1. Intrinsic
2. Along the plane of the main trunk and pes anserinus
3. Aggressive–indistinct margins
4. Adenoidcystic carcinoma, perineural spread

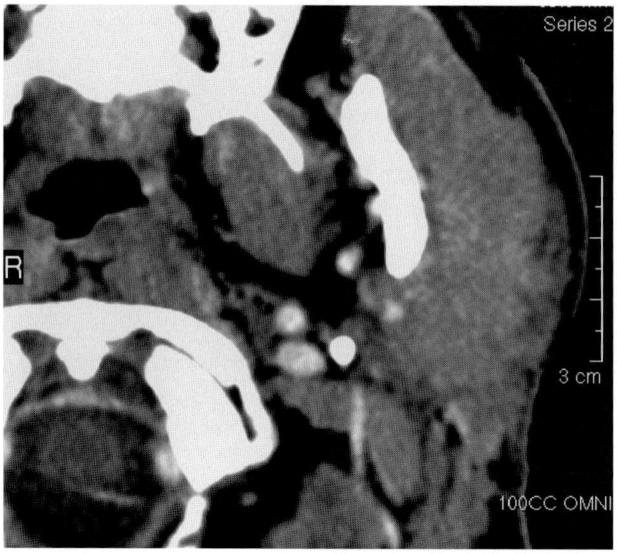

Figure 63E. Patient 1 with undifferentiated carcinoma of the parotid gland, showing an infiltrative mass extensively involving the superficial and deep portion of the parotid gland, including the expected position of the main trunk of the facial nerve. Axial computed tomography image.

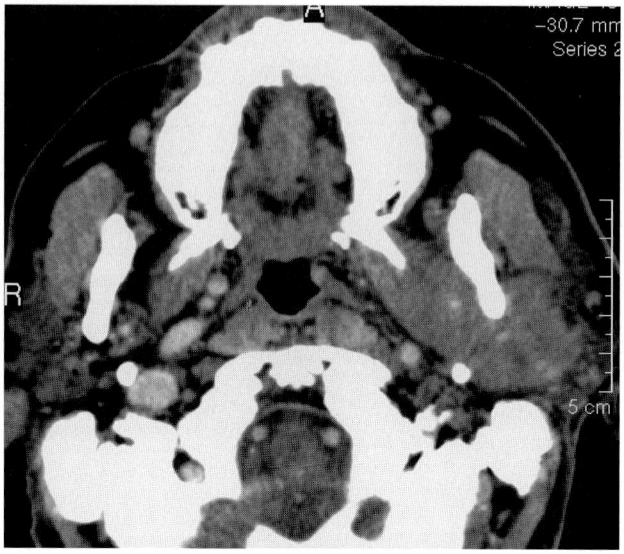

Figure 63F. Patient 2 with high-grade mucoepidermoid carcinoma, showing an infiltrative mass extending along the expected course of the auriculotemporal nerve into the proximal cranial nerve V3 and inferior alveolar nerve (suggested by loss of fat plane in the masticator space). Contrast-enhanced computed tomography image.

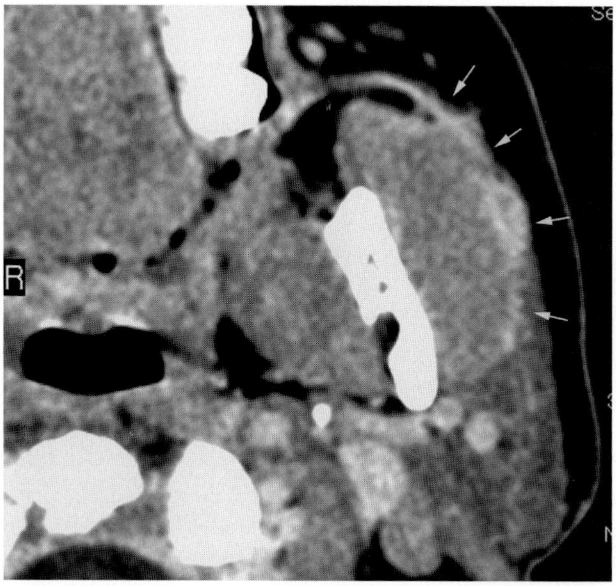

Figure 63G. Patient 3 with a history of resection of skin cancer, presenting with the facial nerve weakness. Contrast-enhanced axial computed tomography image showing linear-shaped enhancing tissue superficial to the masseter muscle along the expected course of the buccal branch of the facial nerve, representing surgically proved perineural tumor spread.

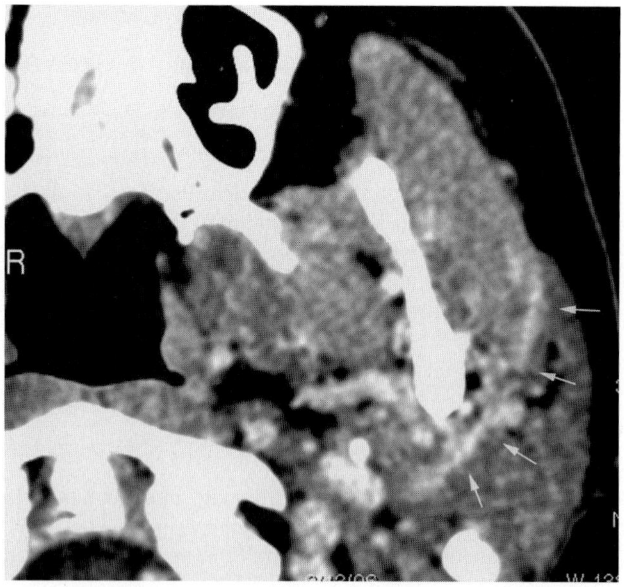

Figure 63H. Patient 3 with history of resection of skin cancer, presenting with the facial nerve weakness. Contrast-enhanced computed tomography image superior to Fig. 63G showing linear enhancement along the expected course of the intraparotid segment of the facial nerve.

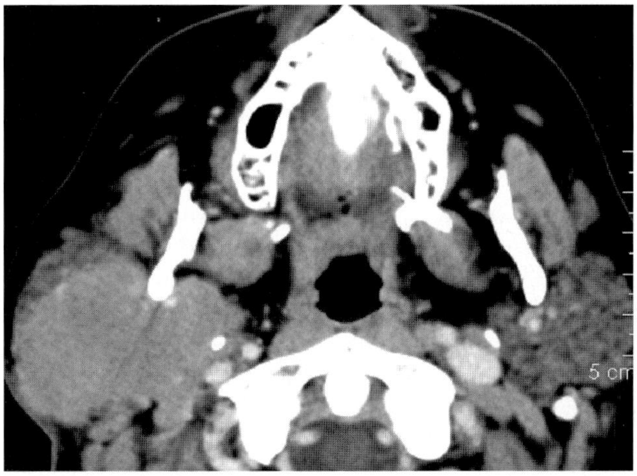

Figure 63I. Patient 4 with Sjögren's syndrome, presenting with non-Hodgkin's lymphoma as a parotid mass. Contrast-enhanced computed tomography image showing a solid mass of homogeneous internal architecture involving the right parotid gland. The spared left parotid gland reveals a typical micronodular pattern of chronic punctate sialoadenitis.

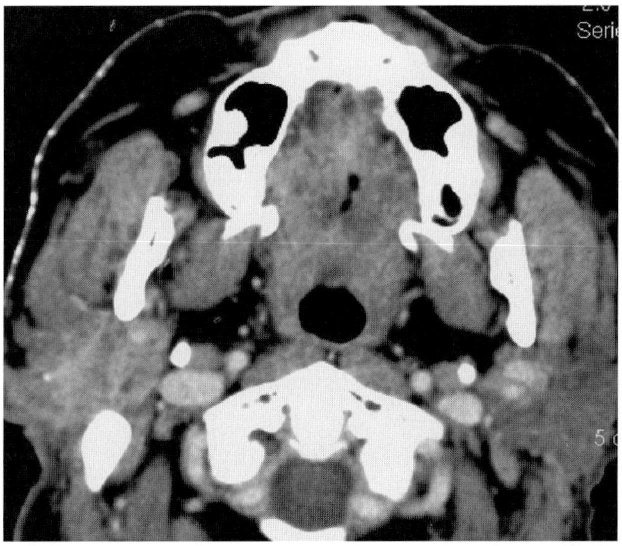

Figure 63J. Patient 5 with adenoid cystic carcinoma of the parotid gland, showing a diffuse, infiltrative mass of the right parotid gland involving the expected position of the main trunk of the facial nerve.

CASE 64

Clinical History: A 55-year-old woman presents with a mass in the parotid region. Because deep margins of the mass could not be appreciated on physical examination, a computed tomography (CT) study was requested.

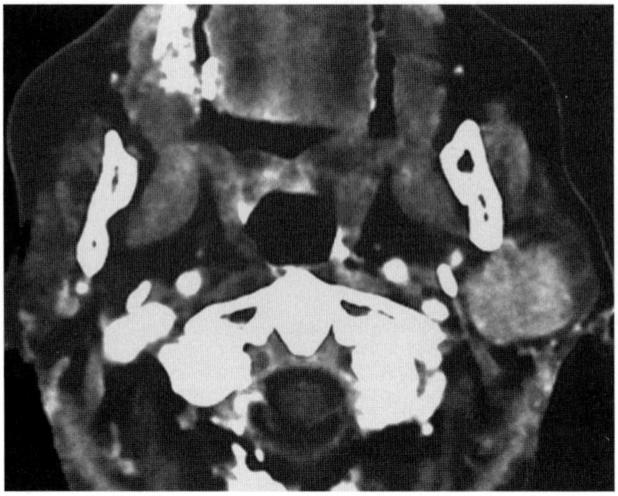

Figure 64A

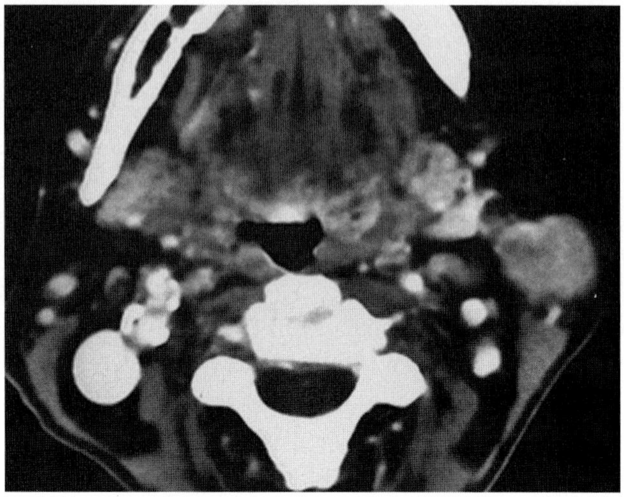

Figure 64B

1. Is the mass intrinsic or extrinsic to the parotid gland?
2. If it is intrinsic, what is its relationship to the main trunk of the facial nerve?
3. Is the mass morphologically aggressive or nonaggressive? What are two imaging signs (besides infiltrating margins) that indicate an aggressive, potentially malignant, lesion?
4. Give the two most likely histologic diagnoses.
5. How is a parotid mass "biopsied" by clinicians (other than needle biopsy)?

Findings

A lobulated, soft tissue mass within the left parotid gland, involving the parotid tail and both the superficial and deep portions of the gland. Its margins are partly irregular.

Problem

A middle-aged adult with a parotid mass

Anatomy

A. Parotid gland: deep and superficial portions, tail, capsule
B. Facial nerve: position of buccal, mandibular, and cervical divisions in the parotid gland (see Fig. 63C)
C. Parotid region lymph nodes: usual locations
D. Retromandibular vein and external carotid artery

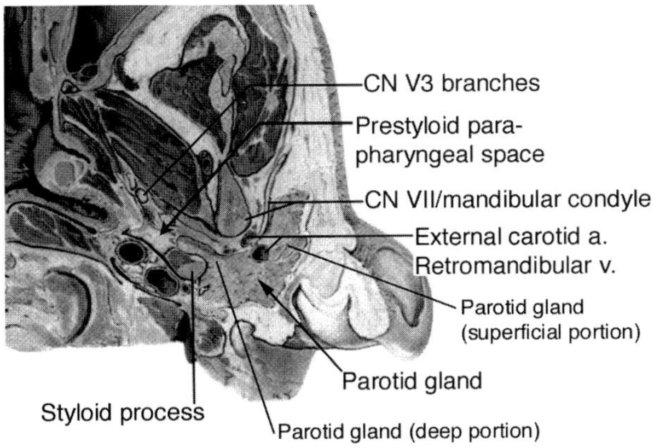

Figure 64C

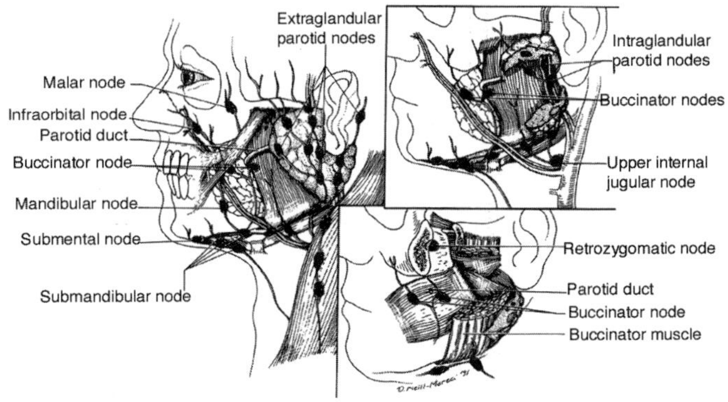

Figure 64D

Differential Diagnosis

Benign epithelial origin parotid lesions: benign mixed tumor (pleomorphic adenoma), Warthin's tumor; malignant epithelial parotid lesions: various carcinomas; metastatic cancer to intraparotid node: usually from a skin primary tumor (squamous cell carcinoma, melanoma, Merkel cell tumor); nodal pathology: lymphoma, reactive

Diagnosis

Warthin's tumor (papillary cystadenoma lymphomatosum) centered in the tail of the parotid gland but involving both its deep and superficial portions

Diagnostic Imaging Approach

A. Intrinsic or extrinsic to the parotid gland?
B. Relationship to the facial nerve?
C. Any signs of the mass being aggressive?
D. Solitary, multiple, or bilateral?
E. Evaluate the internal morphology of mass(es): density, T1- or T2-weighted signal intensity, vascularity, enhancement, calcification.
F. Is there spread beyond the parotid gland?

Clinical Points Of Importance And Supplemental Information

If the referring clinician cannot determine the origin or extent of a parotid region mass by palpation, it must be imaged before any definitive surgical procedure (i.e., needle biopsy can precede imaging, but imaging should precede excision).

Answers To Questions

1. Intrinsic
2. Inferior to the main trunk
3. Hard to determine. Perineural spread, nodal metastases
4. If nonaggressive, benign mixed tumor, Warthin's tumor
5. Superficial parotidectomy: excision, including a margin of normal parotid tissue

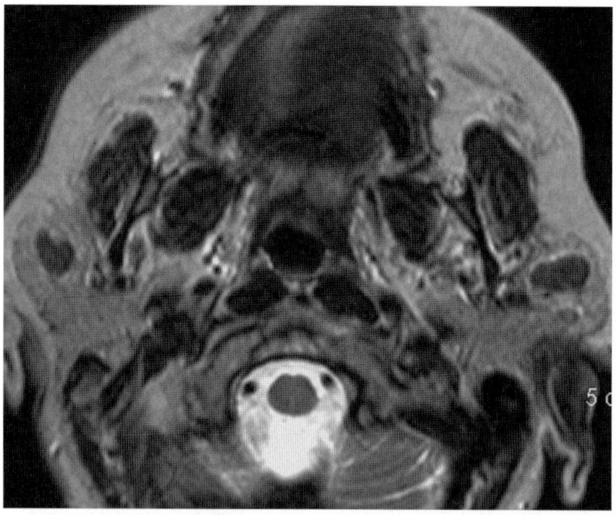

Figure 64E. Patient 1 with Warthin's tumor, showing multiple parotid nodules on both sides. T2-weighted axial image.

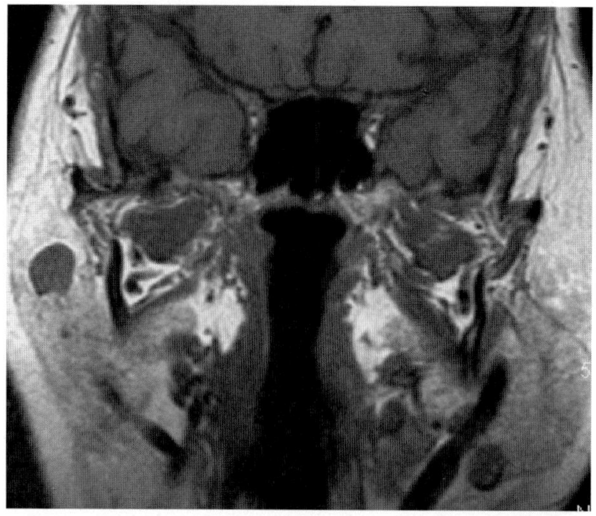

Figure 64F. Patient 1 with Warthin's tumor. T1-weighted coronal image also showing multiple parotid nodules on both sides.

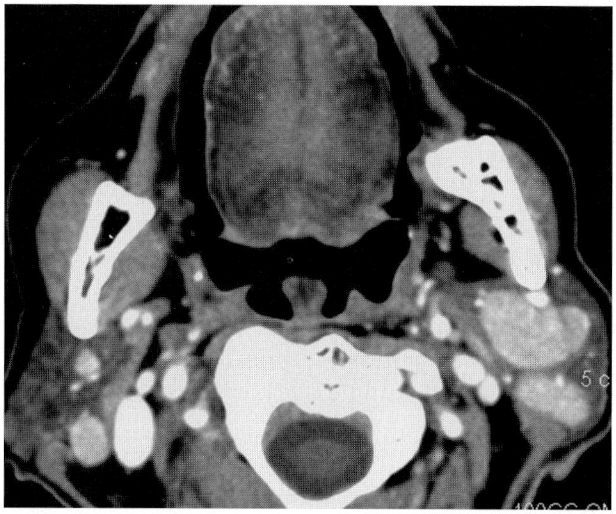

Figure 64G. Patient 2 presenting with left parotid mass, showing multiple, enhancing nodular lesions caused by Warthin's tumors in the parotid tail on both sides. Smaller one in the right parotid tail was not palpable.

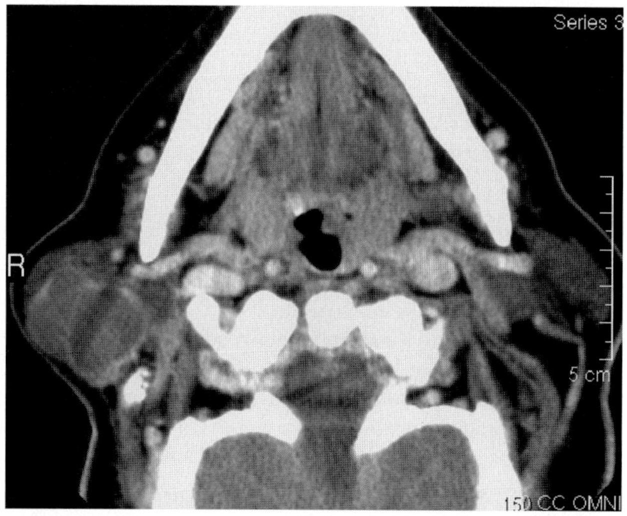

Figure 64H. Patient 3 with Warthin's tumor, showing mainly a cystic mass centered in the tail of the right parotid gland. Computed tomography image with contrast.

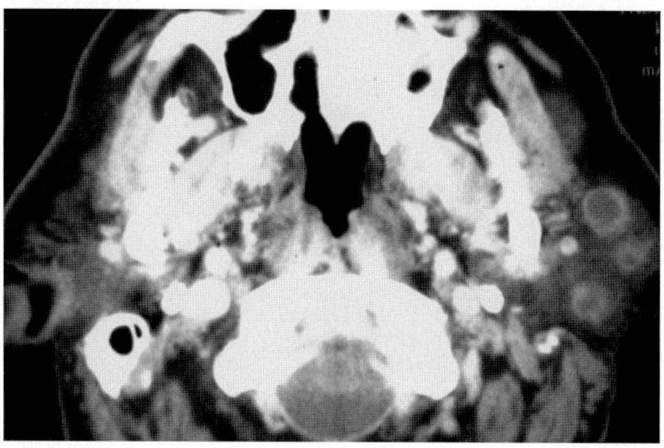

Figure 64I. Patient 4 with squamous cell carcinoma of the skin, with metastases to the parotid nodes. Multiple rim-enhancing nodules are noted randomly distributing in the left parotid gland on contrast-enhanced computed tomography image.

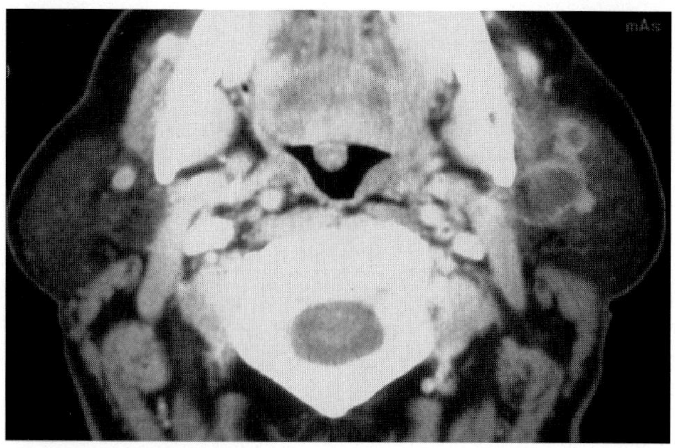

Figure 64J. Patient 5 with squamous cell carcinoma of the skin, with metastases to the parotid nodes. Contrast-enhanced computed tomography image inferior to Fig. 64I.

CASE 65

Clinical History: A 14-year-old girl presents with a mass in the parotid region.

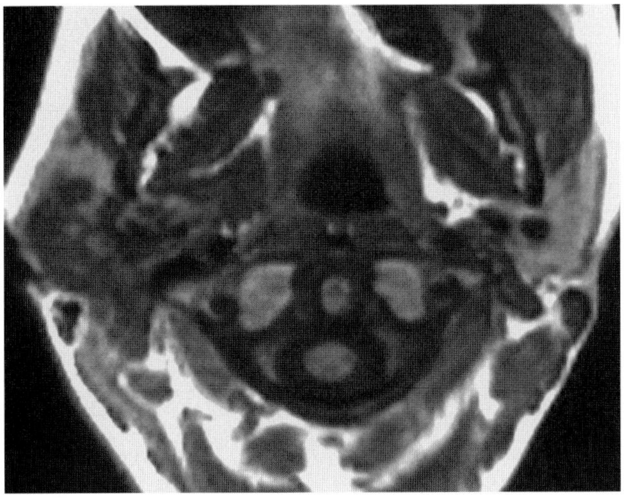

Figure 65A

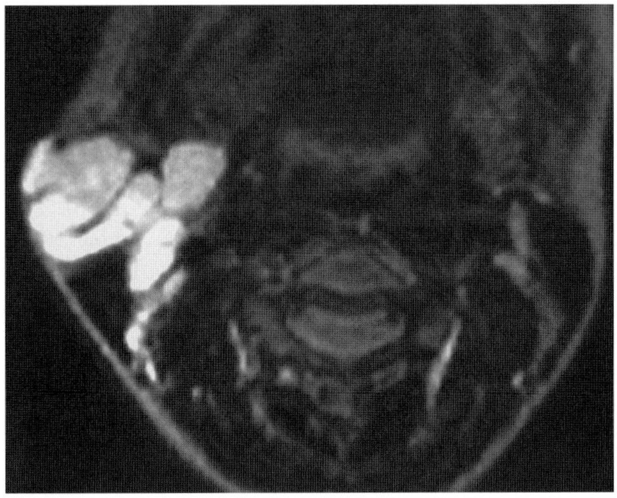

Figure 65B

1. Is the mass intrinsic or extrinsic to the parotid gland?
2. What is the most likely diagnosis?
3. Can epithelial neoplasms of the parotid gland have a similar appearance to this lesion (hint: its not an epithelial lesion) on T2-weighted images? If so, why?

Findings

A multiloculated cystic mass mainly involving the right parotid gland. The lesion protrudes into the prestyloid parapharyngeal space through the stylomandibular tunnel and extends into the posterior triangle. No evident fluid–fluid level noted in its chambers.

Problem

A teenager with a parotid mass

Anatomy

A. Parotid gland: capsule and attachments to external auditory canal
B. Prestyloid parapharyngeal space: limits (see Fig. 64C)
C. Spinal accessory nerve in the upper neck

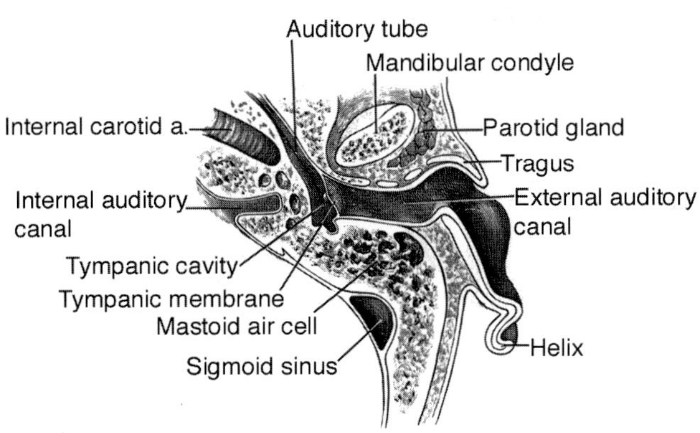

Figure 65C

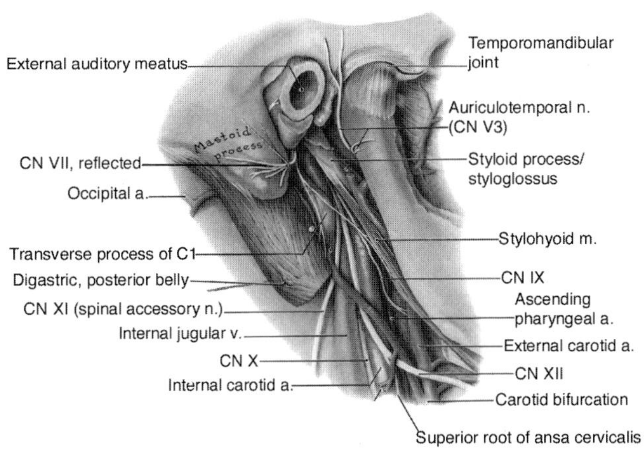

Figure 65D

Differential Diagnosis (For A Child Or Teenager)

Lymphangioma or cystic hygroma, hemangioma, epithelial neoplasm of parotid origin (benign mixed tumor)

Diagnosis

Cystic hygroma (lymphangioma) of the parotid gland, upper posterior triangle, and prestyloid parapharyngeal space

Diagnostic Imaging Approach

A. Parotid or nonparotid gland origin?
B. Relationship of the lesion to the facial nerve?
C. Spread beyond the parotid gland?
D. Solitary, multiple, or bilateral?
E. Evaluate the internal morphology of the mass(es): density, T1- or T2-weighted signal intensity, vascularity, enhancement pattern, calcification.
F. Any signs of aggressive behavior?

Clinical Points Of Importance And Supplemental Information

A. Differential diagnosis of masses in the parotid gland region differs markedly in the pediatric and adult population.
B. Lymphangiomas or cystic hygromas frequently have hemangiomatous components.
C. Branchial cleft cysts are almost never multilocular and do not demonstrate the insinuating growth pattern seen in this case.

Answers To Questions

1. Intrinsic
2. Lymphangioma
3. Yes. Both can contain relatively large fluid-filled spaces or be microcystic.

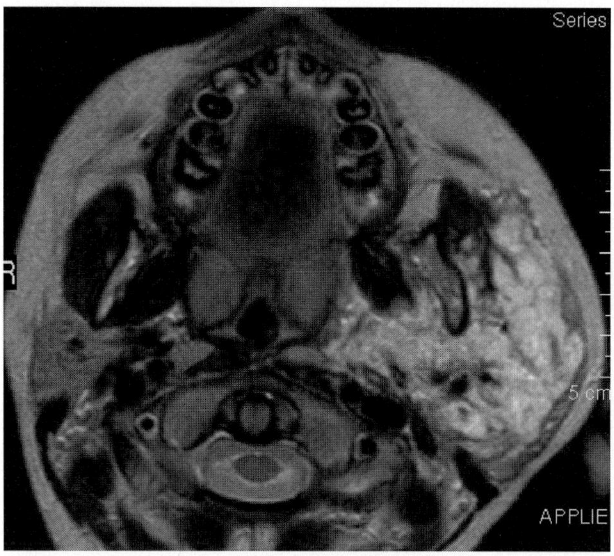

Figure 65E. Patient 1 (1 y/F) with cavernous type vascular malformation of the parotid gland. T2-weighted axial image showing holoparotid involvement of the multilobulated high-intensity mass with direct involvement of adjacent masseter and pterygoid muscles and parapharyngeal space.

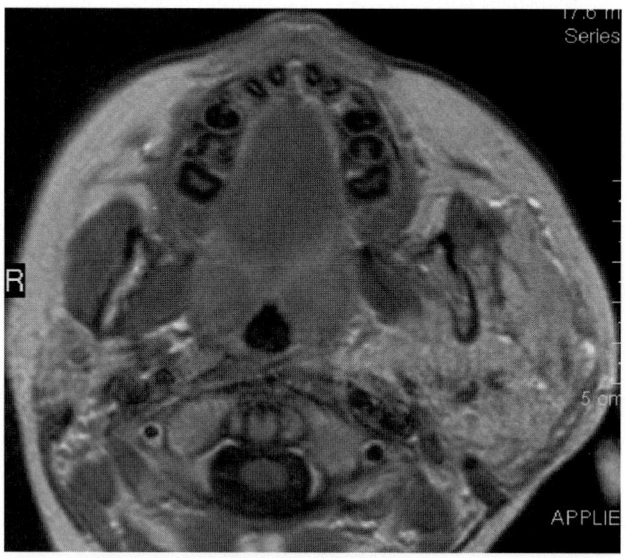

Figure 65F. Patient 1 (1 y/F) with cavernous type vascular malformation of the parotid gland. T1-weighted with contrast showing diffuse enhancement of the mass.

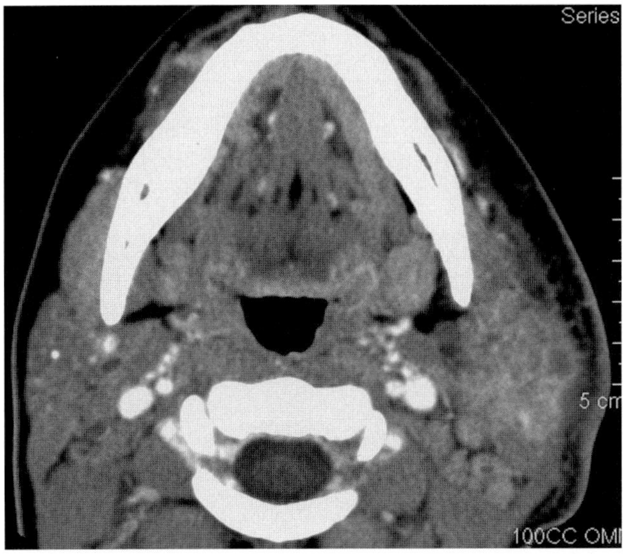

Figure 65G. Patient 2 (11 y/F) with chronic recurrent parotitis in childhood. Contrast-enhanced axial computed tomography image showing a cystic area in the swollen left parotid tail with extensive inflammatory edema in the surrounding soft tissue. Sialoadenitis is noted in the somewhat prominent right parotid tail with diffuse increase in the density due to contrast enhancement.

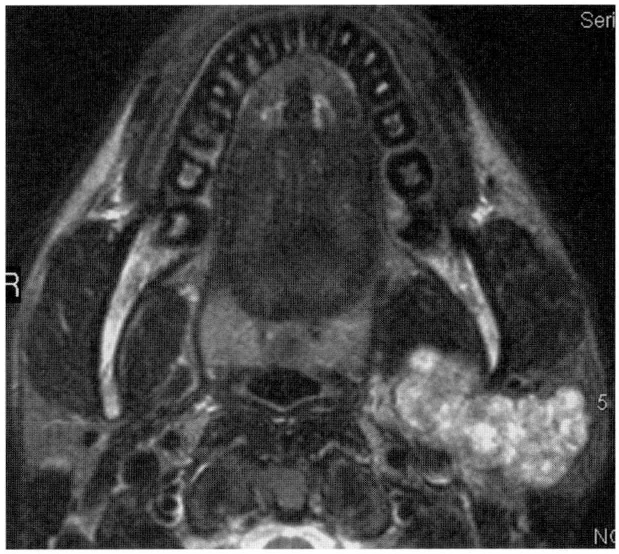

Figure 65H. Patient 3 (18 y/M) with pleomorphic adenoma, showing a lobulated high-intensity mass with cystic components involving both deep and superficial portions of the left parotid gland and extending medially into the prestyloid compartment of the parapharyngeal space.

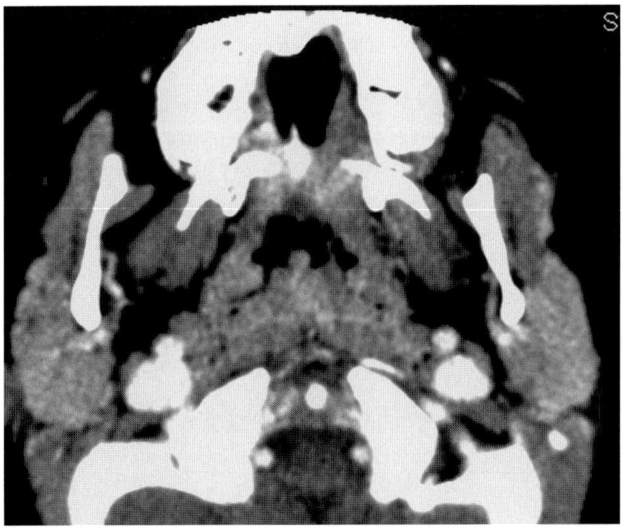

Figure 65I. Patient 4 (10 y/F) with presumed viral parotitis, showing diffuse enlargement of the parotid gland on both sides, which enhances more than usual.

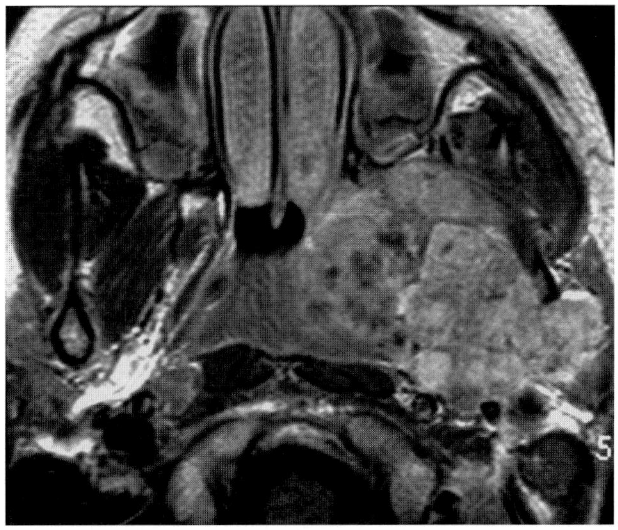

Figure 65J. Patient 5 (14 y/F) with undifferentiated sarcoma, showing an infiltrative mass involving the left parotid gland, masticator space, and prestyloid parapharyngeal space.

CASE 66

Clinical History: A 65-year-old man presents with a solitary parotid gland region mass on physical examination. Facial nerve function is normal.

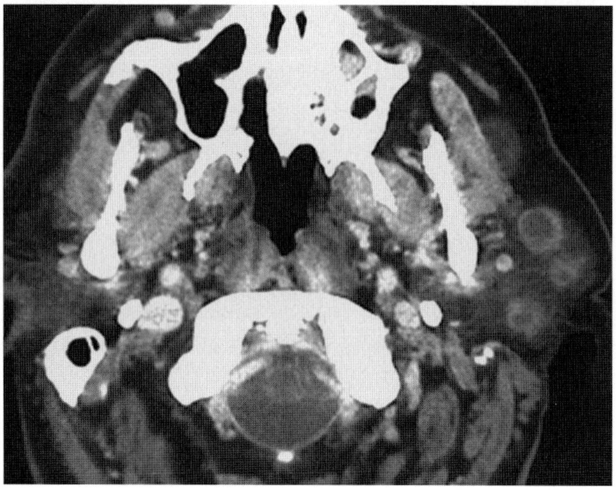

Figure 66A

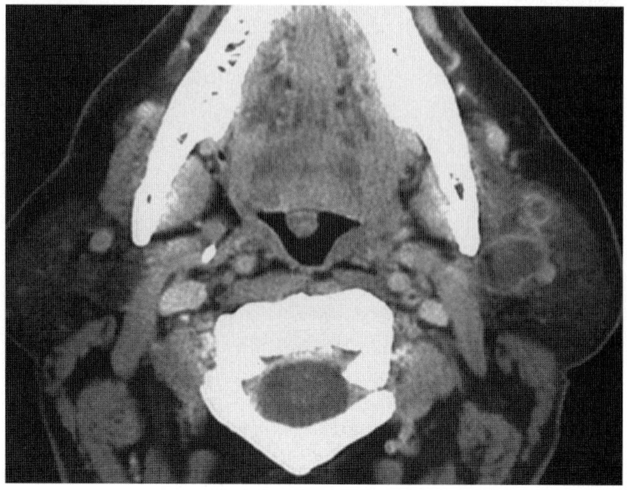

Figure 66B

1. Is the mass intrinsic or extrinsic to the parotid gland?
2. What is the relationship of the mass to the facial nerve?
3. Are there any signs that suggest this may be an aggressive (malignant) rather than benign disease process?
4. List three causes of multiple, *unilateral intra*parotid masses, and three causes of multiple bilateral *intra*parotid masses.
5. If a needle biopsy of the mass indicates a squamous cell carcinoma, what question would you like to ask the patient?

Findings

Multiple rim-enhancing nodules randomly distributing in the left parotid gland

Problem

An elderly man with multiple, unilateral parotid masses

Anatomy

A. Parotid lymph nodes: intraparotid, subcapsular, and periparotid
B. Posterior neck nodes: retromastoid, occipital
C. Level V (spinal accessory nodes)
D. Facial lymph nodes: infraorbital, zygomatic, retrozygomatic, buccal, mandibular

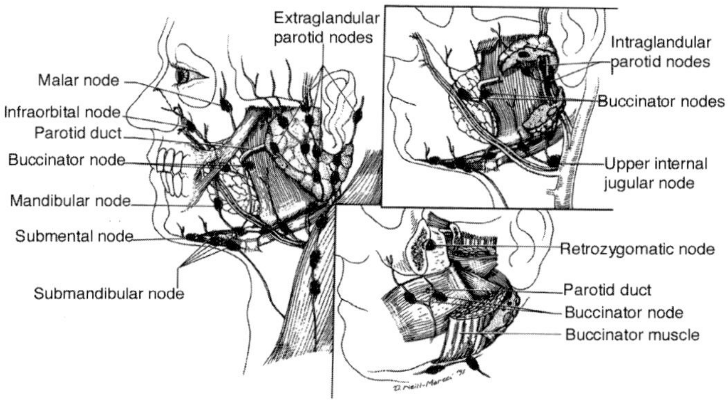

Figure 66C

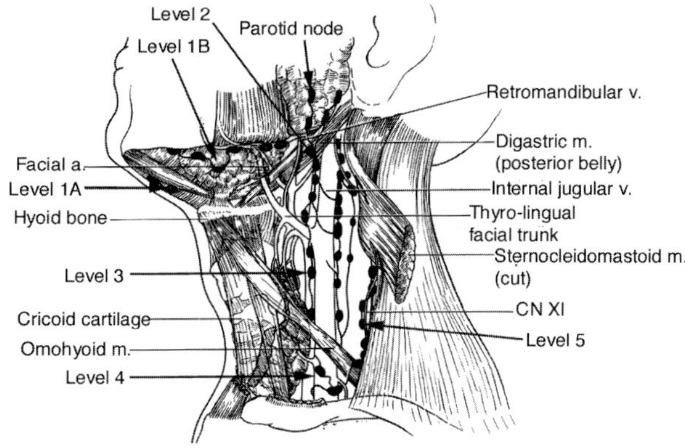

Figure 66D

Differential Diagnosis

1. Multiple unilateral masses: Warthin's tumor, epithelial parotid primary tumor with nodal metastases; metastatic skin cancer, lymphoma, reactive nodes, multiple lymphoepithelial lesions (usually bilateral), autoimmune disease
2. Multiple bilateral masses: Warthin's tumor, multiple lymphoepithelial lesions (human immunodeficiency virus [HIV]); lymphoma; reactive nodes, metastases (rare); autoimmune disease

Diagnosis

Squamous cell carcinoma of the skin (removed 2 years before) metastatic to parotid lymph nodes

Diagnostic Imaging Approach

A. Is the mass(es) intrinsic or extrinsic to the parotid gland?
B. Relationship to the facial nerve?
C. Any evidence of aggressive behavior?
D. Solitary, multiple, or bilateral?
E. If multiple, unilateral masses intrinsic to the gland are noted, is there a dominant mass that suggests a parotid gland primary tumor?
F. Evaluate the internal morphology of the mass(es): density, T1- or T2-weighted signal intensity, vascularity, enhancement pattern, calcification.

Clinical Points Of Importance And Supplemental Information

A. Triad of multiple lymphoepithelial parotid lesions, cervical adenopathy, and adenoidal hypertrophy strongly suggests HIV infection.
B. Multiple nodes containing focal defects strongly suggests metastatic skin cancer; ask for a history of removal of a skin lesion because sometimes a patient is not aware that the lesion was cancerous.

Answers To Questions

1. Intrinsic
2. Not relevant
3. Probable multiple metastatic parotid gland nodes
4. Unilateral: metastatic nodes, primary parotid tumor with nodes, Warthin's tumor, reactive nodes; bilateral: lymphoma, lymphepithelial lesions of HIV, Warthin's tumor
5. Have you ever had a skin lesion removed?

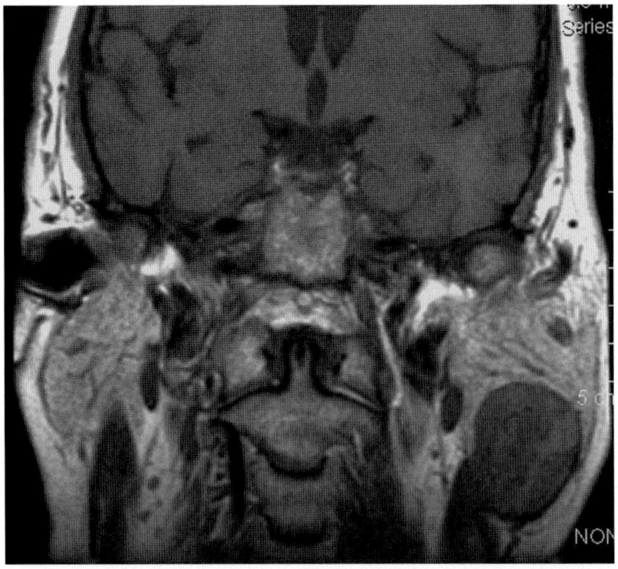

Figure 66E. Patient 1 with Warthin's tumor, showing a well-circumscribed mass centered in the left parotid tail and another smaller nodule in the upper portion, which was not palpable by physical examination. T1-weighted axial image without contrast.

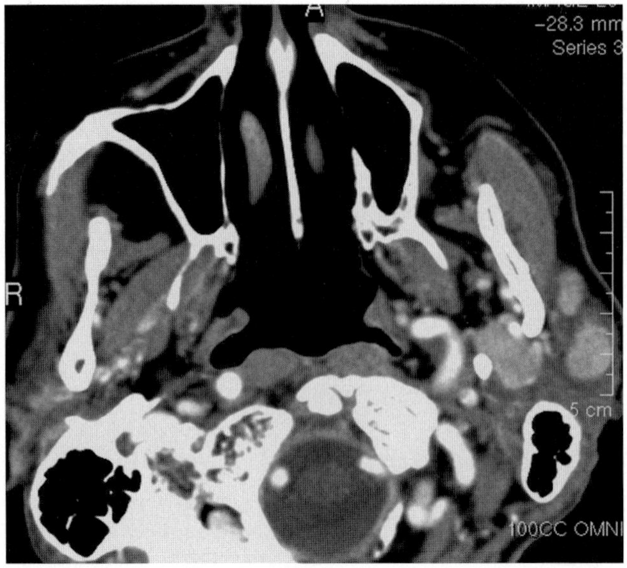

Figure 66F. Patient 2 with Warthin's tumor, showing multiple enhancing tumors in the left parotid gland.

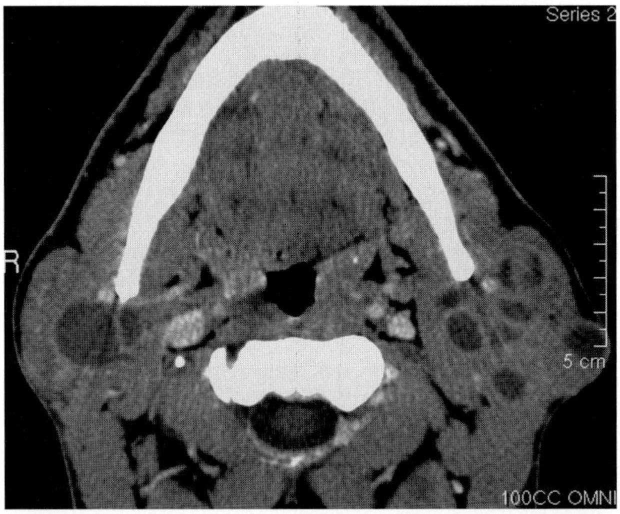

Figure 66G. Patient 3 who is HIV-positive, showing multiple cystic lesions in the enlarged parotid gland on both sides, representing lymphoepithelial cysts. Contrast-enhanced computed tomography image.

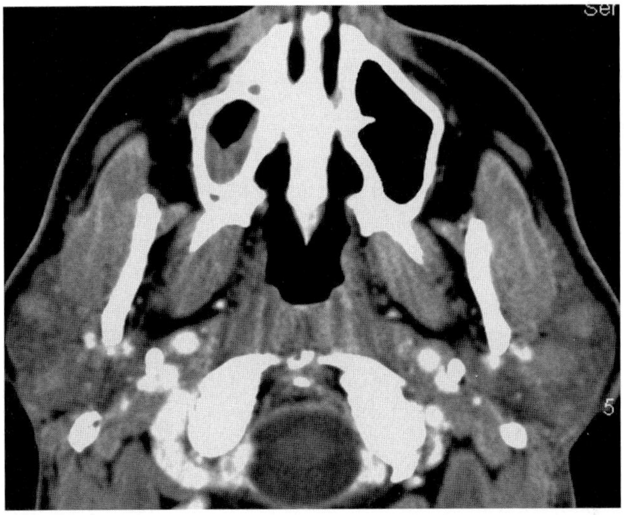

Figure 66H. Patient 4 with chronic myelogenic leukemia, showing multiple parotid lymph nodes bilaterally. Contrast-enhanced computed tomography study.

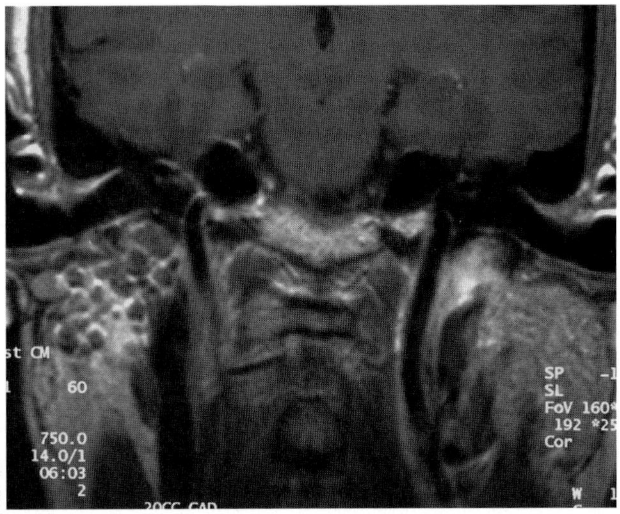

Figure 66I. Patient 5 with recurrent pleomorphic adenoma. T1-weighted coronal image with contrast showing numerous recurrent nodules in the right parotid gland.

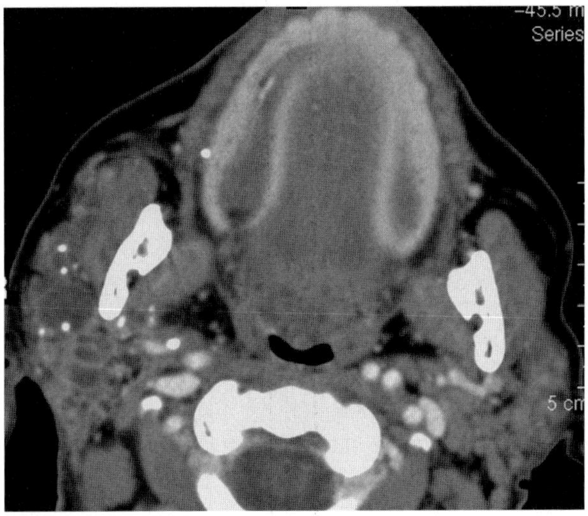

Figure 66J. Patient 6 with Sjögren's syndrome, showing multiple cystic areas in an enlarged right parotid gland, which contains multiple sialolithiases, which is consistent with cystic change caused by chronic punctate sialoadenitis. A diffuse increase in density with the micronodular pattern is noted in the opposite parotid gland. Contrast-enhanced computed tomography image.

CASE 67

Clinical History: A 46-year-old man presents with a history of a right-sided mass near the angle of the mandible. After physical examination, the mass was believed to arise in the submandibular region and possibly be an abnormal lymph node. Some vague tenderness to palpation was noted and he had a history of possible intermittent swelling.

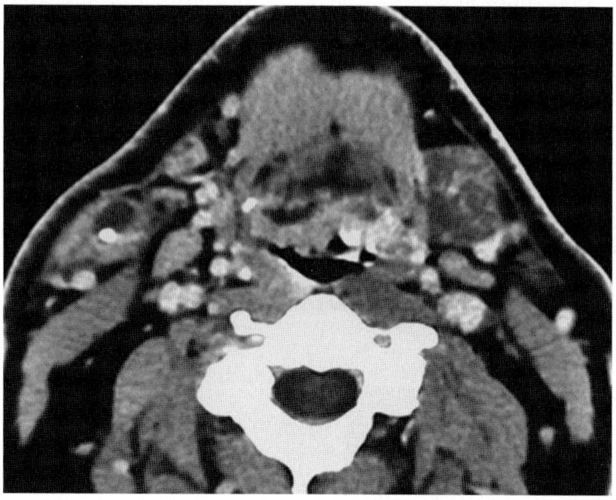

Figure 67A

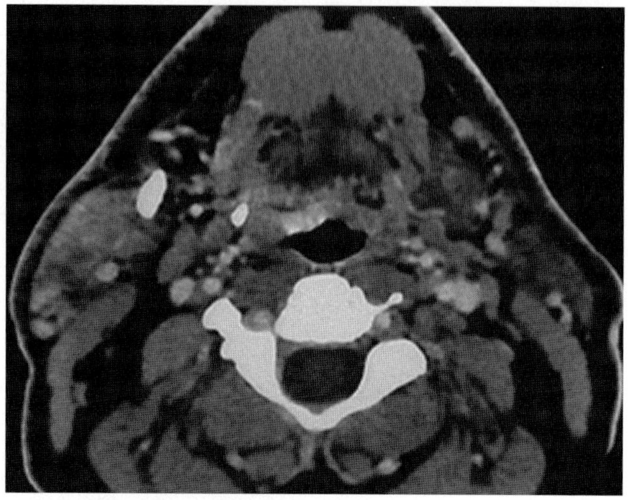

Figure 67B

1. What is the site of origin of the mass?
2. Give as complete a diagnosis as possible.
3. Is sialography useful for diagnosis or management during an episode of acute sialadenitis?

Findings

The tail of the right parotid gland enhances diffusely. A unilocular 1-cm cystic lesion containing calcific focus is centered in the parotid tail. Mild skin thickening and stranding in subcutaneous tissue around it suggests a possible inflammatory process. The right submandibular gland is atrophic.

Problem

An adult with a mass arising in the tail of the parotid gland and a history suggesting a possible inflammatory cause

Anatomy

A. Parotid gland: tail
B. Submandibular space: group I nodes, submandibular gland, platysma
C. Mylohyoid and anterior belly of digastric muscles

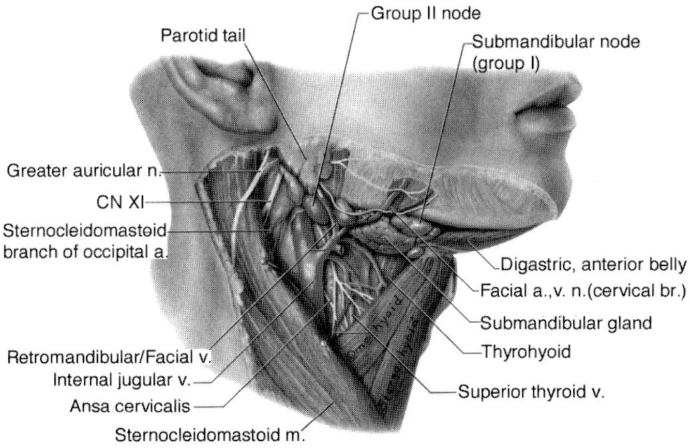

Figure 67C

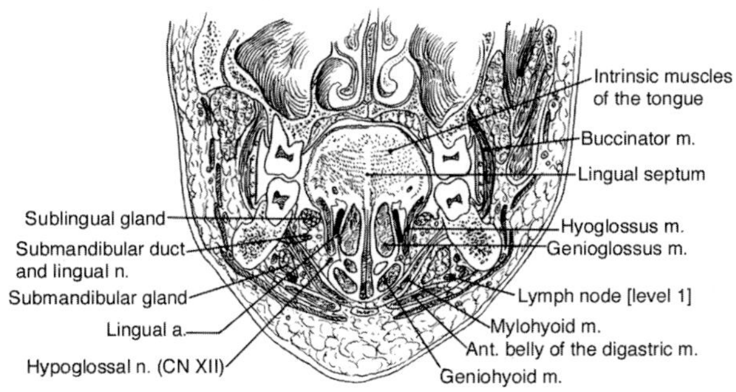

Figure 67D

Differential Diagnosis

Sialocele, mucocele, first branchial cleft cyst (when in parotid or periparotid), node (inflammatory or neoplastic), cystic parotid neoplasm

Diagnosis

Low grade parotid sialadenitis, with sialolithiasis and a probable sialocele or mucocele

Diagnostic Imaging Approach

A. What is the site of origin (i.e., mandible, parotid, submandibular gland, nodal, other)?
B. If a salivary gland is the site of origin, is there evidence of sialadenitis (e.g., enhancement, stones, ductal dilatation)?
C. Unilateral or bilateral?
D. Is more than one salivary gland involved (choices: parotid, submandibular gland, sublingual)?

Clinical Points Of Importance And Supplemental Information

Sialography should be avoided in patients with acute sialadenitis because it can potentially worsen the disease. Sialography remains the best examination for evaluating the parotid and submandibular ductal system.

Answers To Questions

1. Parotid tail
2. Sialocele, sialolithiasis, and focal sialoadenitis
3. No–it is contraindicated

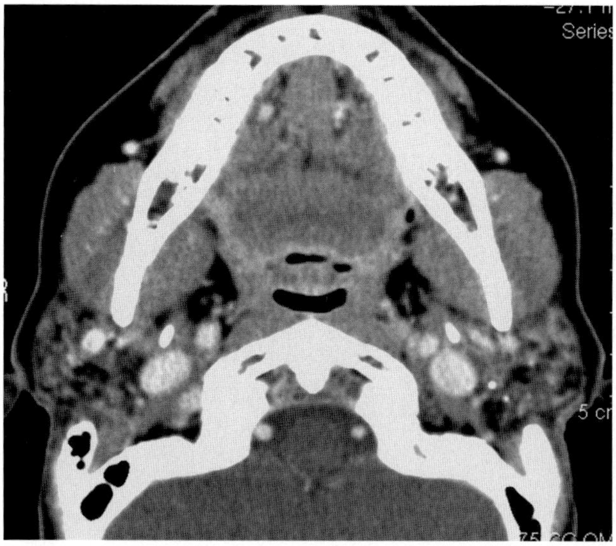

Figure 67E. Patient 1 with Sjögren's syndrome, showing a micronodular pattern throughout the parotid gland bilaterally, consistent with chronic punctate sialoadenitis. Several calcific foci are noted, which is suggestive of sialolithiasis. Contrast-enhanced computed tomography image.

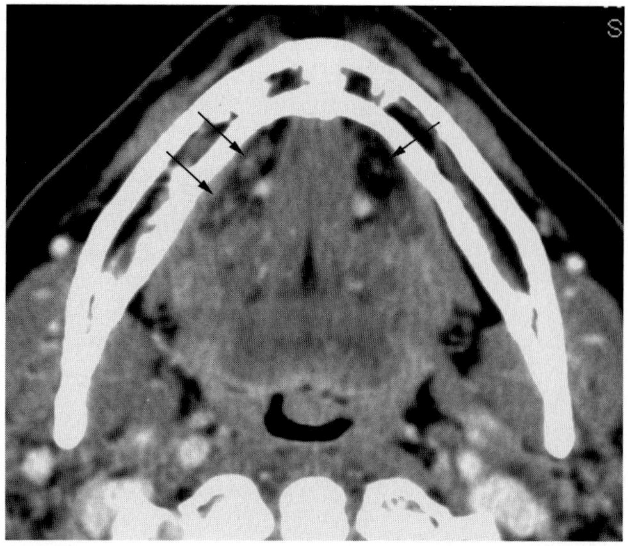

Figure 67F. Patient 1 with Sjöogren's syndrome. Contrast-enhanced computed tomography image inferior to Fig. 67E showing a micronodular pattern in the expected position of the sublingual gland bilaterally, which is suggestive of involvement of the chronic punctate sialoadenitis.

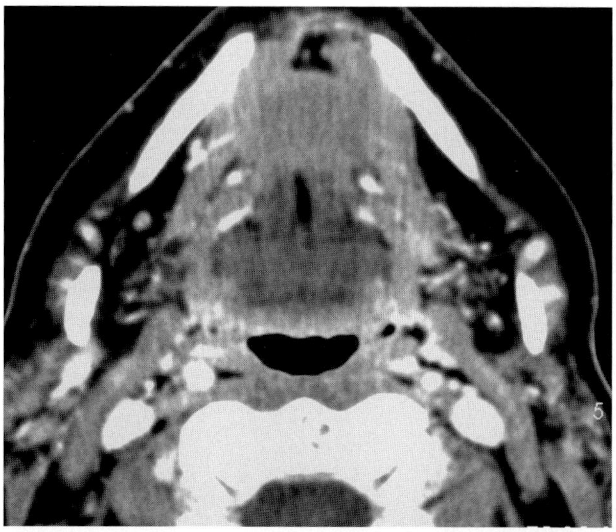

Figure 67G. Patient 1 with Sjögren's syndrome, with the submandibular gland and parotid tail also showing atrophy and a micronodular pattern bilaterally. Contrast-enhanced computed tomography image inferior to Fig. 67F.

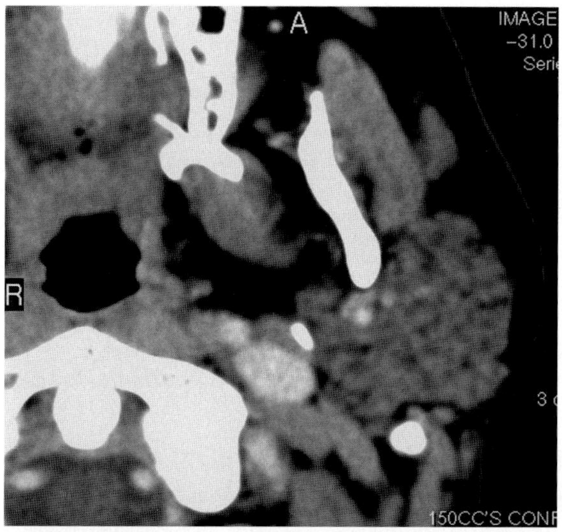

Figure 67H. Patient 2 with Sjögren's syndrome, showing a micronodular pattern throughout the parotid gland, which is consistent with chronic punctate sialoadenitis caused by an autoimmune disease.

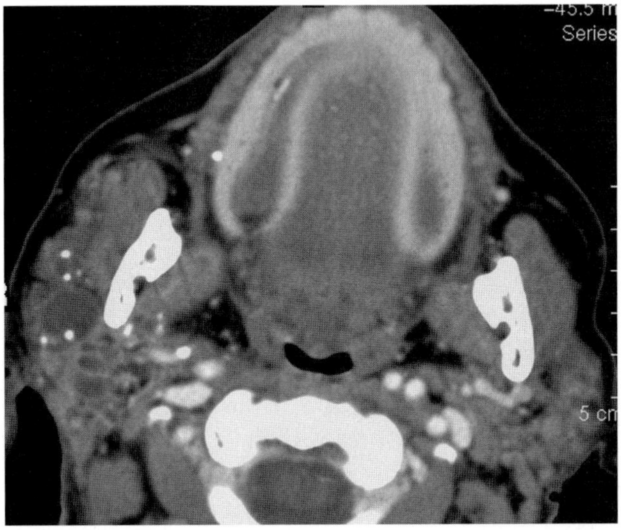

Figure 67I. Patient 3 with Sjögren's syndrome, showing multiple cystic areas in an enlarged right parotid gland that contains multiple sialolithiases, which is consistent with a cystic change caused by chronic punctate sialoadenitis. A diffuse increase in density is noted with micronodular pattern in the opposite parotid gland. Contrast-enhanced computed tomography image.

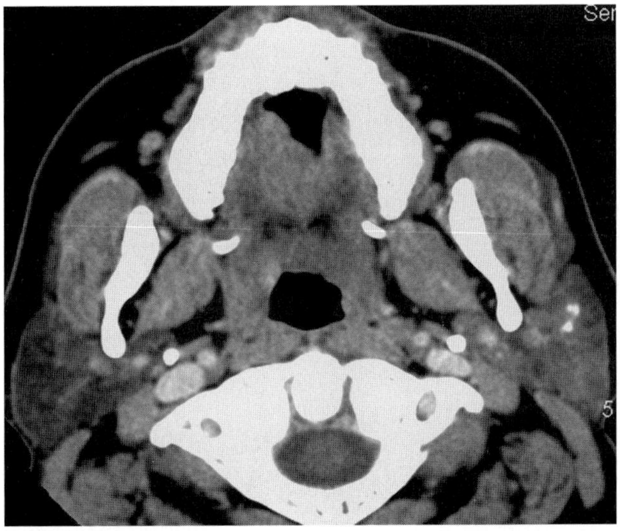

Figure 67J. Patient 4 with chronic inflammation of the parotid gland, showing an infiltrative process with calcified foci in the left parotid gland, mimicking high-grade malignancy. (Biopsy specimen reveals chronic inflammatory change with intraductal calculus.) Contrast-enhanced computed tomography image.

CASE 68

Clinical History: A 26-year-old woman presents with a parotid gland region mass.

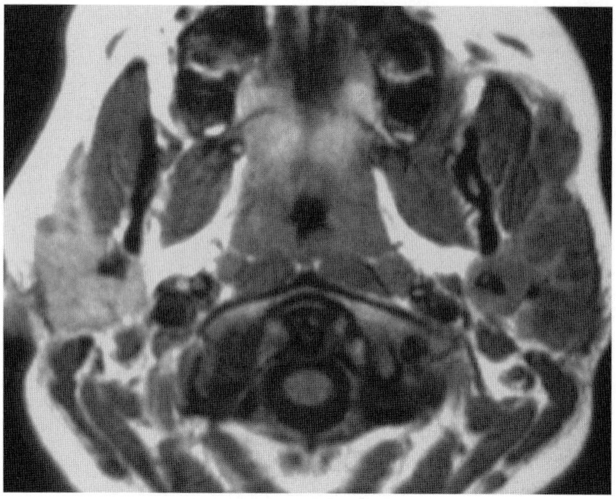

Figure 68A

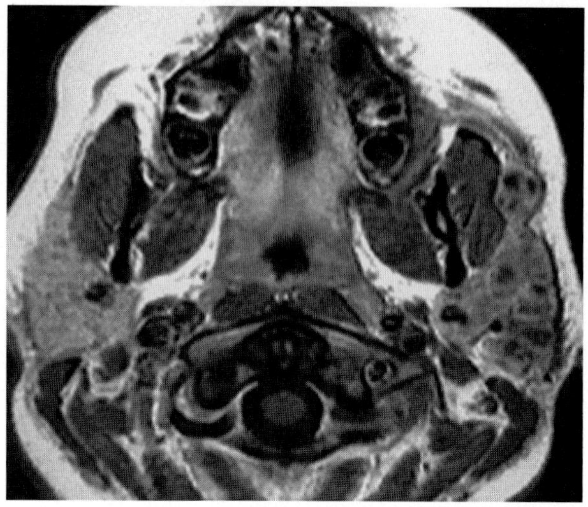

Figure 68B

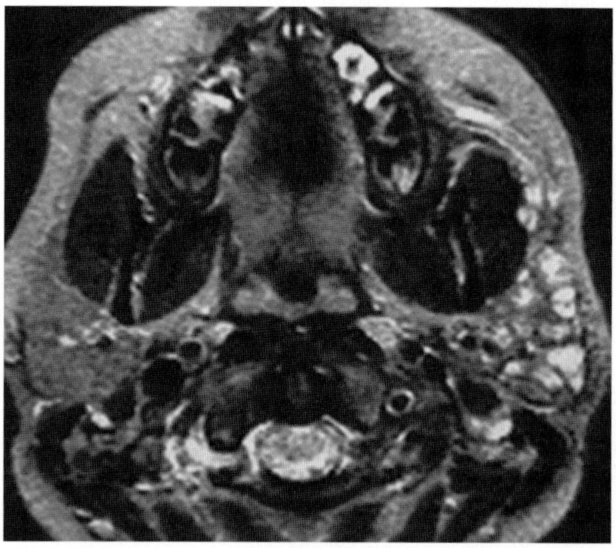

Figure 68C

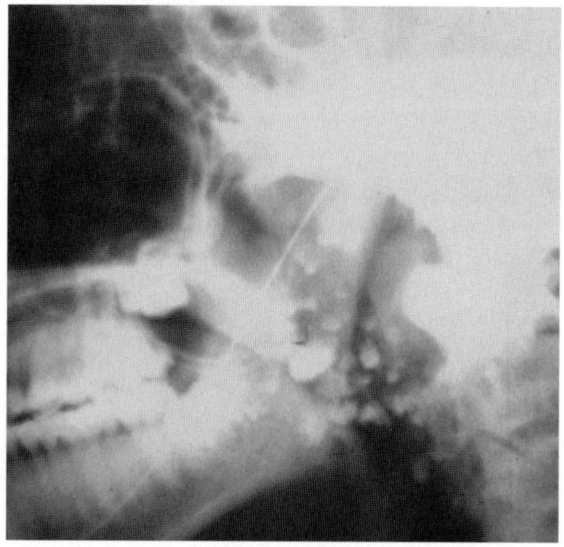

Figure 68D

1. Is a definable mass present?
2. What generic term best describes the findings in the parotid gland?
3. What additional medical (laboratory) work-up would you suggest based on the imaged findings?

Findings

Multicystic areas throughout an enlarged left parotid gland. Right parotid gland is seemingly normal in configuration and signal intensity. Lateral view of the sialogram (delayed view) shows multiple cystic areas filled with contrast in the parotid gland.

Problem

A young adult with a parotid "mass," which is actually caused by a diffuse, multinodular, cystic process

Anatomy

A. Parotid gland: main duct, gland capsule
B. Buccal space: buccinator muscle, fat pad, buccal nodes, minor salivary tissue

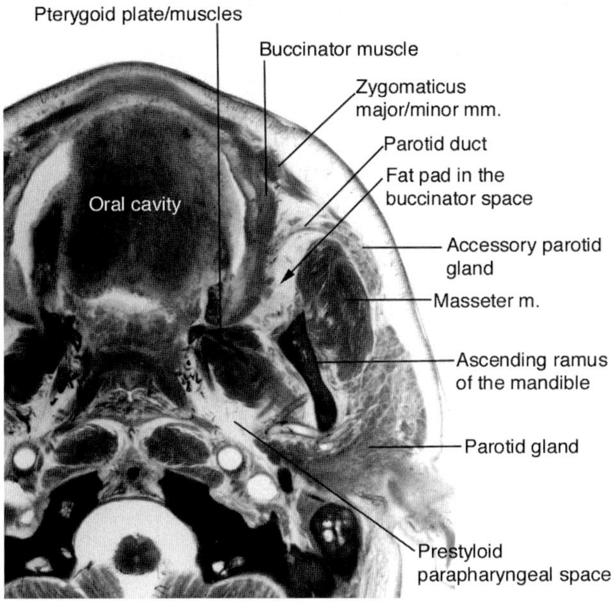

Figure 68E

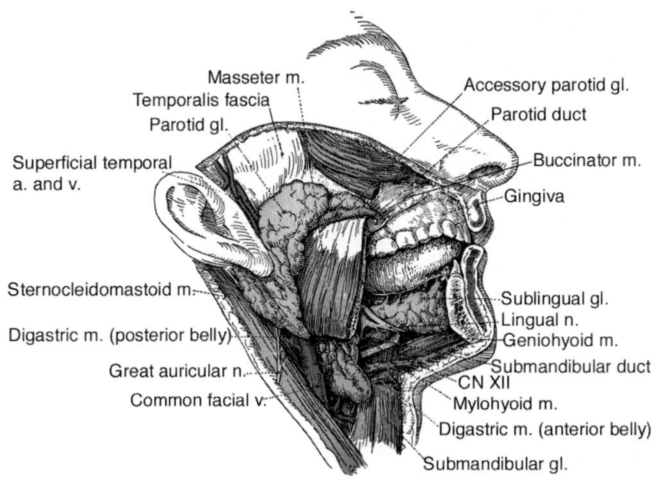

Figure 68F

Differential Diagnosis

Chronic punctate sialadenitis is a generic description of a condition that may be present in chronic infectious or obstructive disease as well as in immune-mediated disease; more subtle multinodular infiltrative patterns may be seen in sarcoidosis.

Diagnosis

Immune-mediated, chronic, punctate sialadenitis of the parotid gland (Sjögren's syndrome)

Diagnostic Imaging Approach

A. Is the mass intrinsic or extrinsic to the parotid gland? If intrinsic, is it a secondary change or a primary parotid pathology?
B. Relationship of the pathology to the facial nerve?
C. Any evidence of aggressive behavior? Any morphologic features that suggest inflammatory pathology?
D. Solitary, multiple, diffuse, bilateral changes?
E. Is more than one salivary gland involved?

Clinical Points Of Importance And Supplemental Information

A. Neither sialography nor imaging has a proved predictive value in the matter of screening for immune-mediated sialadenitis.
B. Whenever coarsely nodular, bilateral changes in the parotid glands are noted on computed tomography or magnetic resonance imaging, the treating physician should be made aware of the possibility that these changes are caused by autoimmune disease or sarcoidosis.

Answers To Questions

1. No. Not a *solitary* mass
2. Multicystic: chronic, punctate sialoadenitis
3. Sedimentation rate, autoimmune workup lip biopsy

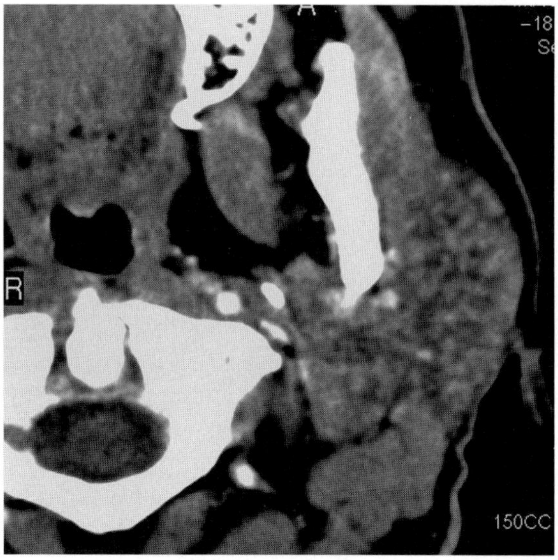

Figure 68G. Patient 1 with sarcoidosis, showing micronodular densities throughout the parotid gland, identical to chronic, punctate sialoadenitis. Contrast-enhanced computed tomography image.

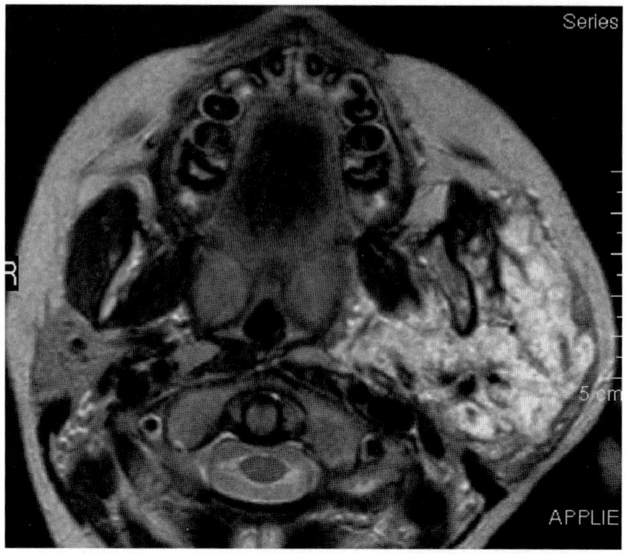

Figure 68H. Patient 2 with cavernous type vascular malformation, showing a high-intensity mass involving almost the entire left parotid gland, with direct invasion into the masticator space and the prestyloid compartment of the parapharyngeal space. T2-weighted axial image.

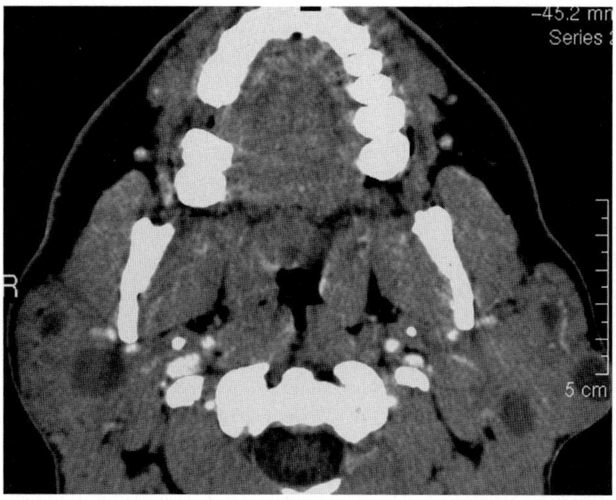

Figure 68I. Patient 3 who is human immunodeficiency virus-positive, showing multiple cystic lesions in the parotid gland bilaterally, which is consistent with lymphoepithelial cysts. Contrast-enhanced computed tomography image.

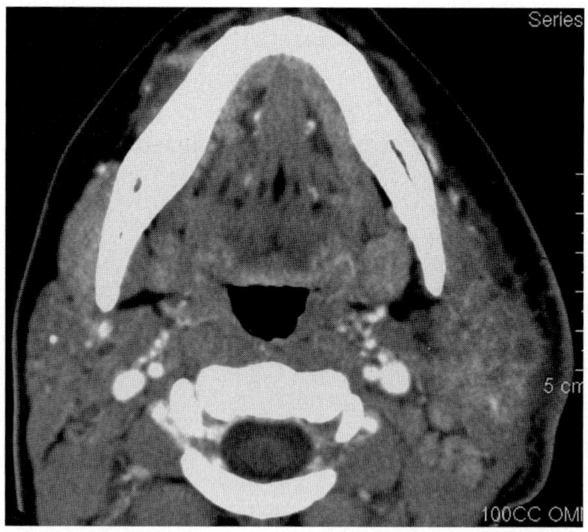

Figure 68J. Patient 4 with chronic recurrent parotitis, showing a swollen left parotid gland with a cystic component and inflammatory edema of the surrounding soft tissue, which enhances more than usual. A diffuse increase in density is noted and sialolithiasis of the right parotid gland. Contrast-enhanced computed tomography image.

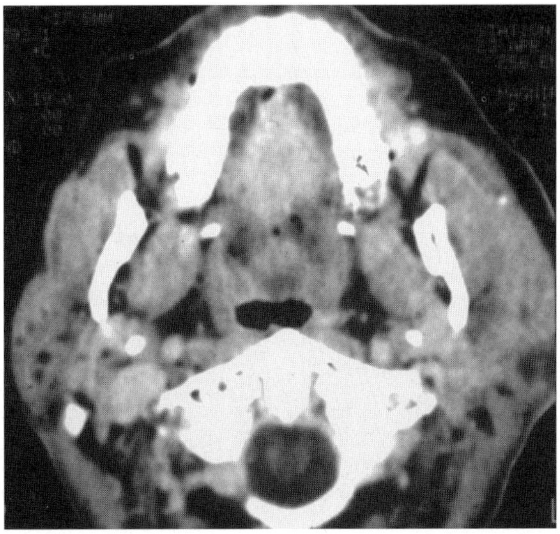

Figure 68K. Patient 5 with chronic inflammation with sialolithiasis of the parotid gland, showing a calcified stone near the orifice of the parotid duct on the left and dilatation of the proximal portion of the duct containing another stone. Diffuse increase in density of the parotid gland on both sides and multiple cystic areas in the left parotid tail represent chronic inflammatory change with a sialocele that was actually a small abscess. Contrast-enhanced computed tomography image.

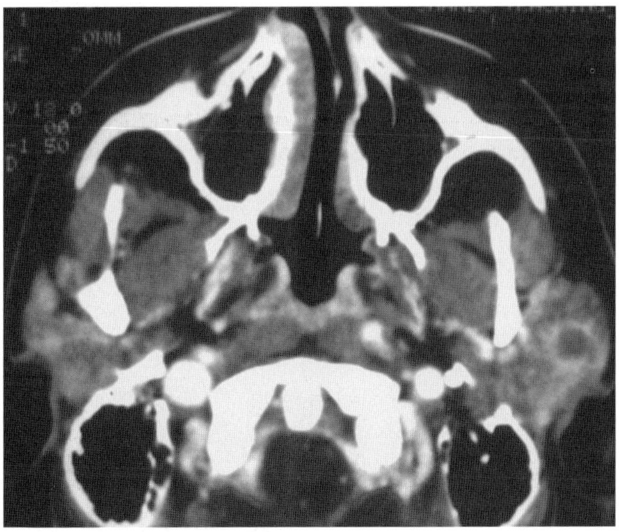

Figure 68L. Patient 6 with tuberculous lymphadenitis in an intraglandular parotid node, showing a cystic lesion with rim-enhancement in the superficial portion of the left parotid gland. Contrast-enhanced computed tomography image.

CASE 69

Clinical History: A 4-year old girl presents with intermittent parotid gland region swelling and tenderness. A palpable fullness is seen in her upper neck, but no discrete mass was noted in the parotid gland.

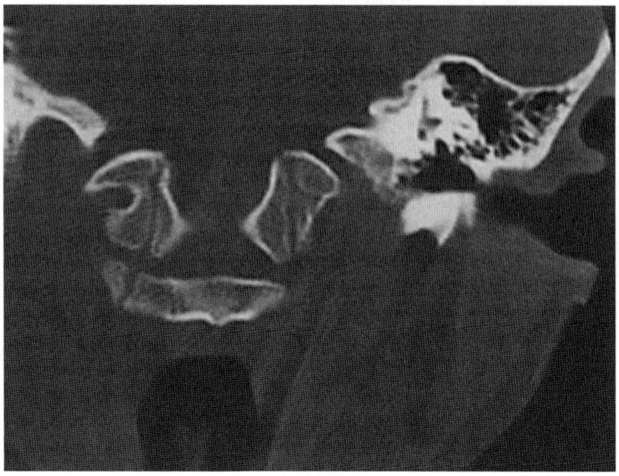

Figure 69A

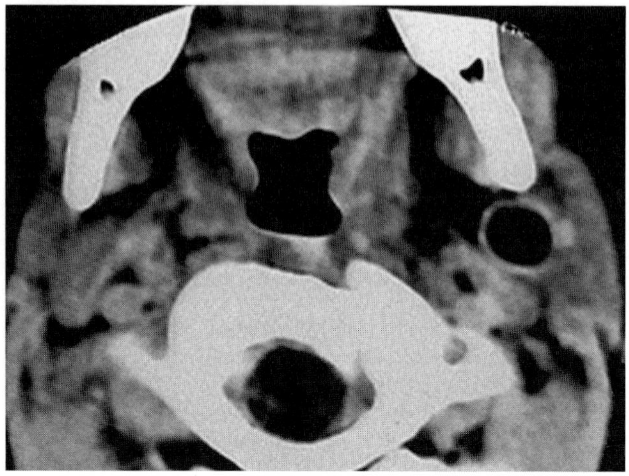

Figure 69B

1. What is the relationship of the mass to the facial nerve? To the external auditory canal?
2. What is the diagnosis (be specific)?

Findings

A rim-enhancing, unilocular cystic mass in the deep portion of the left parotid gland, which is just deep to the retromandibular vein and external carotid artery. The lesion is associated with the sinus tract to inferior aspect of the bone-cartilage junction of the external auditory canal.

Problem

A child with swelling in the parotid gland region and a cystic mass in the deep portion of the parotid gland

Anatomy

A. Parotid gland: superficial and deep portions, relationship of the parotid gland capsule to the external auditory canal
B. External auditory canal: bony and cartilaginous portions

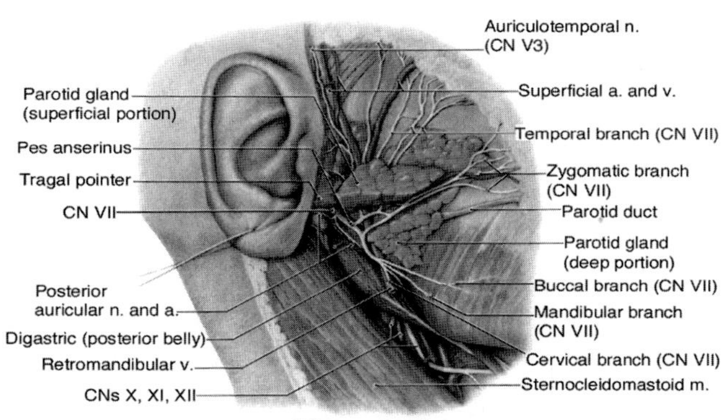

Figure 69C

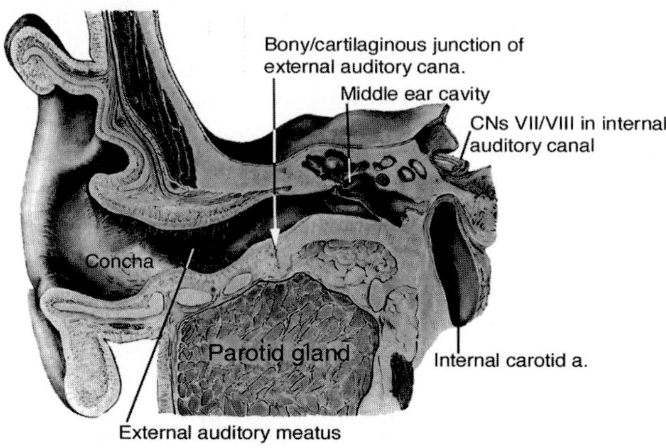

Figure 69D

Differential Diagnosis

None in this case because of the sinus tract association. For the cystic mass, one could consider an isolated first branchial cleft cyst, abscess, infected sialocele or mucocele, cystic neoplasm.

Diagnosis

Type 2 first branchial cleft cyst with a sinus tract through the bony external auditory canal

Diagnostic Imaging Approach

A. Is the mass intrinsic or extrinsic to the parotid gland?
B. Relationship to the facial nerve?
C. Any signs of aggressive behavior?
D. Solitary, multiple, or bilateral?
E. Evaluate internal morphology: density, T1- or T2-weighted signal intensity, enhancement pattern, vascularity, calcifications.
F. Does the mass extend beyond the parotid gland; in this case, is there a tract?
G. Any associated abnormalities?

Clinical Points Of Importance And Supplemental Information

A. The differential diagnosis of masses in the parotid gland in children differs markedly from that of adults.
B. Type 2 *first* branchial cleft cysts have a component deep to the facial nerve and this affects the surgical approach. Look for associated abnormalities (e.g., epidermoids) and study the temporal bone carefully in these anomalies.

Answers To Questions

1. Deep to the facial nerve. Tract from the cyst to the bony cartilaginous junction.
2. Type 2 first branchial cleft cyst

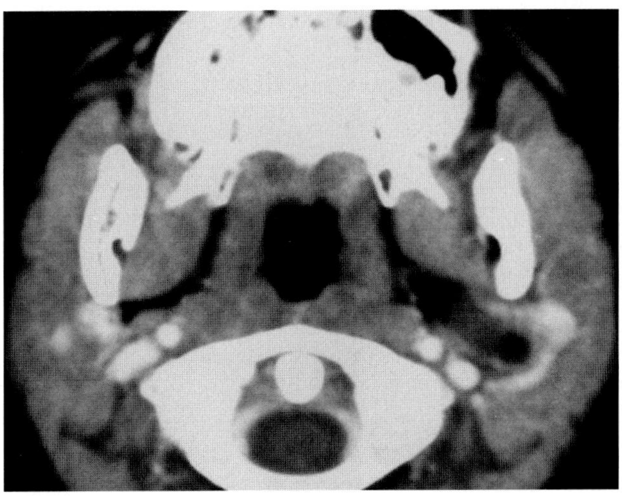

Figure 69E. Patient 1 with first branchial cleft cyst, showing an oblong cystic mass in the deep portion of left parotid gland, extending into the prestyloid parapharyngeal space. Contrast-enhanced computed tomography image.

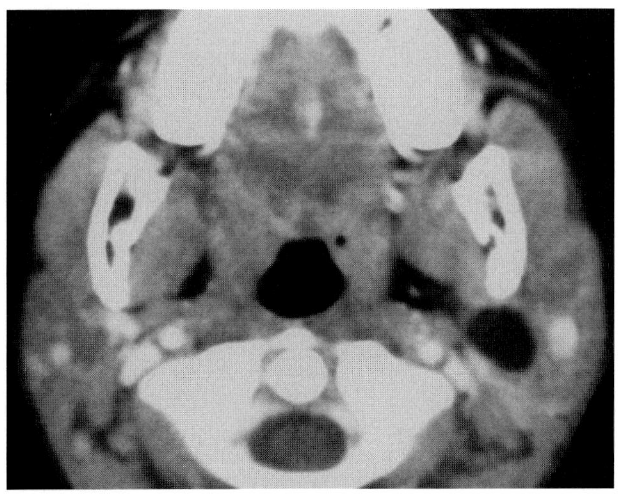

Figure 69F. Patient 1 with first branchial cleft cyst, showing a unilocular cystic mass in the deep portion of the left parotid gland.

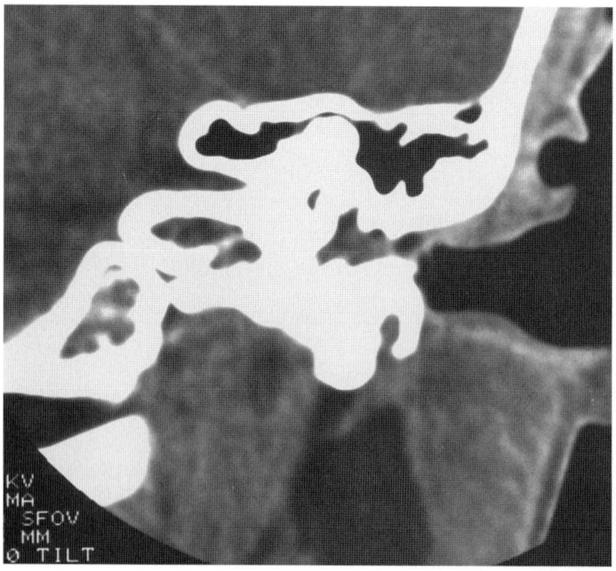

Figure 69G. Patient 1 with first branchial cleft cyst. Coronal computed tomography image showing a bony defect extending toward the external auditory canal, superior to the cystic mass.

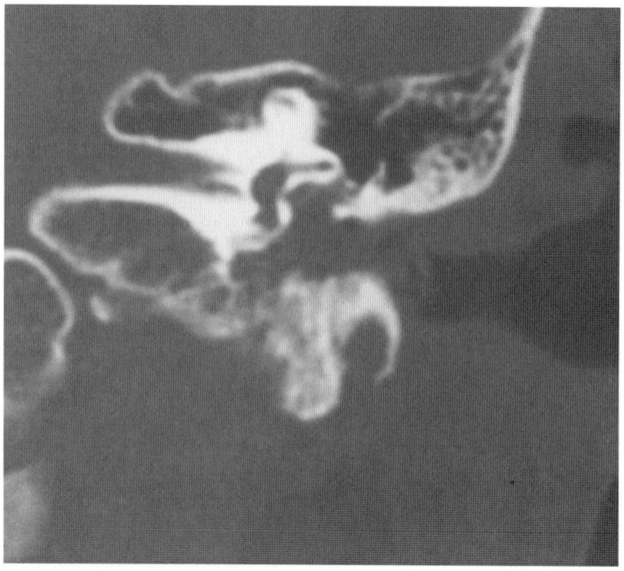

Figure 69H. Patient 1 with first branchial cleft cyst. Coronal computed tomography image at bone window setting showing a bone defect under the external auditory canal. The middle ear cavity and bony portion of the external auditory canal are filled with soft tissue density, which is suggestive of cholesteatoma.

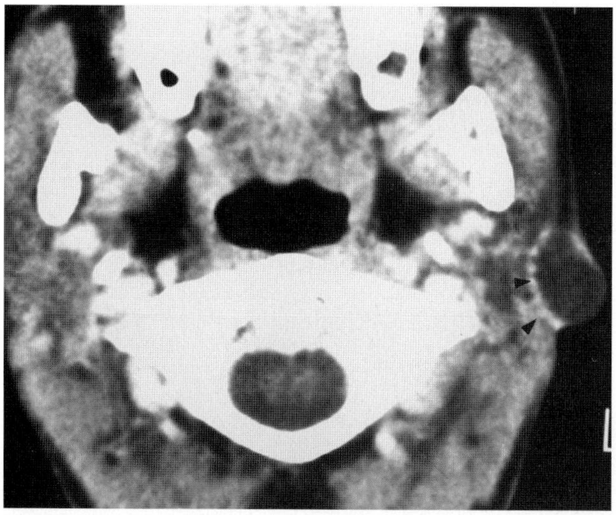

Figure 69I. Patient 2 with first branchial cleft cyst, showing a unilocular cystic mass superficial to the superficial portion of the left parotid gland.

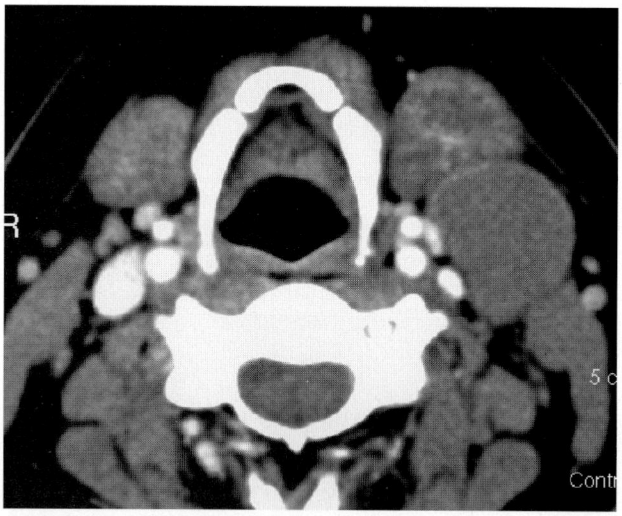

Figure 69J. Patient 3 with second branchial cleft cyst, showing a unilocular cystic mass between the submandibular gland and the sternocleidomastoid muscle on the left.

CHAPTER 7

NASOPHARYNX, OROPHARYNX, AND RELATED SPACES

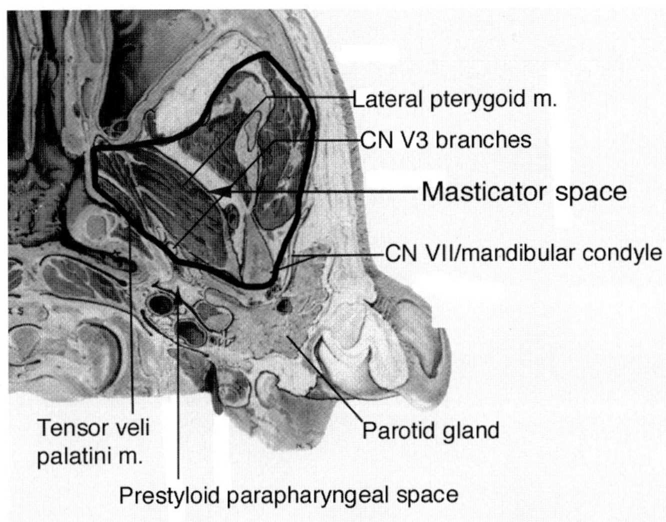

CASE 70

Clinical History: A 50-year-old woman whose dentist discovered a submucosal mass displacing the left tonsil presents with no other symptoms or physical findings.

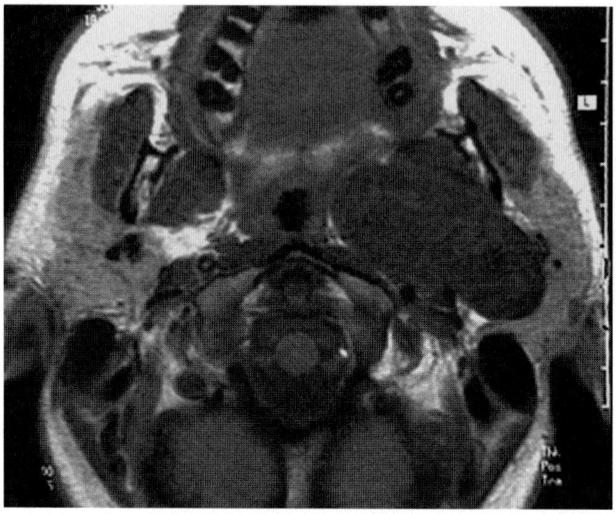

Figure 70A

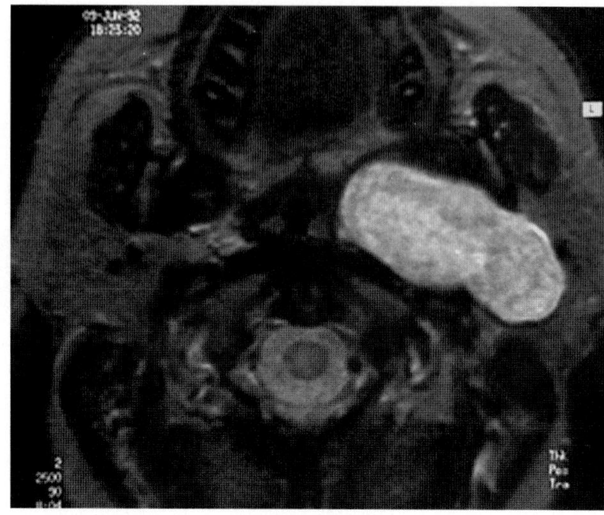

Figure 70B

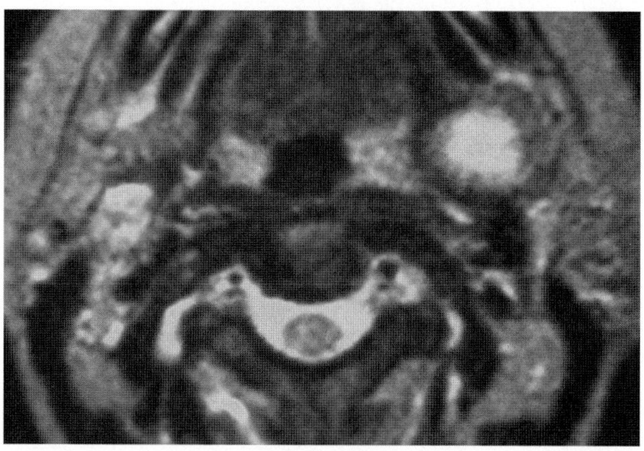

Figure 70C

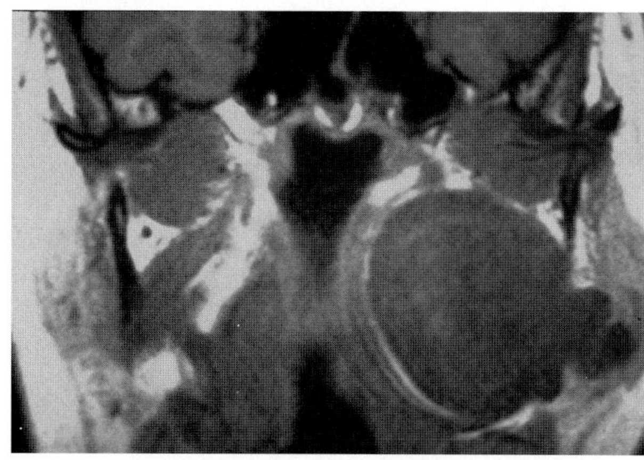

Figure 70D

1. Should such a mass be biopsied before imaging to help plan the diagnostic imaging approach?
2. What are the two potential sites of origin of the mass?
3. What is the most likely diagnosis and cite two important factors to a surgeon considering resection of the lesion.

Findings

A well-demarcated mass displacing fat of the parapharyngeal space centrifugally. The lesion results in anterior distortion of adjacent left pterygoid muscle and remodeling of the left ascending ramus of the mandible. The retromandibular vein lies lateral and adjacent to the lesion. The carotid sheath structures and the styloid musculature are displaced posteriorly. The bottom of the mass enters the superior aspect of the submandibular space. The signal intensity of the lesion is slightly inhomogeneous on both T1- and T2-weighted images.

Problem

An adult with a submucosal mass arising in the parapharyngeal space

Anatomy

A. Prestyloid parapharyngeal space: all boundaries and contents
B. Poststyloid parapharyngeal space: all boundaries and contents
C. Masticator space: relationship to parapharyngeal space

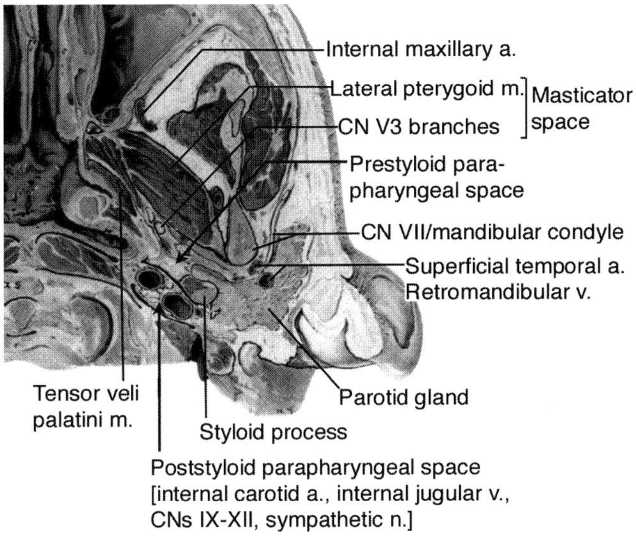

Figure 70E

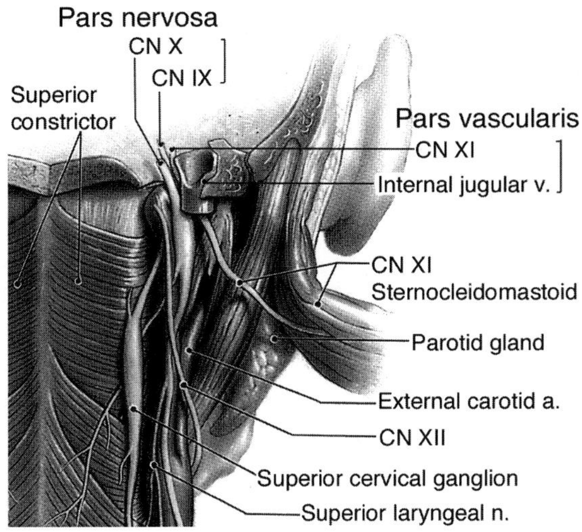

Figure 70F

Differential Diagnosis

Benign mixed tumor (90% to 95% of the time) arising from accessory salivary gland tissue or deep portion of the parotid; malignant minor salivary gland tumor (e.g., adeno- or adenoidcystic carcinoma); second branchial cleft cyst, sarcoma, leiomyoma, and rhabdomyoma, all of which are rare

Diagnosis

Benign mixed tumor (pleomorphic adenoma) centered in the prestyloid parapharyngeal space and inseparable from the deep portion of the parotid gland

Diagnostic Imaging Approach

A. Establish space of origin: parapharyngeal, masticator, retropharyngeal vs. mucosal origin (e.g., eustachian tube origin might explain a submucosal mass on clinical examination).
B. If parapharyngeal space origin, is it prestyloid or poststyloid?
C. If prestyloid, is it separable from the deep portion of the parotid gland?
D. Establish the proximity to the skull base, inferior extent, and relationship to superior constrictor muscle.
E. Evaluate margins for signs of aggressive behavior.
F. Evaluate internal morphology: density, T1- or T2-weighted signal intensity, enhancement pattern, vascularity, blood products, calcifications, and matrix.

Clinical Points Of Importance And Supplemental Information

A submucosal mass producing a bulge of the pharyngeal wall should *never* be biopsied before imaging.

Answers To Questions

1. *Never* biopsy a submucosal mass before imaging!
2. Parotid and prestyloid parapharyngeal space
3. Pleomorphic adenoma (benign mixed tumor). The relationship to the deep portion of the parotid (facial nerve) and proximity to the skull base.

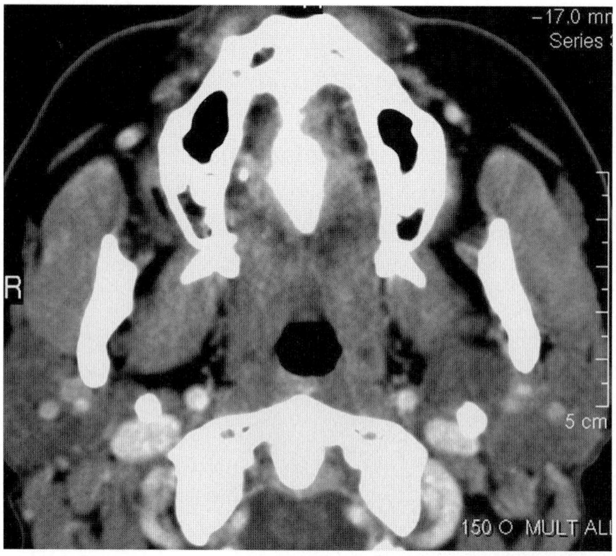

Figure 70G. Patient 1 with pleomorphic adenoma arising from the deep portion of the parotid gland, showing a well-defined mass centered in the lateral aspect of the prestyloid parapharyngeal space, with widening of the stylomandibular tunnel. The mass is inseparable from the deep portion of the left parotid gland. Contrast-enhanced computed tomography image.

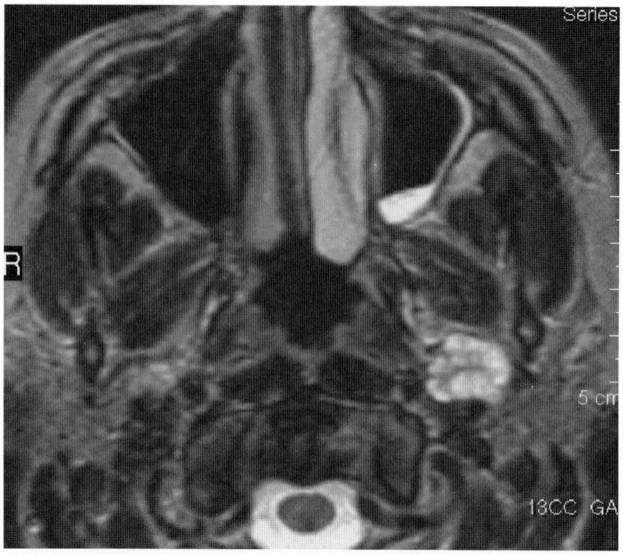

Figure 70H. Patient 1 with pleomorphic adenoma arising from the deep portion of the parotid gland. T2-weighted axial image showing a high-intensity mass of lobular contour in the prestyloid parapharyngeal space on the left.

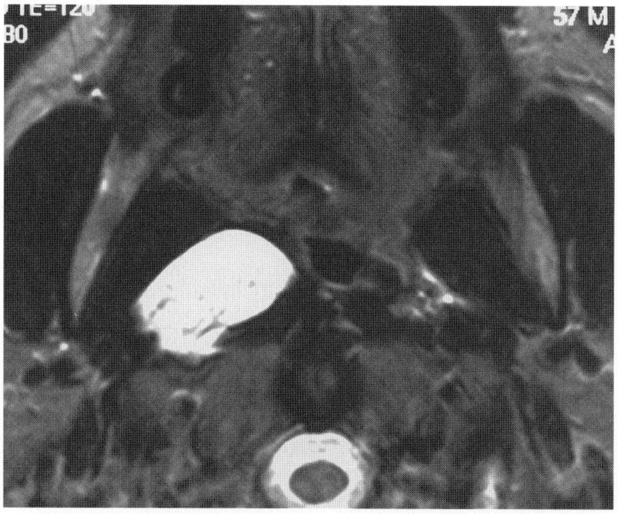

Figure 70I. Patient 2 with cavernous type vascular malformation. T2-weighted image showing well-circumscribed, high-intensity mass in the prestyloid of the right parapharyngeal space.

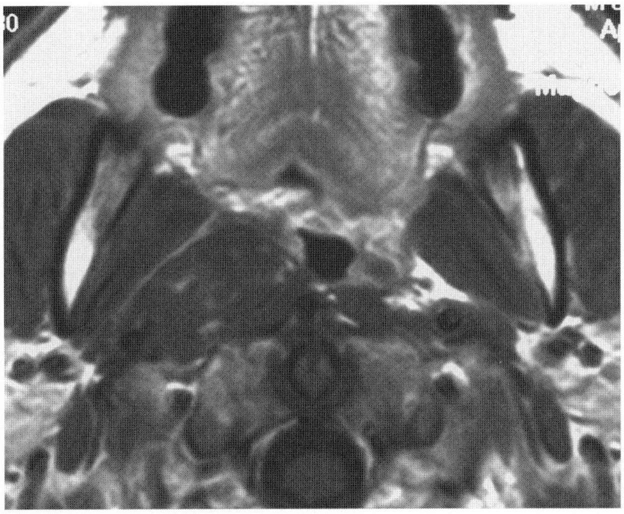

Figure 70J. Patient 2 with cavernous type vascular malformation. T1-weighted axial image with contrast showing speckled areas of enhancement in the mass.

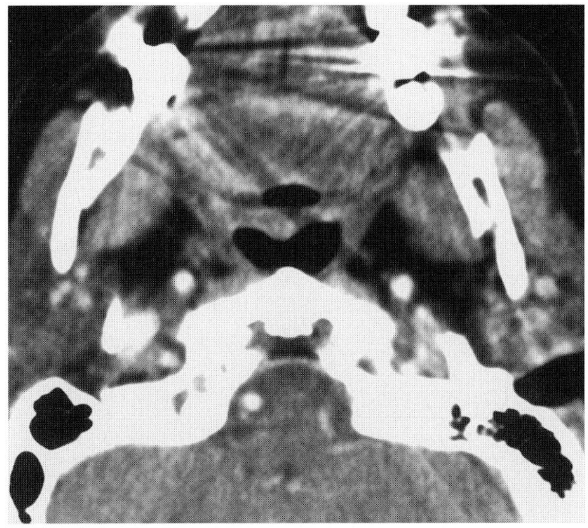

Figure 70K. Patient 3 with lung carcinoma, showing a small nodular lesion in the prestyloid parapharyngeal space on the right. Contrast-enhanced axial computed tomography image.

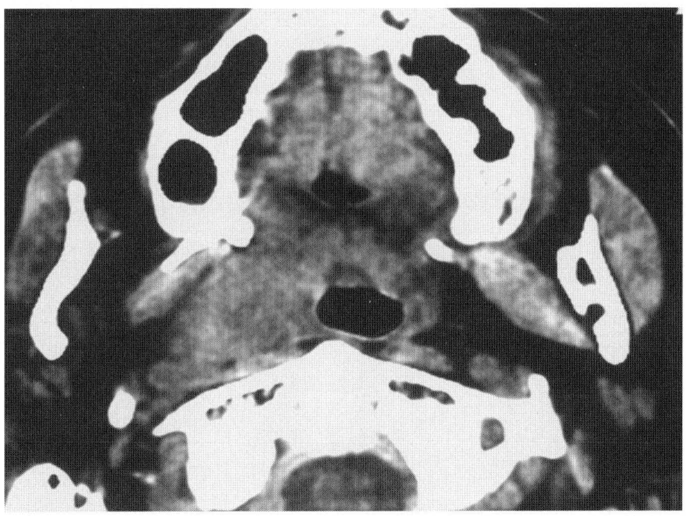

Figure 70L. Patient 3 with lung carcinoma. Computed tomography study 3 months after Fig. 70K, showing a rapid growth of the lesion in the prestyloid parapharyngeal space, which is consistent with metastatic disease.

CASE 71

Clinical History: A 51-year-old woman presents after her dentist noted a pharyngeal wall bulge during a routine visit.

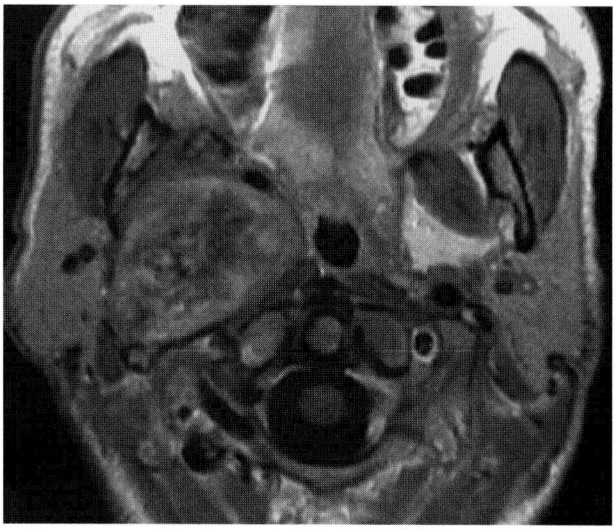

Figure 71A

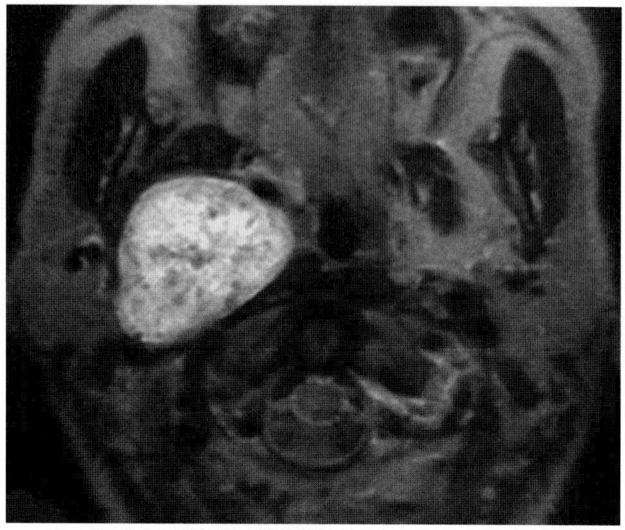

Figure 71B

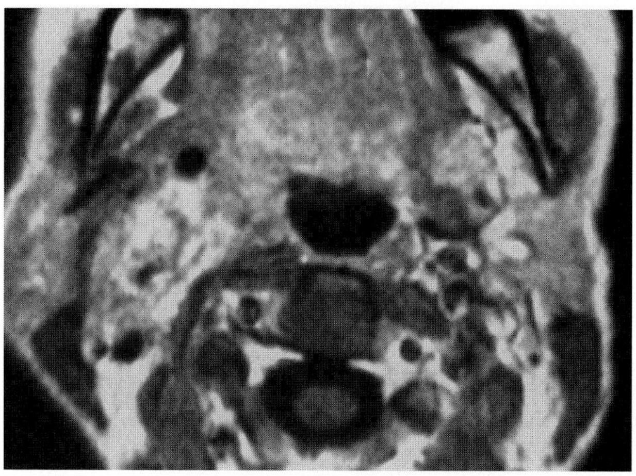

Figure 71C

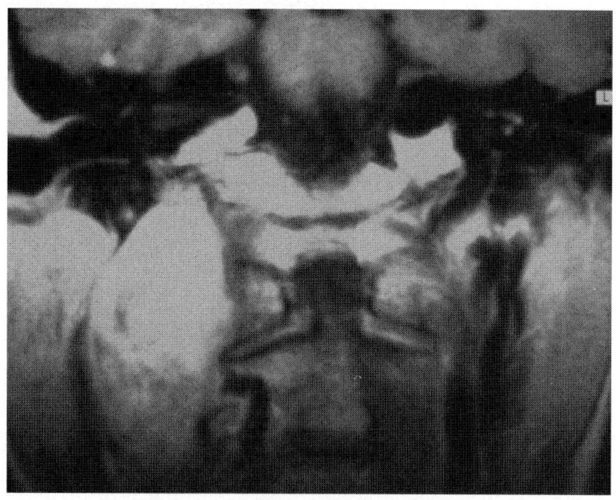

Figure 71D

1. What is the space of origin of the lesion? What are the two most common lesions arising in this space?
2. How does the overall and internal morphology of the lesion help with the differential diagnosis?
3. Is angiography *necessary* for the diagnosis? As an adjunct to surgery (i.e., preoperative embolotherapy)?

Findings

A well-demarcated mass in the right parapharyngeal space. The lesion intervenes between the anteromedially displaced internal carotid artery and posterolaterally displaced internal jugular vein. Remodeling is noted at the posterior aspect of the right ramus of the mandible. The lesion inhomogeneously enhances after administration of contrast material. No obvious flow void is seen in the lesion, but a single vascular pedicle may be present.

Problem

A middle-aged woman with a submucosal mass arising within the parapharyngeal space

Anatomy

A. Parapharyngeal space: prestyloid and poststyloid divisions and their contents; styloid process and related musculature (see Fig. 70E)
B. Retropharyngeal space and nodes
C. Relationship of the masticator space to the parapharyngeal space

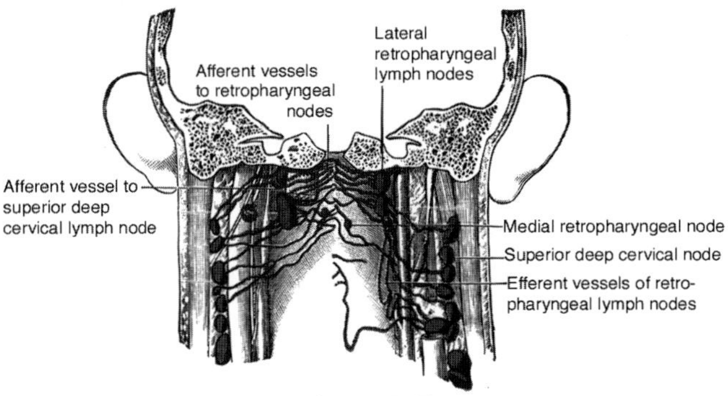

Figure 71E

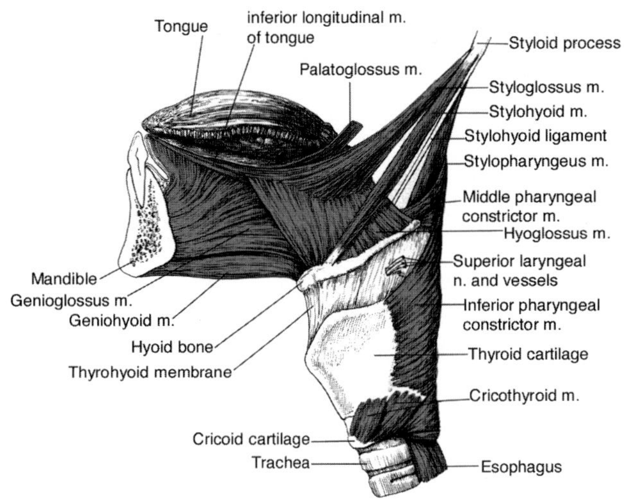

Figure 71F

Differential Diagnosis

Schwannoma or neurofibroma (vagal, sympathetic origin most common), paraganglioma (glomus vagale, jugulare, or carotid body tumor), abnormal retropharyngeal node (reactive, lymphoma, metastatic), cervical neuroblastoma, carotid artery aneurysm, meningioma, hemangiopericytoma

Diagnosis

Schwannoma of the poststyloid parapharyngeal space

Diagnostic Imaging Approach

A. Determine the site (space) of origin: parapharyngeal, masticator vs. mucosal origin (e.g., eustachian tube, skull base, or even intracranial origin might explain a submucosal mass in the nasopharynx seen on physical examination).
B. If parapharyngeal space origin, is it prestyloid or poststyloid?
C. If poststyloid, is it medial or lateral to the carotid artery?
D. Establish the proximity to the skull base, inferior extent, and relationship to parotid gland and facial nerve.
E. Is the carotid artery displaced or enveloped by the mass? Does the mass originate in the carotid artery?
F. Evaluate margins for signs of aggressive behavior.
G. Evaluate internal morphology: density, T1- or T2-weighted signal intensity, enhancement pattern, vascularity, blood products, calcification, matrix.

Clinical Points Of Importance And Supplemental Information

A. A submucosal mass producing a bulge of the pharyngeal wall should never be biopsied before imaging.
B. Always consider carotid aneurysm as a possible cause (it is almost always possible to exclude this on the basis of high-quality computed tomography scan or magnetic resonance image).
C. Angiography may be necessary for confirmation of diagnosis and planning embolotherapy. Embolotherapy is a useful adjunct to surgery for paragangliomas and some neurogenic tumors.

Answers To Questions

1. Poststyloid parapharyngeal. Nerve sheath tumor and paraganglioma.
2. Lack of obvious flow voids make nerve sheath tumor virtually certain.
3. Not for diagnosis, except in unusual circumstances. As an adjunct, it can be helpful to the surgeon. Magnetic resonance angiography is of no real help.

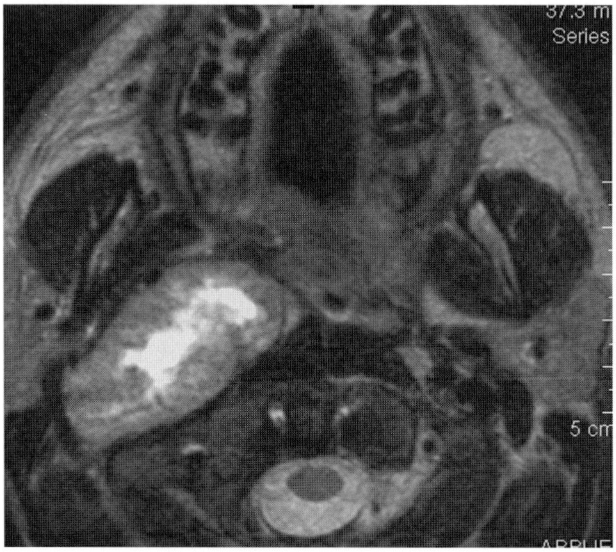

Figure 71G. Patient 1 with schwannoma of the vagus nerve, showing a mass centered in the poststyloid parapharyngeal space displacing the internal carotid artery and styloid musculature anteriorly. Irregularly shaped high-intensity area in the mass is a cystic component. T2-weighted axial image.

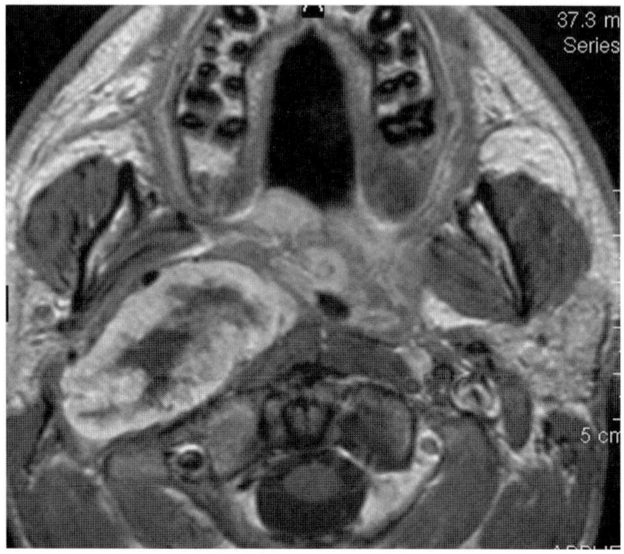

Figure 71H. Patient 1 with schwannoma of the vagus nerve. T1-weighted axial image with contrast.

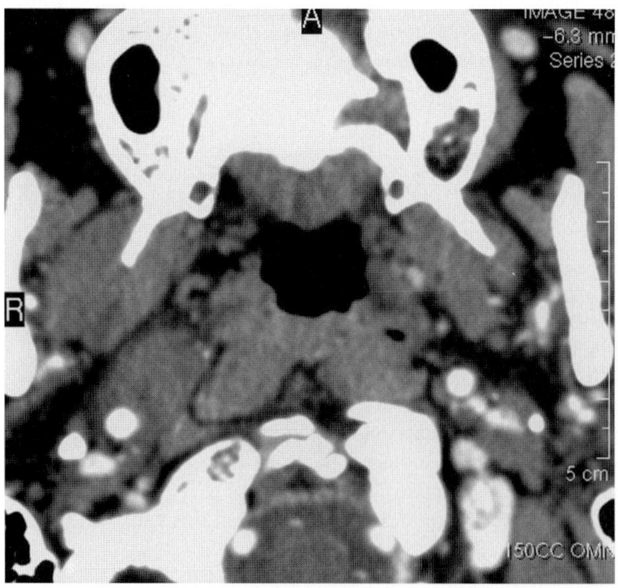

Figure 71I. Patient 2 with schwannoma of the sympathetic trunk, showing a soft tissue mass in the poststyloid parapharyngeal space on the right, which lies medial to the internal carotid artery. Early phase of a contrast-enhanced computed tomography image; late phase showed the mass to enhance.

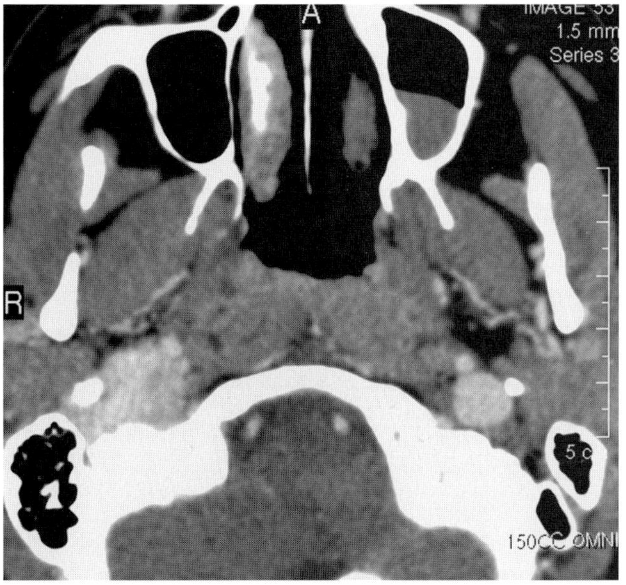

Figure 71J. Patient 3 with glomus jugulare type of paraganglioma, showing intensely enhancing mass in the poststyloid parapharyngeal space just below the jugular foramen. Contrast-enhanced computed tomography image.

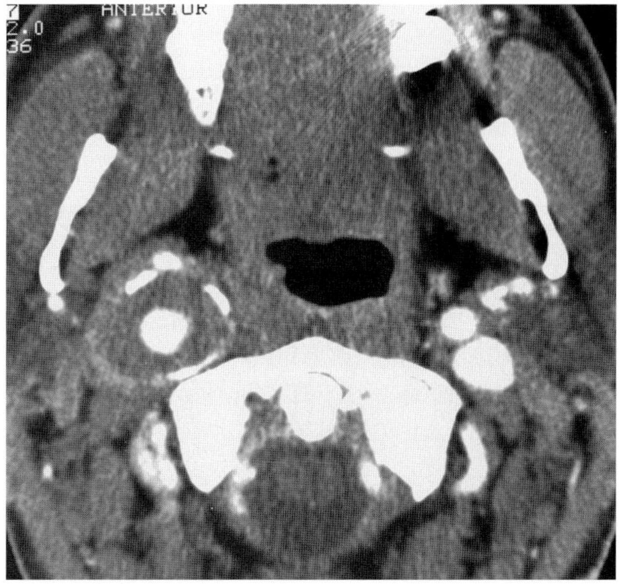

Figure 71K. Patient 4 with aneurysm of the internal carotid artery, showing a partially rim-calcified mass surrounding the right internal carotid artery in the poststyloid parapharyngeal space.

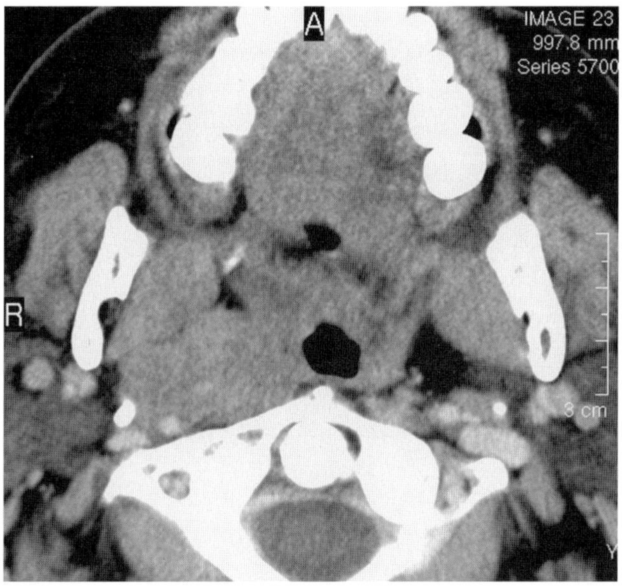

Figure 71L. Patient 5 with tonsillar carcinoma, showing a mass mainly involving the poststyloid parapharyngeal space, which is consistent with metastasis to the lateral retropharyngeal lymph node (see normal lateral retropharyngeal lymph node on the left).

CASE 72

Clinical History: A 7-year-old girl who is HIV positive and has facial pain.

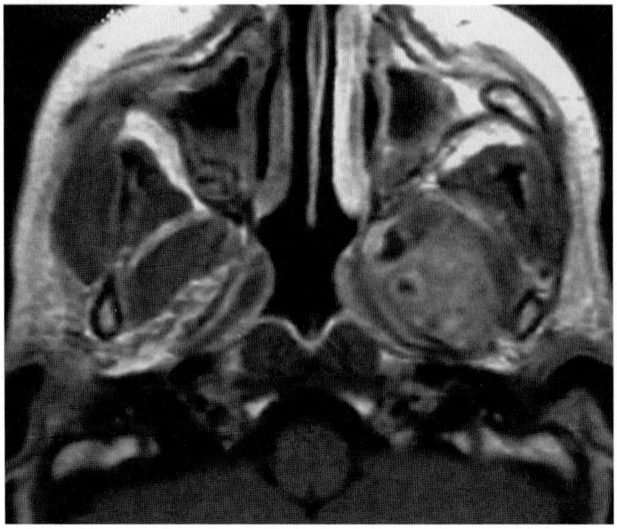

Figure 72A

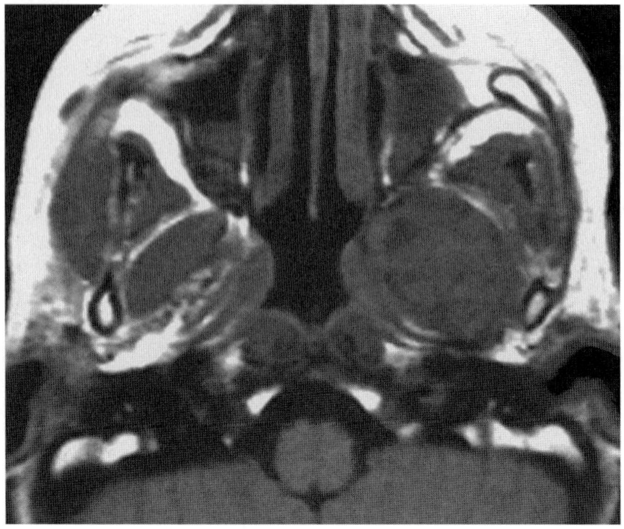

Figure 72B

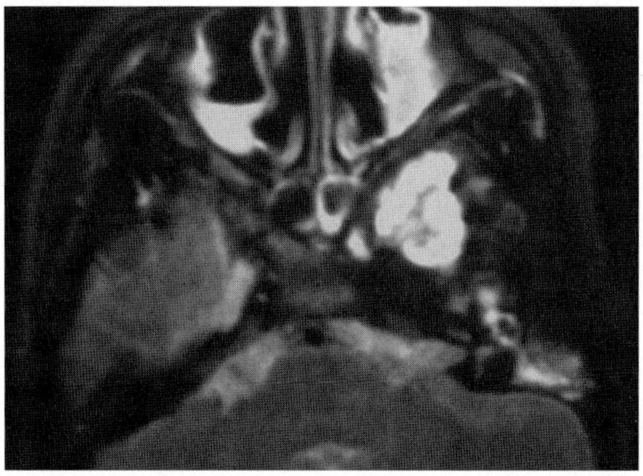

Figure 72C

1. What is the space of origin?
2. What neoplastic lesions commonly involve this space? (by the way, all are uncommon)
3. What is the most likely diagnosis?

Findings

There is an inhomogeneously enhancing mass in the left masticator space that involves the pterygoid muscles. Fat tissue in the parapharyngeal space is displaced medially. Several cystic (necrotic) areas are present in the lesion. The mass appears to invade the fat of the prestyloid parapharyngeal space.

Problem

An HIV-positive child with a mass arising in the masticator space

Anatomy

A. Masticator space - boundaries, contents
B. Mandibular division of trigeminal nerve (V3) - from trigeminal ganglion to its terminal branches
C. Central skull base and floor of middle cranial fossa - foramen ovale and foramen spinosum

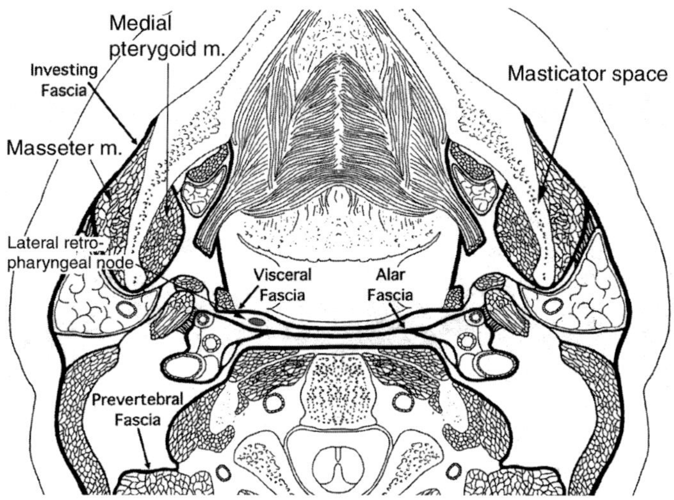

Figure 72D

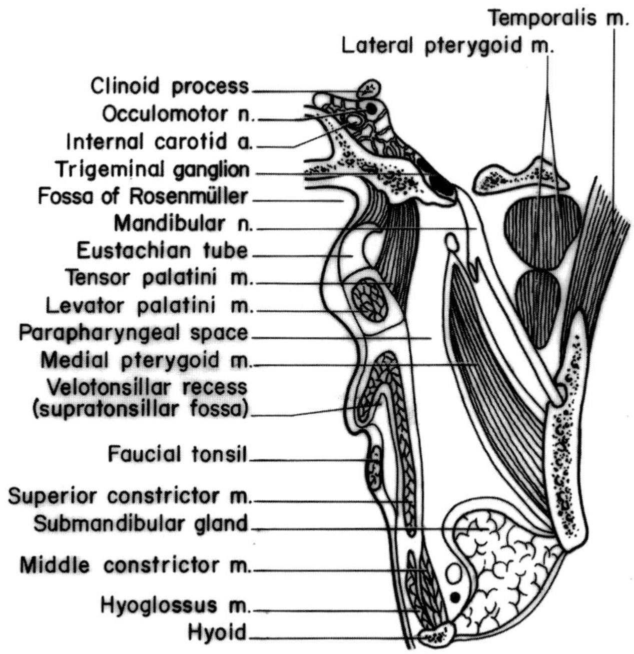

Figure 72E

Differential Diagnosis

Schwannoma or neurofibroma, meningioma, hemangiopericytoma, sarcoma, lymphoma, pseudotumor; masticator space abscess; bony and dental lesions arising from the mandible

Diagnosis

Hemangiopericytoma of the masticator space

Diagnostic Imaging Approach

A. Establish the space of origin—parapharyngeal, masticator, retropharyngeal
B. Establish the proximity to the skull base, inferior extent, relationship to tensor veli palatini fascia and superior constrictor muscle.
C. If the masticator space is the origin, is it arising from V3, muscle or the mandible?
D. Is there intracranial spread—dural and/or perineural?
E. Evaluate margins for signs of aggressive behavior.
F. Evaluate internal morphology—density, T1-/T2- signal intensity, enhancement pattern, vascularity, blood products, calcification, matrix.

Clinical Points Of Importance And Supplemental Information

A. Masticator space masses are approached much differently than those in the prestyloid parapharyngeal space; it is essential to establish the true space of origin.
B. Trismus is frequently not present in even very large masticator space masses.

Answers To Questions

1. Masticator space
2. Nerve sheath tumors, transcranial meningioma and variants, sarcoma
3. Considering the history hemangiopericytoma

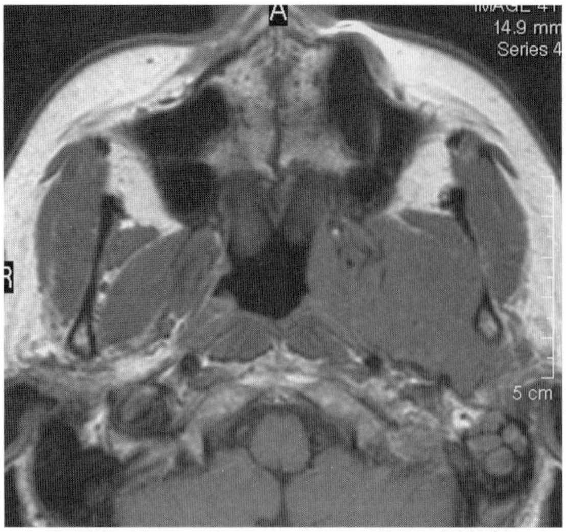

Figure 72F. Patient 1 with extranodal involvement of non-Hodgkin's lymphoma showing diffuse infiltrative process involving the masticator space and the prestyloid parapharyngeal space on the left. There is fluid collection in the left mastoid air cells due to eustachian tube involvement. T1-weighted axial image.

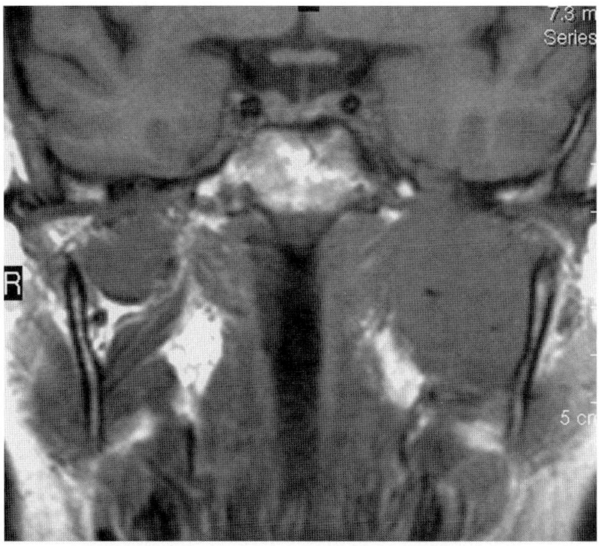

Figure 72G. Patient 1 with extranodal involvement of non-Hodgkin's lymphoma. T1-weighted coronal image.

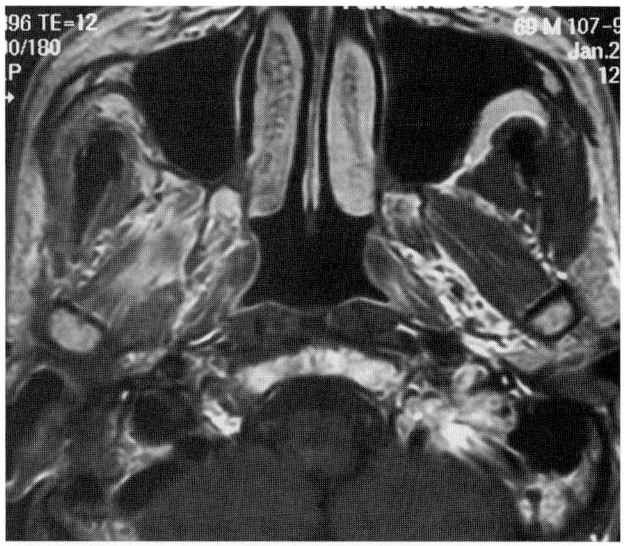

Figure 72H. Patient 2 with history of undifferentiated carcinoma of the parotid gland perineural tumor spread along CN V3 showing enhancing mass at expected position of the right CN V3 and denervation atrophy of the muscles within the masticator space. T1-weighted axial image with contrast.

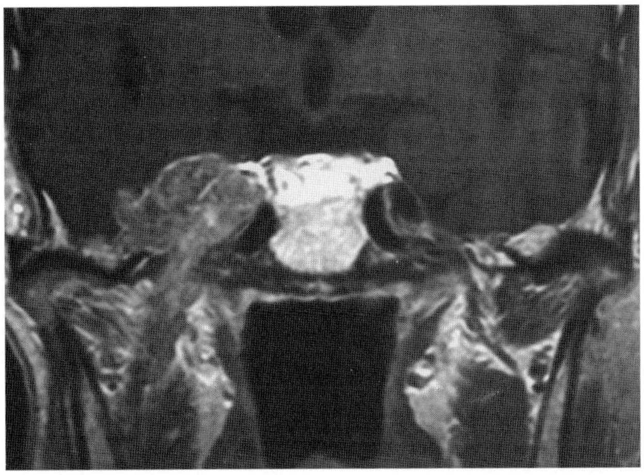

Figure 72I. Patient 2 with history of undifferentiated carcinoma of the parotid glandperineural tumor spread along CN V3. T1-weighted axial image with contrast showing enhancing mass extending along CN V3 into the area of the trigeminal ganglion through the enlarged foramen ovale (see normal CN V3 on the left).

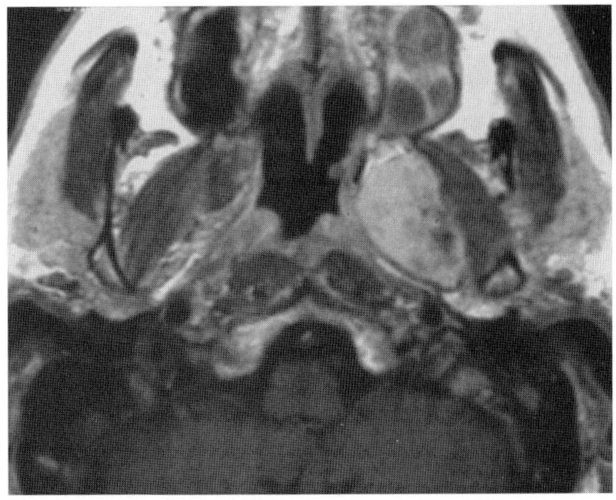

Figure 72J. Patient 3 with schwannoma arising from CN V3 showing well-defined mass centered in the expected position of CN V3, displacing the pterygoid muscle anterolaterally and fat in the prestyloid parapharyngeal space with the fascia of the masticator space posteromedially. T1-weighted axial image with contrast.

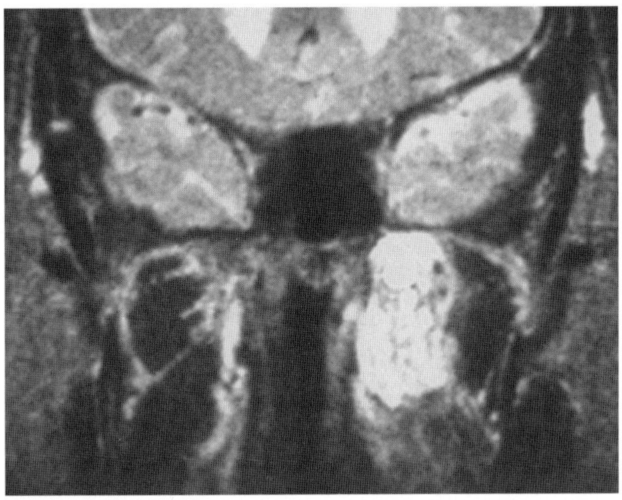

Figure 72K. Patient 3 with schwannoma arising from CN V3. T2-weighted coronal image showing an oblong high intensity mass medial to the lateral pterygoid muscle on the left.

CASE 73

Clinical History: A 16-year-old boy presents with swelling and periauricular pain in the parotid gland region. Based on findings of a computed tomography (CT) study at another institution, he had been told he had a sarcoma of the deep face. He presented to our institution for cancer management. Percutaneous CT-guided biopsy was requested by our referring clinical service.

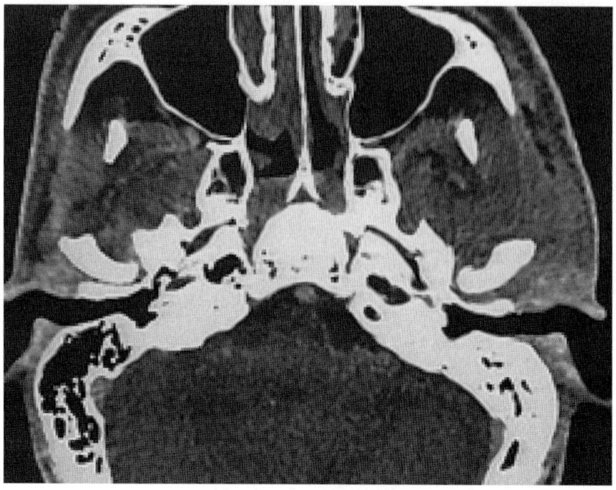

Figure 73A

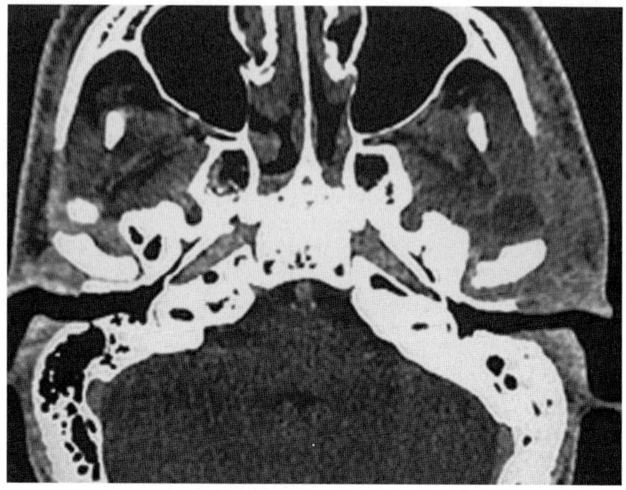

Figure 73B

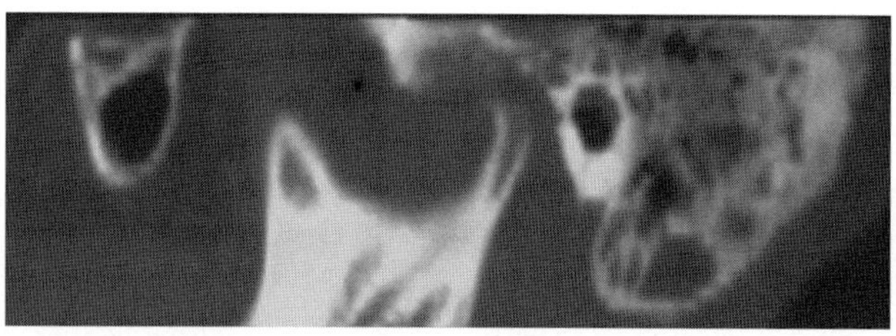

Figure 73C

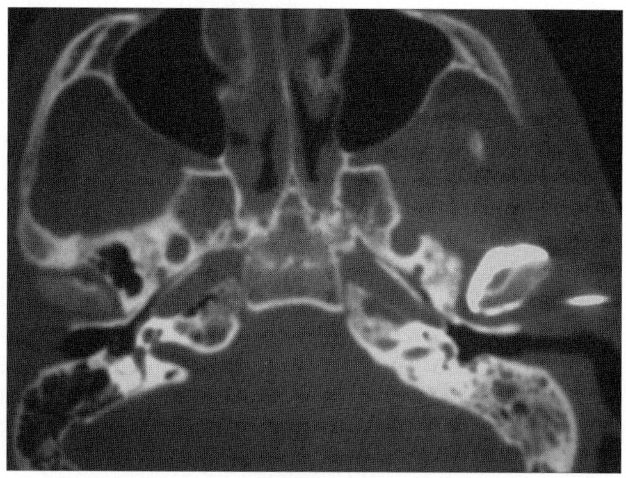

Figure 73D

1. Is the morphology of the mass helpful in the differential diagnosis?
2. How would you approach the requested tissue sampling, based on the findings in these two images (i.e., sampling method, sampling sites; analysis of these samples)?

Findings

An ill-defined mass around the condylar head of the mandible on the left. Tissue planes in this area are obscured. The lesion is associated with a rim-enhancing cystic area within the soft tissue swelling. Noted are increased density within the subcutaneous fat and thickening of skin in this area. Arthrogram (CT) shows the joint space to be normal and not communicating with the pathology. Bone windows show mastoiditis tracking forward with air cells over the condylar fossa and into the root of the zygoma.

Problem

A teenager with an infiltrating, possibly inflammatory mass of the upper masticator space temporomandibular joint (TMJ) region

Anatomy

A. Upper masticator space
B. Relationship of parotid gland to:
   1. Masticator space (parotidomasseteric fascia)
   2. External auditory canal
C. Mandibular condyle and TMJ

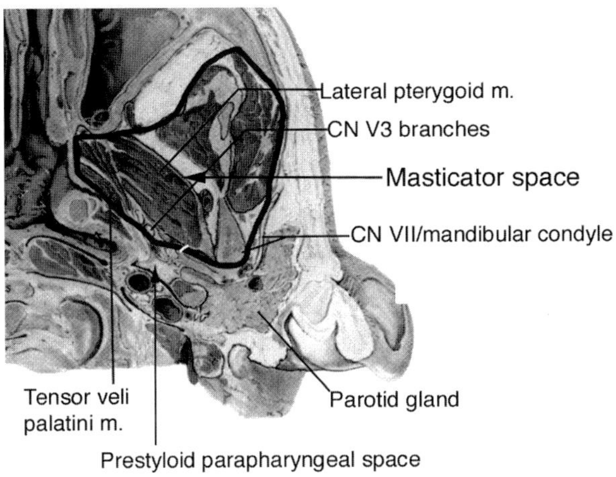

Figure 73E

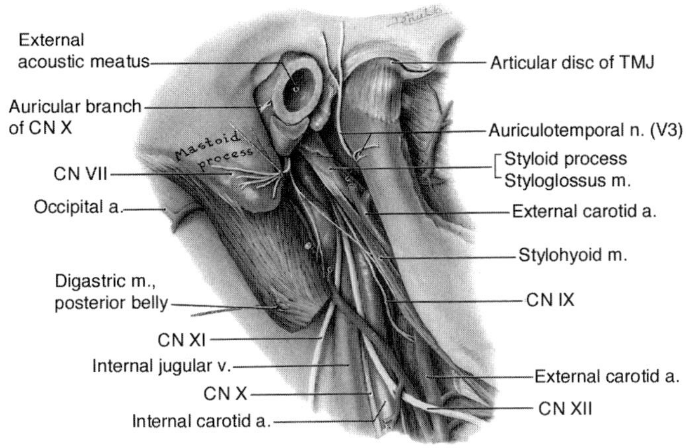

Figure 73F

Differential Diagnosis

1. Tumor: rhabdomyosarcoma, synovial sarcoma, lymphoma
2. Inflammatory: abscess and cellulitis; pseudotumor, histiocytosis

Diagnosis

Masticator space abscess or cellulitis secondary to mastoiditis

Diagnostic Imaging Approach

A. Identify the space of origin.
B. Is the disease focal, multifocal, or diffuse?
C. Any evidence seen of aggressive behavior (e.g., infiltrating margins, bone destruction, perineural spread, nodal metastases)?
D. Is the gross morphology more suggestive of inflammatory or neoplastic disease?
   1. For abscess: rim-enhancing fluid collection.
   2. For cellulitis: diffuse infiltrating pattern with associated edema.

Clinical Points Of Importance And Supplemental Information

A. Lesions believed clinically to be parotid in origin frequently arise from other sites.
B. Recognizing an "inflammatory" rather than "neoplastic" morphology of a lesion as seen on magnetic resonance imaging or CT scan helps reorganize the diagnostic process.

Answers To Questions

1. Yes; edema and fluid area suggest inflammatory rather than a neoplastic origin.
2. CT arthrography or aspiration of fluid to start, then Gram stain, culture, and cytology.

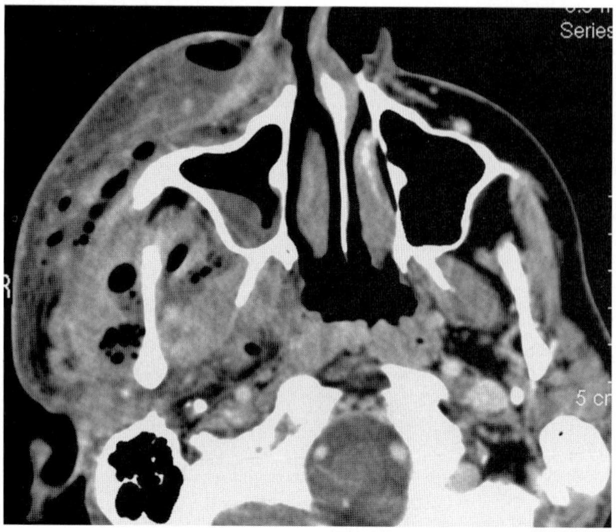

Figure 73G. Patient 1 with necrotizing fascitis, showing diffuse inflammatory edema and air collection in the masticator space and subcutaneous tissue in the cheek on the right, with skin thickening and some enhancement of the muscles in the masticator space. Contrast-enhanced computed tomography image.

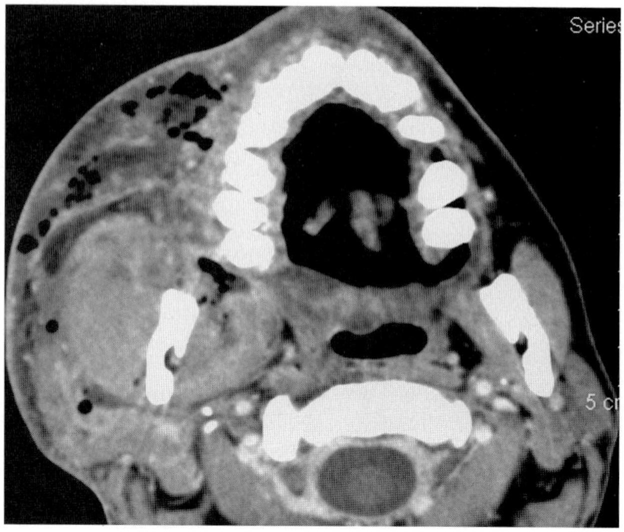

Figure 73H. Patient 1 with necrotizing fascitis. Contrast-enhanced computed tomography image inferior to Fig. 73G showing extensive inflammatory change involving the masticator space and subcutaneous tissue and skin in the right upper neck.

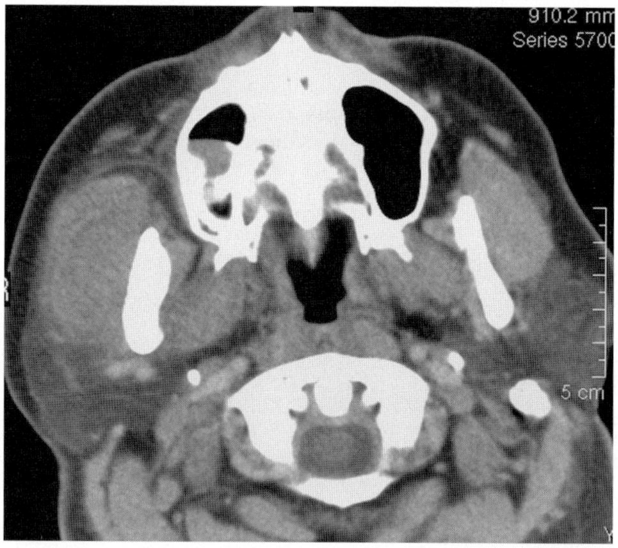

Figure 73I. Patient 2 with sclerosing osteomyelitis of the mandible, showing diffuse soft tissue swelling around the ascending ramus of the mandible on the right, mainly involving the masseter muscle. Contrast-enhanced computed tomography image.

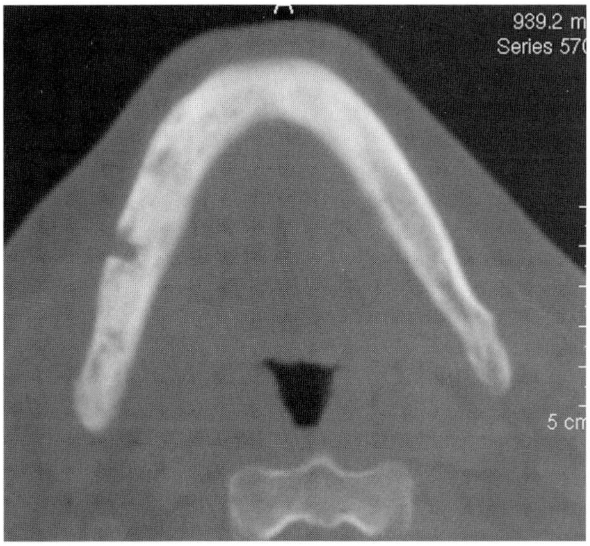

Figure 73J. Patient 2 with sclerosing osteomyelitis of the mandible. Computed tomography image inferior to Fig. 73I at bone window setting showing sclerotic change of the mandible, with cortical disruption in the external aspect of the body of mandible.

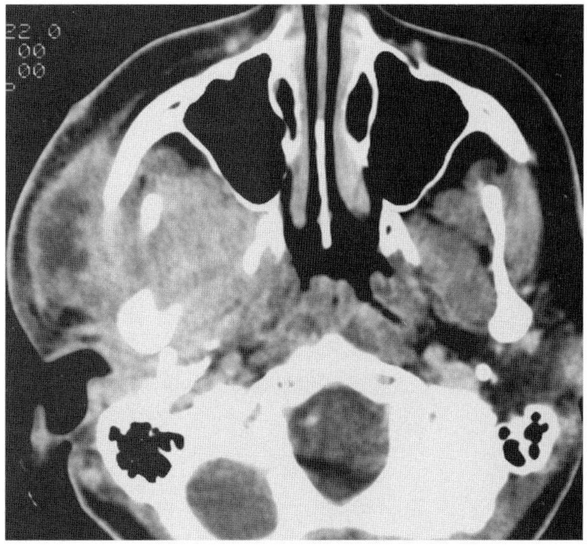

Figure 73K. Patient 3 with actinomycosis infection, showing extensive soft tissue swelling and abnormal enhancement mainly involving the masticator space on the right, with abscess superficial to the masticator space under the superficial musculoaponeurotic system. Contrast-enhanced computed tomography image.

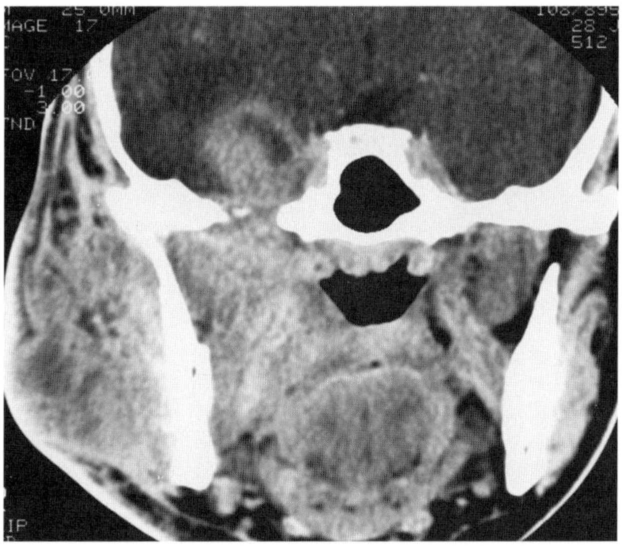

Figure 73L. Patient 3 with actinomycosis infection. Contrast-enhanced coronal computed tomography image showing transcranial extension via the foramen ovale leading to more widespread bone enhancement with the destruction of the floor of the middle cranial fossa.

CASE 74

Clinical History: A 25-year-old man presents with difficulty swallowing.

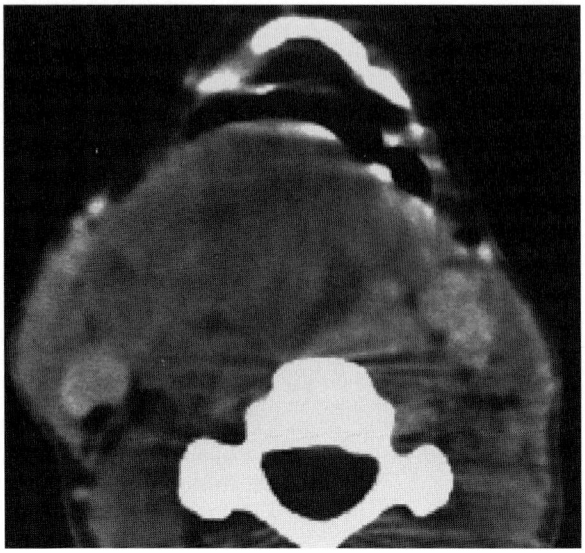

Figure 74A

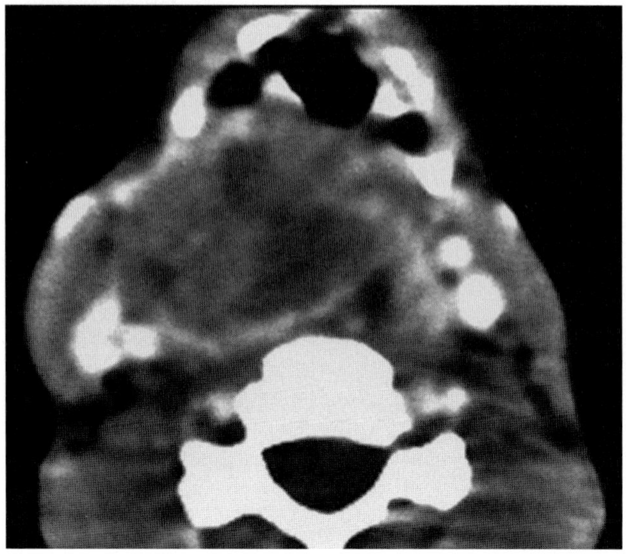

Figure 74B

1. What is the space of origin?
2. Is the process more likely inflammatory or neoplastic?
3. List three neoplasms that might arise primarily in this space.

Findings

A bulky retropharyngeal soft tissue mass. The prevertebral muscles intervene between the mass and the cervical vertebrae. The supraglottic larynx and pyriform sinuses are displaced anteriorly by the lesion. The lesion shows minimal heterogeneous enhancement.

Problem

An adult with difficulty swallowing and a retropharyngeal mass

Anatomy

A. Spaces of the neck
   1. Suprahyoid (see Fig. 70E): visceral space, parapharyngeal space (pre- and poststyloid); retropharyngeal space, prevertebral space
   2. Infrahyoid: visceral, lateral, and posterior compartments

B. Sympathetic trunk

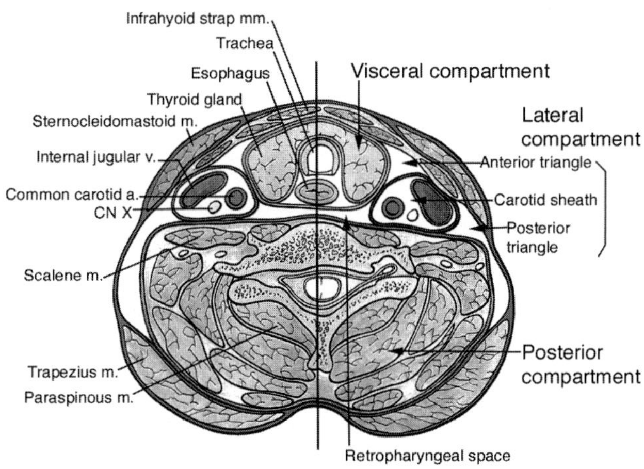

Figure 74C

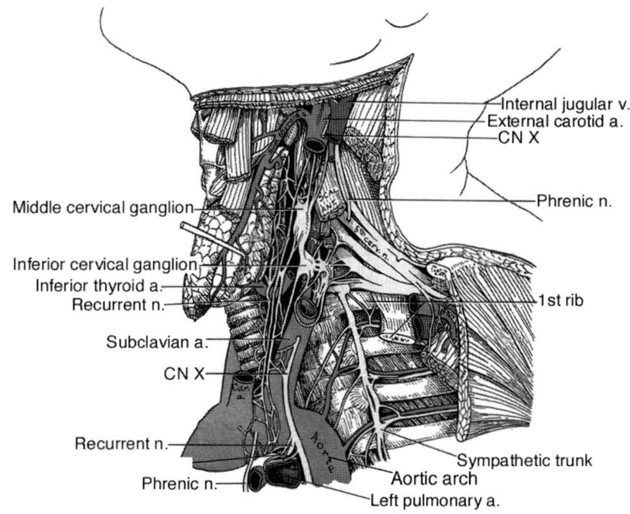

Figure 74D

Differential Diagnosis

Neurogenic tumor, mesenchymal lesion (sarcoma or benign variant), benign mixed tumor, lymphoma

Diagnosis

Benign mixed tumor arising in the retropharyngeal space

Diagnostic Imaging Approach

A. What is the space of origin (center-vector)?
B. Is the lesion transcompartmental?
C. Is there an inflammatory morphology (infiltrative margins, edema)?
D. Any other morphology: density, T1- or T2-weighted signal intensity, enhancement, hypervascularity, blood products?

Clinical Points Of Importance And Supplemental Information

A. Lesions clinically believed to be parotid in origin frequently arise from other sites.
B. Recognizing an "inflammatory" rather than a "neoplastic" morphology of a lesion as seen on magnetic resonance imaging or computed tomography scan can help reorganize the diagnostic process.

Answers To Questions

1. Retropharyngeal
2. Neoplastic
3. Neurogenic, minor salivary gland origin, mesenchymal

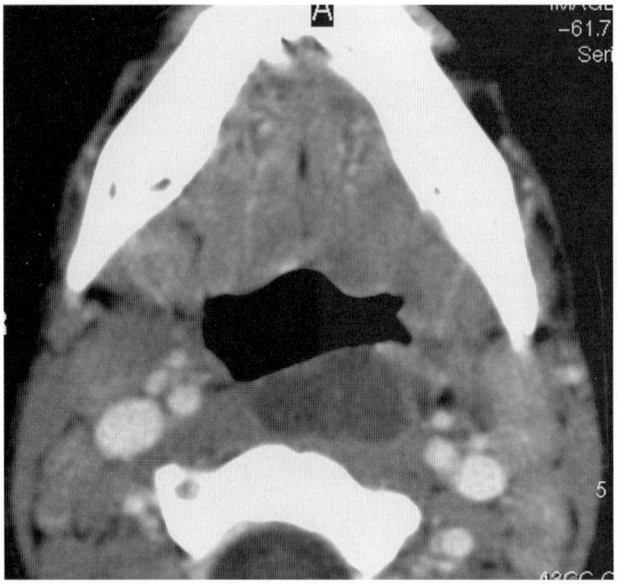

Figure 74E. Patient 1 with cystic hygroma (a variety of venolymphatic malformation), showing a cystic mass involving the retropharyngeal space without enhancement of the wall. Contrast-enhanced computed tomography image.

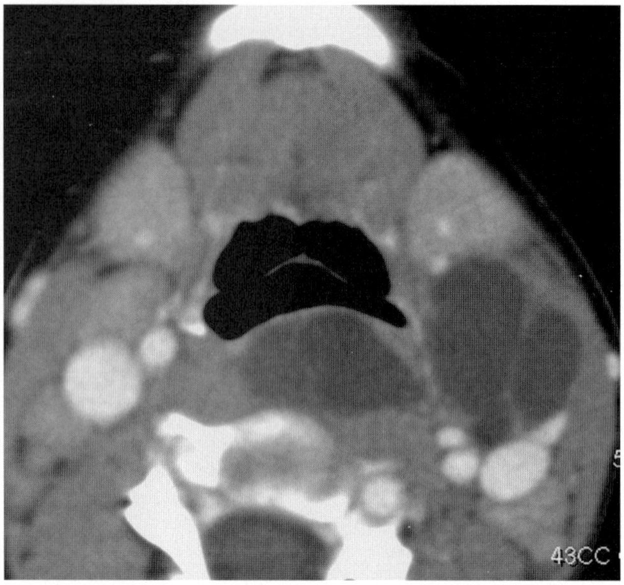

Figure 74F. Patient 1 with cystic hygroma (a variety of venolymphatic malformation), showing a loculated cystic mass in the retropharyngeal and submandibular space.

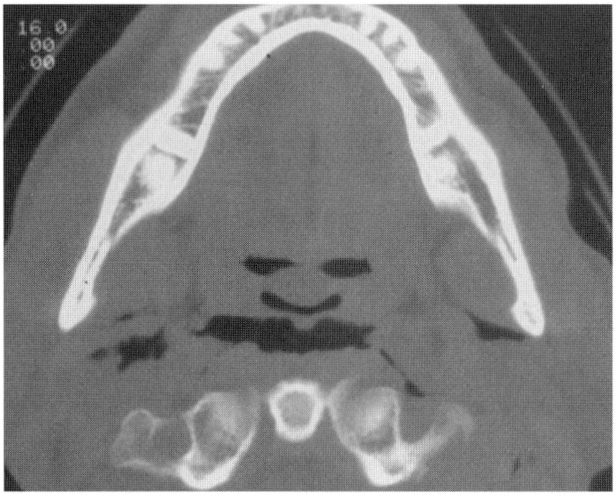

Figure 74G. Patient 2 with soft tissue emphysema, showing extraluminal air collection in the retropharyngeal space and lower prestyloid parapharyngeal space on both sides. Computed tomography image at wide window setting.

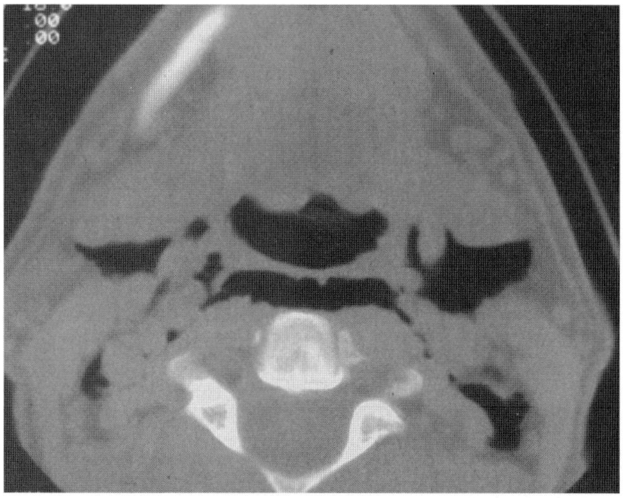

Figure 74H. Patient 2 with soft tissue emphysema. Computed tomography image at wide window setting inferior to Fig. 74G showing air collection in the retropharyngeal and submandibular space on both sides and extending into the posterior triangle.

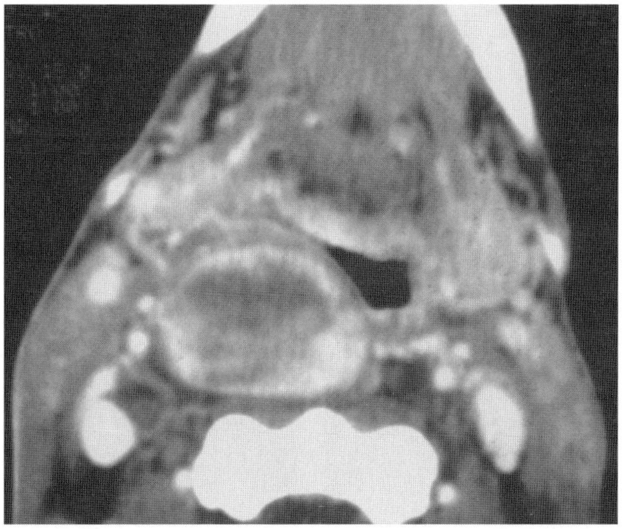

Figure 74I. Patient 3 with neurofibromatosis type I, showing a well-circumscribed mass in the retropharyngeal space distorting the oropharyngeal lumen. Contrast-enhanced computed tomography image.

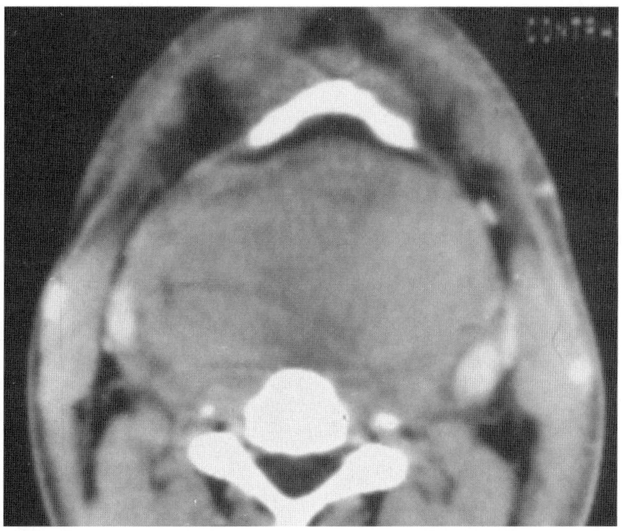

Figure 74J. Patient 4 with spontaneous (cause never was found) hematoma in the retropharyngeal space, showing a bulky mass centered in the retropharyngeal space resulting in airway collapse and displacement of the common carotid artery and internal jugular vein laterally. Contrast enhanced computed tomography image.

CASE 75

Clinical History: A 1-year-old girl presents with a 3-day history of lethargy, poor feeding, air hunger, and signs of possible meningeal irritation. Lumbar puncture finding was negative.

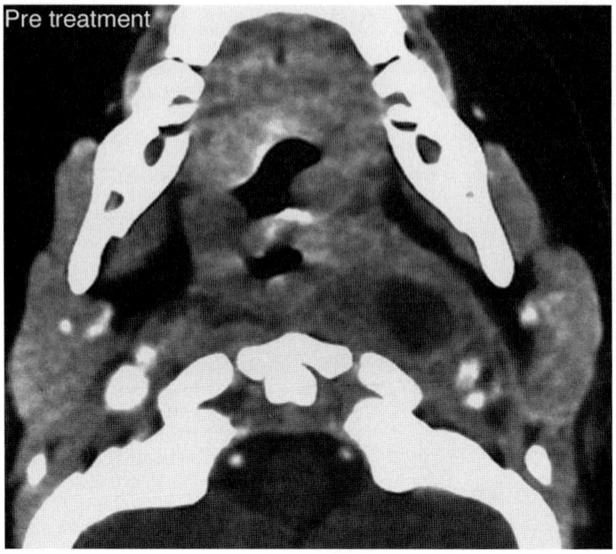

Figure 75A

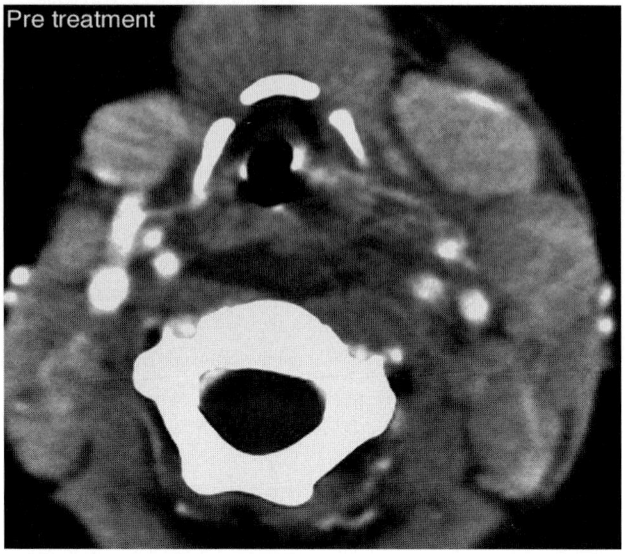

Figure 75B

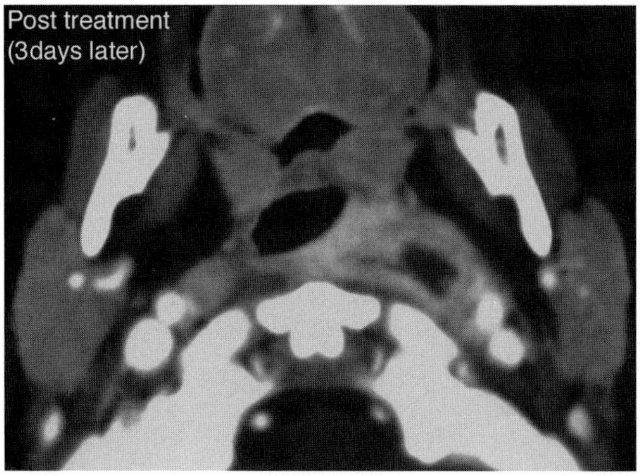

Figure 75C

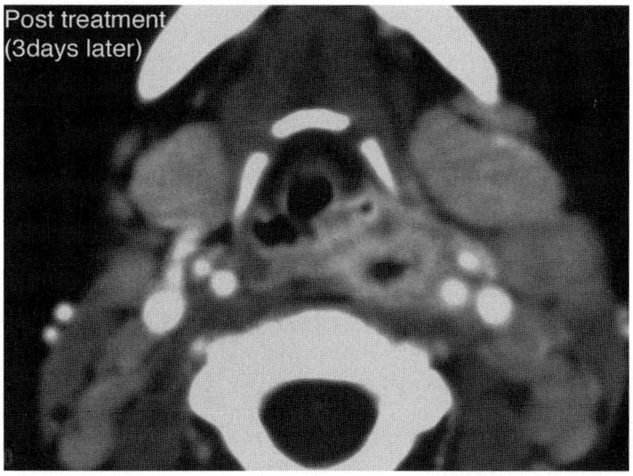

Figure 75D

1. Is there a retropharyngeal abscess?
2. What is the diagnosis?
3. Does the disease require surgical drainage for cure?

Findings

A slightly rim-enhancing cystic mass anterior to the prevertebral muscles and medial to the internal carotid artery at the expected site of the lateral retropharyngeal lymph node on the left. Soft tissue swelling obliterates the poststyloid parapharyngeal fat and displaces the prestyloid parapharyngeal fat anterolaterally. Left lateral wall (tonsillar fossa) of the oropharynx is thickened. The retropharyngeal space is distended, with fluid density without rim enhancement at the level of the hypopharynx. Multiple enlarged level 2 and 5 nodes are present on the left. Following treatment with antibiotics, the symptoms are improving markedly.

Problem

An infant with retropharyngeal abnormalities and symptoms suggestive of an inflammatory cause

Anatomy

A. Visceral space: nasopharynx and oropharynx
B. Retropharyngeal space: visceral, alar, and prevertebral fasciae (see 74C)
C. Retropharyngeal lymph nodes
D. Poststyloid parapharyngeal space (see Figs. 70E and 70F)

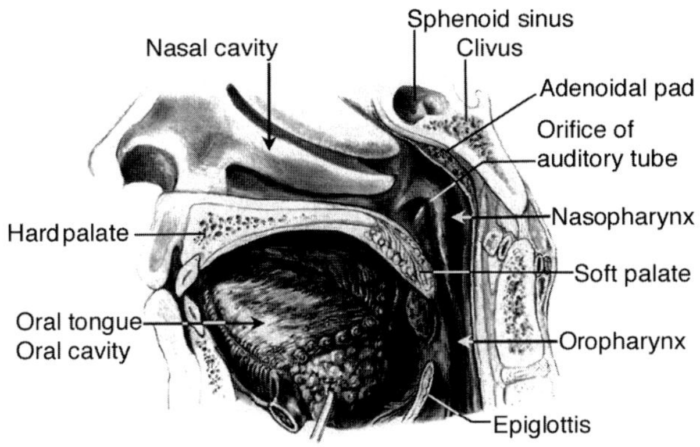

Figure 75E

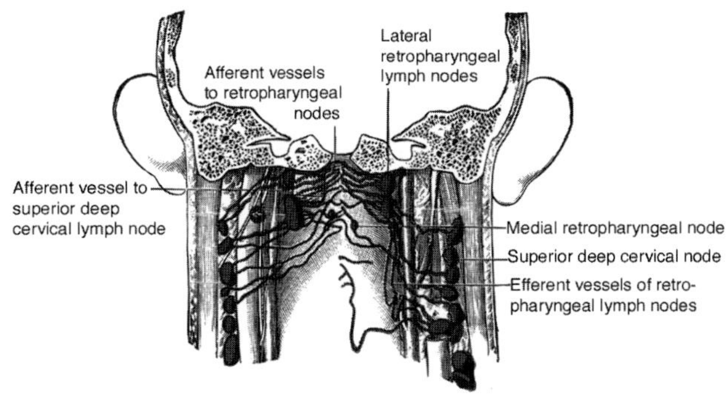

Figure 75F

Differential Diagnosis

None, in this clinical setting

Diagnosis

Pyogenic, suppurative retropharyngeal adenitis with retropharyngeal edema; *no* retropharyngeal abscess noted

Diagnostic Imaging Approach

A. Space of origin?
B. Is the lesion transcompartmental (i.e., is more than one contiguous space involved)? Which spaces?
C. Is there an inflammatory morphology?
   1. Edema or phlegmon?
   2. Abscess?
   3. Adenitis: suppurative or reactive?
   4. Combination of 1–3?
D. If inflammatory and more than one space is involved, define the nature of disease in *each* space (i.e., abscess vs. edema).
E. If inflammatory, is a complication or source (e.g., aneurysm, jugular thrombophlebitis, osteomyelitis) present?
F. If another cause is likely, evaluate the internal morphology: density, T1- or T2-weighted signal intensity, enhancement, vascularity, blood products, calcifications.

Clinical Points Of Importance And Supplemental Information

A. Suppurative retropharyngeal adenitis is a medical disease. Surgical drainage of infected nodes is not necessary except in cases of airway compromise, the disease is not responsive to intravenous antibiotics, or some other compelling clinical circumstances exist.
B. Retropharyngeal edema such as that seen here is frequently misdiagnosed as abscess. Recognizing the morphologic differences between abscess and edema in the retropharyngeal space can lead to more accurate treatment decisions.
C. Abnormal retropharyngeal "collections" must always be traced to their most inferior extent (i.e., into the chest, as necessary).

Answers To Questions

1. No
2. Suppurative retropharyngeal adenitis and retropharyngeal edema
3. No

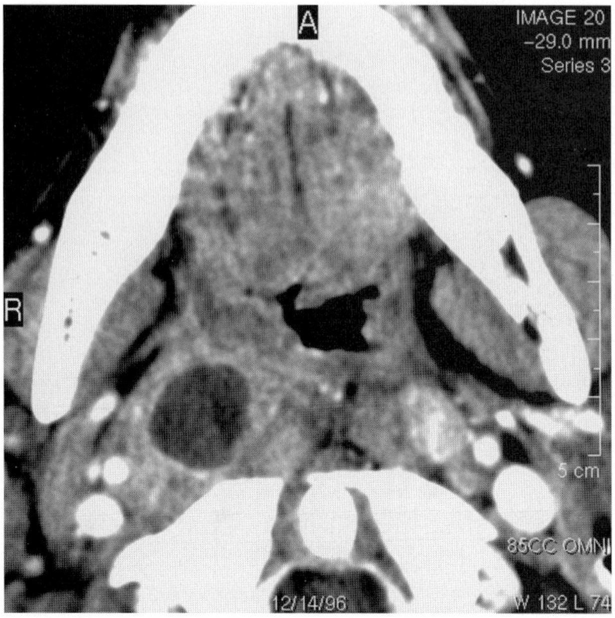

Figure 75G. Patient 1 (8 y/M) with suppurative retropharyngeal lymphadenitis, showing a cystic mass localized in the expected position of the right lateral retropharyngeal lymph node, which is surrounded by soft tissue swelling. A reactive lymphadenopathy of the left lateral retropharyngeal node suggested by enhancement is greater than is usual.

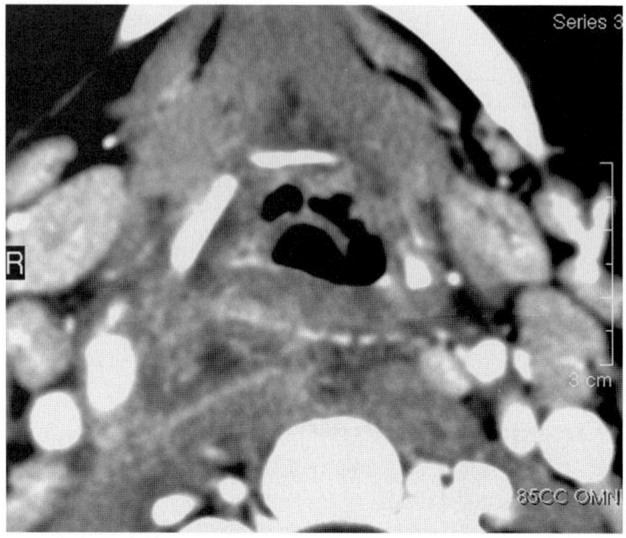

Figure 75H. Patient 1 (8 y/M) with suppurative retropharyngeal lymphadenitis. Contrast-enhanced computed tomography image inferior to Fig. 75G showing edematous swelling of the retropharyngeal space, with enhancement of the prevertebral and alar fascial layers. The swelling resolved on intravenous antibiotics without drainage.

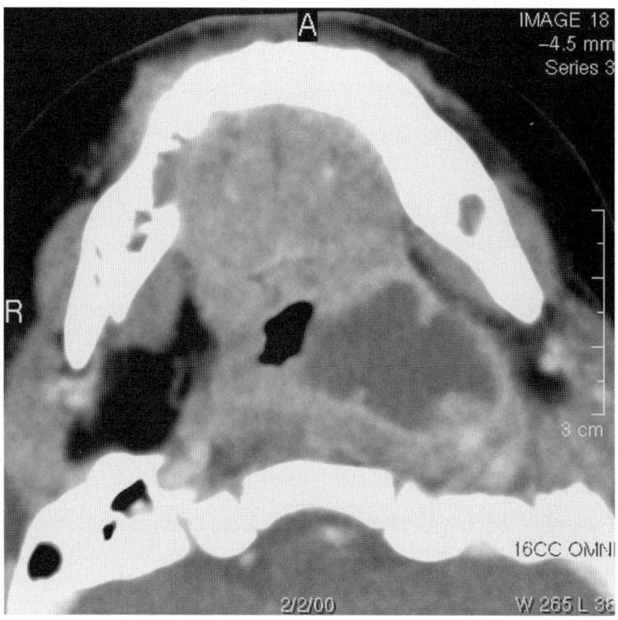

Figure 75I. Patient 2 (8 m/M) with suppurative retropharyngeal lymphadenitis, showing a cystic mass centered in the expected position of the left lateral retropharyngeal lymph node, which is larger than in 75A–D. This resolved on intravenous antibiotics alone without drainage.

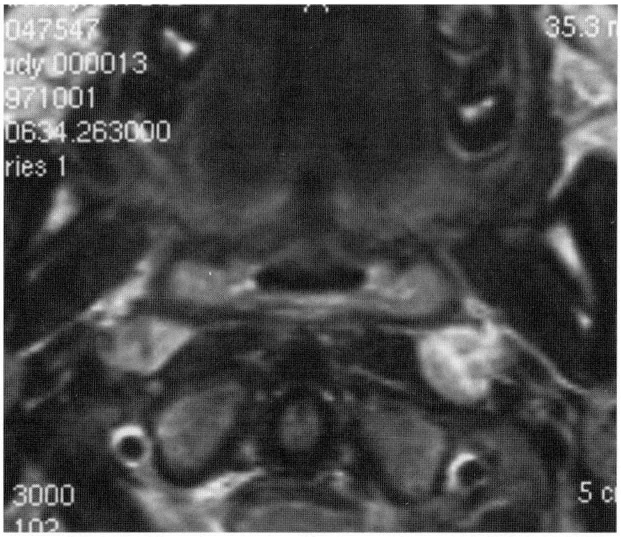

Figure 75J. Patient 3 with presumed early suppurative (vs. just reactive) retropharyngeal lymphadenitis. T2-weighted axial image showing irregularly shaped, high-intensity focus in the enlarged left lateral retropharyngeal lymph node.

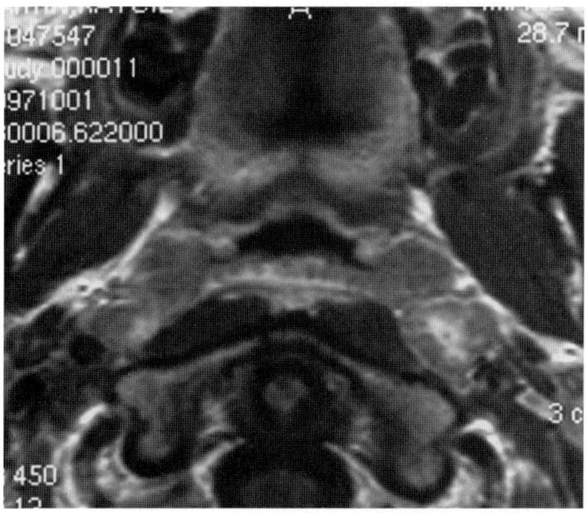

Figure 75K. Patient 3 with presumed early suppurative (vs. just reactive) retropharyngeal lymphadenitis. T1-weighted axial image with contrast showing enhancing area in the left lateral retropharyngeal lymph node.

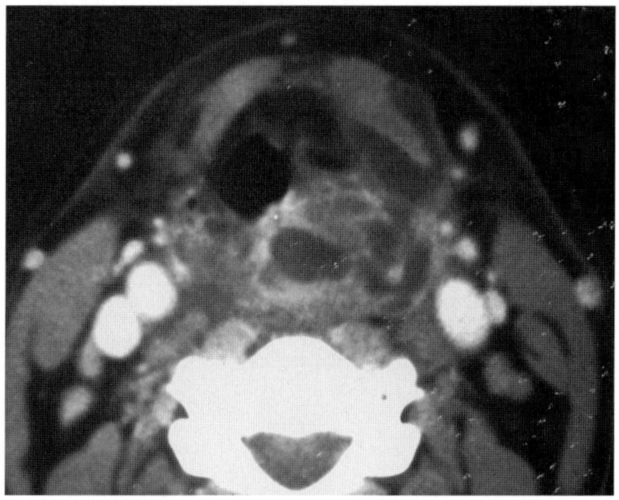

Figure 75L. Patient 4 with retropharyngeal abscess, showing multiloculated fluid collection, with enhancement of the wall and septa involving the retropharyngeal space and visceral space.

CASE 76

Clinical History: A 9-month-old girl presents with difficulty breathing and a nasopharyngeal mass.

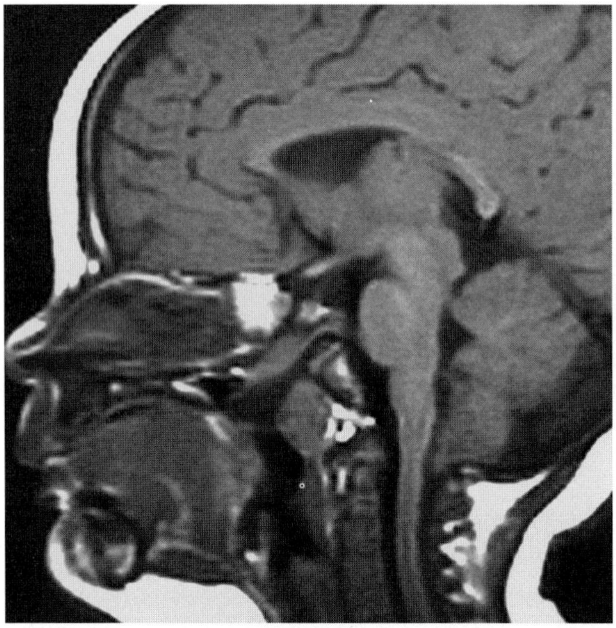

Figure 76A

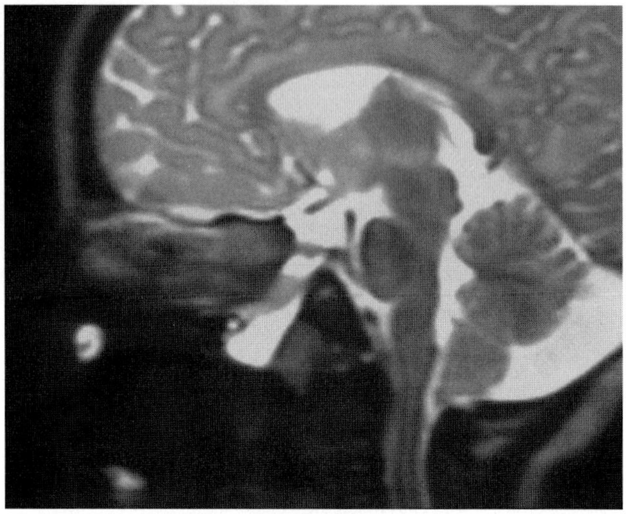

Figure 76B

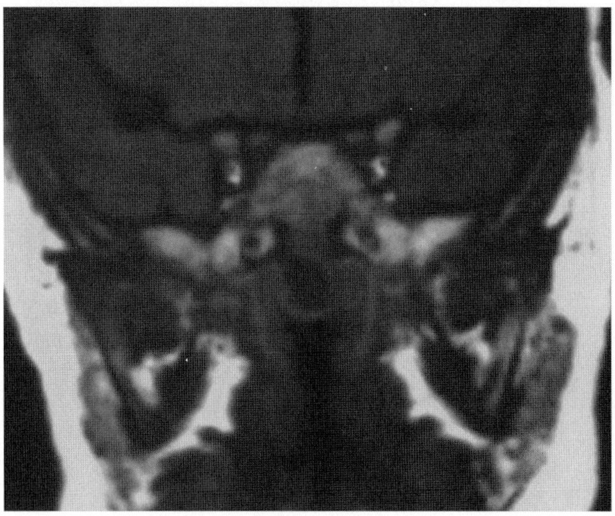

Figure 76C

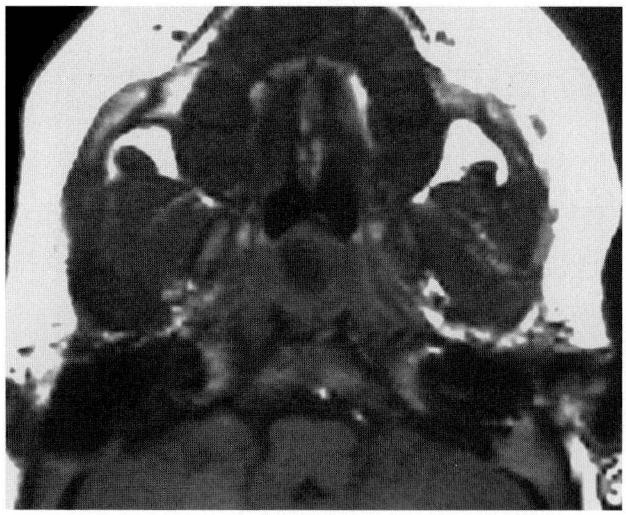

Figure 76D

1. Is the mass in the nasopharynx normal or abnormal?
2. Would you recommend a biopsy?
3. Name the three types of nasopharyngeal cysts and state the significance of each.

Findings

Partially cystic mass protrudes into the nasopharynx, which is seemingly contiguous with the prepontine cistern through a defect of the clivus

Problem

An infant with airway obstruction and a nasopharyngeal mass that appears partially cystic and is extending through the central skull base

Anatomy

A. Nasopharynx: anatomic limits, lymphoid tissue (adenoids, pharyngeal tonsil), pharyngeal bursa
B. Central skull base: basisphenoid, basiocciput, sphenooccipital synchondrosis

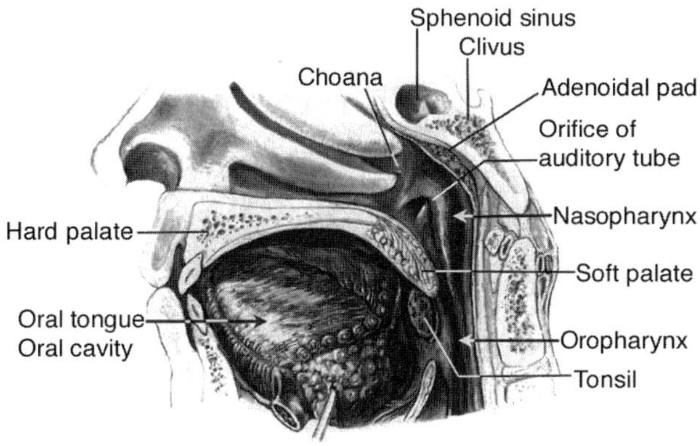

Figure 76E

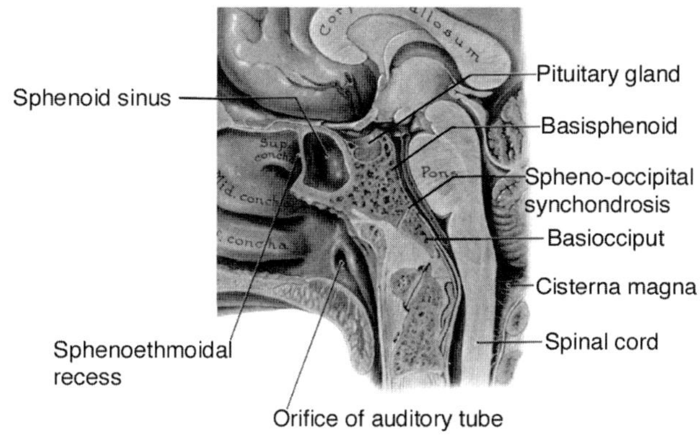

Figure 76F

Differential Diagnosis

1. None in this case
2. For a submucosal cystic mass in the nasopharynx: retention cyst, Tornwaldt's cyst, Rathke's cleft cyst, branchial cleft cyst, adenitis with localized abscess

Diagnosis

Basal meningoencephalocele

Diagnostic Imaging Approach

A. Is the "mass" abnormal or a normal variant (e.g., prominent lymphoid tissue?
B. What is the site of origin: visceral compartment (nasopharynx), skull base, deep spaces (e.g., parapharyngeal), central nervous system (CNS)?
C. Are there signs of aggressive behavior: invasive margins, deep space invasion, nodal metastases, perineural spread, skull base invasion?
D. If of CNS origin, is it attached to intracranial structures and are there associated developmental abnormalities?
E. Evaluate internal morphology: density, T1- or T2-weighted signal intensity, enhancement, vascularity, blood products, calcifications.

Clinical Points Of Importance And Supplemental Information

A. A submucosal mass anywhere in the pharynx *must* be imaged before it is biopsied.
B. Discovery of one CNS developmental abnormality requires a diligent search for other craniofacial or CNS abnormalities.

Answers To Questions

1. Abnormal
2. No!
3. Retention: none; Tornwaldt's: usually none; branchial cleft: infection; Rathke's: rare, potentially connected intracranially.

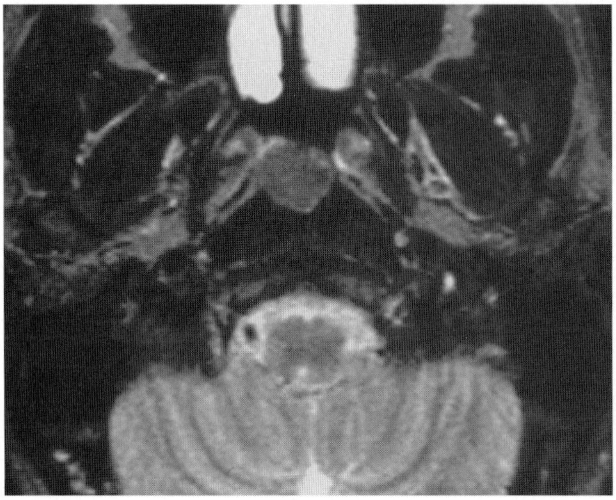

Figure 76G. Patient 1 with Tornwaldt's cyst. T2-weighted axial image showing a relatively low-intensity mass in the midline of nasopharynx.

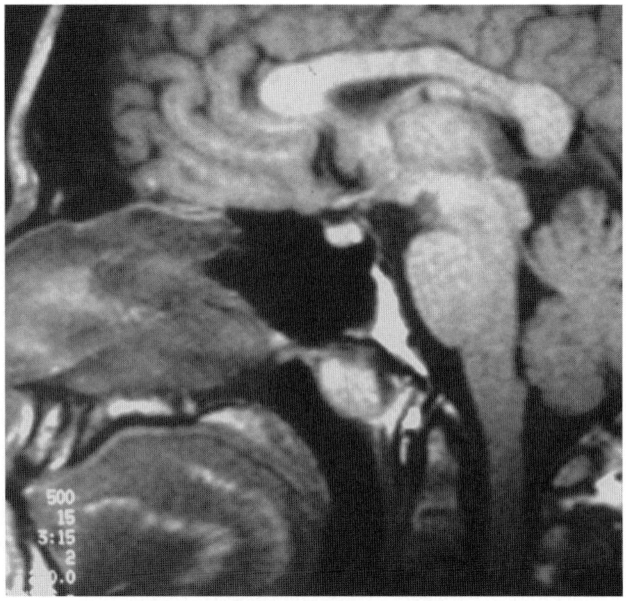

Figure 76H. Patient 1 with Tornwaldt's cyst. T1-weighted sagittal image without contrast showing a relatively high-intensity mass in the roof of the nasopharynx without connection with intracranial space.

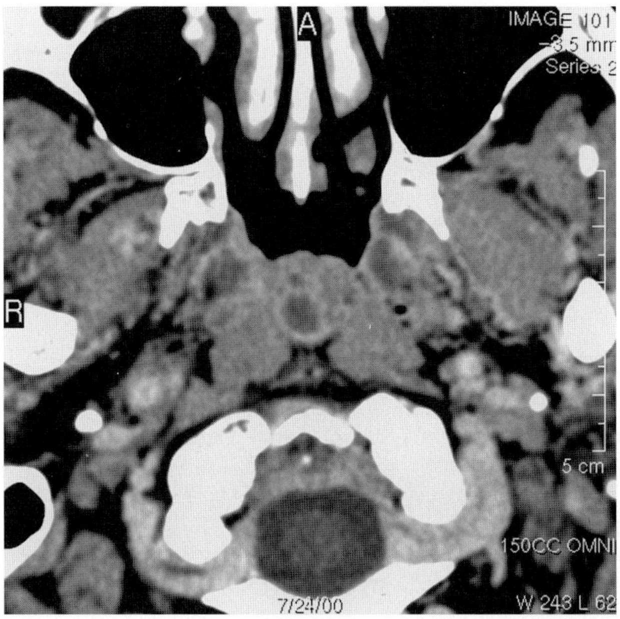

Figure 76I. Patient 2 with Tornwaldt's cyst, showing a unilocular cystic lesion in the midline of posterior nasopharyngeal wall. Contrast-enhanced computed tomography image.

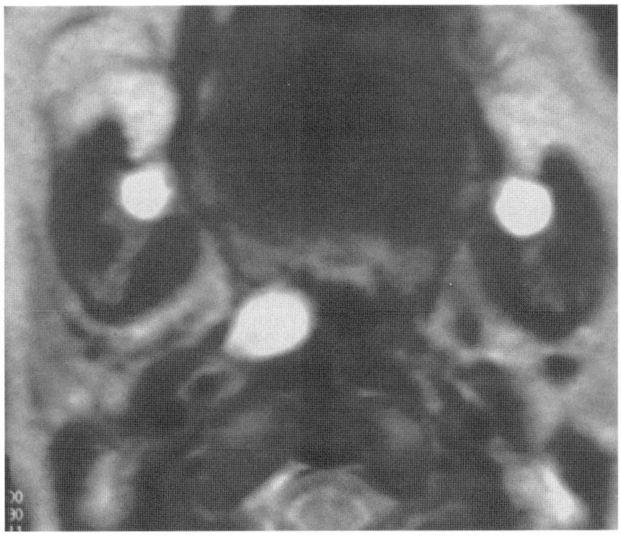

Figure 76J. Patient 3 with second branchial cleft cyst, showing a submucosal cystic mass of the lateral wall of nasopharynx on the right. T2-weighted axial image.

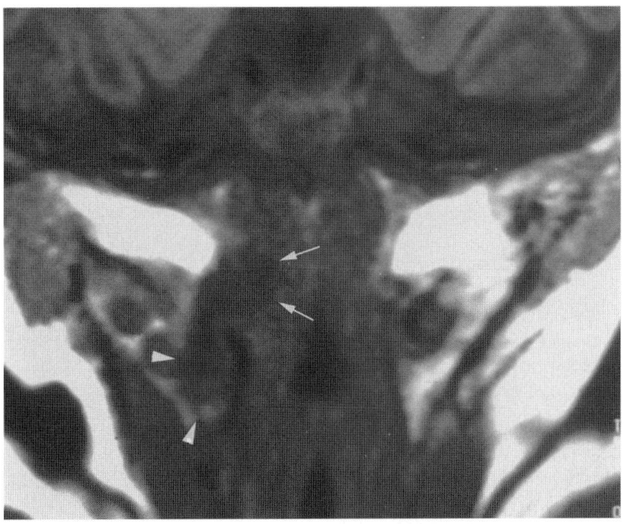

Figure 76K. Patient 3 with second branchial cleft cyst. T1-weighted coronal image without contrast showing an bilobed cystic mass with one component (*arrow heads*) in the parapharyngeal space and a second (*arrows*) within the lateral wall of the nasopharynx.

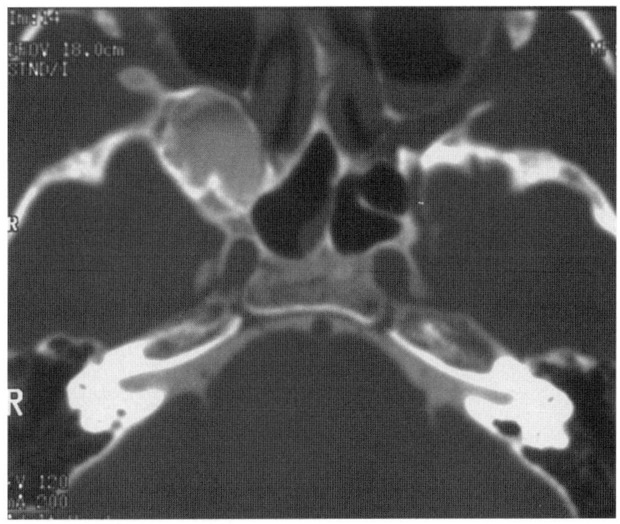

Figure 76L. Patient 4 with transsphenoidal meningoencephalocele. Computed tomography cisternography showing a cystic mass centered in medial aspect of the greater wing of sphenoid bone on the right, which enhances with intrathecally injected contrast.

CASE 77

Clinical History: A 15-year-old boy presents with nosebleeds.

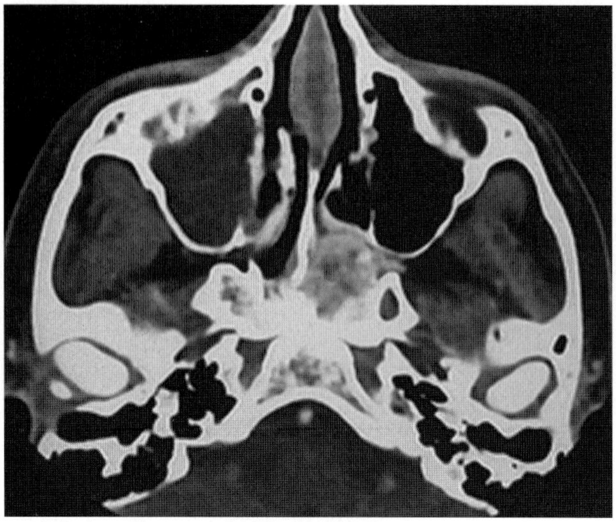

Figure 77A

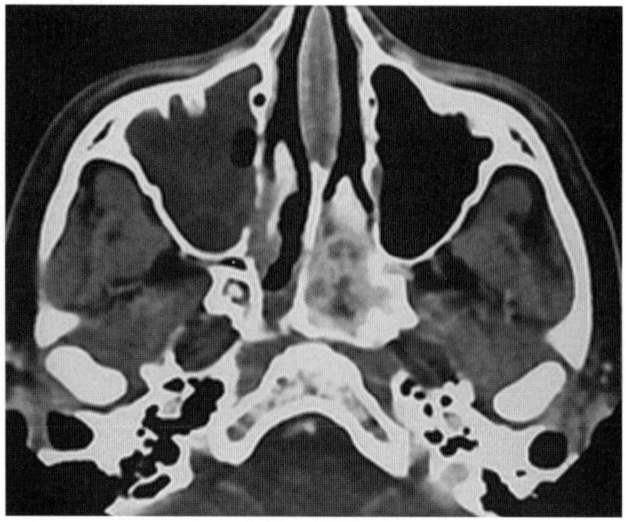

Figure 77B

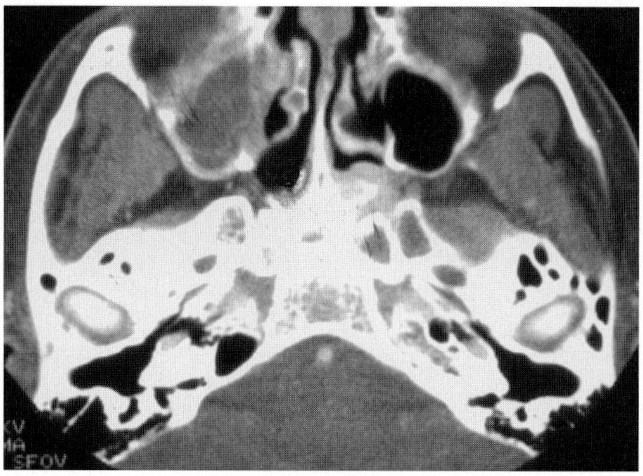

Figure 77C

1. What is the diagnosis?
2. Does the patient need an angiogram before or after the biopsy?
3. Would you predict a blood supply from the internal carotid artery?

Findings

An intensely enhancing mass in the nasopharynx and posterior nasal cavity, bridging the posterior choana. The mass is contiguous with a widened left pterygopalatine fossa through the sphenopalatine foramen. The base of left pterygoid process is eroded. Incidental right maxillary sinusitis is noted.

Problem

A teenaged boy with nosebleeds and an enhancing nasopharyngeal mass

Anatomy

A. Nasopharynx: anatomic limits
B. Posterior choana and posterior nasal cavity
C. Skull base
   1. Palatine bone and pterygoid process or plates of the sphenoid bone, pterygoid fossa
   2. Sphenopalatine foramen, pterygopalatine fossa, pterygomaxillary fissure
   3. Vidian canal
   4. Distal maxillary artery
D. Infratemporal fossa (see Fig. 57F)

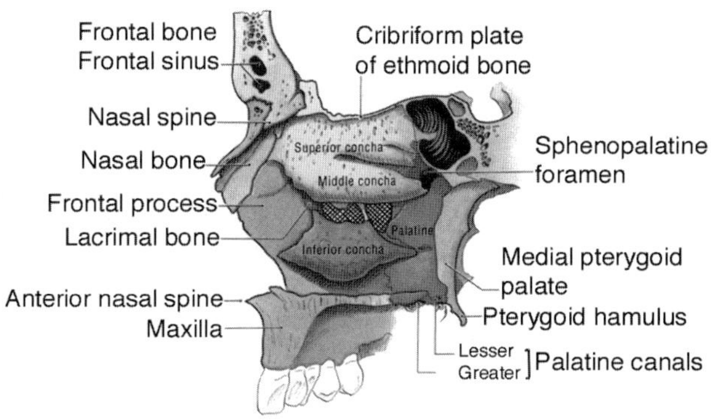

Figure 77D

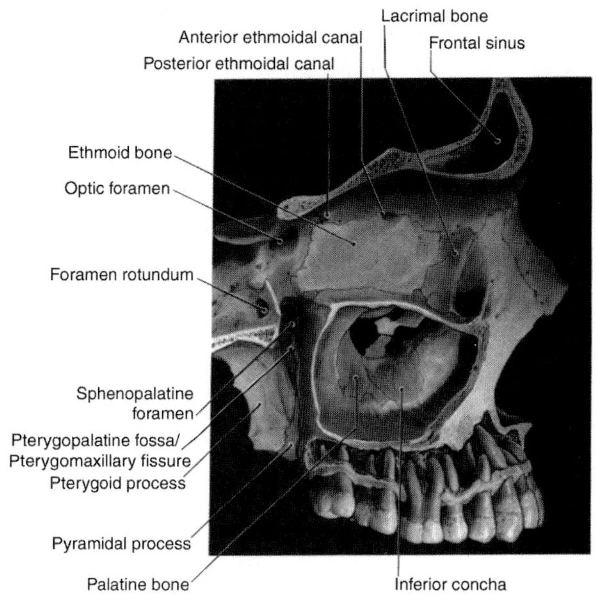

Figure 77E

Differential Diagnosis

Juvenile angiofibroma, angiomatous polyps, hypervascular malignancy, metastases

Diagnosis

Juvenile angiofibroma

Diagnostic Imaging Approach

A. Where is the lesion centered?
B. Where does the lesion extend (e.g., pterygopalatine fossa, skull base, intracranially, orbit, sinonasal)?
C. Evidence of hypervascularity: enhancement, flow voids, enlarged maxillary or ascending pharyngeal vessels?
D. Is angiography required? For diagnosis? For management?
E. Any features atypical for juvenile angiofibroma (JAF) (location, extent, pattern of bone destruction, enlarged retropharyngeal lymph nodes)?

Clinical Points Of Importance And Supplemental Information

A. The clinical setting is virtually always typical for JAF (i.e., pubescent male with nosebleeds and nasal stuffiness). However, not all "typical" clinical situations are caused by JAF.
B. If in doubt of diagnosis, angiography (not magnetic resonance angiography) should be done before biopsy.
C. It is essential to exclude the internal carotid supply if surgery is contemplated.
D. These lesions are easily and permanently controlled with radiation therapy (3,500 cGy).

Answers To Questions

1. Juvenile angiofibroma
2. Before, if at all
3. Possibly from the artery of the pterygoid canal (Vidian a.) if limited to the areas on the views submitted

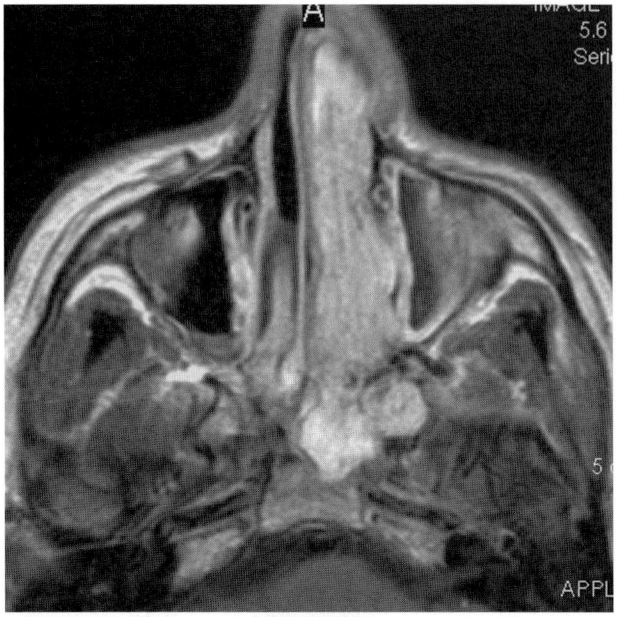

Figure 77F. Patient 1 (15 y/M) with juvenile angiofibroma, showing an intensely enhancing mass filling the left nasal cavity and dilated distal maxillary as a feeding vessel. T1-weighted axial image with contrast.

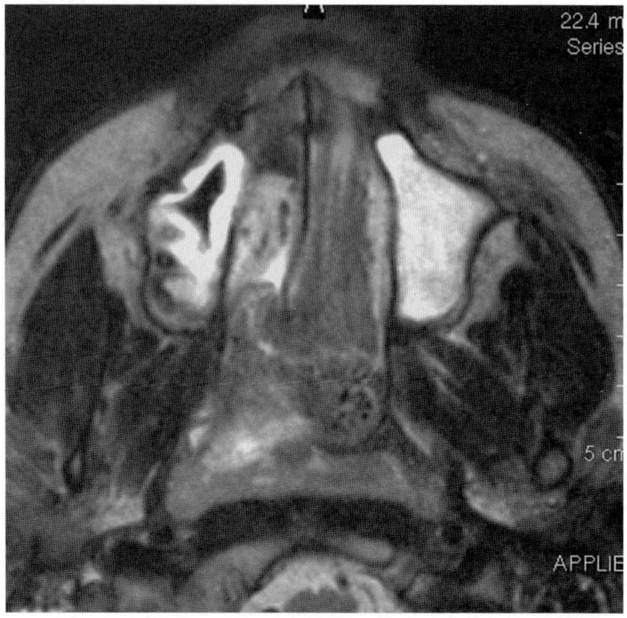

Figure 77G. Patient 1 (15 y/M) with juvenile angiofibroma, showing the mass containing multiple areas of flow void mainly in the left nasal cavity and the nasopharyngeal lumen. The mass shows lower signal intensity than edematous mucosal thickening and secretion in the maxillary sinus.

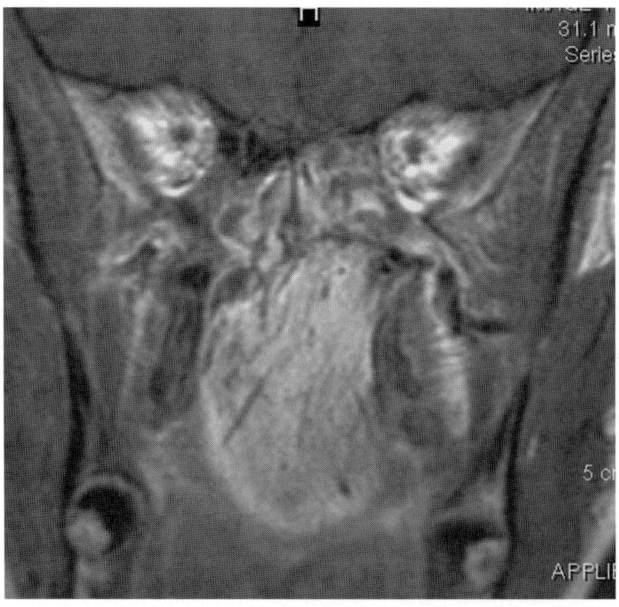

Figure 77H. Patient 1 (15 y/M) with juvenile angiofibroma. T1-weighted coronal image with contrast showing an enhancing mass and a dilated maxillary artery as a vascular pedicle of the mass and obvious flow voids in the enhancing tumor.

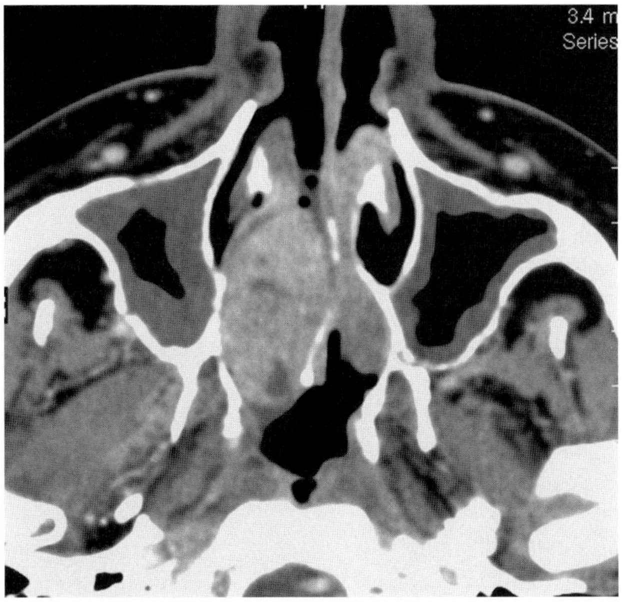

Figure 77I. Patient 2 with olfactory neuroblastoma, showing an avidly enhancing mass in the right nasal cavity and mucosal thickening in the maxillary sinus on both sides. Contrast-enhanced axial computed tomography image.

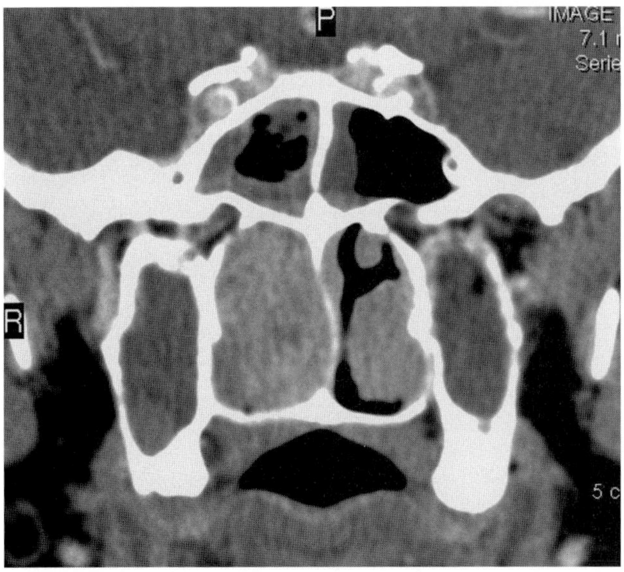

Figure 77J. Patient 2 with olfactory neuroblastoma, showing a mass in the right nasal cavity, although the adjacent sphenopalatine foramen and pterygopalatine fossa are intact. Contrast-enhanced coronal computed tomography image with contrast.

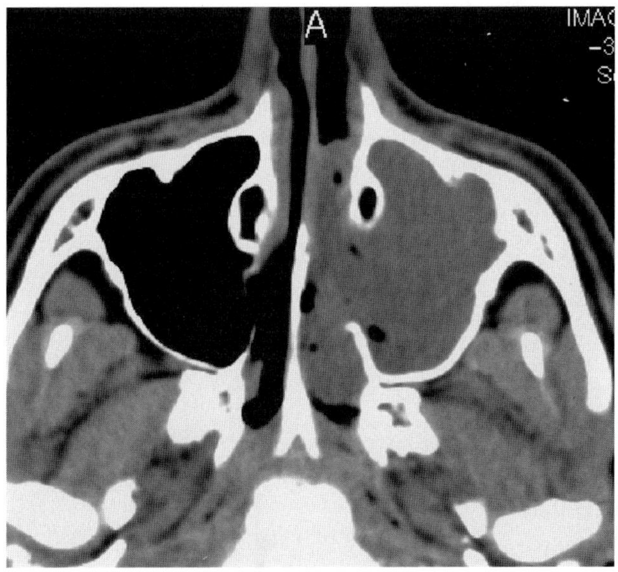

Figure 77K. Patient 3 with antrochoanal polyp, showing a relatively low-attenuation mass filling the left maxillary sinus, with extension into the left nasal cavity via the secondary ostium. No disease extent is noted in the pterygopalatine fossa. Axial computed tomography image.

CASE 78

Clinical History: A 32-year-old man presents with a 2-year history of left-sided otalgia, and a 1-year history of left eustachian tube dysfunction unresponsive to medical management. Two prior computed tomography (CT) studies over the last 18 months, done at other institutions, were read as "normal."

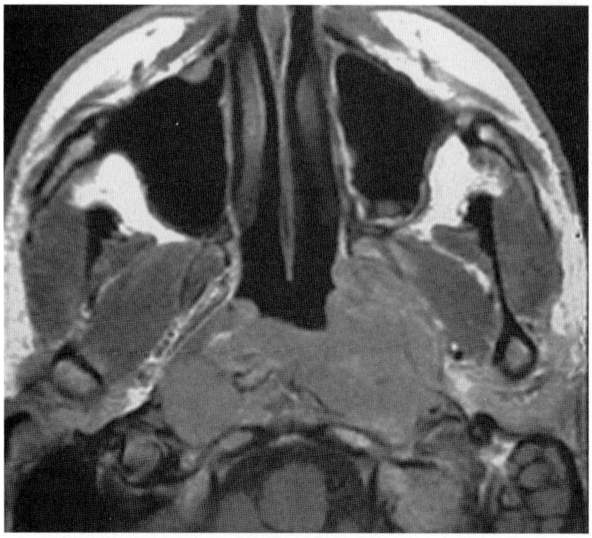

Figure 78A

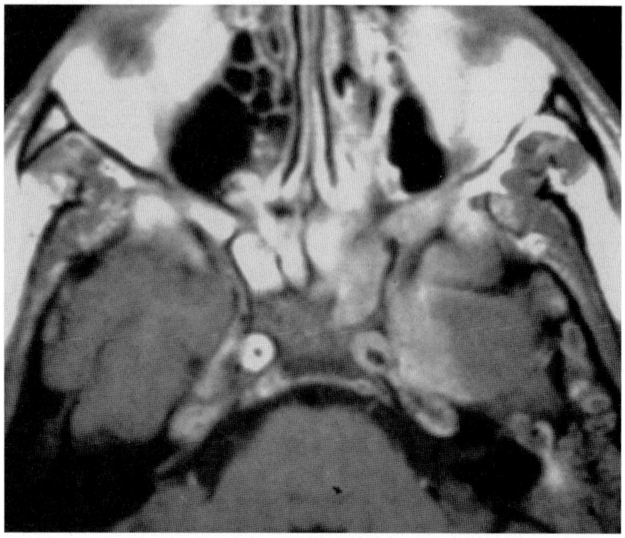

Figure 78B

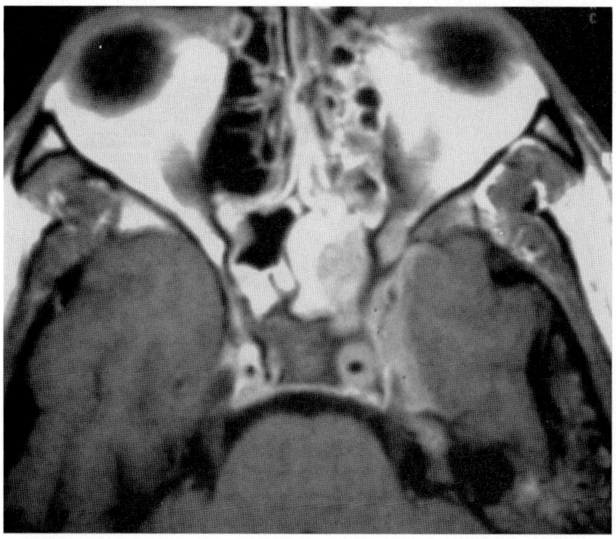

Figure 78C

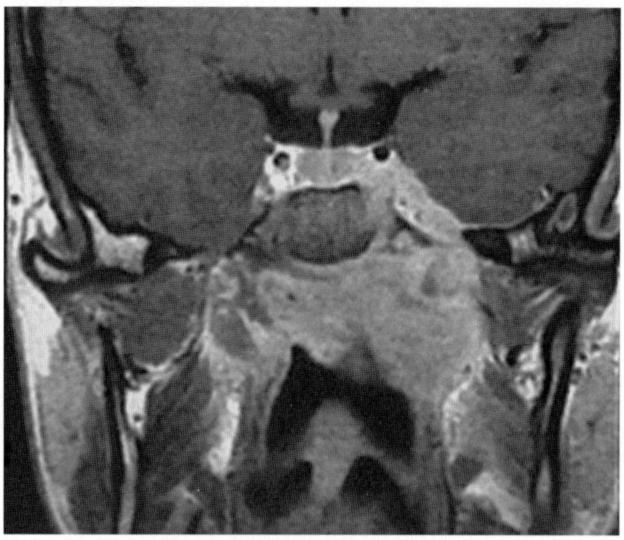

Figure 78D

1. What is the diagnosis?
2. Is there skull base invasion?
3. Is there intracranial spread? If so, by what route(s)?
4. Can intracranial spread of aggressive disease processes occur in the absence of skull base destruction?

Findings

An invasive soft tissue mass in the nasopharynx that spreads along the entire course of the left eustachian tube. The lesion extends into the middle cranial fossa, with involvement of the left cavernous sinus partly via the enlarged left foramen ovale and trigeminal cistern as well as along the carotid canal. The lesion directly involves the left parapharyngeal space laterally and the retropharyngeal and prevertebral spaces posteriorly. The medial aspect of the masticator space is also minimally involved. Secondary left otomastoid disease is noted, and the retropharyngeal lymph nodes are involved.

Problem

An adult with unilateral serous otitis media and ear pain for 1 to 2 years and an infiltrating mass in the nasopharynx

Anatomy

A. Nasopharynx: eustachian tube orifice, torus tubarius, fossa of Rosenmüller, palatine muscles, pharyngobasilar fascia (see Fig. 70F)
B. Prestyloid parapharyngeal space
C. Masticator space
D. Central skull base: clivus, foramen lacerum, foramen ovale, middle cranial fossa floor
E. Cavernous sinus, trigeminal nerve (mandibular division), cavernous carotid (see Fig. 54E)

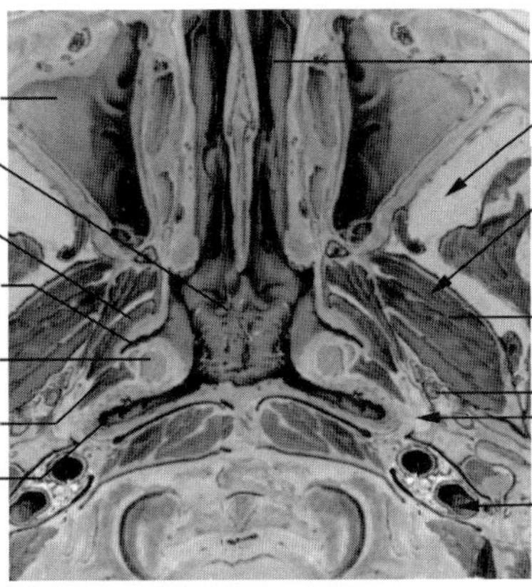

Figure 78E

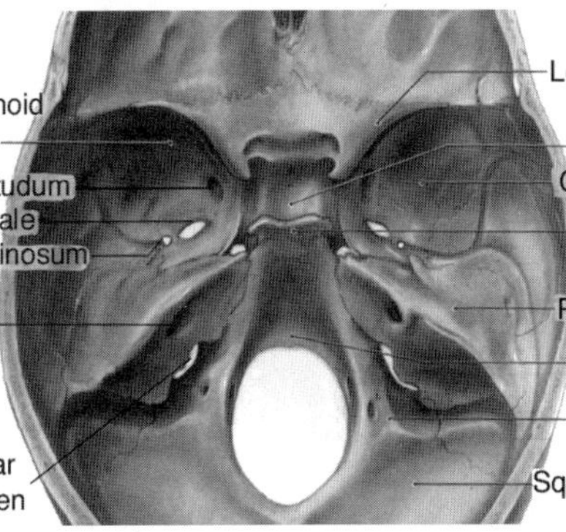

Figure 78F

Differential Diagnosis

1. Nasopharyngeal malignancy: carcinoma (85%), lymphoma (5% to 10%); others (5%), including sarcomas, plasmacytoma; rhabdomyosarcoma common in young children
2. Inflammatory lesions: Wegener's granulomatosis, sarcoidosis, histiocytosis, actinomycosis, pseudotumor, adenitis (all unusual or rare, compared with carcinoma)

Diagnosis

Squamous cell carcinoma of the nasopharynx, with skull base invasion and intracranial spread to the cavernous sinus

Diagnostic Imaging Approach

A. Where is the mass centered (arising)?
B. Any infiltrating or well-circumscribed margins seen?
C. Is the morphology more likely inflammatory or neoplastic?
D. Is there spread to skull base, cavernous sinus, or other intracranial area?
E. Is there perineural spread?
F. Any abnormal retropharyngeal nodes?
G. Define the precise margins in all directions.

Clinical Points Of Importance And Supplemental Information

A. Any adult with unilateral serous otitis media unresponsive to medical management for 3 to 6 months must have a high-resolution CT or magnetic resonance imaging study to exclude a lesion obstructing the eustachian tube.
B. The infiltrating neoplastic and inflammatory diseases of the nasopharynx cannot be distinguished on the basis of their imaging characteristics. Repeated negative or "inflammatory tissue only" biopsies require a workup for a nonmalignant etiology (e.g., antineutrophil cytoplasmic antibodies for Wegener's granulomatosis).

Answers To Questions

1. Nasopharyngeal malignant tumor
2. Yes
3. Yes; direct invasion at the petroclival fissure and along V3.
4. Yes, mainly via perineural spread. Meningeal and hematogenous spread is also possible.

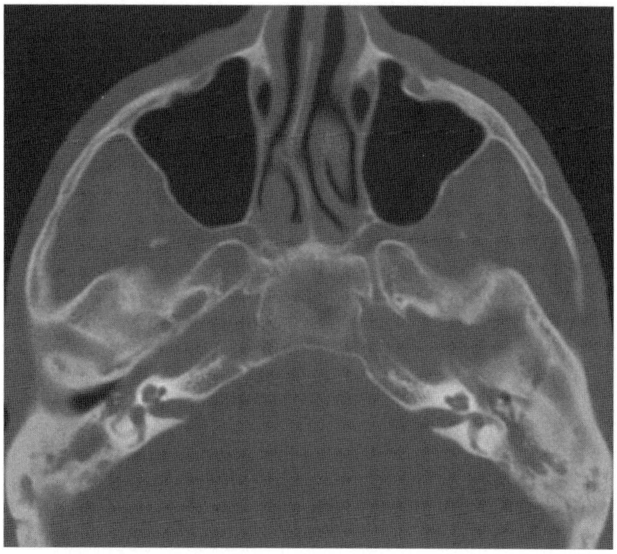

Figure 78G. Patient 1 with non-Hodgkin's lymphoma of the nasopharynx, presenting with bilateral otomastoiditis, showing mucosal thickening or fluid collection in the middle ear and mastoid air cells bilaterally. Axial computed tomography image at bone window setting.

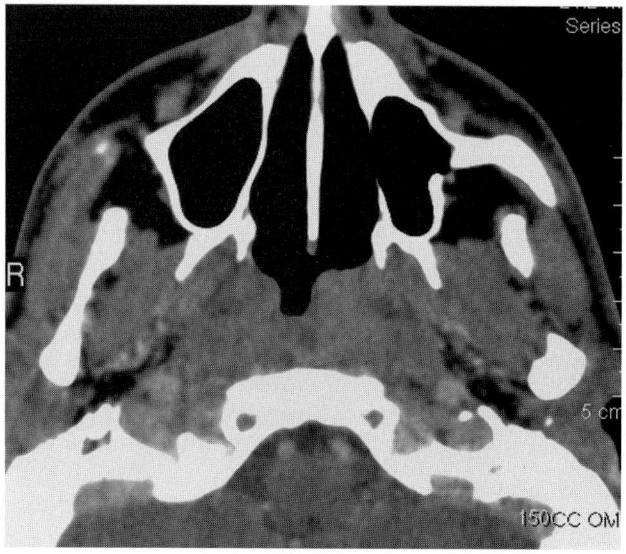

Figure 78H. Patient 1 with non-Hodgkin's lymphoma of the nasopharynx, presenting with bilateral otomastoiditis. Contrast-enhanced computed tomography image inferior to Fig. 78G showing infiltrative mass of the nasopharynx, involving expected course (along the levator veli palatini muscle) of the eustachian tube on either side.

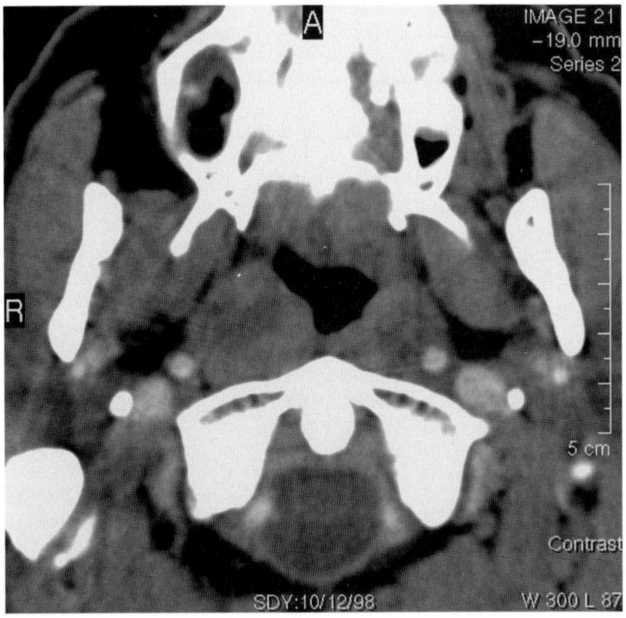

Figure 78I. Patient 2 with otomastoiditis believed to be caused by a cystic mass of undetermined origin adjacent to the distal eustachian tube. Axial computed tomography image showing soft tissue fullness in the right posterolateral aspect of the nasopharynx, involving the expected course of the right eustachian tube.

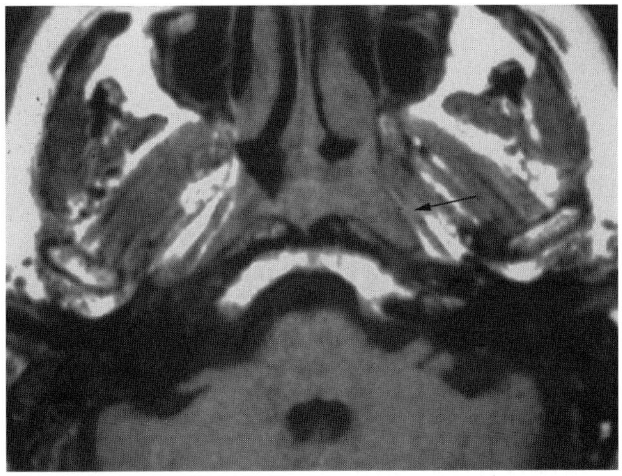

Figure 78J. Patient 3 with early nasopharyngeal carcinoma presenting with unilateral serous otitis media. T1-weighted axial image without contrast showing subtle invasive process of the nasopharynx involving the prestyloid parapharyngeal space on the left.

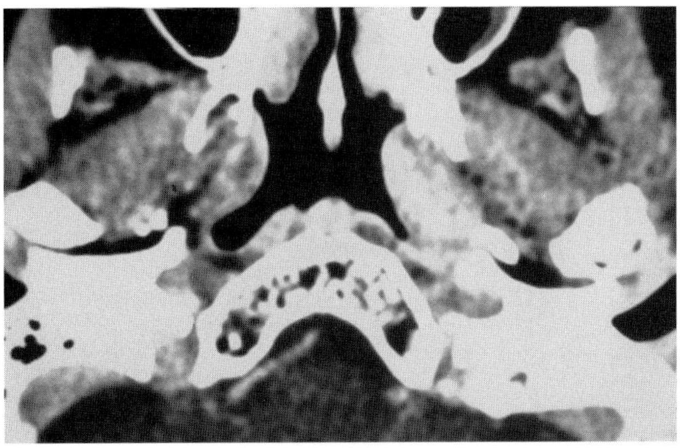

Figure 78K. Patient 4 with Wegener's granulomatosis (presenting as unilateral serous otitis media, the mass was originally thought to be an early carcinoma) showing an infiltrative process involving the left lateral wall of nasopharynx. Contrast-enhanced computed tomography axial image.

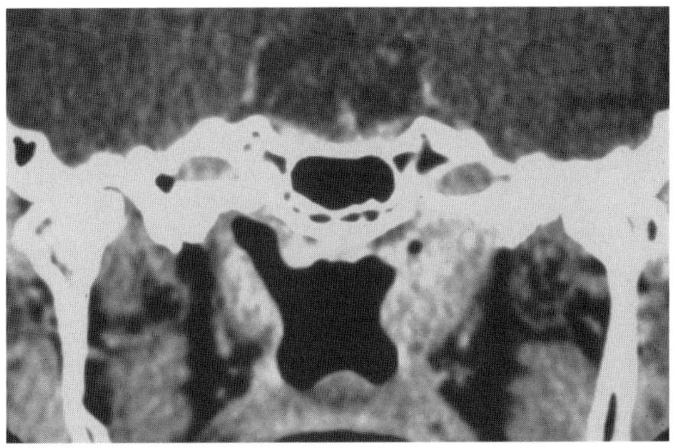

Figure 78L. Patient 4 with Wegener's granulomatosis. Contrast-enhanced coronal computed tomography image.

CASE 79

Clinical History: A 2-week-old infant boy presents with a submucosal nasopharyngeal and oropharyngeal mass. The stated reason for the study is "R/O meningoencephalocele."

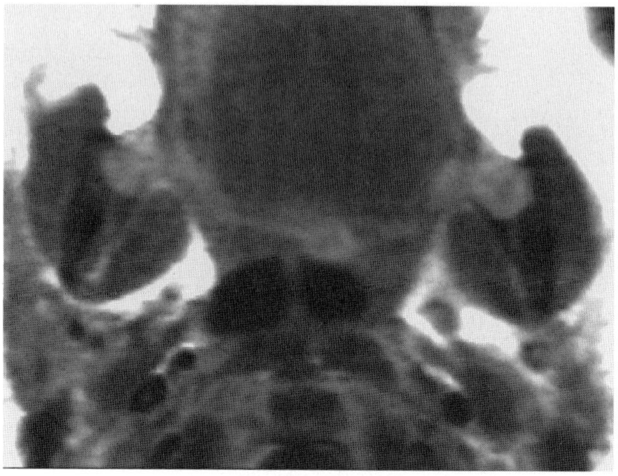

Figure 79A

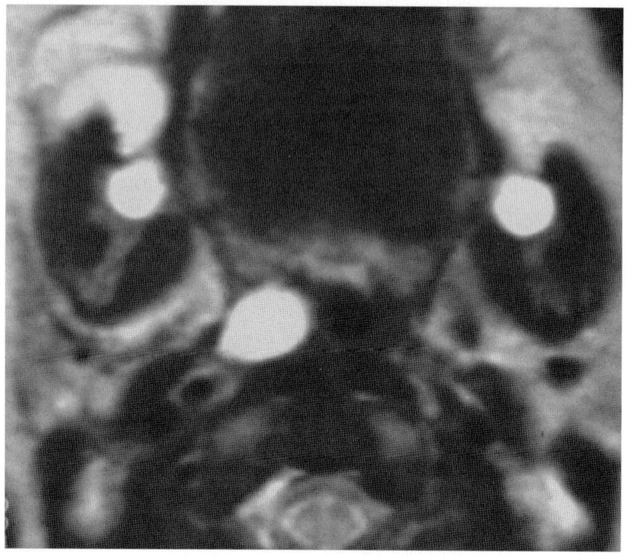

Figure 79B

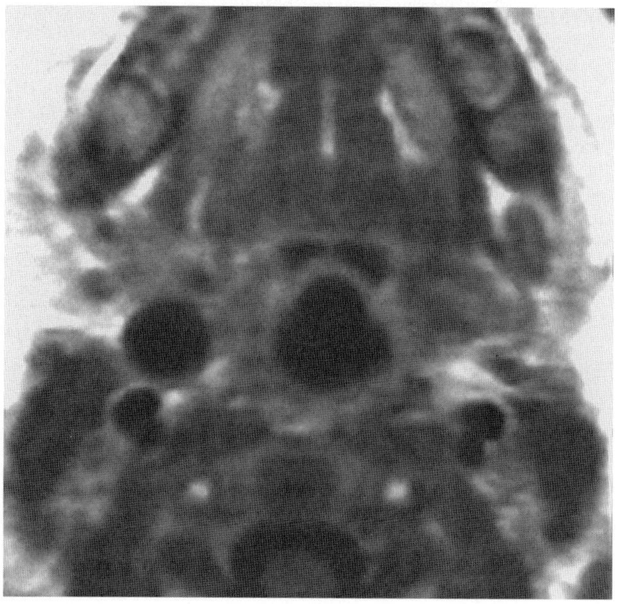

Figure 79C

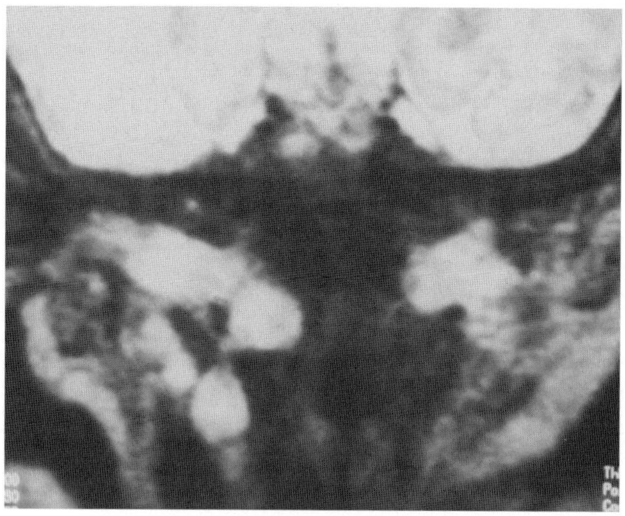

Figure 79D

1. Is this mass of central nervous system origin?
2. A specific diagnosis is possible; can you make it from these two images?
3. Name three causes of cystic masses in the tonsillar region or upper pharynx of a child.
4. Give three reasons why a mass might be "transcompartmental" or "transspatial" (i.e., why it might cross from the visceral compartment to the neck or parapharyngeal space)?

Findings

A bilobular (dumbbell) cystic mass in the right prestyloid parapharyngeal space and paratonsillar space, which bridges the superior pharyngeal constrictor muscle.

Problem

An infant with a cystic appearing submucosal mass involving the pharyngeal wall and deep neck

Anatomy

A. Oropharynx: soft palate, anterior and posterior tonsillar pillars, palatine tonsil, superior constrictor muscle
B. Parapharyngeal space: prestyloid and poststyloid (see Fig. 48F)

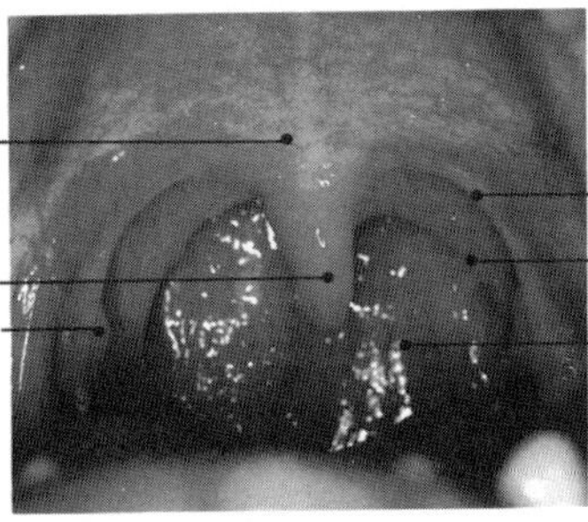

Figure 79E

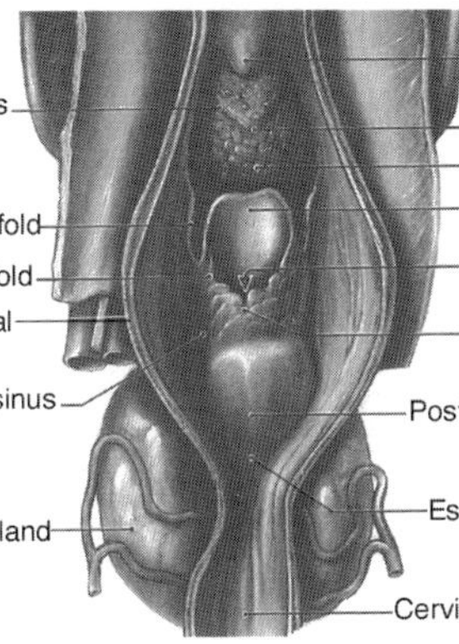

Figure 79F

Differential Diagnosis

Second branchial cleft cyst, cystic hygroma

Diagnosis

Second branchial cleft cyst

Diagnostic Imaging Approach

A. What is the site of origin: pharyngeal mucosa, muscular wall, parapharyngeal space, other extrinsic structures (e.g., carotid artery)?
B. Any signs of aggressive behavior?
C. Is the lesion confined to one compartment (space) or is it transcompartmental (spatial)?
D. Evaluate the morphology: density, T1- or T2-weighted signal intensity, enhancement, vascularity, blood products, calcifications, wall thickness or enhancement (when cystic).

Clinical Points Of Importance And Supplemental Information

A. Lesions become transcompartmental (spatial) for several reasons, including developmental cause, aggressiveness, spread along structures that cross compartments (e.g., lymphatics, nerves, arteries, veins, muscle bundles), multifocal disease, existing pathway of least resistance (e.g., sublingual to submandibular space over the posterior edge of the mylohyoid muscle).
B. A submucosal pharyngeal mass must *always* be imaged before biopsy or definitive treatment.

Answers To Questions

1. No
2. Second branchial cleft cyst
3. Meningoencephalocele, branchial cleft cyst, cystic hygroma
4. Aggressive: does not respect tissue boundaries; developmental pathway follows a transcompartmental structure (e.g., veins in lymph [hemangioma]); growth along nerves.

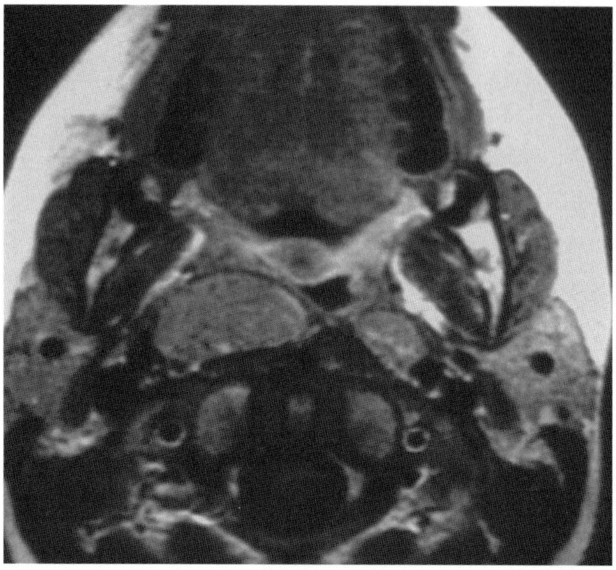

Figure 79G. Patient 1 is a child with surgically proved Castleman's disease, presenting as a submucosal pharyngeal mass, showing the enlarged lateral retropharyngeal lymph node on the right. T1-weighted axial image with contrast.

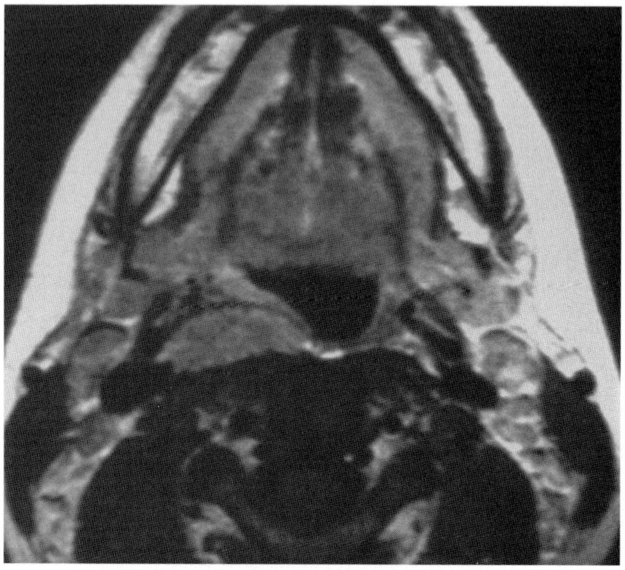

Figure 79H. Patient 1 with Castleman's disease. T1-weighted axial image with contrast inferior to Fig. 79G.

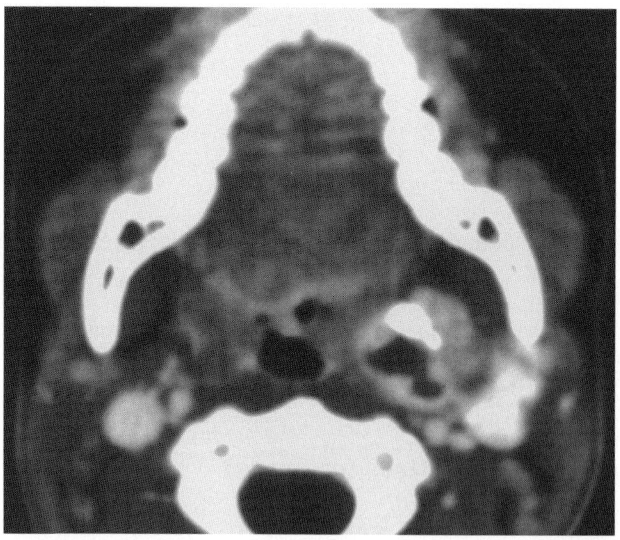

Figure 79I. Patient 2 is a young adult woman with leiomyosarcoma, showing a partially cystic mass, with focal calcification in the prestyloid parapharyngeal space, clinically presenting as a submucosal mass in the area of the left tonsil. Contrast-enhanced computed tomography image.

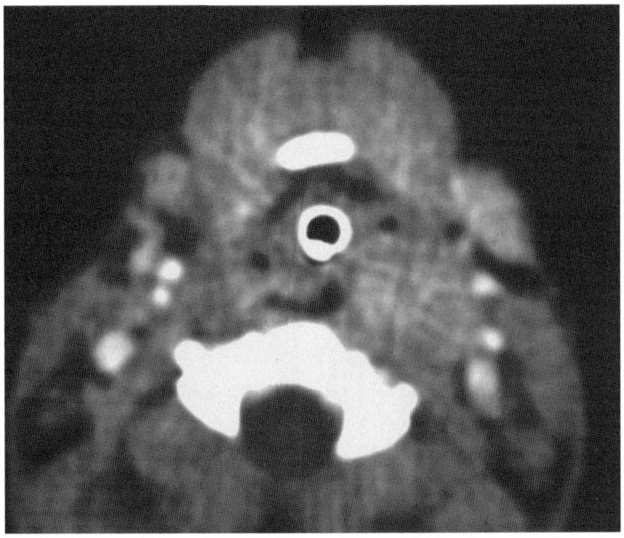

Figure 79J. Patient 3 with primary cervical neuroblastoma presenting with opsoclonus. The submucosal mass in the oropharynx on the left was appreciated after computed tomography (CT) study. Contrast-enhanced CT image.

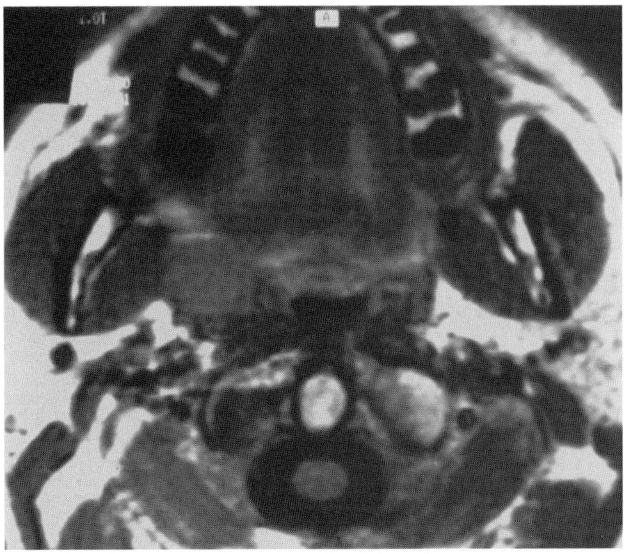

Figure 79K. Patient 4 with metastatic neck disease of unknown primary, showing a totally submucosal tumor deep to the tonsillar fossa on the right, which was appreciated on physical examination only after its discovery on magnetic resonance imaging. T1-weighted axial image.

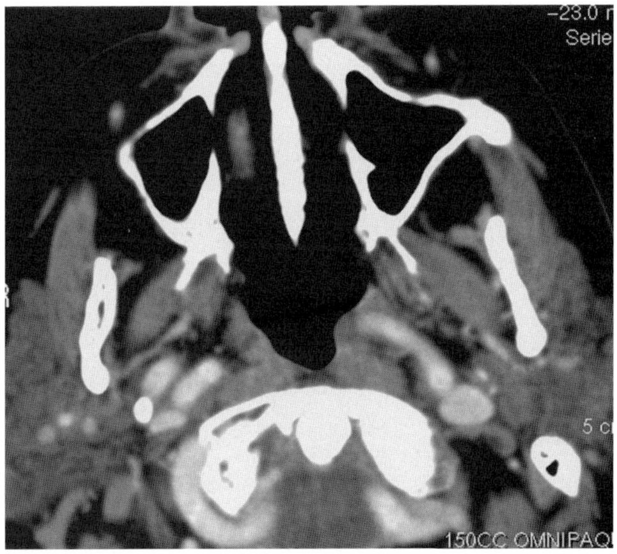

Figure 79L. Patient 5 clinically suspected of having a submucosal mass of the nasopharynx, showing tortuous left internal carotid artery indenting the left lateral wall of the nasopharynx and presenting as a submucosal mass.

CASE 80

Clinical History: A 52-year-old man presents with squamous cell carcinoma of the palatine (faucial) tonsil. No clinical evidence is noted of spread to the nasopharynx.

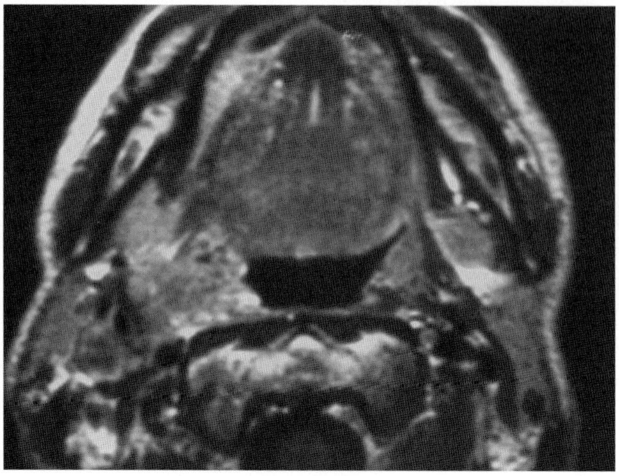

Figure 80A

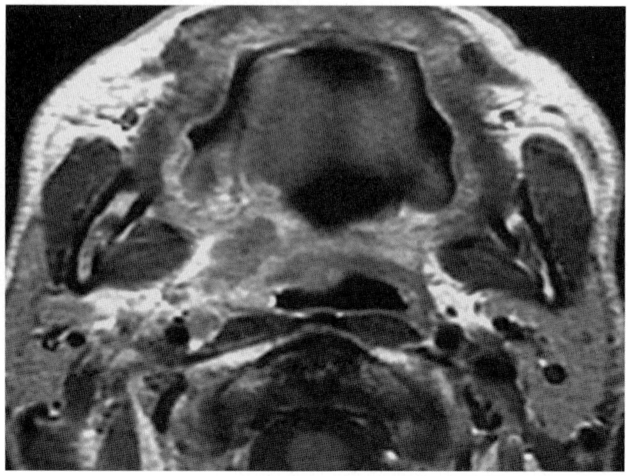

Figure 80B

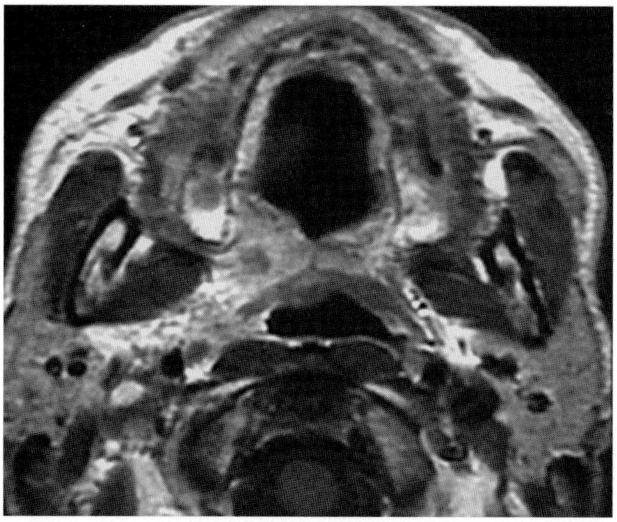

Figure 80C

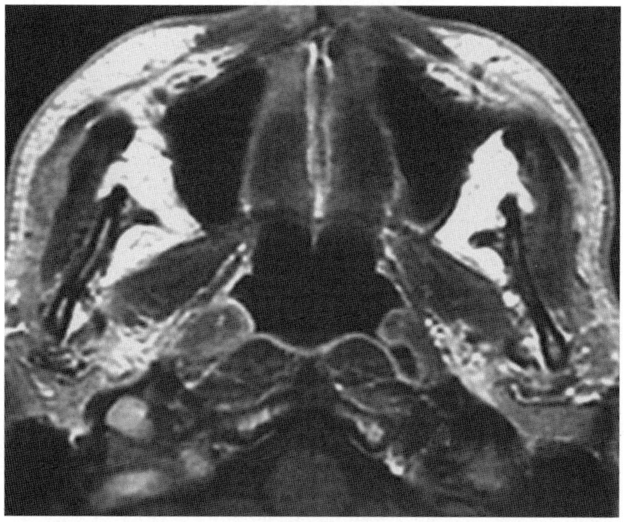

Figure 80D

1. If this tumor has spread to the level of the eustachian tube orifice, curative surgery is not possible; has it spread there? The surgeon will act only on the basis of your opinion.
2. Any abnormal retropharyngeal nodes seen?
3. What is the "T" stage, and why?

Findings

An infiltrative mass centered in the right palatine tonsil. The lesion involves the prestyloid parapharyngeal space laterally, the right lateral wall of the nasopharynx superiorly, and the soft palate via the palatopharyngeal muscle. The lesion has invaded the superior pharyngeal constrictor and levator veli palatini muscles in this area. Although the lesion involves the orifice of the right eustachian tube, no secondary otomastoiditis is seen. A small necrotic lateral retropharyngeal lymph node is seen on the right and a smaller reactive retropharyngeal node on the opposite side. Pterygomandibular raphe is involved.

Problem

A man with tonsillar squamous cell carcinoma whose treatment will be based on an assessment of the extent of the tumor

Anatomy

A. Oropharynx: tonsillar fossa, anterior and posterior tonsillar pillars, tensor and levator muscles of the soft palate, superior constrictor muscle
B. Nasopharynx: muscular wall, tensor and levator muscles of the palate, eustachian tube (in detail)
C. Retropharyngeal lymph nodes (see 75F)

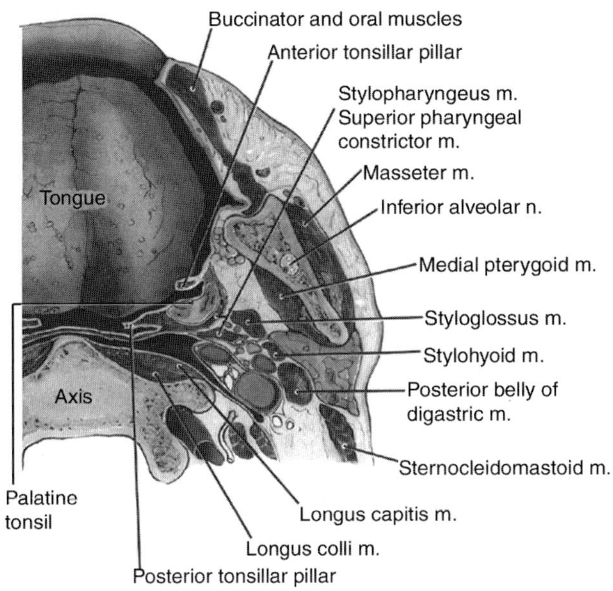

Figure 80E

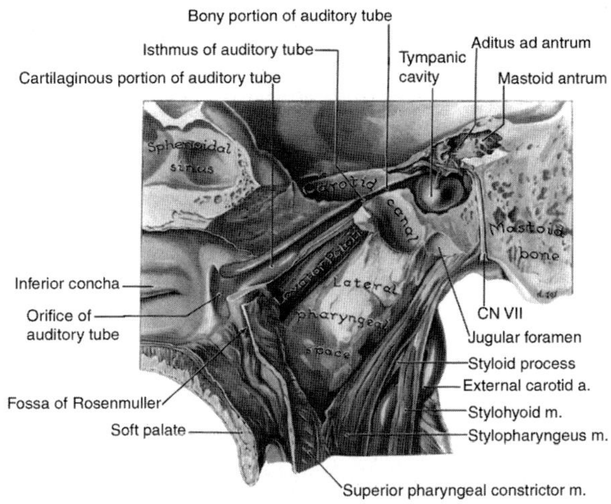

Figure 80F

Differential Diagnosis

Not applicable

Diagnosis

Tonsillar carcinoma spreading submucosally along the pharyngeal musculature to the eustachian tube orifice and metastasis to a retropharyngeal node

Diagnostic Imaging Approach

A. Know potential routes of local spread for particular primary site and evaluate each potential pathway in detail.
B. Know potential routes of perineural spread and evaluate each in detail.
C. Know potential routes of capillary lymphatic drainage (first and second echelon nodal sites) for the primary site and evaluate these nodes for size and presence of focal defects.
D. Know risk of bone invasion and establish its likelihood.
E. Determine the relationship of the primary and the nodal disease to the carotid artery.

Clinical Points Of Importance And Supplemental Information

The third dimension (deep margins) of many pharyngeal malignancies can only be assessed with imaging. The radiologist must know the routes of spread to accurately assess the full extent of the cancers. The imaging findings can markedly alter treatment and prognosis.

Answers To Questions

1. Yes
2. Yes, on the right
3. T3 or T4, depending on system; nasopharyngeal involvement

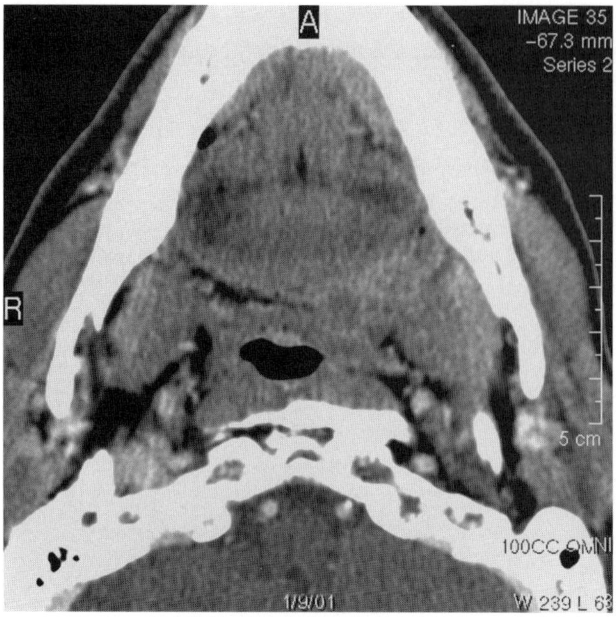

Figure 80G. Patient 1 with submucosal extent of tonsillar carcinoma along the pterygomandibular raphe, showing an infiltrative mass involving the palatine tonsil and anterior tonsillar pillar on the left.

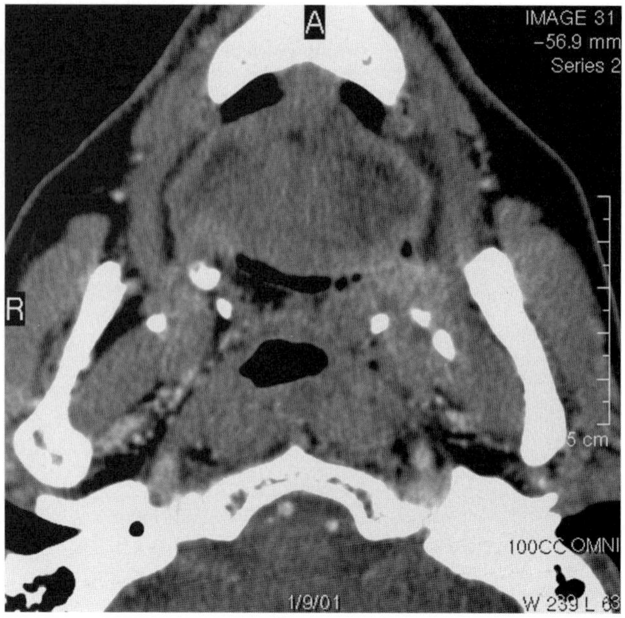

Figure 80H. Patient 1 with submucosal extent of tonsillar carcinoma along the pterygomandibular raphe. Contrast-enhanced computed tomography image superior to Fig. 80G showing an infiltrative mass around hamulus of the pterygoid plate on the left, where the pterygomandibular raphe attaches.

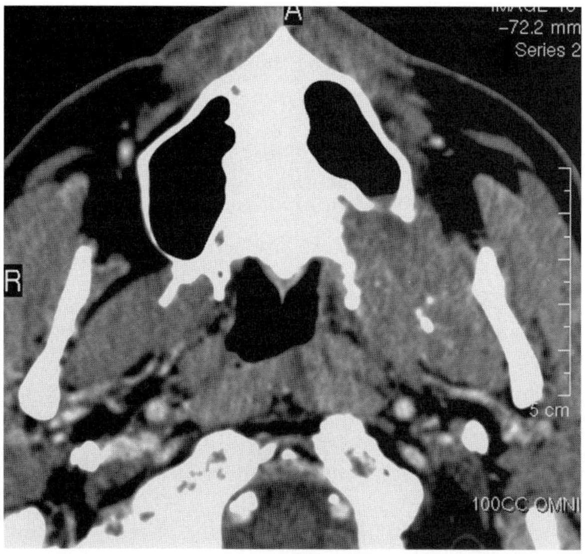

Figure 80I. Patient 1 with submucosal extent of tonsillar carcinoma along the pterygomandibular raphe. Contrast-enhanced computed tomography image superior to 80H showing an infiltrative mass involving the pterygoid muscles, with destruction of the pterygoid plate and posterior aspect of the maxillary sinus, which is a potential risk of perineural tumor spread along the greater or lesser palatine and posterior inferior alveolar neurovascular bundles.

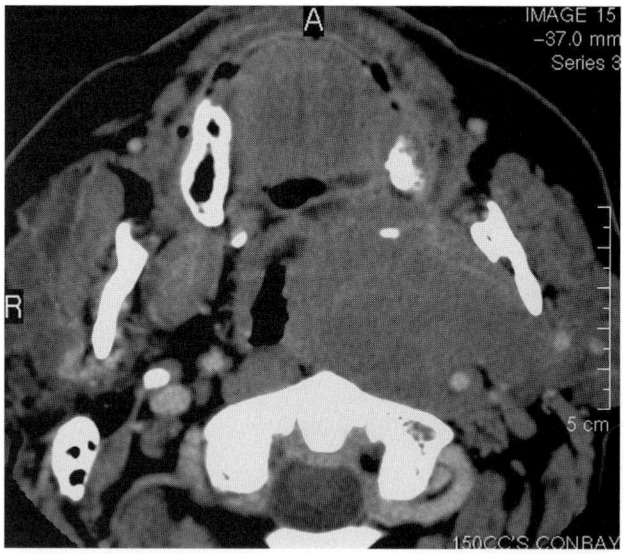

Figure 80J. Patient 2 with advanced tonsillar carcinoma extensively involving the nasopharynx, showing an infiltrative mass centered in the left palatine tonsil involving the parapharyngeal space, masticator space, and the prevertebral muscles. Contrast-enhanced computed tomography image.

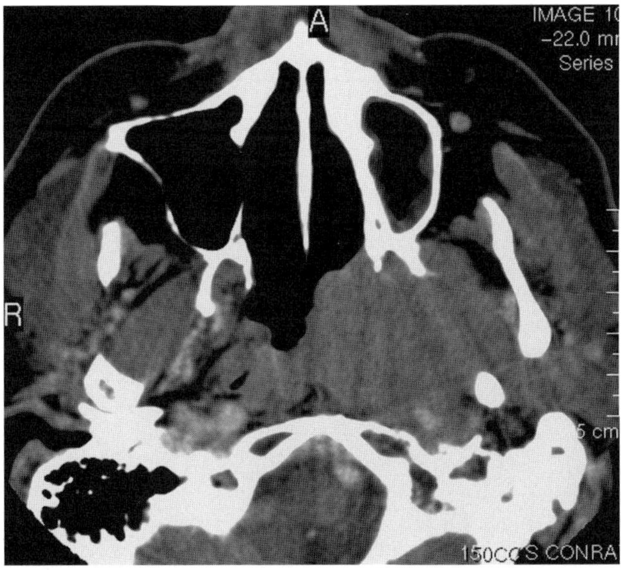

Figure 80K. Patient 2 with advanced tonsillar carcinoma extensively involving the nasopharynx. Contrast-enhanced computed tomography image at the level of the nasopharynx, superior to 80J, showing an infiltrative mass involving the left lateral and posterior aspect of the nasopharynx, with direct invasion to the parapharyngeal space and longus colli muscle. It is impossible to differentiate primary nasopharyngeal carcinoma from nasopharyngeal involvement of the tonsillar carcinoma based only on this image.

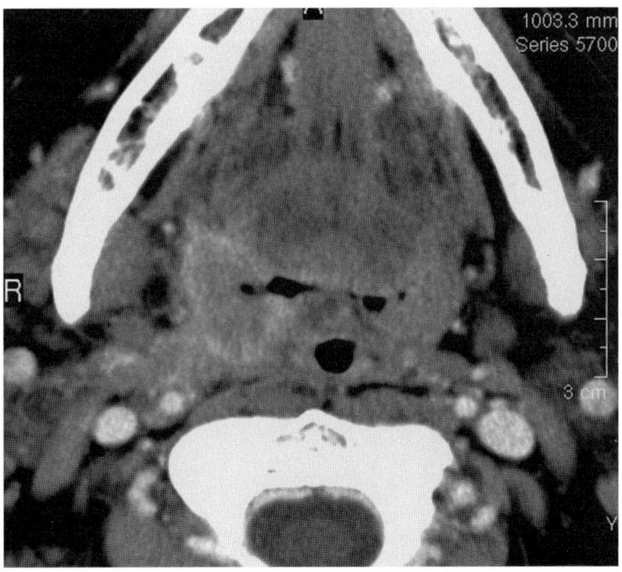

Figure 80L. Patient 3 with tonsillar carcinoma, showing an infiltrative mass centered in the right palatine tonsil, contiguously extending into the area of the right retropharyngeal lymph node and along the styloid musculature.

CASE 81

Clinical History: A 32-year-old man presents with severe throat pain and fever. This study was done to "R/O abscess."

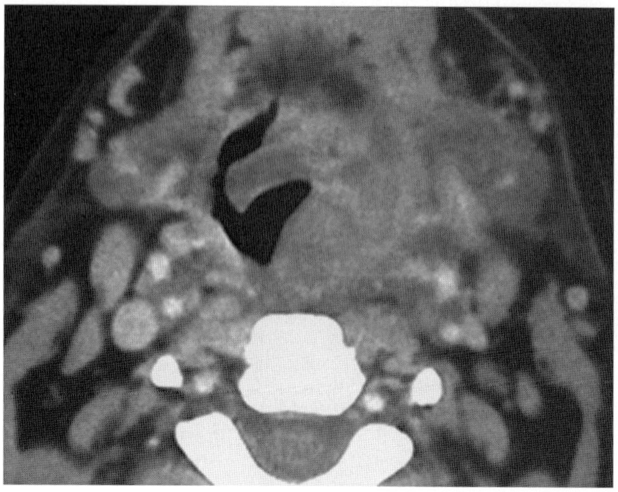

Figure 81A

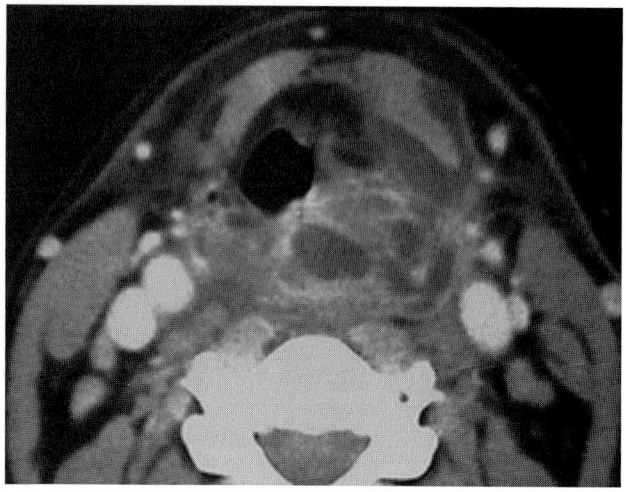

Figure 81B

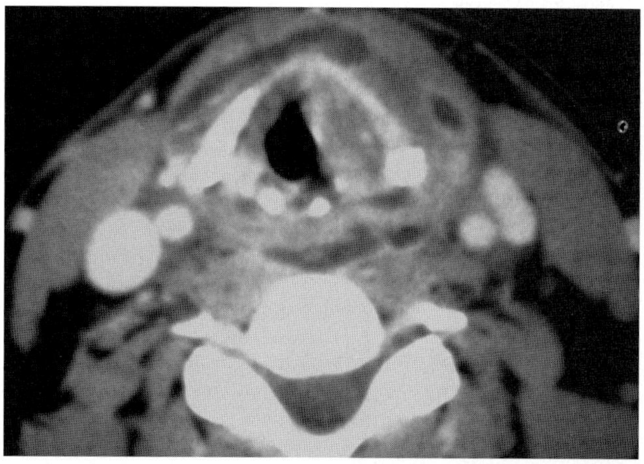

Figure 81C

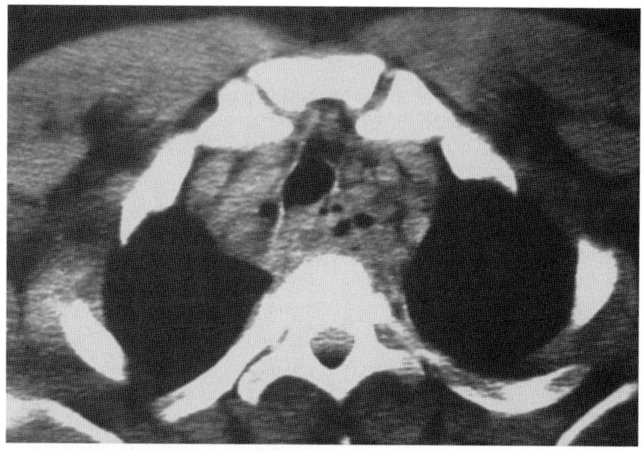

Figure 81D

1. What is the likely basic disease process?
2. What space(s) or compartment(s) does the abscess involve?
3. List the radiologist's three main responsibilities in this clinical setting.

Findings

An obvious soft tissue swelling of lower oropharynx and hypopharynx, mainly at the left lateral and posterior aspects. Multiloculated fluid collections with rim-enhancement are noted in the visceral space, spreading along the infrahyoid strap muscles. The left pyriform sinus and paraglottic spaces are severely distorted. An edematous change is noted of the retropharyngeal space at some levels, with multiloculated frank abscess formation at others. Tissue planes of bilateral carotid and left submandibular spaces are obliterated. Slight thickening of the platysma muscle is seen. The pus extends into the middle mediastinum.

Problem

A 32-year-old man with fever and a multiloculated, aggressive mass involving the pharynx

Anatomy

A. Visceral compartment (space): oropharynx, hypopharynx, infrahyoid strap muscles, middle constrictors, visceral fascia
B. Retropharyngeal space
C. Prevertebral space and fascia

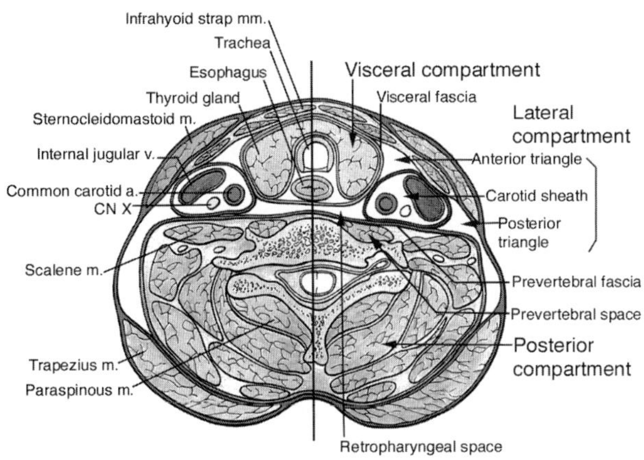

Figure 81E

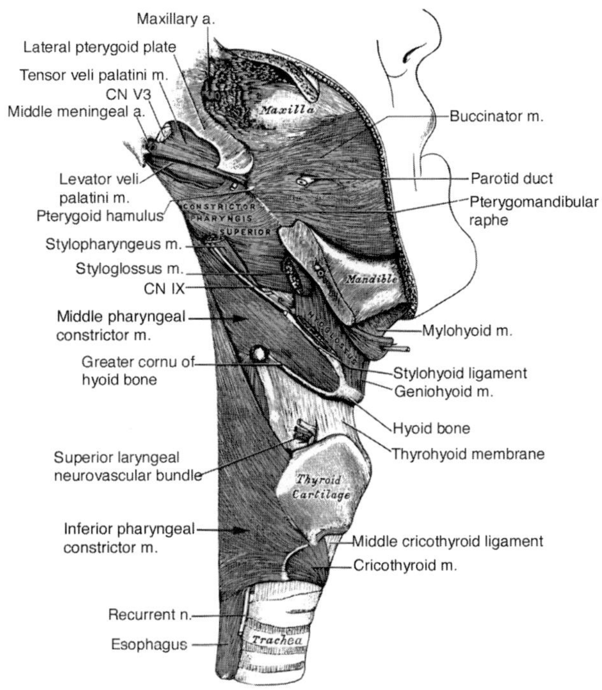

Figure 81F

Differential Diagnosis

None; consider infected tumor, when appropriate.

Diagnosis

Lingual tonsillitis, with multiloculated abscess confined to the visceral compartment; more inferior sections show abscess spreading to the retropharyngeal space and the mediastinum.

Diagnostic Imaging Approach

A. Establish the compartment (space) of origin.
B. Is there transcompartmental (spatial) spread?
C. Is the morphology more likely inflammatory or neoplastic?
   1. If inflammatory morphology, is it abscess, edema?
D. If inflammatory disease:
   1. Establish precise upper and lower limits and determine which compartments (spaces) are involved.
   2. Distinguish between drainable and nondrainable abnormalities.
   3. Determine the extent of loculation.
   4. Try to establish the cause (e.g., look for perforations, foreign bodies).
   5. Exclude complications (e.g., carotid endarteritis).

Clinical Points Of Importance And Supplemental Information

A. Well-done imaging (most experience is with computed tomography) can virtually always distinguish between drainable and nondrainable collections. In the rare questionable case, an indeterminate area can be tapped.
B. The full extent of drainable collections must be accurately established by the radiologist. In retropharyngeal abscesses, this frequently requires continuing the study to include the chest.

Answers To Questions

1. Pharyngeal abscess
2. Pharyngeal wall, visceral
3. Determine origin of the abscess; map its full extent; and look for foreign body, complications.

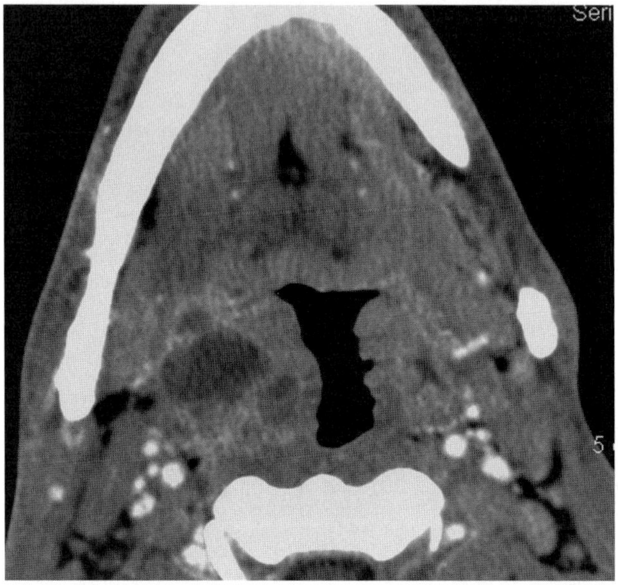

Figure 81G. Patient 1 with tonsillar infection, showing a loculated fluid collection in the enlarged right palatine tonsil with surrounding soft tissue swelling, which is consistent with tonsillar or peritonsillar abscess. Contrast-enhanced computed tomography image.

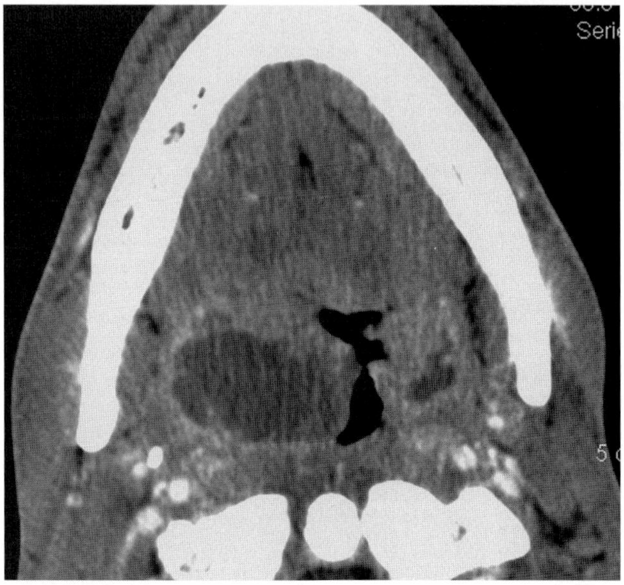

Figure 81H. Patient 1 with tonsillar infection. Contrast-enhanced computed tomography image, superior to Fig. 81G, showing the peritonsillar abscess on the left. A smaller fluid attenuation area localized in the left palatine tonsil represents tonsillar abscess.

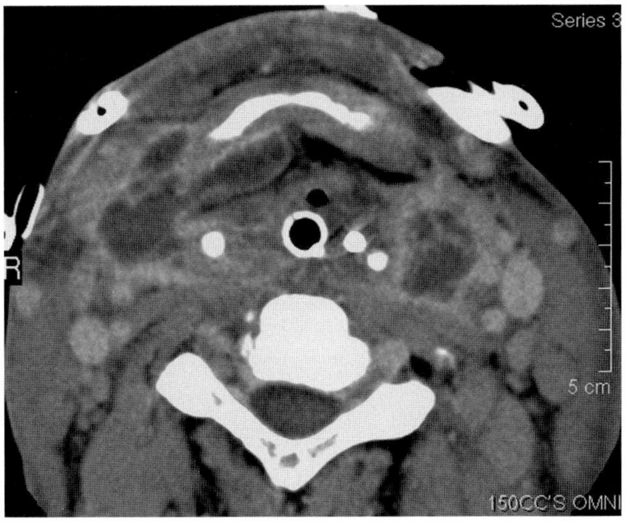

Figure 81I. Patient 2 with deep neck abscess with mediastinal extension. Contrast-enhanced computed tomography image showing an abscess formed in the visceral space, with extension into the paraglottic space resulting in significant narrowness of the airway. Patient has already been intubated.

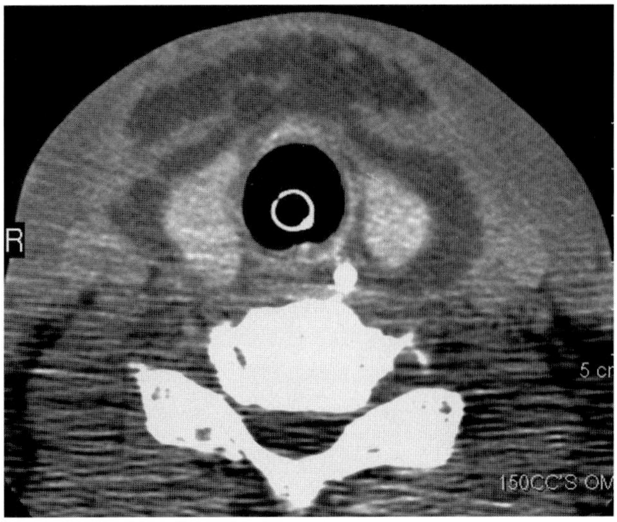

Figure 81J. Patient 2 with deep neck abscess with mediastinal extension. Contrast-enhanced computed tomography image inferior to Fig. 81I showing the abscess spreading within the muscles and viscera of this compartment.

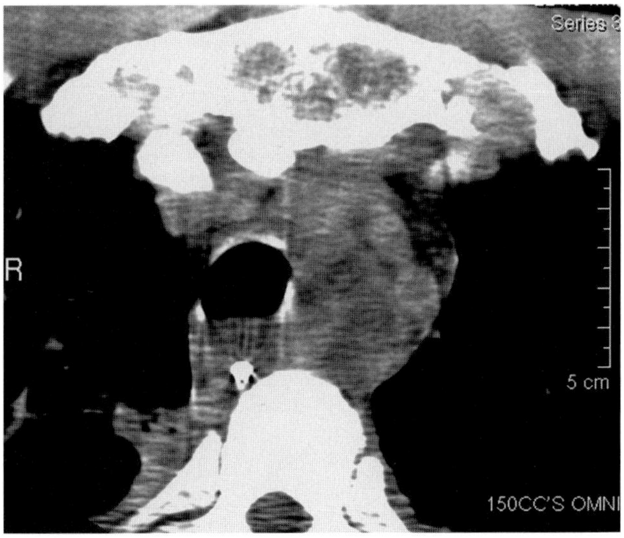

Figure 81K. Patient 2 with deep neck abscess with mediastinal extension. Contrast-enhanced computed tomography image inferior to Fig. 81J showing mediastinal extension of the abscess.

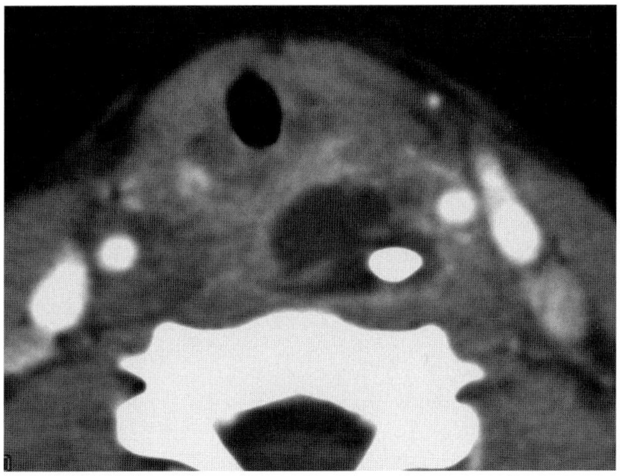

Figure 81L. Patient 3 with retropharyngeal abscess caused by penetrating trauma to the posterior pharyngeal wall, showing abscess formation in the retropharyngeal space, which contains a radiodense foreign body (chicken bone). Contrast-enhanced computed tomography image.

CHAPTER 8

ORAL CAVITY, FLOOR OF MOUTH, AND TONGUE

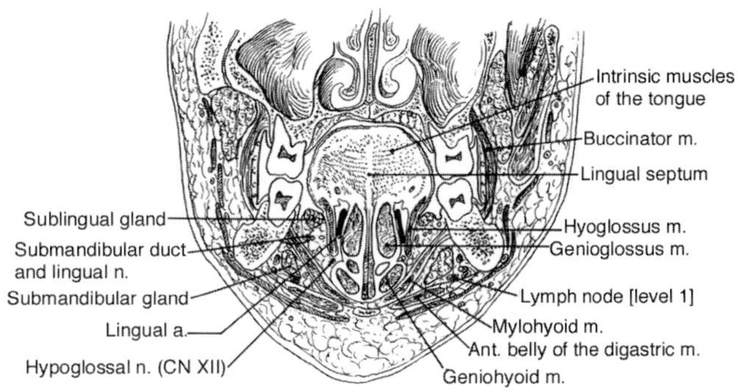

CASE 82

Clinical History: A 19-year-old woman presents with a 4.5-year history of an enlarging submandibular region mass.

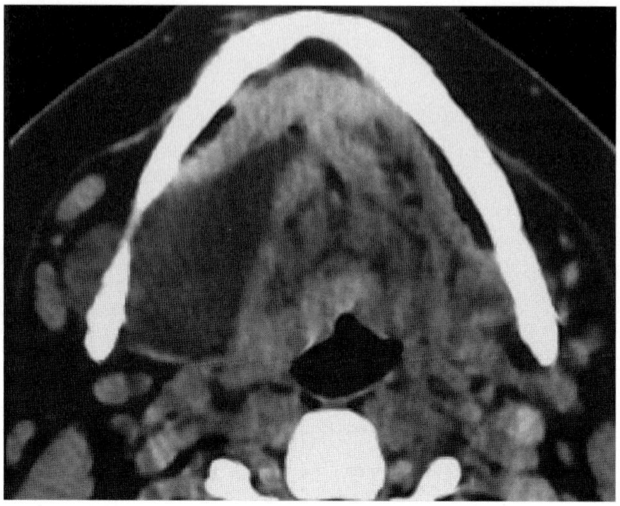

Figure 82A

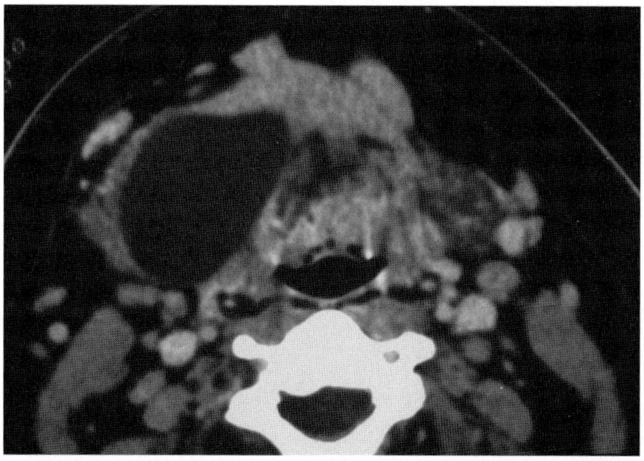

Figure 82B

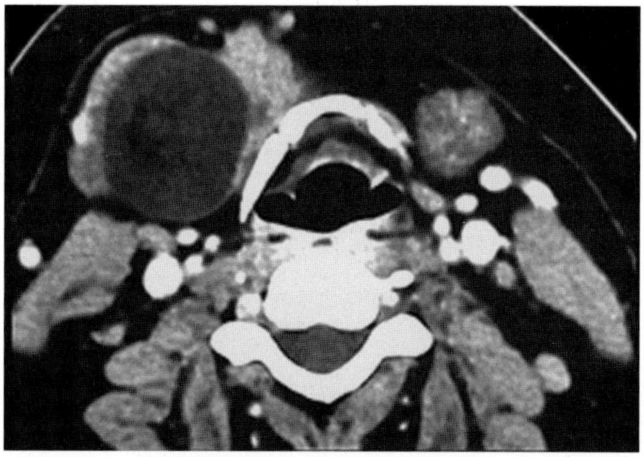

Figure 82C

1. What space does the mass occupy?
2. What are the two most likely diagnoses?
3. Does the internal morphology of the lesion aid in the differential diagnosis?

Findings

A relatively well-defined, mainly fluid, attenuation mass in the submandibular space distorting the sublingual space on the right. Small areas of fat-equivalent attenuation are noted in some areas. It is difficult to tell whether the lesion is displacing the mylohyoid upward or whether it might have components both above and below that muscle. A coronal study would be helpful.

Problem

A young adult with a slowly enlarging, cystic-appearing, submandibular space mass

Anatomy

A. Submandibular space: limits, contents, relationship to the sublingual space and floor of the mouth
B. Floor of the mouth: mylohyoid muscle, limits of the sublingual space, position of the lingual artery, vein, nerve, and hypoglossal nerve (relative to hyoglossus muscle)

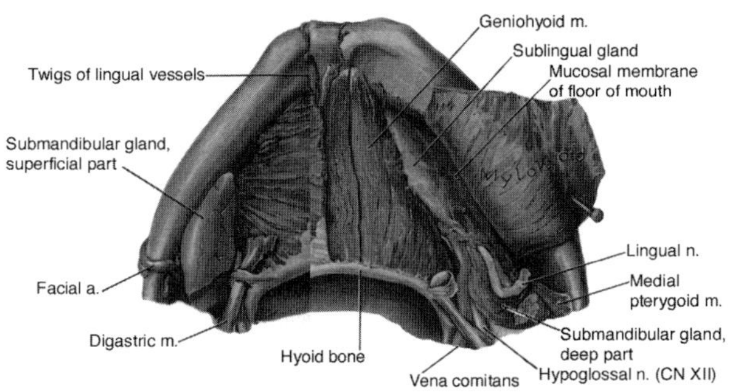

Figure 82D

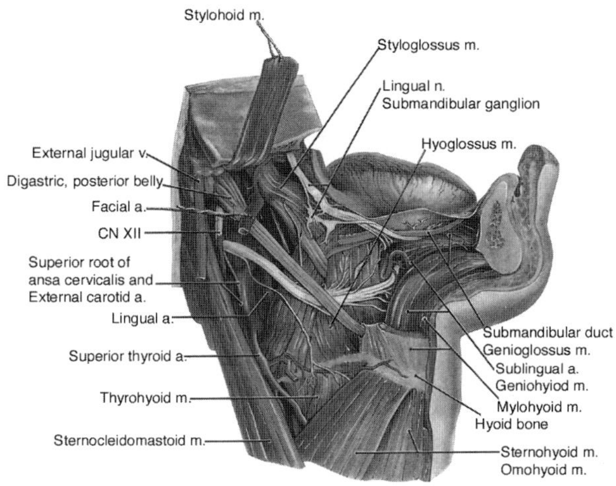

Figure 82E

Differential Diagnosis

Is heavily dependent on anatomic or developmental origin.

1. Anatomically: consider submandibular gland, node, ranula (submandibular gland), neurogenic or mesenchymal tumor
2. Developmentally: consider epidermoid or dermoid cyst, lymphangioma
3. Specifically (in this case): differential is between ranula and epidermoid or dermoid cyst (notice the fat)

Diagnosis

Dermoid cyst of the submandibular space

Diagnostic Imaging Approach

A. Establish the space (region, compartment) or structure of origin.
B. Is it intrinsic, extrinsic, or indeterminate in its relationship to the submandibular gland?
C. Is the lesion transspatial (compartmental)?
D. Any evidence of aggressive behavior?
E. Is there an inflammatory morphology?
F. Evaluate internal morphology: density, T1- or T2-weighted signal intensity, enhancement, vascularity, calcifications, blood products.

Clinical Points Of Importance And Supplemental Information

Midline and paramedian cystic lesions in the head and neck region and central nervous system frequently will be caused by an epidermoid or dermoid cyst.

Answers To Questions

1. Submandibular
2. Epidermoid or dermoid cyst; ranula
3. Yes, a fat density zone indicates a dermoid cyst.

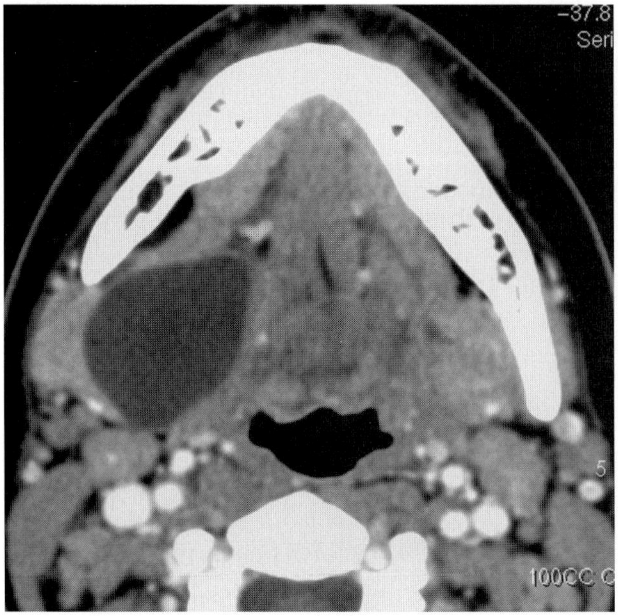

Figure 82F. Patient 1 with an epidermoid cyst in the submandibular space, showing a unilocular cystic mass in the submandibular space displacing the submandibular gland laterally. The sublingual space anterior to the mass is intact. Contrast-enhanced computed tomography image.

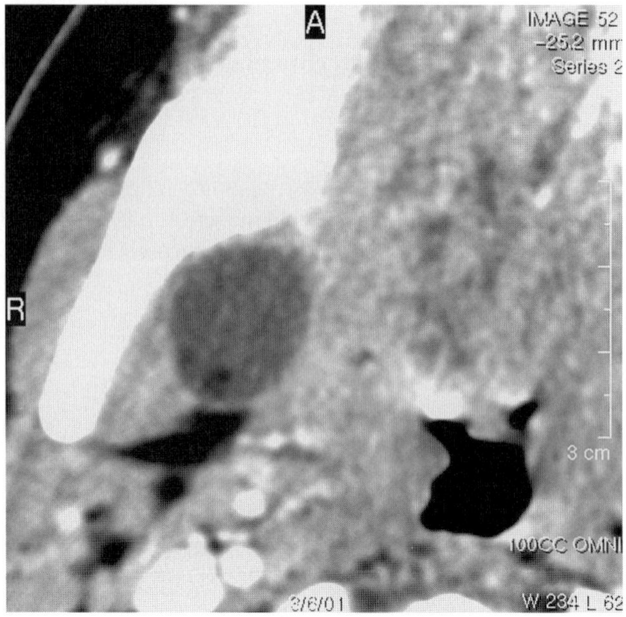

Figure 82G. Patient 1 with an epidermoid cyst in the submandibular space; the mass contains fat globules, which suggests the diagnosis. Contrast-enhanced computed tomography image.

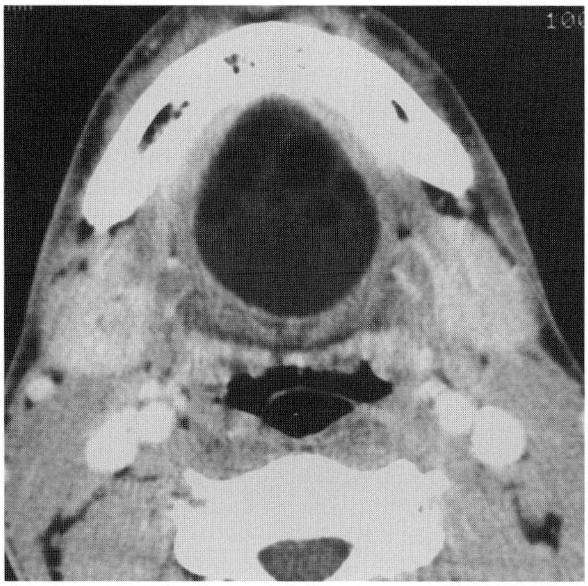

Figure 82H. Patient 2 with a dermoid cyst (sublingual type) in the floor of the mouth, showing a cystic mass centered in the midline of the floor of the mouth, which contains multiple globules of fat attenuation. Contrast-enhanced computed tomography image.

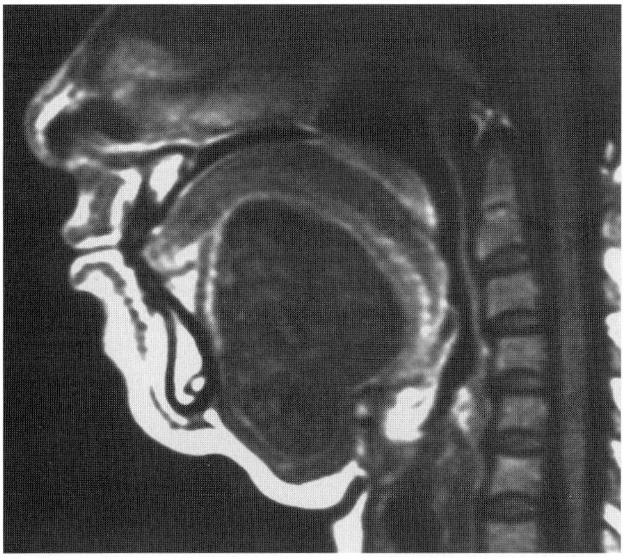

Figure 82I. Patient 2 with a dermoid cyst (sublingual type) in the floor of the mouth. T1-weighted contrast-enhanced sagittal image showing a cystic mass containing multiple high-intensity foci, which are suggestive of fatty contents above the mylohyoid muscle.

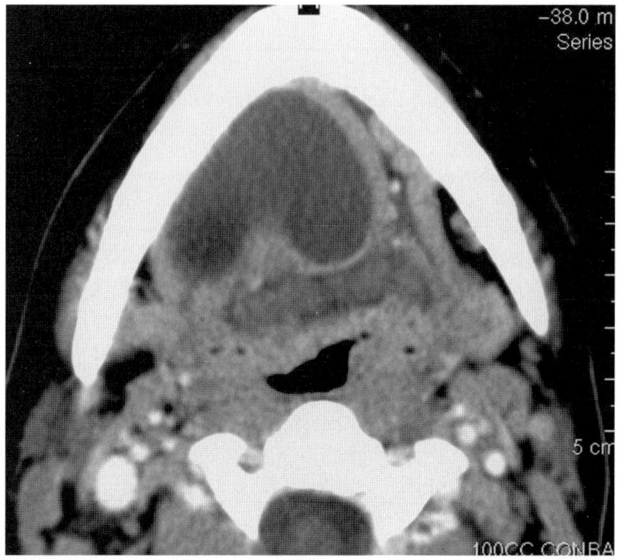

Figure 82J. Patient 3 with a dermoid cyst in the floor of the mouth, also showing a lobulated cystic mass in the floor of the mouth without obvious fat attenuation. Contrast-enhanced computed tomography image.

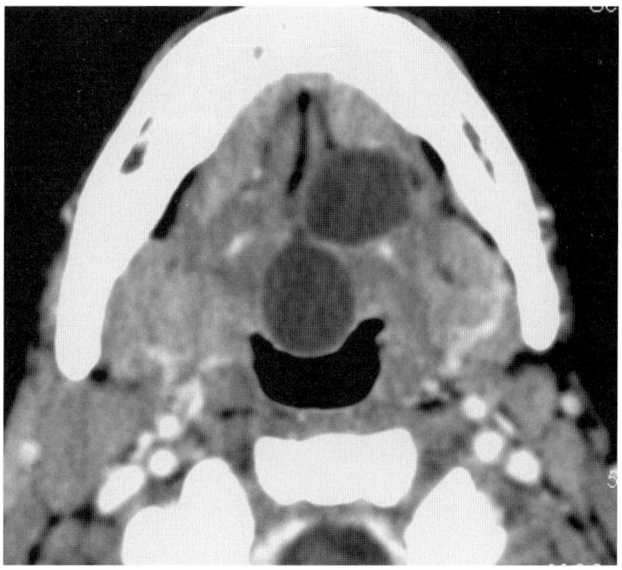

Figure 82K. Patient 4 with mucous retention cyst in the floor of the mouth, showing two cystic masses (no obvious connection is seen between them on any computed tomography image). One mass is midline in the area of the foramen cecum, although it is not possible to differentiate the lesion from thyroglossal duct remnant cyst based on imaging findings, and the other is in the left sublingual space. Contrast-enhanced computed tomography image.

CASE 83

Clinical History: A 24-year-old man presents with a submandibular region mass.

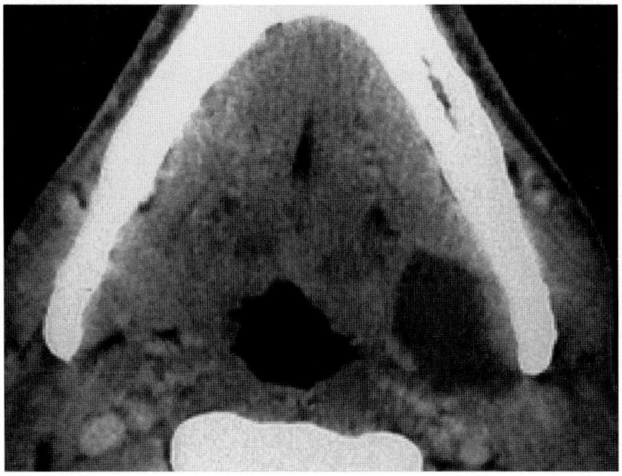

Figure 83A

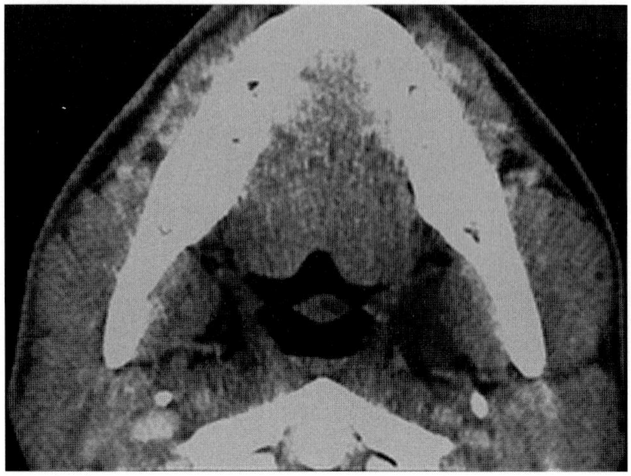

Figure 83B

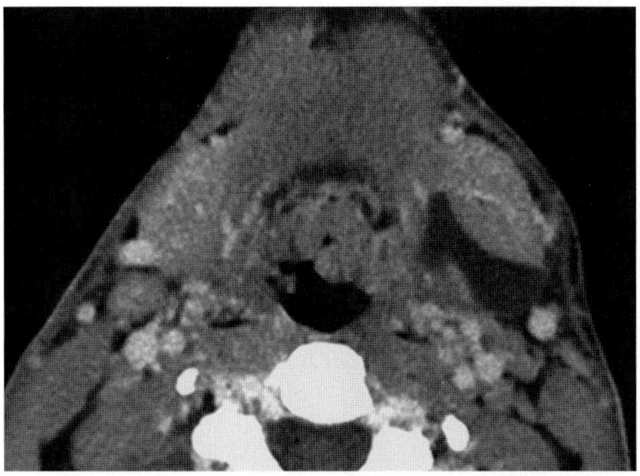

Figure 83C

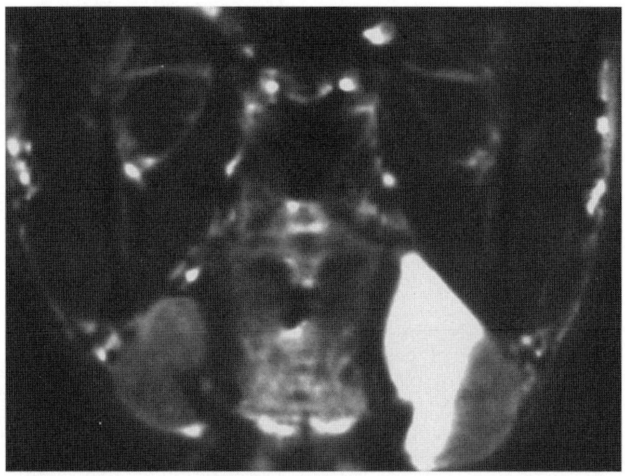

Figure 83D

1. What space(s) does the mass occupy?
2. List the two most likely diagnoses.

Findings

There is a unilocular purely cystic mass in left submandibular space with no definite tail extending toward posterior sublingual space. The lesion superiorly extends into lower parapharyngeal space. The submandibular gland is slightly displaced laterally by the mass.

Problem

A young man with a cystic appearing submandibular space mass

Anatomy

A. Relationship of the prestyloid parapharyngeal space to the submandibular space
B. Relationship of the sublingual and submandibular spaces and glands
C. Course of the submandibular gland duct relative to the hyoglossus and mylohyoid muscles

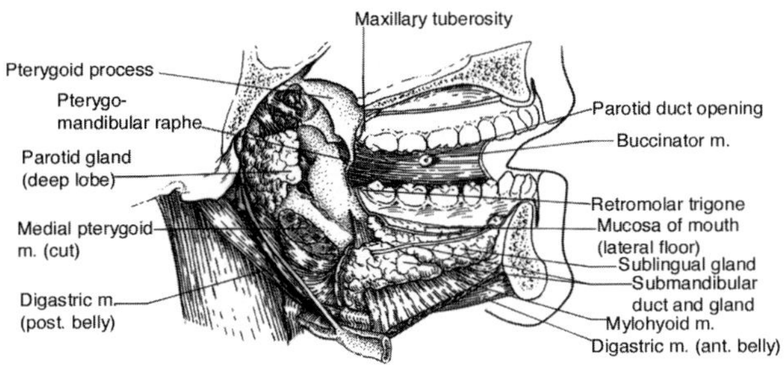

Figure 83E

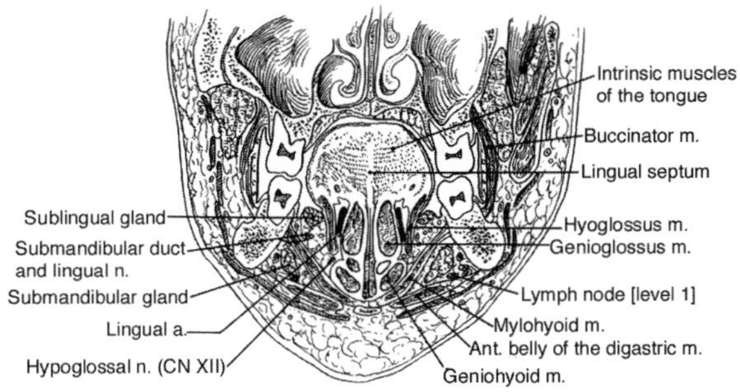

Figure 83F

Differential Diagnosis

Is heavily dependent on anatomic or developmental origin

1. Anatomically, consider—submandibular gland, node, ranula (sublingual gland), neurogenic or mesenchymal lesion
2. Developmentally, consider—epidermoid/dermoid, lymphangioma
3. Specifically (in this case), differential is lymphangioma/cystic hygroma vs. ranula

Diagnosis

Plunging or diving ranula

Diagnostic Imaging Approach

A. Establish the space (region, compartment) or structure (e.g., lymph node submandibular gland) of origin
B. Is it intrinsic, extrinsic or indeterminate in its relationship to the submandibular gland?
C. Is the lesion transpatial?
D. Is there any evidence of aggressive behavior?
E. Is there an inflammatory morphology?
F. Evaluate morphology—density, T1-/T2- signal intensity, internal enhancement, vascularity, calcifications, blood products

Clinical Points Of Importance And Supplemental Information

A. Ranulas are said to "always" leave a tail in the submandibular space—this may not be true, but it is very helpful when present.
B. It is important to establish the full extent of a ranula prior to surgery so that the risk of recurrence due to incomplete excision can be reduced.

Answers To Questions

1. Submandibular space, prestyloid parapharyngeal space
2. Ranula, lymphangioma

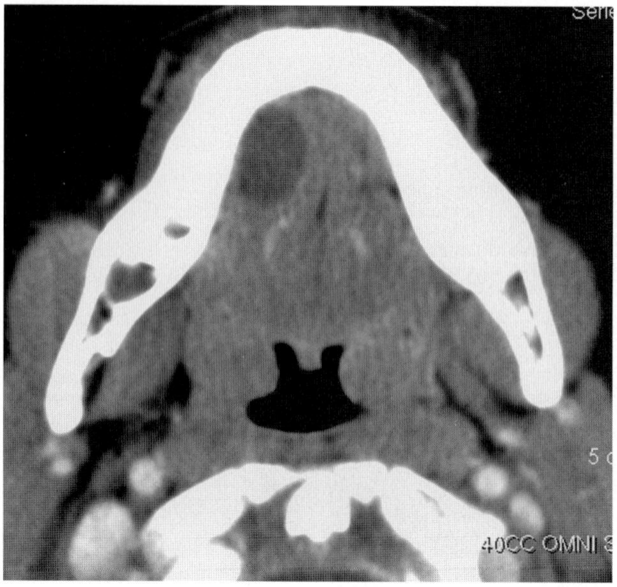

Figure 83G. Patient 1 with simple ranula showing unilocular cystic mass centered in right sublingual space. Contrast-enhanced CT image.

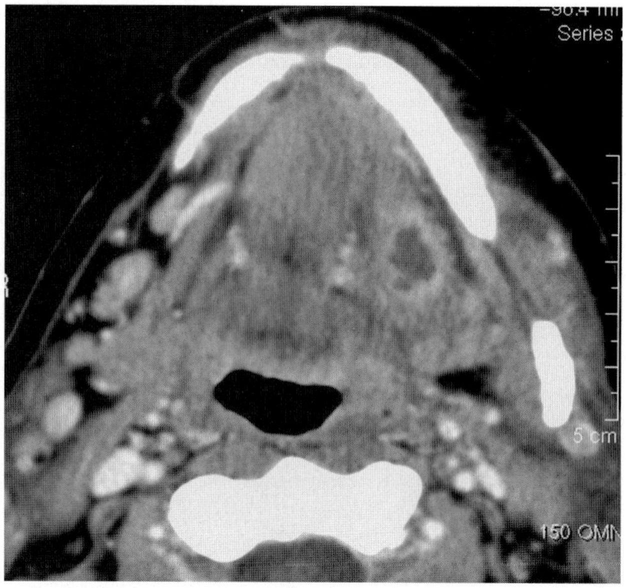

Figure 83H. Patient 2 with presumed suppurative lymph adenitis of the sublingual node showing rim-enhancing fluid attenuation nodule in the sublingual space. Contrast-enhanced CT image.

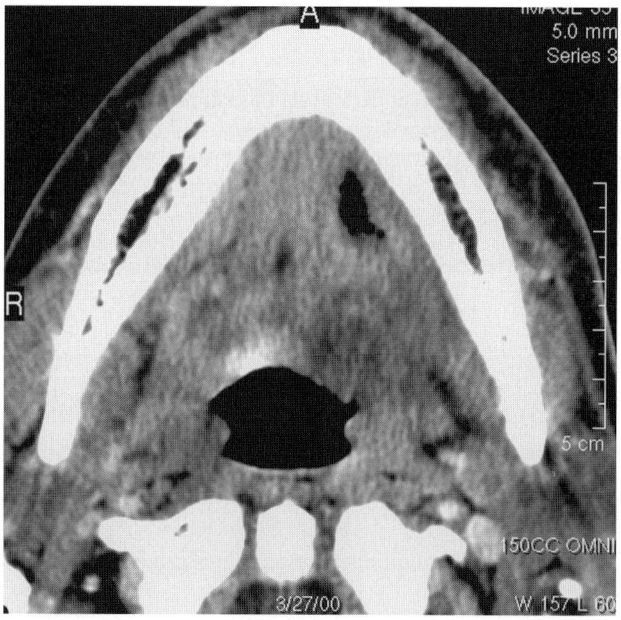

Figure 83I. Patient 3 with gas-producing organism infection in the sublingual space showing air attenuation in the sublingual space on the left. Contrast-enhanced CT image.

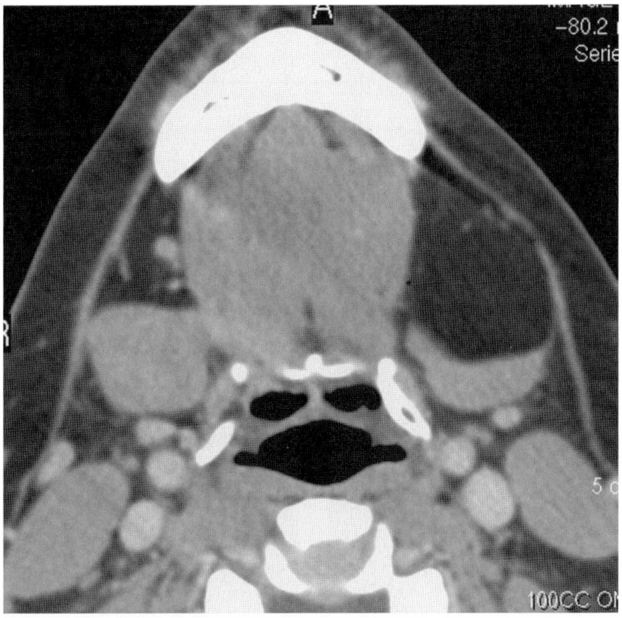

Figure 83J. Patient 4 with lipoma in the submandibular space showing a mass of purely fatty attenuation in the submandibular space on the left, displacing the submandibular gland posteriorly. Contrast-enhanced CT image.

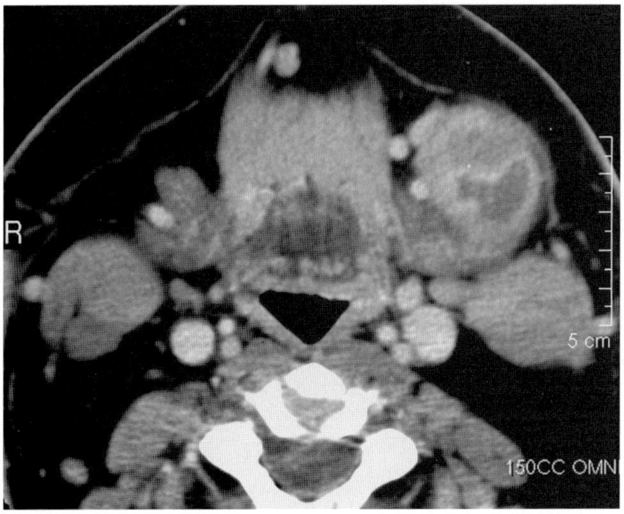

Figure 83K. Patient 5 with nodal involvement of non-Hodgkin's lymphoma showing the enlarged left submandibular lymph node containing cystic component and another enlarged lymph node in the level 2. Contrast-enhanced CT image.

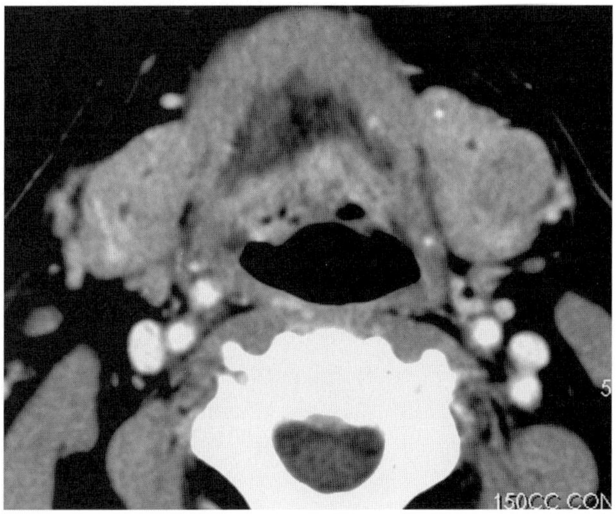

Figure 83L. Patient 6 with pleomorphic adenoma of the submandibular gland showing an intrinsic submandibular gland mass on the left. Contrast-enhanced CT image.

CASE 84

Clinical History: A 51-year-old man presents with squamous cell carcinoma of the floor of the mouth and tongue.

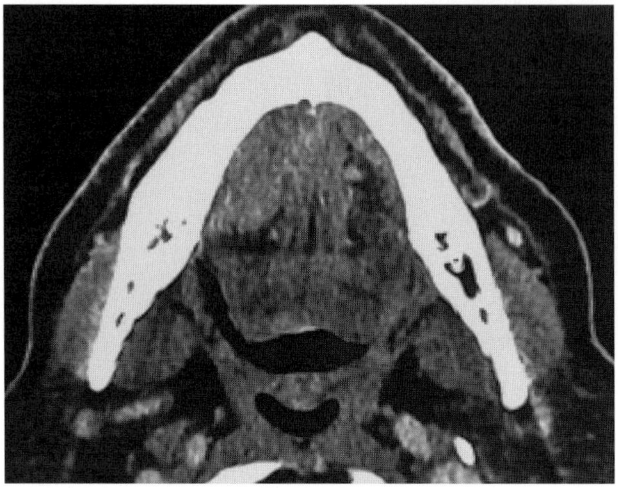

Figure 84A

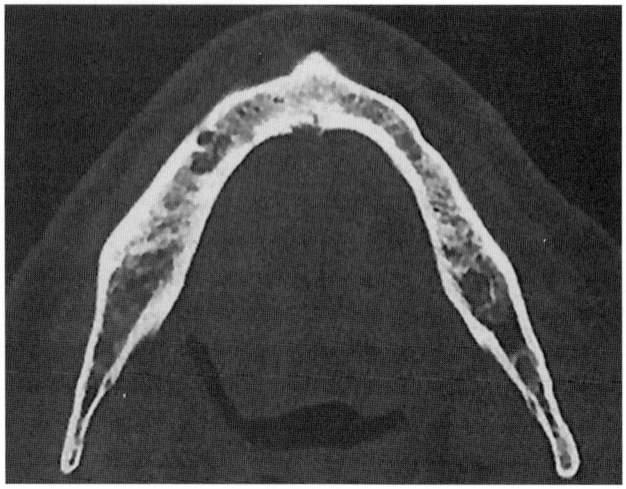

Figure 84B

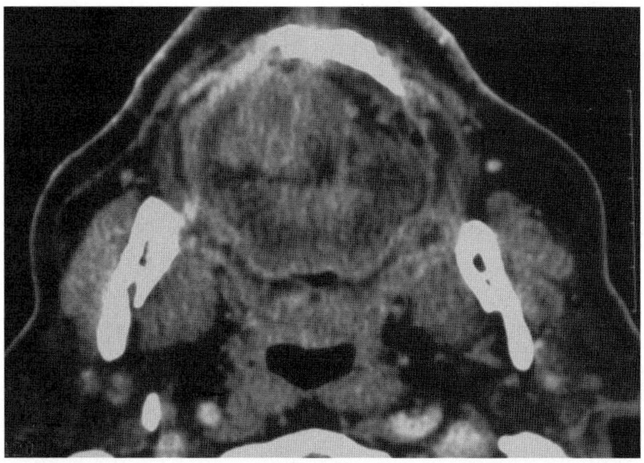

Figure 84C

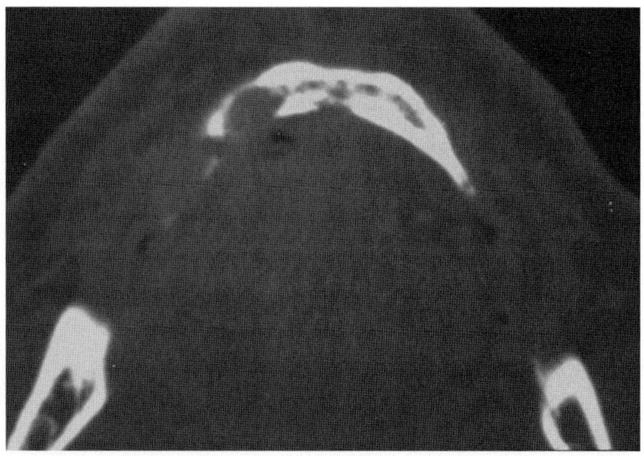

Figure 84D

1. Is the mandible invaded?
2. Would you suggest a magnetic resonance imaging (MRI) study to exclude mandibular invasion and to evaluate the soft tissue extent of the lesion?
3. Is gross (visible on imaging) perineural spread of cancer likely to be present?

Findings

A mass infiltrating the floor of the mouth and tongue on the right. The lesion extends across midline, invading the lingual plate of the mandible as deep as the genial tubercles. It invades the right mylohyoid and genioglossus muscles and the sublingual space; the lingual neurovascular pedicle is likely to be involved as well.

Problem

A man with squamous cell carcinoma of the oral cavity. The decision to resect or preserve the mandible will be based on imaging findings.

Anatomy

A. Mandible: lingual surface, genial tubercles, buccal surface, retromolar trigone, alveolar ridge
B. Pterygomandibular raphe
C. Group I (submandibular or submental) lymph nodes in detail
D. Groups II, III, IV, and V lymph nodes (see Fig. 66D)
E. Intrinsic and extrinsic muscles of the tongue (including the tongue base)
F. Course of the lingual neurovascular bundle and hypoglossal nerve in the neck, tongue and floor of the mouth (see Fig. 82E)

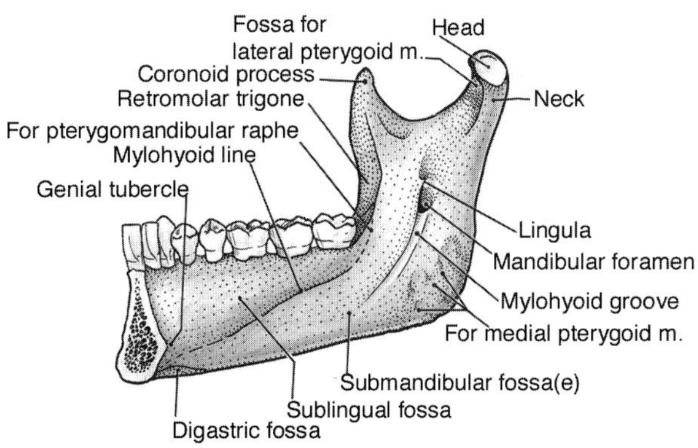

Figure 84E

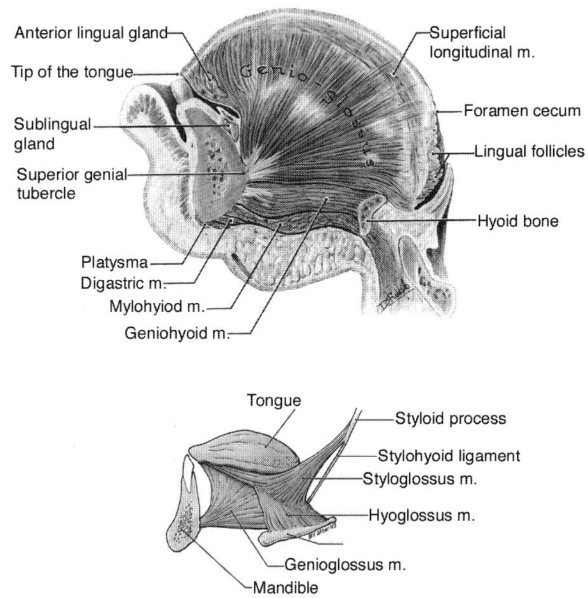

Figure 84F

Differential Diagnosis

Not applicable

Diagnosis

Squamous cell carcinoma of the floor of the mouth, with mandibular invasion

Diagnostic Imaging Approach

A. Determine the local soft tissue extent of the lesion:
   1. Proximity to mandible.
   2. Proximity to midline and contralateral lingual neurovascular bundle.
B. Is the mandible invaded?
   1. Alveolar ridge: dental films.
   2. Buccal or lingual surface: 1- to 2-mm contiguous computed tomography (CT) sections are essential to confidentially *exclude* invasion.
   3. Marrow space (not usually necessary): MRI or CT.
C. Any evidence of spread along the neurovascular bundles?
D. Establish presence and extent of lymph node metastases.

Clinical Points Of Importance And Supplemental Information

A. CT is far superior to MRI for excluding invasion of the *buccal* or lingual surface of the mandible (with 1- to 2-mm sections, small field of view and bone algorithm). This is key to deciding whether mandibular preservation surgery is possible.
B. MRI may map soft tissue extent of oral cavity cancers better than CT in selected cases, assuming high resolution, motion free images are available.

Answers To Questions

1. Yes
2. No
3. Not certain

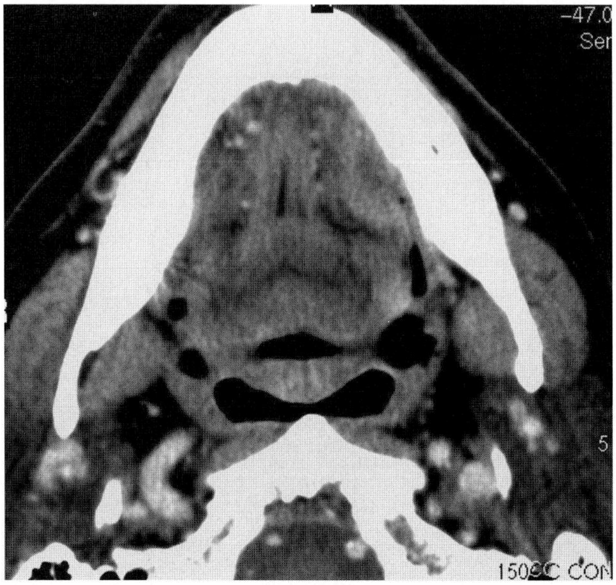

Figure 84G. Patient 1 with squamous cell carcinoma of the floor of the mouth, showing an infiltrative mass involving the anterior floor of the mouth on the left, directly abutting the lingual surface of the mandible. Contrast-enhanced computed tomography image.

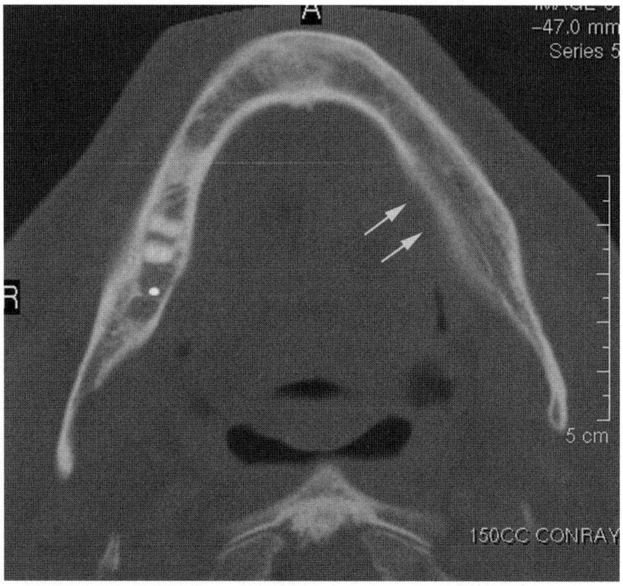

Figure 84H. Patient 1 with squamous cell carcinoma of the floor of the mouth. Computed tomography image at bone window setting shows bone erosion along the mylohyoid line of the mandible.

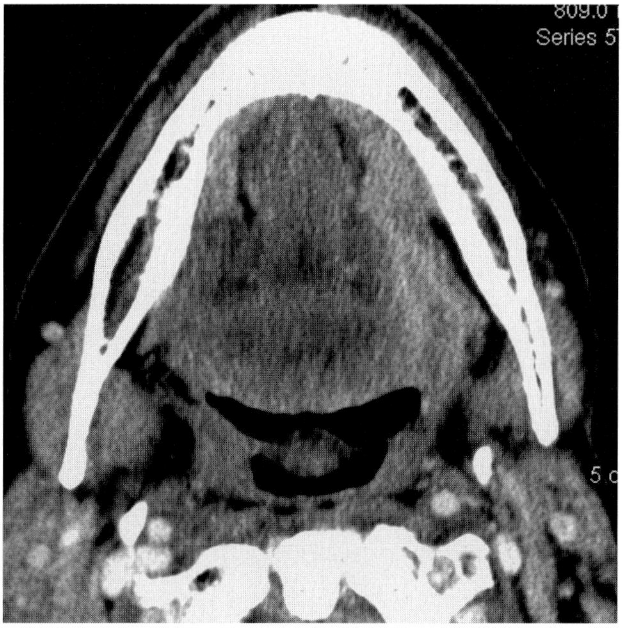

Figure 84I. Patient 2 with squamous cell carcinoma of the floor of the mouth, showing an infiltrative mass extending along the hyoglossus muscle, which is the anatomic landmark of the lingual neurovascular bundle. Contrast-enhanced computed tomography image.

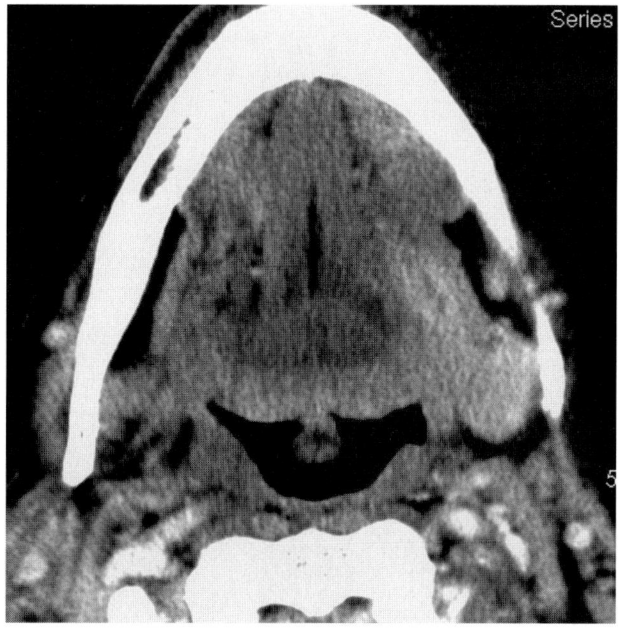

Figure 84J. Patient 2 with squamous cell carcinoma of the floor of the mouth, showing a common aggressive spread pattern into the submandibular gland and out of the floor of the mouth over the back edge of the mylohyoid muscle to the deep neck. Contrast-enhanced computed tomography image inferior to Fig. 84I.

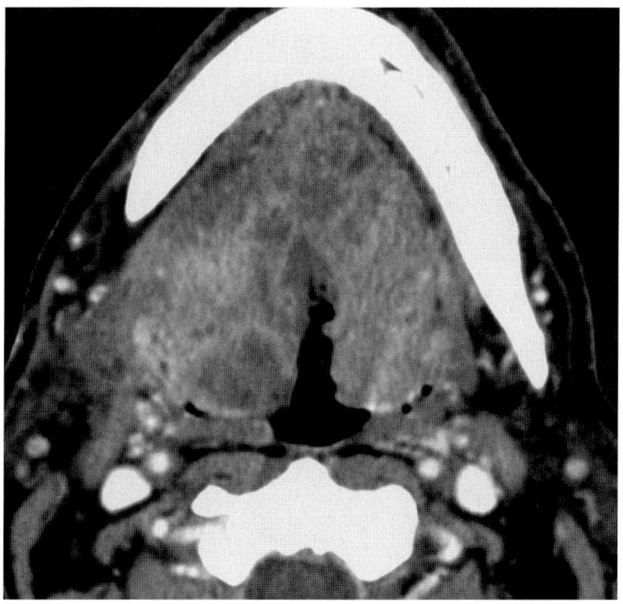

Figure 84K. Patient 3 with advanced tongue carcinoma, showing an infiltrative mass involving the entire tongue and tongue base, with extensive involvement of the floor of the mouth but contained within the attachment of the mylohyoid muscle bilaterally.

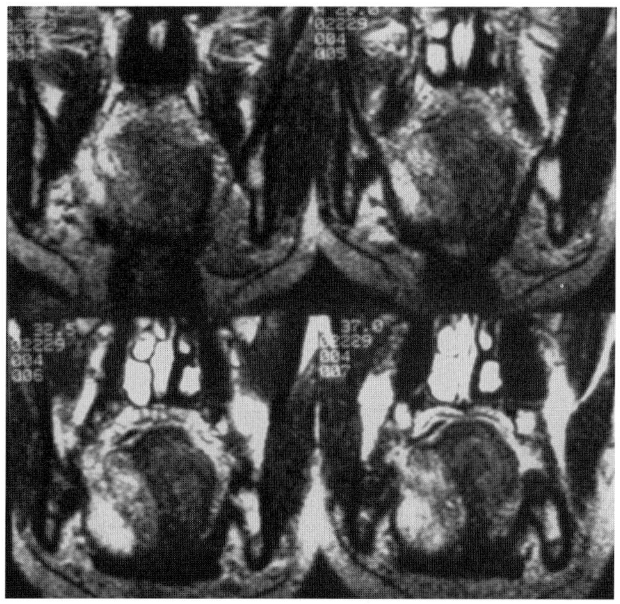

Figure 84L. Patient 4 with squamous cell carcinoma of the floor of mouth. T2-weighted coronal images showing an infiltrative mass involving the right lateral aspect of the tongue, with invasion into the floor of the mouth, but contained by the mylohyoid muscle along the tumor's lateral margin.

CHAPTER 9

INFRAHYOID NECK

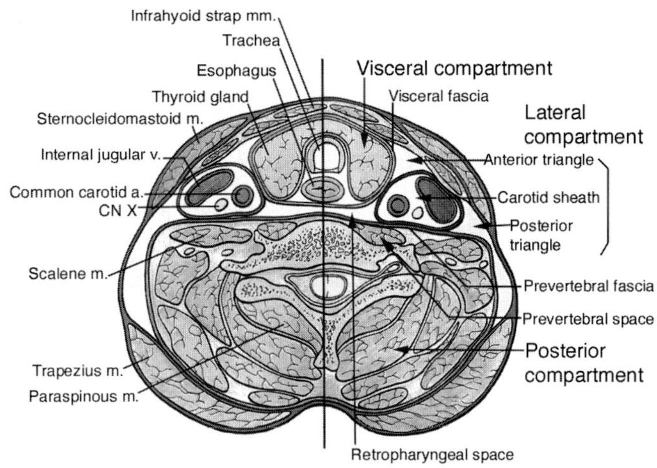

CASE 85

Clinical History: A 70-year-old man presents with a 4-month history of an enlarging upper neck mass. Physical examination suggests either pulsation within the mass or transmitted pulsations.

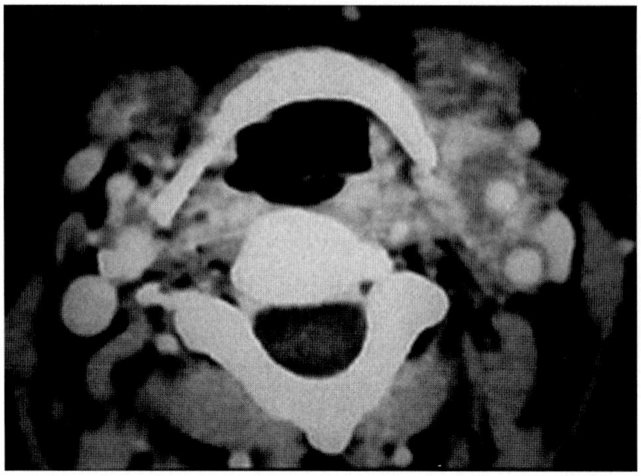

Figure 85A

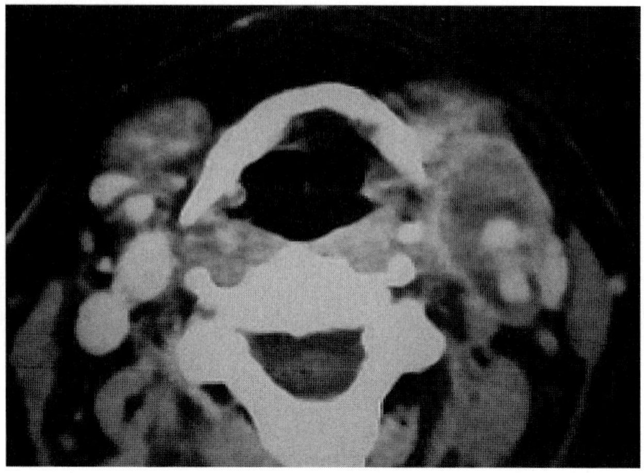

Figure 85B

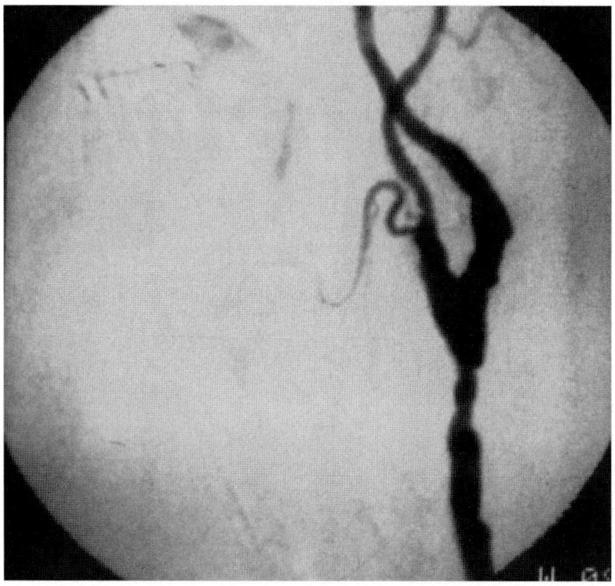

Figure 85C

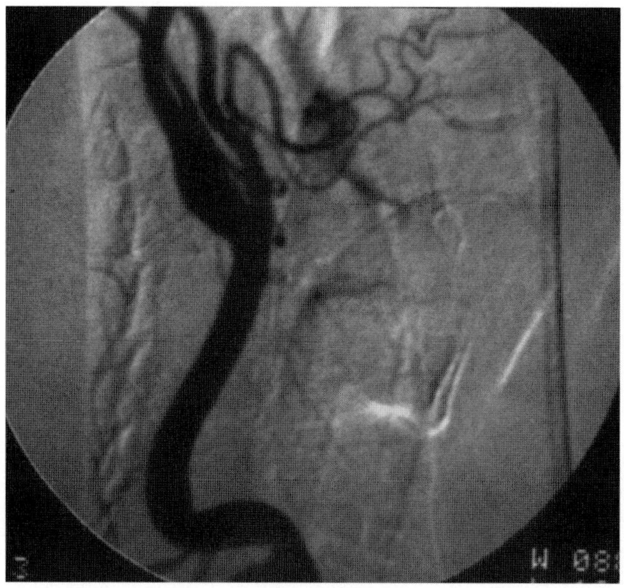

Figure 85D

1. Is imaging required before needle biopsy in this clinical setting? If so, would you choose magnetic resonance imaging (MRI), computed tomography (CT), or ultrasound (US)?
2. What neck compartment(s) is involved? What is your best working diagnosis?
3. What other radiologic study should be done on this patient before a biopsy or definitive management?
4. If the patient had vocal cord paralysis and tongue deviation, would your diagnosis and approach to care change? If so, how?

Findings

An ill-defined mass surrounding the carotid bifurcation, with the vessels retaining what appear to be widely patent lumens. The lesion enhances inhomogeneously mostly at its periphery. The left internal jugular vein and facial vein are displaced centrifugally.

Problem

An elderly man with a pulsatile neck mass and a CT image showing the mass to be inseparable from the carotid artery, possibly a carotid artery aneurysm

Anatomy

A. Neck compartments and contents
   1. Visceral: within visceral fascia
   2. Lateral (paired): within investing layer of deep cervical fascia; carotid artery and branches, jugular vein and tributaries, vagus nerve, lymph nodes (groups II, III, IV, V), fibroadipose tissue, small nerves and vessels, sympathetic trunk, spinal accessory nerve, sternocleidomastoid muscle
   3. Posterior: within prevertebral (deep) layer of deep cervical fascia

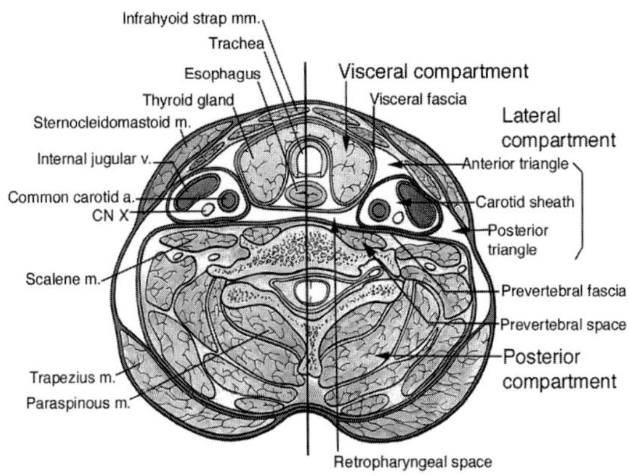

Figure 85E

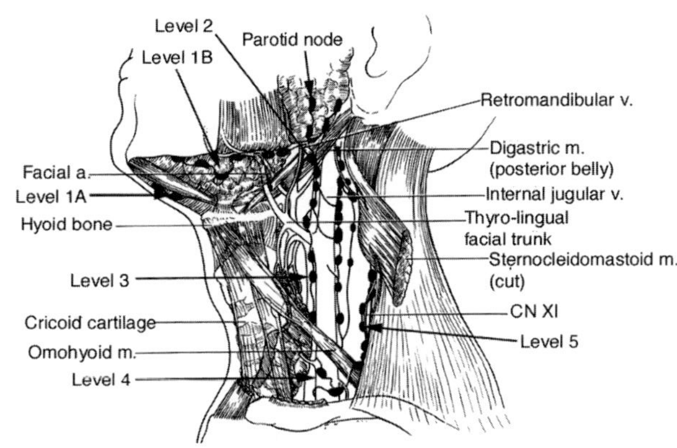

Figure 85F

Differential Diagnosis

Not applicable

Diagnosis

Malignant fibrous histiocytoma encasing the common carotid artery and bifurcation

Diagnostic Imaging Approach

A. Compartment of origin?
B. If the mass is in the lateral compartment *and* pulsatile, is the lesion arising from, involving, or displacing the carotid artery?
C. If the carotid artery does not explain the pulsatile nature, is there some other cause (e.g., arteriovenous malformation, hypervascular mass)?
D. Is an US study, MR angiography, or conventional angiogram necessary?
E. If the mass is not vascular and not of carotid origin, what is causing it?
   1. Anatomic origin: node, vagus, sympathetic trunk, vein, mesenchyma, salivary rest, sternocleidomastoid muscle, visceral or posterior compartment.
   2. Developmental origin: branchial cleft cyst, lymphangioma, thyroglossal duct cyst, thymic.
F. Evaluate morphology: aggressive margins, inflammatory features, related edema, density, T1- or T2-weighted signal intensity, enhancement, vascularity, blood products, calcifications.

Clinical Points Of Importance And Supplemental Information

A. A pulsatile mass *must* be imaged with US, MRI, or CT before biopsy.
B. A target sign (i.e., central, potentially vascular channel with surrounding tissue) is an aneurysm until proved otherwise.

Answers To Questions

1. Yes. Any of the three, but US might not be definitive
2. Lateral compartment. Carotid sheath
3. Angiogram
4. Look for a lesion at the skull base or at least more proximal.

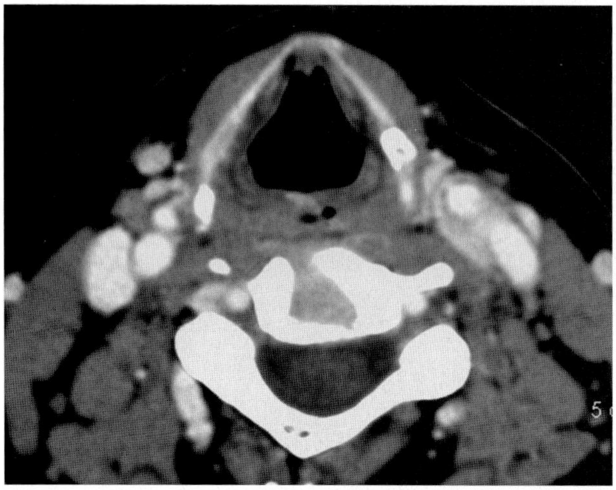

Figure 85G. Patient 1 with carotid body type paraganglioma, showing avidly enhancing mass between and around the carotid bifurcation on the left. Contrast-enhanced computed tomography.

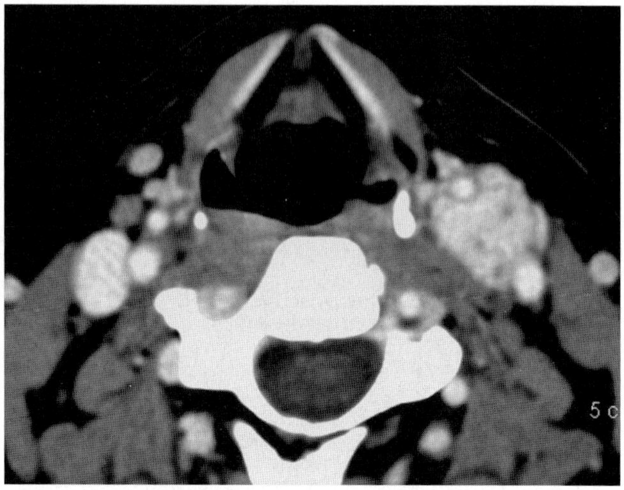

Figure 85H. Patient 1 with carotid body type paraganglioma. Contrast-enhanced computed tomography image, superior to Fig. 85E, showing avidly enhancing mass centered between splayed carotid bifurcation.

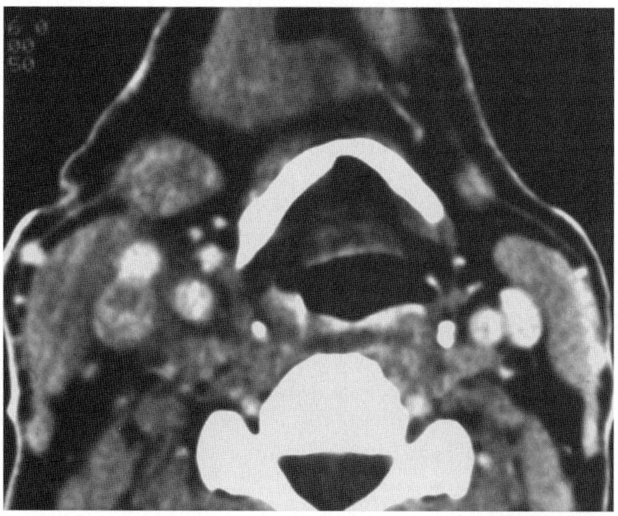

Figure 85I. Patient 2 with acute thrombophlebitis of the internal jugular vein, showing a filling defect in the enlarged right internal jugular vein, with loss of tissue plane around it, mimicking metastasis to the lymph node. Edema in the retropharyngeal space seen here is commonly present in this condition. Contrast-enhanced computed tomography image.

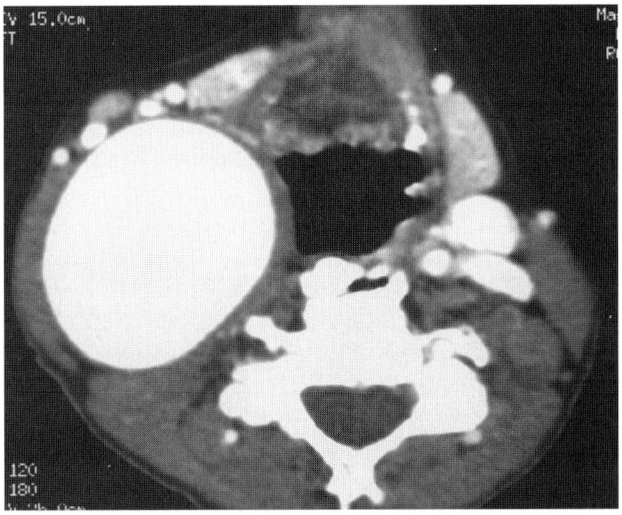

Figure 85J. Patient 3 with pulsatile neck mass, showing a large aneurysm of the right internal carotid artery. Contrast-enhanced computed tomography image.

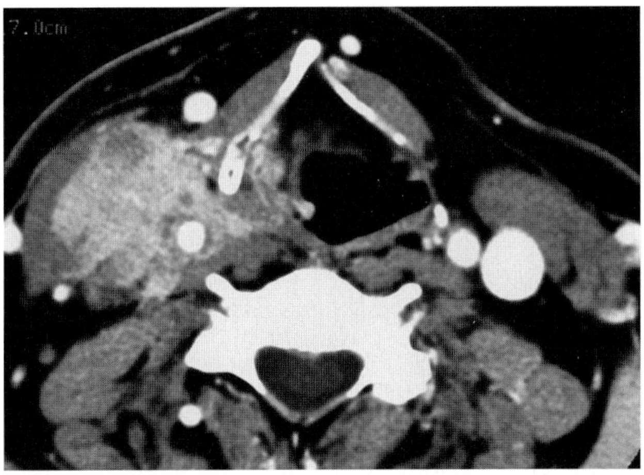

Figure 85K. Patient 4 with pyriform sinus carcinoma with neck metastasis showing an infiltrative mass involving the right pyriform sinus. Extracapsular spread of the metastatic neck disease to the level 3 lymph nodes encases the common carotid artery and invades the sternocleidomastoid muscle. Contrast-enhanced computed tomography image.

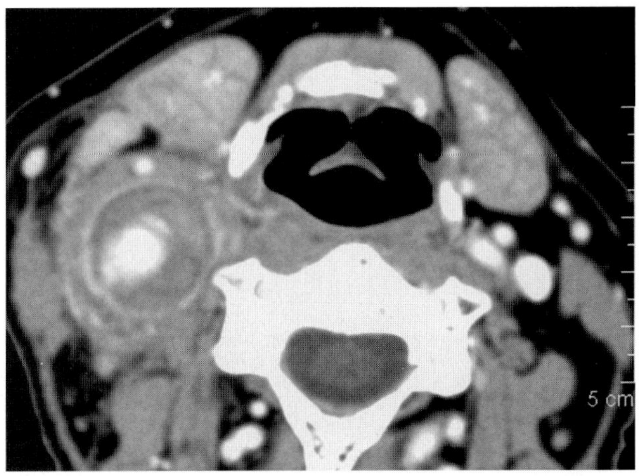

Figure 85L. Patient 5 with ruptured aneurysm, showing a mass centered in the right carotid sheath, which contains an enlarged aneurysmal lumen extending beyond a concentric high attenuation rim (presumed original aneurysmal wall). Contrast-enhanced computed tomography image.

CASE 86

Clinical History: An 18-year-old man presents with a left lower neck mass. A needle biopsy performed at another institution reportedly was not diagnostic; an open biopsy followed, still without the benefit of imaging studies.

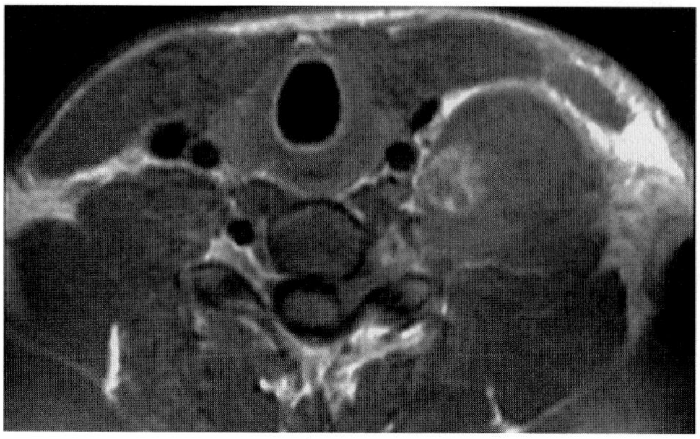

Figure 86A

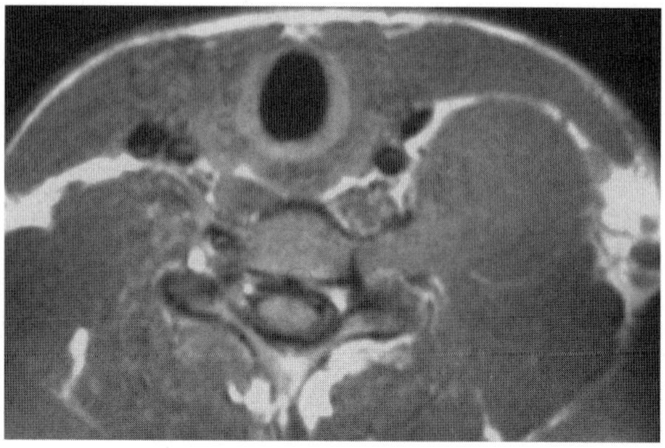

Figure 86B

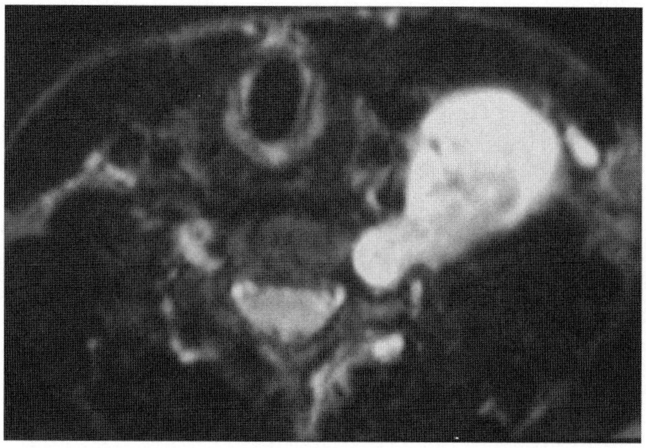

Figure 86C

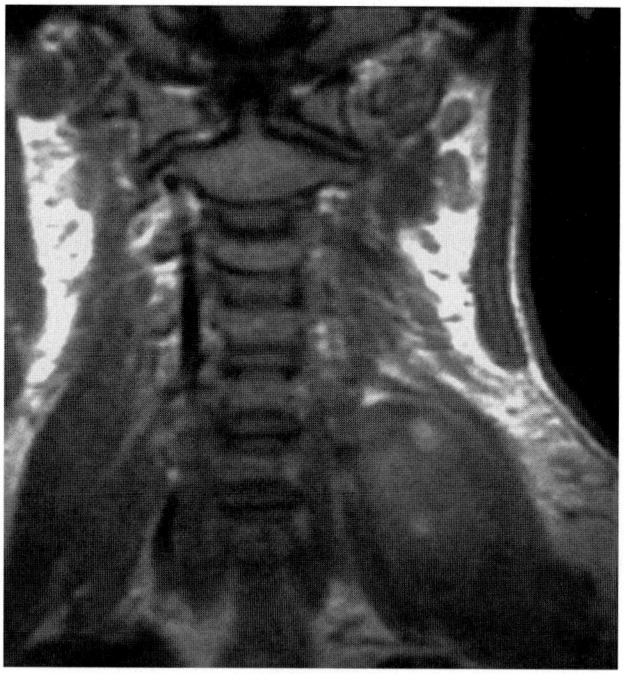

Figure 86D

1. Must imaging precede needle biopsy in the evaluation of a lower neck mass?
2. What imaging study—magnetic resonance imaging (MRI), computed tomography (CT), or ultrasound—would you prefer if the mass is *a*) likely thyroid related; *b*) possibly vascular; *c*) nodal; *d*) associated with neurologic findings; or *e*) inflammatory?
3. List four neurologic deficits that might be associated with a lower neck mass.

Findings

A well-demarcated paravertebral mass in the lower neck on the left. The lesion intervenes between the scalene group muscles and displaces the carotid sheath anteriorly and levator scapula muscle posteriorly. The mass enhances diffusely and then more intensely at some points. The lesion extends through an enlarged left neural foramen and partly protrudes into the spinal canal.

Problem

A young adult with a "lateral" neck mass that appears to be arising in the paravertebral region (posterior neck compartment)

Anatomy

A. Neck compartments and contents
   1. Visceral: within visceral fascia
   2. Lateral (paired): within investing (superficial) layer of the *deep* cervical fascia
   3. Posterior: within the prevertebral (deep) layer of deep cervical fascia—spine, spinal cord, nerve roots (brachial plexus), phrenic nerve, muscles, fat, vertebral artery and other vessels, connective tissue, lymphatics

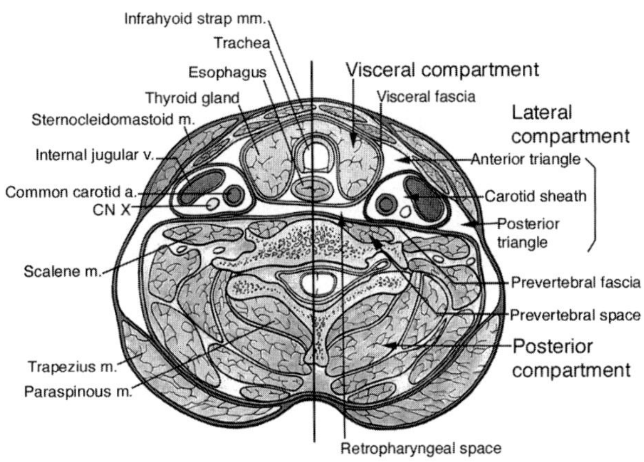

Figure 86E

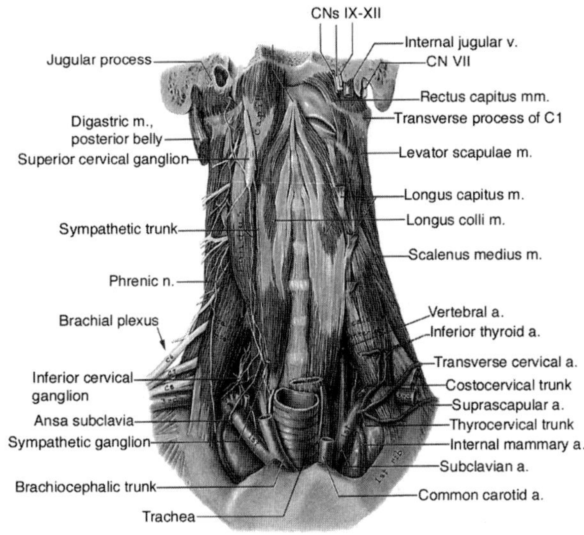

Figure 86F

Differential Diagnosis

Not applicable

Diagnosis

Neurofibroma of the brachial plexus

Diagnostic Imaging Approach

A. Establish the compartment of origin.
B. Determine the specific structure of origin if possible (e.g., nerve root, intervertebral disk, muscle).
C. Specifically exclude a vascular cause or highly vascular lesion. Is an angiogram necessary?.
D. If the mass is not vascular, what is causing it?
   1. Anatomic origin: see number 3 (above) under *Anatomy.*
   2. Developmental origin: vascular malformation, lymphangiomas usually involve posterior compartment secondarily, dermoid or epidermoid cyst.
E. Evaluate morphology: aggressive margins, inflammatory features, related edema, density, T1- or T2-weighted signal intensity, enhancement, vascularity, blood products, calcifications.

Clinical Points Of Importance And Supplemental Information

If a needle biopsy of a neck mass is indeterminate, imaging should be performed before an open surgical procedure in almost all patients.

Answers To Questions

1. Not always, but it is usually wise in cases of any doubt about it being vascular.
2. a. CT; b. Any of the three–your choice; c. CT; d. MRI; e. CT
3. Vocal cord paralysis, Horner's syndrome, sensory and motor deficits (brachial plexus), paralyzed diaphragm

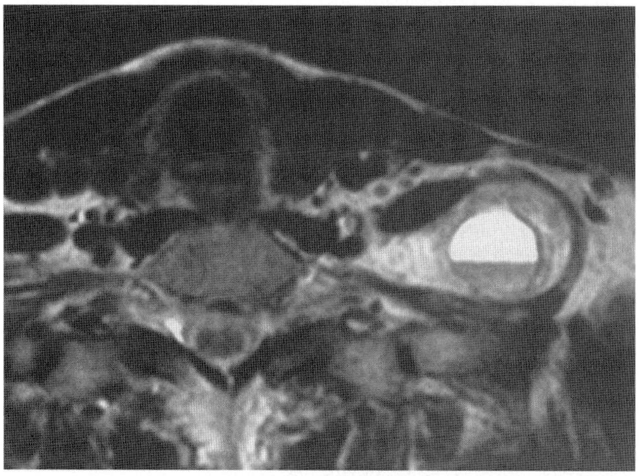

Figure 86G. Patient 1 with schwannoma arising from the brachial plexus, showing cystic mass with fluid–fluid level (likely posthemorrhagic) between the anterior, and middle and posterior scalene muscles. T2-weighted axial image.

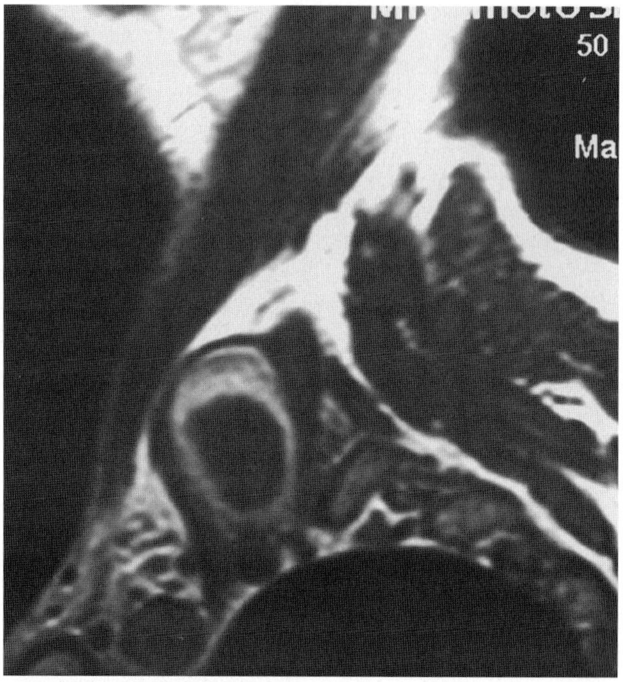

Figure 86H. Patient 1 with schwannoma arising from the brachial plexus. T1-weighted axial image with contrast showing enhancement of the wall of the mass displacing the anterior scalene muscle anteriorly. T1-weighted sagittal image with contrast.

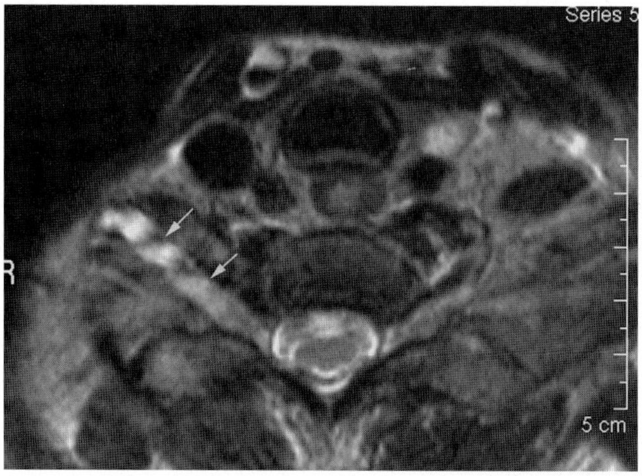

Figure 86I. Patient 2 with postirradiation brachial plexopathy, showing the enlargement of the nerve root (*arrows*) of the brachial plexus on the right. A recurrent tumor is seen surrounding the anterior scalene muscle on the left. T2-weighted axial image.

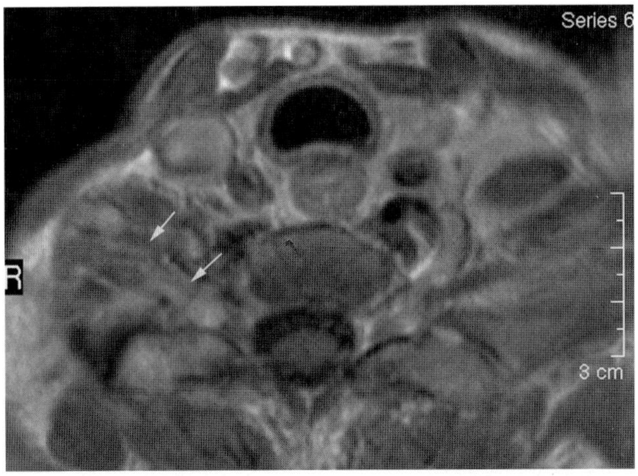

Figure 86J. Patient 2 with postirradiation brachial plexopathy. T1-weighted axial image with contrast showing enhancement of the swollen nerve root (*arrows*).

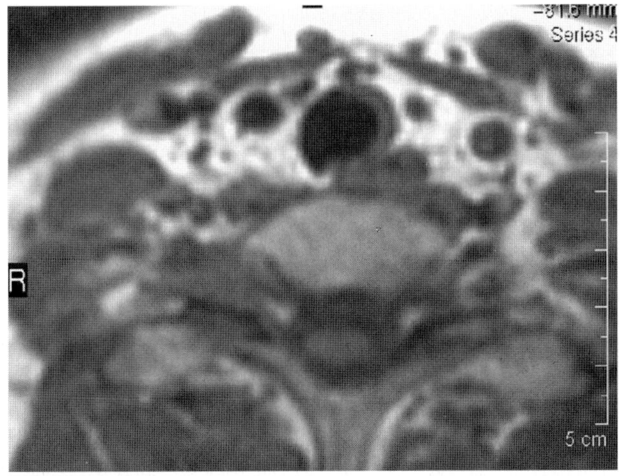

Figure 86K. Patient 3 with "neurotropic" non-Hodgkin's lymphoma, showing an infiltrative mass in the area of the neural foramen on the right. T1-weighted axial image.

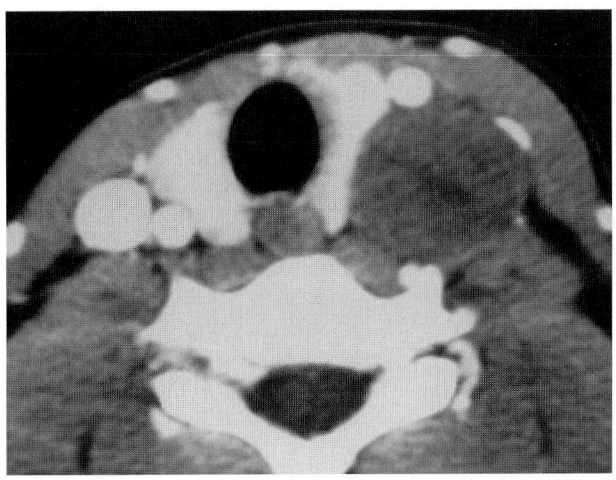

Figure 86L. Patient 4 with schwannoma arising from the sympathetic plexus, showing a well-circumscribed mass anterior to the scalene muscles on the right, displacing both the common carotid artery and internal jugular vein anteriorly. Contrast-enhanced computed tomography image.

CASE 87

Clinical History: A 20-year-old man presents with cervical adenopathy.

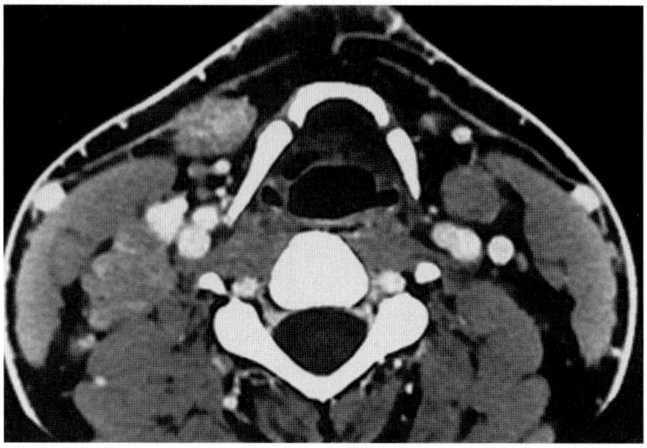

Figure 87A

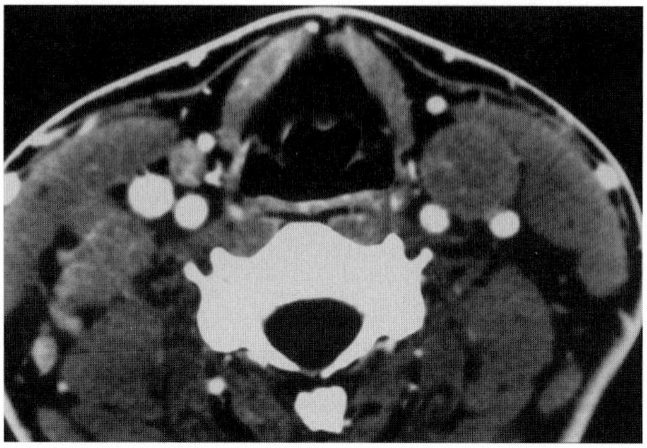

Figure 87B

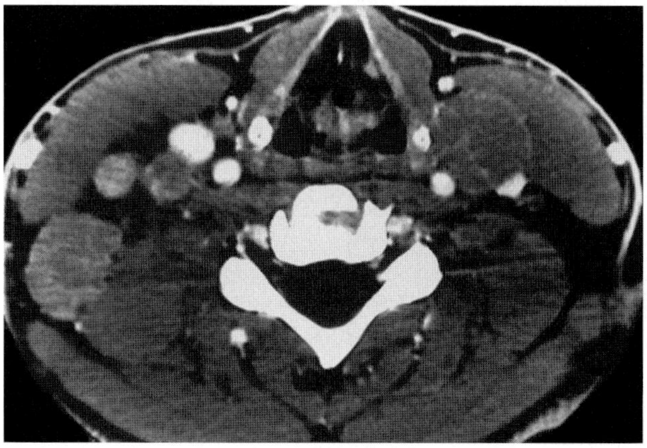

Figure 87C

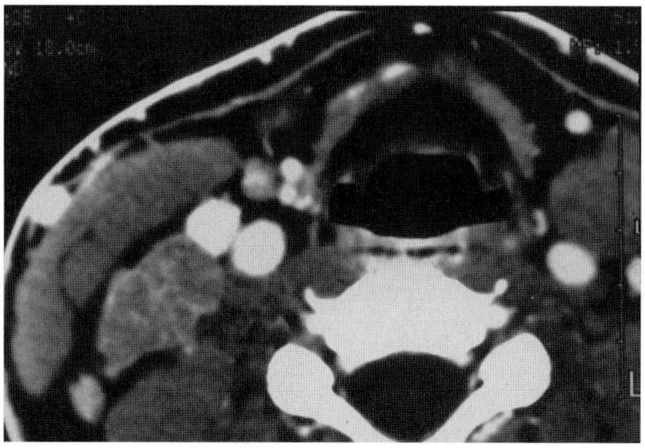

Figure 87D

1. What nodal group(s) is involved?
2. What causative factors do the nodal morphology and distribution suggest?
3. Can the clinicians anticipate a "clean" excisional biopsy (rather than an incisional biopsy)?

Findings

Multiple enlarged solid lymph nodes bilaterally along the internal jugular vein and in the right posterior triangle. The capsule of some larger nodes enhances minimally without frank extracapsular spread. In some areas, extracapsular spread may be "matting" the nodes together. Neither a cystic area nor calcification is seen in the nodes.

Problem

A young man with generalized cervical adenopathy confirmed on computed tomography (CT)

Anatomy

A. Cervical lymph node groups: limits of each group or appearance and size of normal nodes (pediatric and adult age groups).
   1. Group I: submandibular or submental
   2. Group II: upper internal jugular
   3. Group III: middle internal jugular
   4. Group IV: lower internal jugular
   5. Group V: spinal accessory
   6. Others: pretracheal, paratracheal, prethyroid, laryngeal, tracheoesophageal groove.

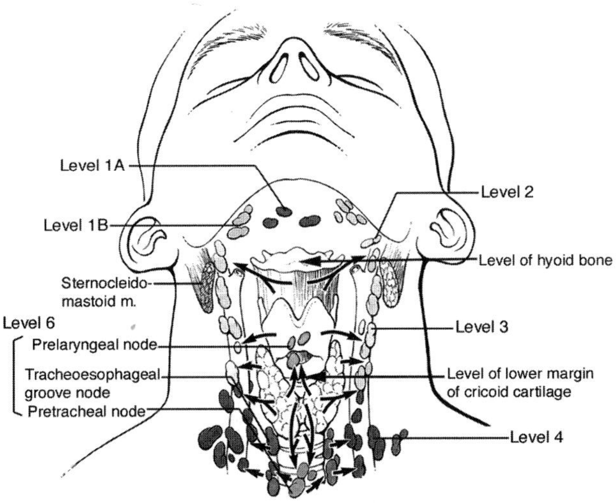

Figure 87E

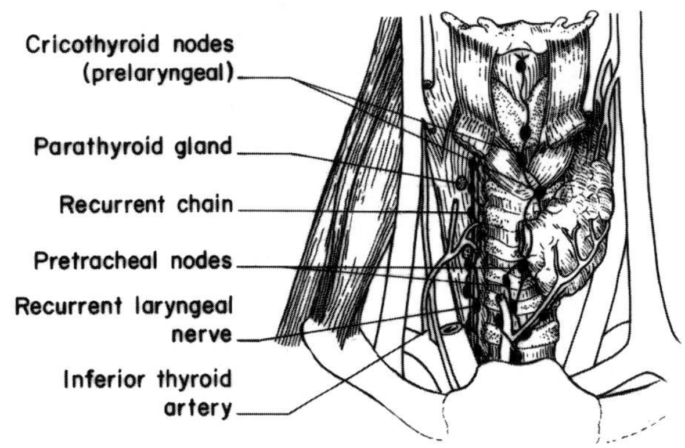

Figure 87F

Differential Diagnosis

1. Nodal: metastatic from head and neck primary or infraclavicular primary, lymphoma, reactive, generalized lymphatic system disease (e.g., sarcoidosis), tuberculosis, suppurative adenitis
2. Nonnodal: branchial cleft cyst, neurogenic tumor, other more rare tumors (e.g., benign mixed) that happen to occur in lymph node-bearing areas

Diagnosis

Lymphoma

Diagnostic Imaging Approach

A. Is the mass of lymph node origin?
B. Is the node solitary, one of multiple abnormal nodes, or is there generalized adenopathy?
C. What specific neck groups are involved? Are there other groups (retropharyngeal, facial, parotid) involved?
D. Nodal morphology:
   1. Solid, minimal capsular and hilar enhancement point to lymphoma (nonspecific), reactive adenopathy, sarcoid, and so on.
   2. Focal peripheral defects in normal or enlarged nodes point to metastases from "solid" neoplasms (usually squamous cell carcinoma).
   3. Large fluid areas in nodes indicate gross necrotic metastases or infectious disease (pyogenic, tuberculosis).
   4. Any capsular involvement or extracapsular spread (important to note extent of spread)?
   5. Does the extranodal spread involve the carotid, jugular, prevertebral fascia, sternocleidomastoid muscle, and so on?
E. Does the nodal morphology suggest an inflammatory rather than neoplastic cause of the adenopathy?
F. Another abnormality present that might be associated with the adenopathy (e.g., primary site, Waldeyer's ring lymphoma, lymphoepithelial parotid lesions, or human immunodeficiency virus [HIV])?

Clinical Points Of Importance And Supplemental Information

A. If needle biopsy shows squamous cell carcinoma, a scan must include the entire pharynx and neck and a careful search made for a clinically occult primary tumor. The groups involved will suggest the most likely primary sites.
B. Discrete nodes without evidence of capsular penetration can be safely and completely excised for diagnosis; *incisional* biopsy of cervical nodes should be avoided.

Answers To Questions

1. Groups 2, 3, and 5
2. Lymphoma, reactive (viral), sarcoid, HIV
3. Yes

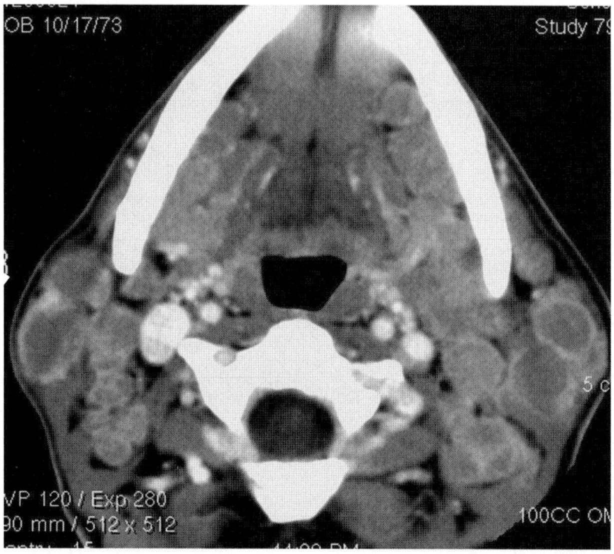

Figure 87G. Patient 1 with non-Hodgkin's lymphoma, showing multiple enlarged lymph nodes with capsular hyperemia involving multiple lymph node levels bilaterally. Contrast-enhanced computed tomography image.

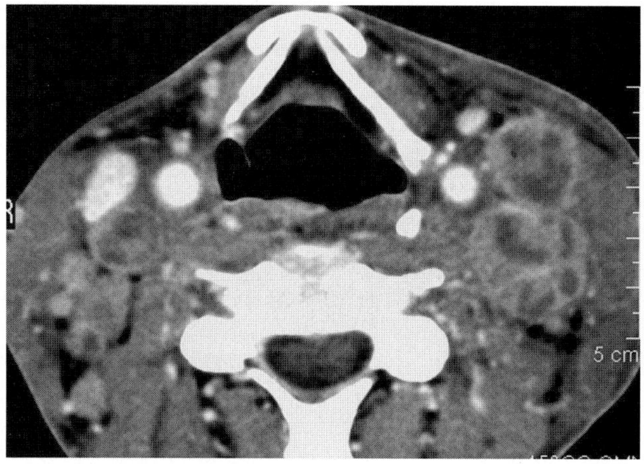

Figure 87H. Patient 2 with high-grade, non-Hodgkin's lymphoma, showing multiple enlarged lymph nodes containing cystic areas in multiple lymph node levels bilaterally.

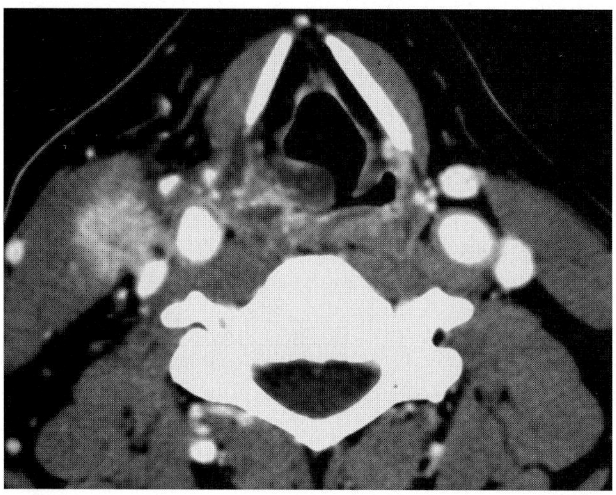

Figure 87I. Patient 3 with pyriform sinus carcinoma, showing metastasis to the level 3 lymph node with extracapsular spread directly invading the sternocleidomastoid muscle. Contrast-enhanced computed tomography image.

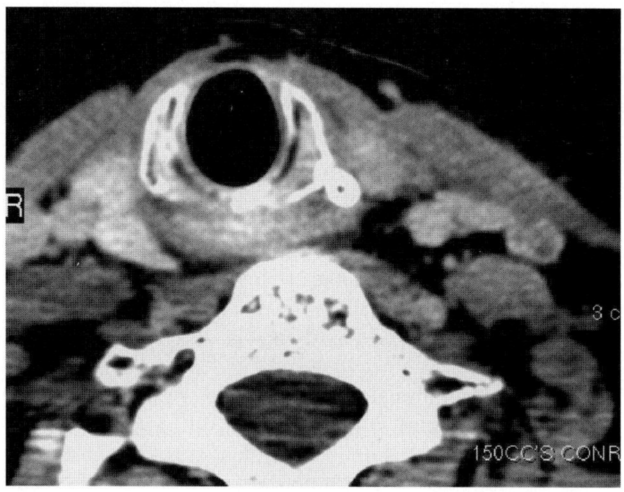

Figure 87J. Patient 4 with supraglottic carcinoma, showing a level 3 lymph node with focal areas of low attenuation strongly suggestive of metastatic deposits. Contrast-enhanced computed tomography image.

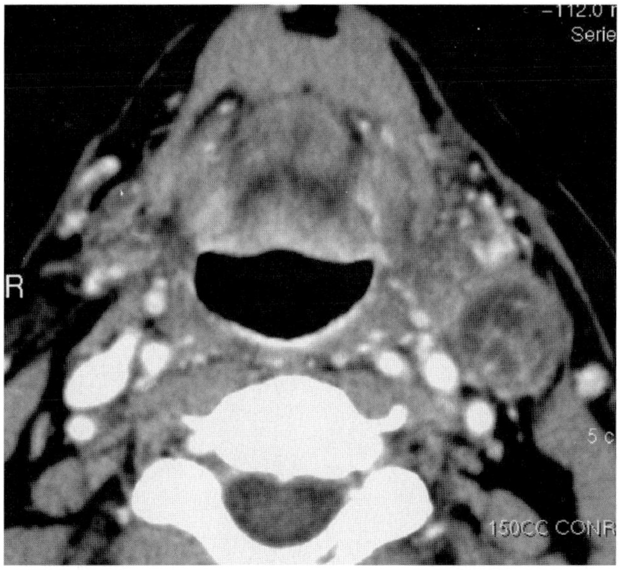

Figure 87K. Patient 5 with squamous cell carcinoma of the glossotonsillar sulcus, showing the enlarged level 2 lymph node containing multiple foci of metastatic deposit on the left. Contrast-enhanced computed tomography image.

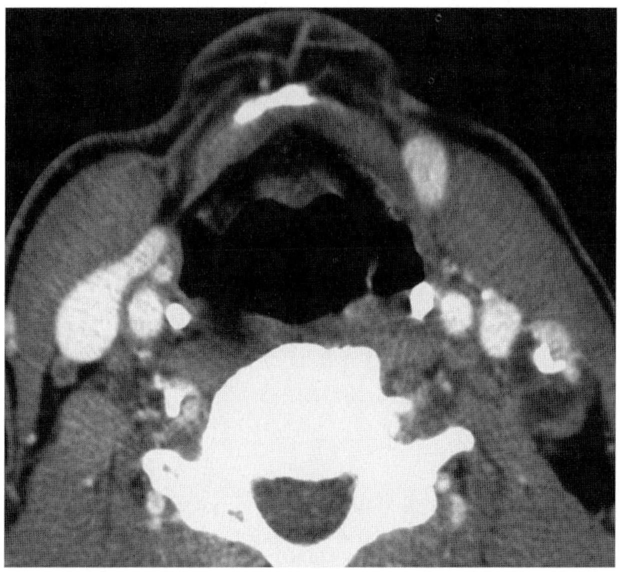

Figure 87L. Patient 6 with cervical lymph node metastases from thyroid carcinoma, showing a cystic level 3 lymph node containing an enhancing solid component and a focal area of calcification. Note smaller metastatic lymph node on the right. Contrast-enhanced computed tomography image.

CASE 88

Clinical History: A 22-year-old man presents with a neck mass.

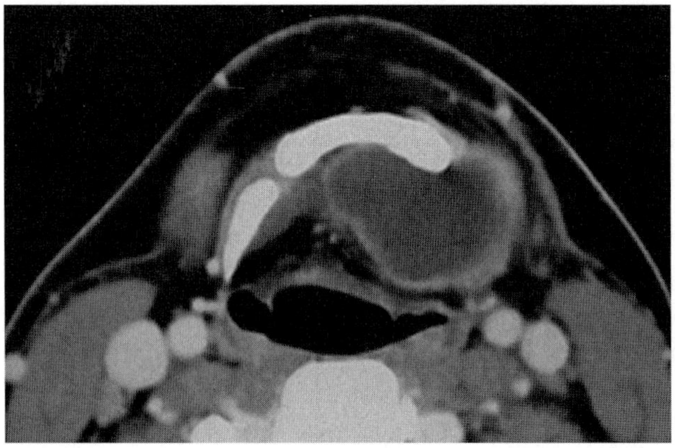

Figure 88A

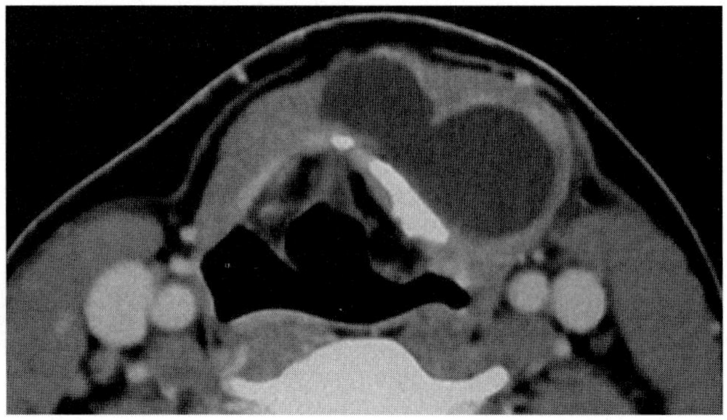

Figure 88B

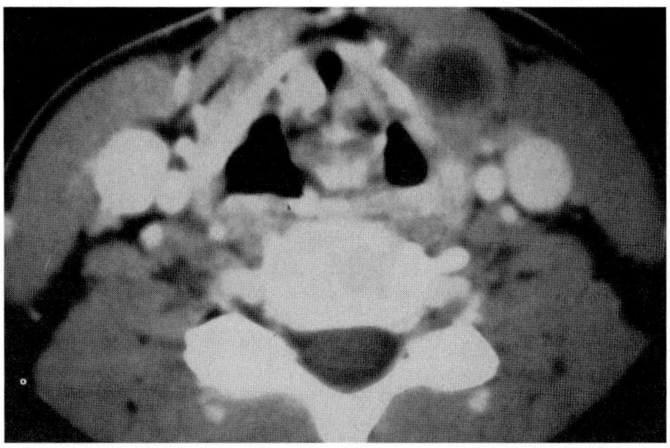

Figure 88C

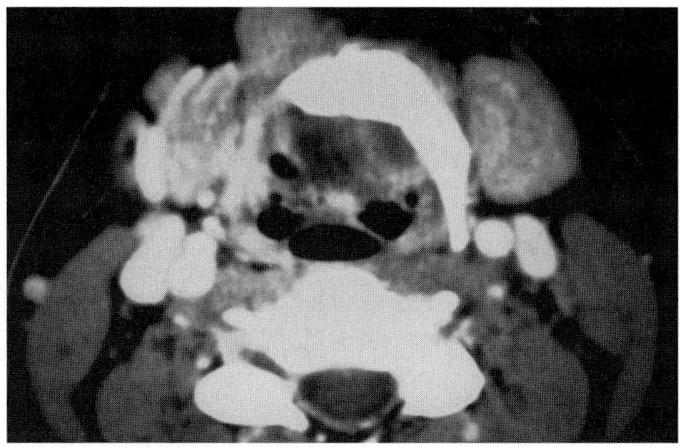

Figure 88D

1. What is the compartment of origin?
2. What is the diagnosis? Give one other reasonable differential choice based on these two images.
3. What are the radiologist's three main responsibilities in evaluating this specific entity?

Findings

A paramedian cystic mass at the level of hyoid and infrahyoid neck. The lesion is deep to the infrahyoid strap muscles. Although the lesion compresses preepiglottic space, no true extension into the supraglottic larynx is noted. No nodular or papillary component is seen in the lesion. Relatively thick wall of the mass and thickening of adjacent platysma muscle suggest past inflammatory episodes.

Problem

A young adult with a paramedian neck mass arising from the visceral compartment

Anatomy

A. Compartments of the neck
   1. Visceral (within visceral fascia): larynx, hypopharynx, trachea, thyroid, parathyroids, esophagus, recurrent laryngeal nerve, lymph nodes associated with viscera, infrahyoid strap muscles
   2. Lateral (paired): within investing (superficial) layer of deep cervical fascia
   3. Posterior: within prevertebral (deep) layer of deep cervical fascia

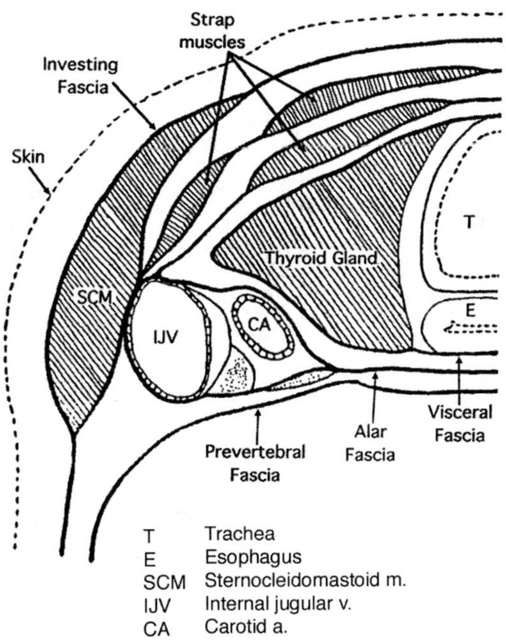

Figure 88E

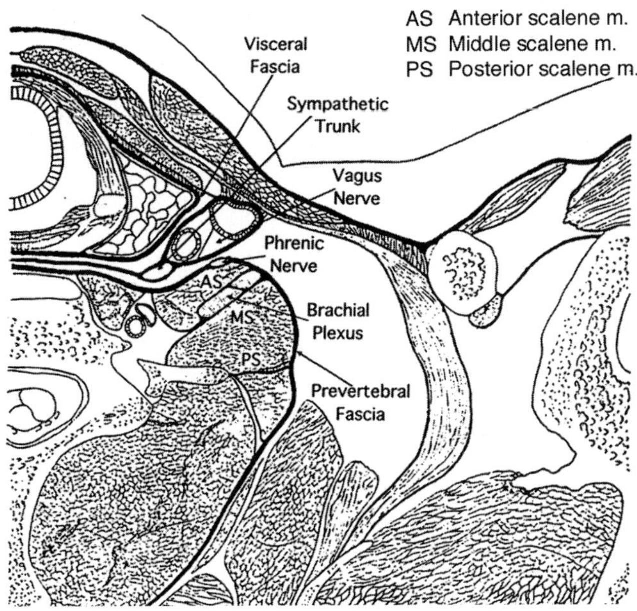

Figure 88F

Differential Diagnosis

Not applicable

Diagnosis

Thyroglossal duct cyst

Diagnostic Imaging Approach

A. Establish the compartment of origin.
B. Determine the specific structure or organ of origin.
C. Specifically exclude a vascular cause or highly vascular lesion; is an angiogram necessary?
D. If a mass is not vascular, what is causing it?
   1. Anatomic origin: see number 1 (above) under *Anatomy*; some specific examples would include laryngocele, pyriform sinus cancer, Zenker's diverticulum.
   2. Developmental origin: thyroglossal duct cyst, dermoid or epidermoid cyst, lymphangioma (usually are spreading to rather than arising from the visceral compartment).
E. Evaluate morphology: aggressive margins, inflammatory features, related edema, density, T1- or T2-weighted signal intensity, enhancement, vascularity, blood products, calcifications.

Clinical Points Of Importance And Supplemental Information

A. These lesions are typically midline or paramedian and are easily diagnosed clinically. Imaging is done to evaluate the full extent (study from the foramen cecum to the thoracic inlet) to choose Sistrunk or modified Sistrunk procedure for removal.
B. Incidental, small thyroglossal duct cysts are frequently seen on computed tomography and magnetic resonance imaging studies done for other purposes.
C. Whenever a developmental abnormality of thyroid migration is evaluated, the normal thyroid gland tissue must be localized.

Answers To Questions

1. Visceral
2. Thyroglossal duct cyst. Laryngocele.
3. Proper diagnosis: extent from tongue base (foramen cecum to thyroid gland); any signs of cancer arising in a benign thyroglossal duct cyst (very rare); presence of a normal thyroid.

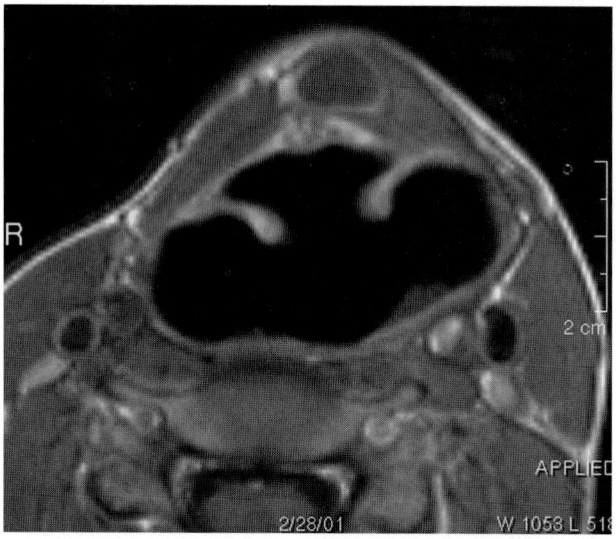

Figure 88G. Patient 1 with infrahyoid thyroglossal duct cyst, showing a cystic mass anterior to the thyrohyoid membrane and deep to the infrahyoid strap muscle. T1-weighted axial image with contrast.

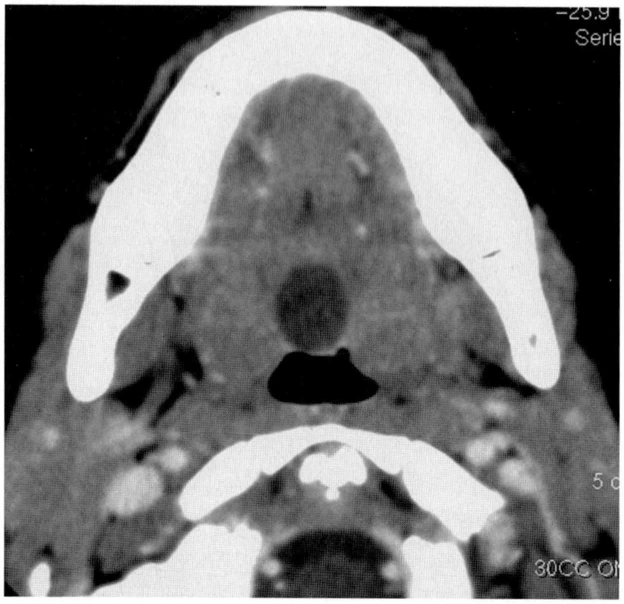

Figure 88H. Patient 2 with suprahyoid thyroglossal duct cyst, showing unilocular cystic mass in the midline of the tongue base, centered in the expected position of the foramen cecum. Contrast-enhanced computed tomography image.

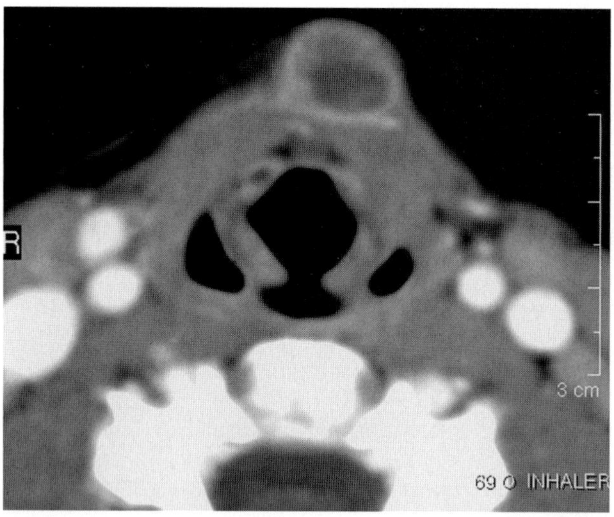

Figure 88I. Patient 3 with surgically proved ruptured thyroglossal duct cyst, showing a cystic mass with rim enhancement superficial to the infrahyoid strap muscle.

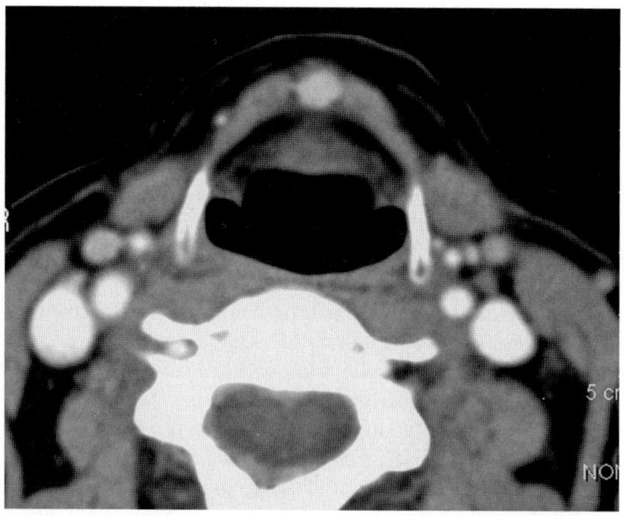

Figure 88J. Patient 4 with ectopic thyroid tissue along the course of the thyroglossal duct, showing high attenuation structure in the midline of the anterior neck, superficial to the thyrohyoid membrane. Contrast-enhanced computed tomography image.

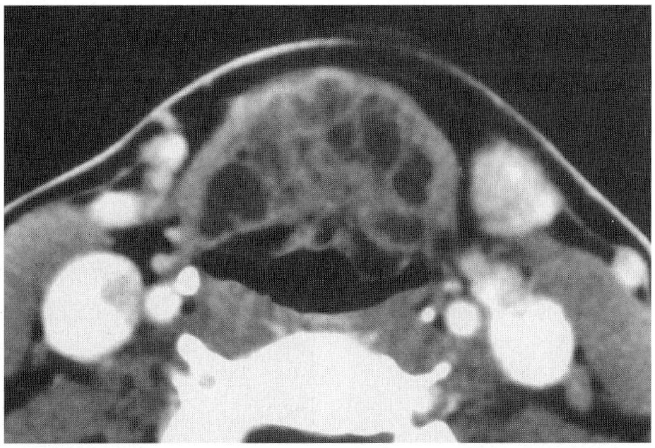

Figure 88K. Patient 5 with unusual presentation of the infrahyoid thyroglossal duct cyst, showing a multiloculated cystic mass superficial to the thyrohyoid membrane and deep to the infrahyoid strap muscle.

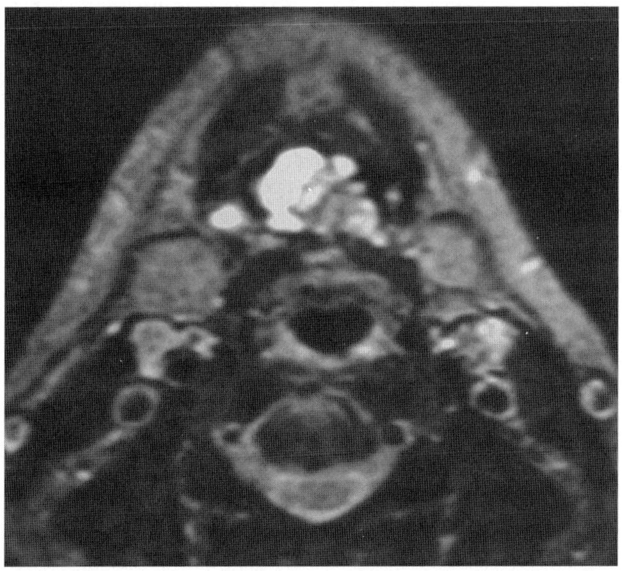

Figure 88L. Patient 6 with papillary carcinoma arising from a thyroglossal duct cyst, showing a cystic mass containing a solid component in the submental region. T2-weighted axial image.

CASE 89

Clinical History: A 3-year-old male presents with a neck mass.

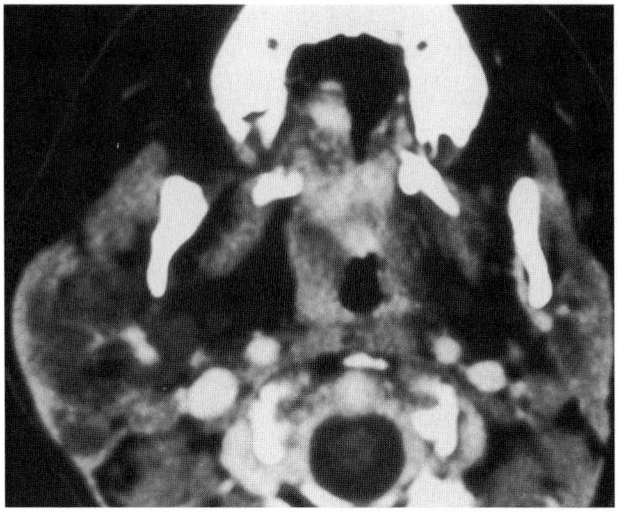

Figure 89A

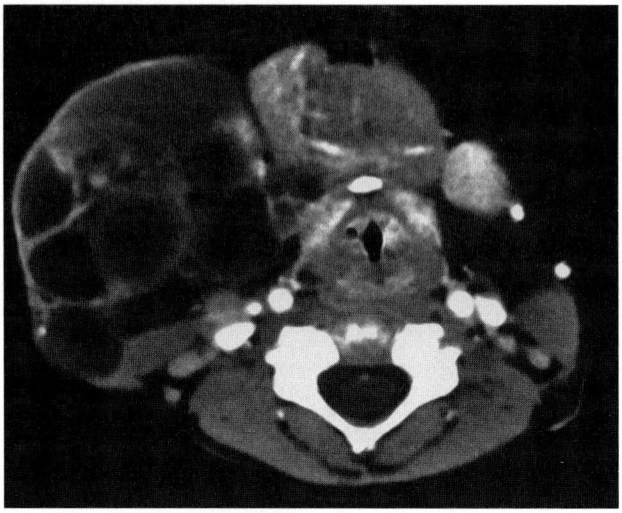

Figure 89B

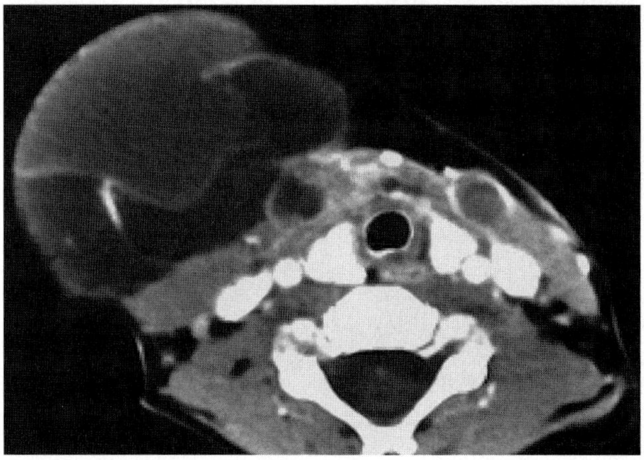

Figure 89C

1. What is the relationship of the mass to the investing layer of the cervical fascia?
2. Give a complete diagnosis.
3. Give two reasons a mass such as this might enlarge acutely.
4. What is the more common location of this category of disease?

Findings

An extensive multiloculated cystic mass at right anterolateral aspect of the infrahyoid neck. Some solid areas and septations enhance on postcontrast images. The lesion stays centered in the carotid triangle of the anterior cervical triangle. The mass spreads primarily by surrounding the expected position of the superficial fascia. The mass is bilateral and extends deeper into the parotid gland and parapharyngeal space superiorly.

Problem

A young child with a multiloculated, predominantly cystic neck mass in the anterior cervical triangle

Anatomy

A. Superficial layer of the cervical fascia (platysma)
B. Investing layer of the cervical fascia (also known as superficial layer of the *deep* cervical fascia)
C. Prevertebral layer (also known as deep layer of the deep cervical fascia)

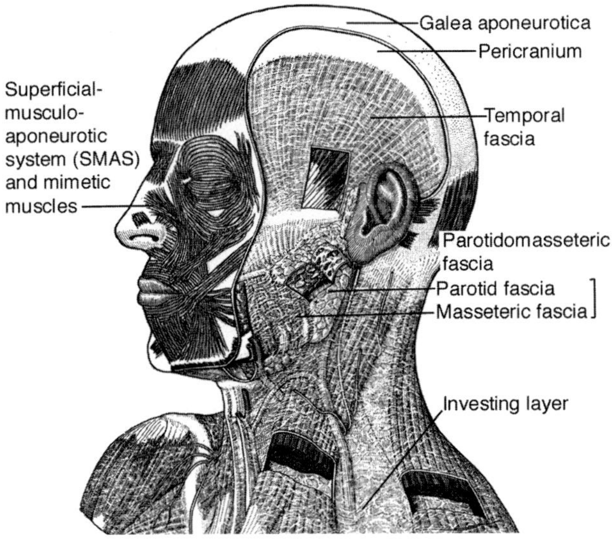

Figure 89D

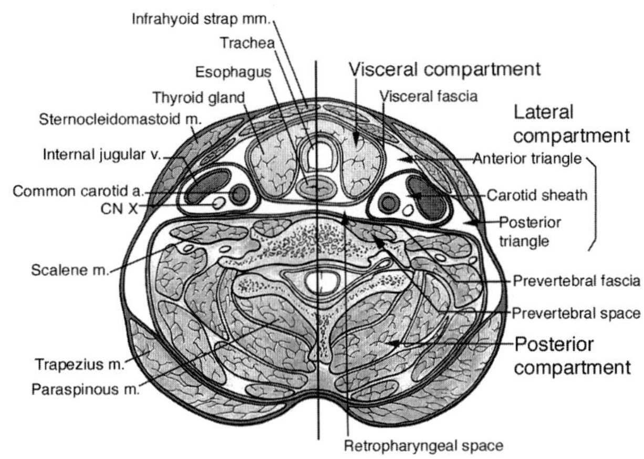

Figure 89E

Differential Diagnosis

None

Diagnosis

Bilateral, mixed lymphangioma or hemangioma (venolymphatic malformation) of the superficial anterior triangle regions (with acute bleeding as an explanation for the rapid enlargement)

Diagnostic Imaging Approach

A. Establish the compartment of origin.
B. Determine the specific structure or organ of origin, if any.
C. Exclude a vascular (e.g., carotid artery) origin or highly vascular tumor as a cause; is an angiogram necessary?
D. Evaluate morphology:
   1. If cystic: wall thickness, wall enhancement, cyst contents, degree of loculation or separation.
   2. Other features: aggressive margins, inflammatory features, related edema, density, T1- or T2-weighted signal intensity, enhancement, vascularity, blood products, calcifications.
   3. Growth pattern: insinuating vs. discrete mass, with displacement rather than growth around normal structures.

Clinical Points Of Importance And Supplemental Information

A. Removal of these lesions is usually related to functional and cosmetic issues. Because of their often insinuating growth around critical structures (e.g., carotid artery, vagus nerve), gross total excision is frequently not possible.
B. These lesions frequently enlarge rapidly because of hemorrhage or reactive lymphoid hyperplasia caused by upper respiratory infections (the lesions arise from the lymphatic system and contain immune competent cells). If their presence was unknown before such an incident, this presentation might mimic a more aggressive process. This is especially common in the supraclavicular fossa in adults.

Answers To Questions

1. Superficial to the investing layer–deep to the superficial layer (platysma)
2. Bilateral mixed heme-lymphangioma
3. Reaction to inflammation because it contains immune-competent cells and bleeding
4. Posterior triangle, face

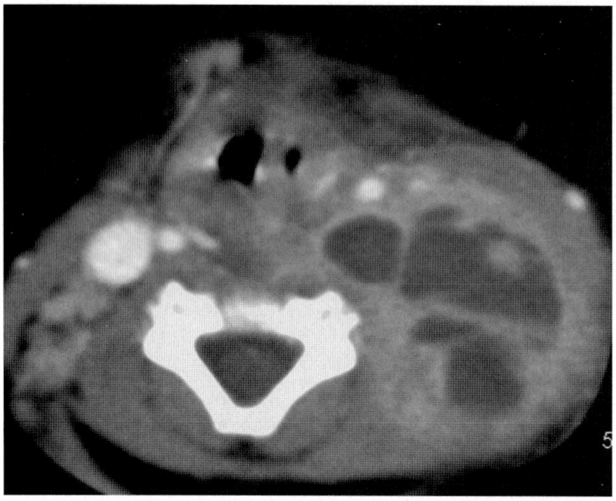

Figure 89F. Patient 1 (10 m/M) with infected cystic hygroma (venolymphatic malformation), showing a loculated cystic mass with enhancement of the wall and septa and soft tissue swelling around it, centered in the posterior triangle on the left. Contrast-enhanced computed tomography image.

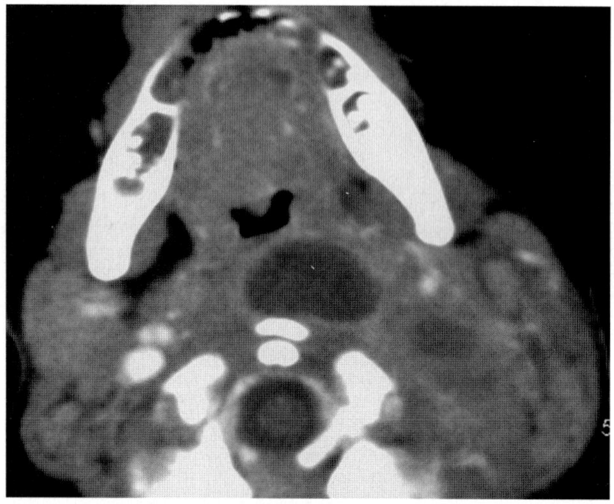

Figure 89G. Patient 1 (10 m/M) with infected cystic hygroma (venolymphatic malformation). Contrast-enhanced computed tomography image, superior to Fig. 89F, showing the process insinuating into the retropharyngeal space.

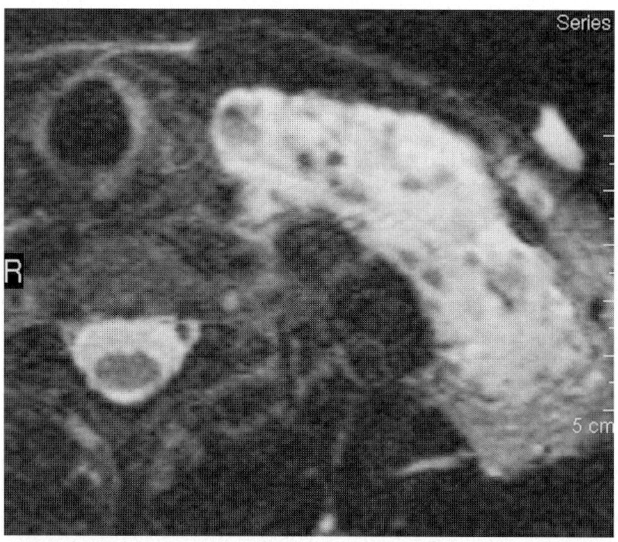

Figure 89H. Patient 2 (12 y/F) with cavernous type vascular malformation. T2-weighted axial image showing a high-intensity mass of the left lateral neck, mainly involving the posterior triangle.

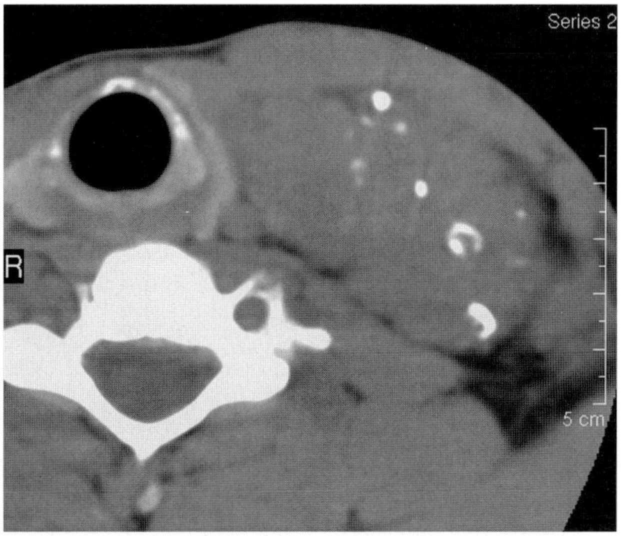

Figure 89I. Patient 2 (12 y/F) with cavernous type vascular malformation. Computed tomography image without contrast showing multiple phlebolith in the mass, which is suggestive of the diagnosis.

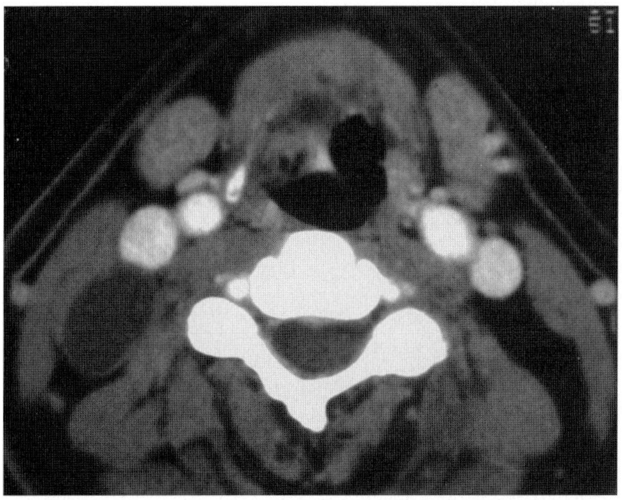

Figure 89J. Patient 3 with a second branchial cleft cyst, showing a unilocular cystic mass in a less typical posterior triangle location on the right. Contrast-enhanced computed tomography image.

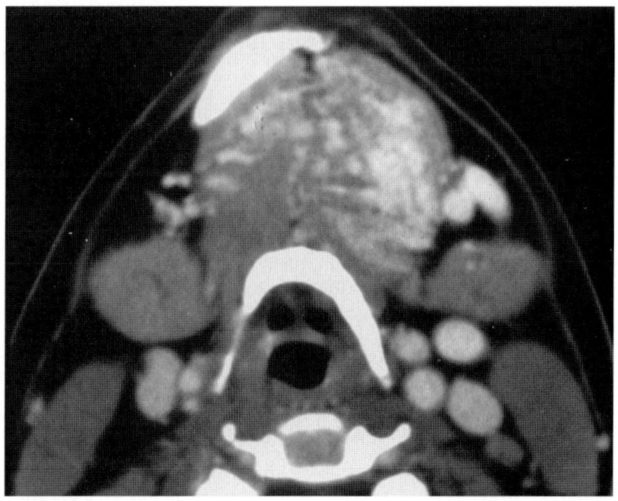

Figure 89K. Patient 4 with a high-flow vascular malformation involving the mouth floor and submandibular space, showing avidly enhancing tortuous vessels between the anterior belly of the digastric muscle and musculature of the mouth floor, with enlarged facial vessels on the left.

CASE 90

Clinical History: A 41-year-old man presents with a slightly tender right upper neck mass believed to be a nodal metastasis. The computed tomography study was done to determine the cause of the mass and the possible presence of an occult pharyngeal primary tumor as a source of the metastatic disease.

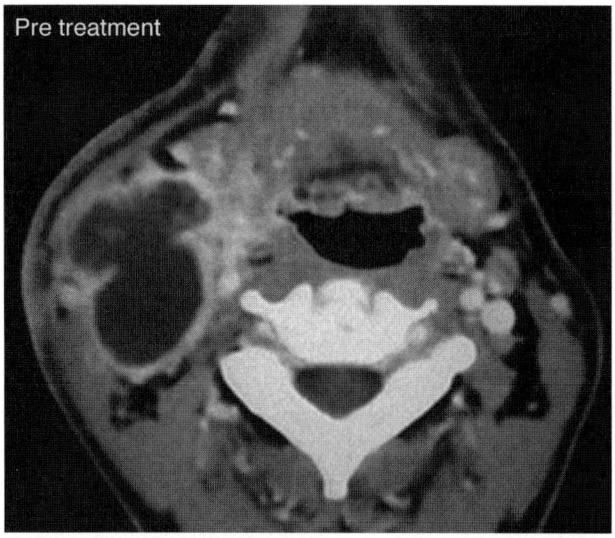

Figure 90A

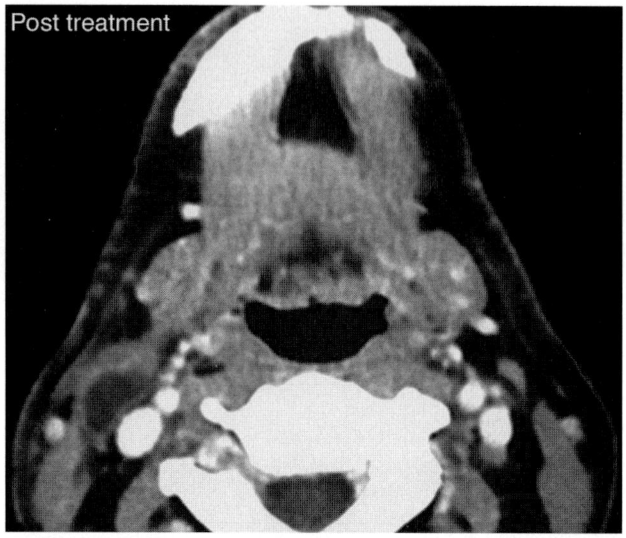

Figure 90C

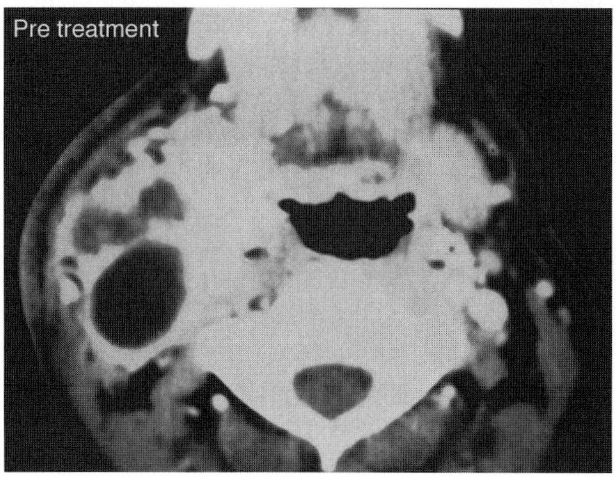

Figure 90B

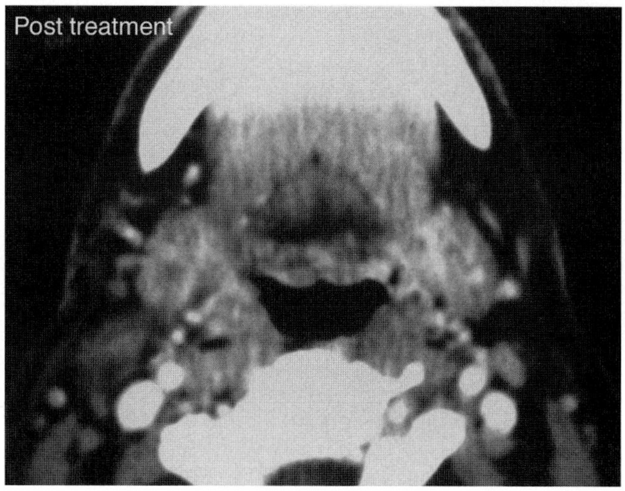

Figure 90D

1. What neck compartment is the site of origin?
2. Is the morphology more likely inflammatory or neoplastic?
3. What course of action was recommended, based on the first image? What was the result (see second study)? What is the diagnosis?

Findings

A cystic mass in the right carotid triangle of the anterior cervical triangle. The lesion displaces the sternocleidomastoid muscle posterolaterally and the submandibular gland anteromedially. Its wall is generally thick, which enhances on post-contrast images. No evident sinus tract communicating with the tonsillar fossa or skin. Thickening of adjacent platysma muscle and the skin and increased density of subcutaneous fat suggest an inflammatory process. The mass drastically decreased in size on the second study done 10 days after nonsurgical treatment.

Problem

A middle-aged man with a lateral compartment neck mass that appears cystic, with a thick enhancing margin and surrounding edema

Anatomy

A. Compartments of the neck
   1. Visceral: within visceral fascia
   2. Lateral: paired and within investing (superficial) layer of deep cervical fascia; contains carotid, jugular, vagus nerve, nodes, spinal accessory nerve, sternocleidomastoid muscle, fat, connective tissue, sympathetic trunk
   3. Posterior: within prevertebral (deep) layer of deep cervical fascia

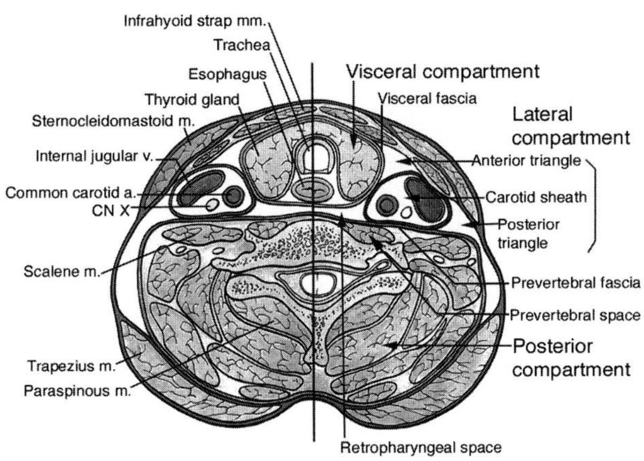

Figure 90E

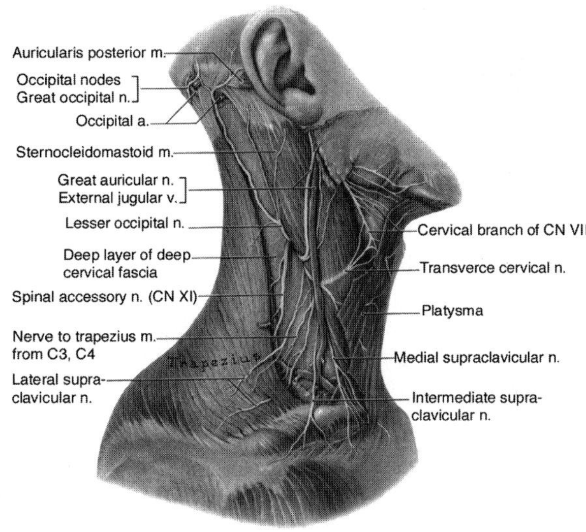

Figure 90F

Differential Diagnosis

Not applicable

Diagnosis

Infected second branchial cleft cyst before and after antibiotics

Diagnostic Imaging Approach

A. Establish the compartment and, if possible, structure or organ of origin.
B. Is the mass transcompartmental?
C. Do margins or associated findings (e.g., edema) suggest an aggressive lesion? An inflammatory lesion?
D. Differential diagnosis on the basis of imaging is driven by anatomic or developmental considerations:
   1. Anatomic: see number 2 (above) under *Anatomy*; the differential is easily developed by considering anatomic options.
   2. Developmental: branchial apparatus links the neck to the pharyngeal development; venous system gives rise to lymph or hemangiomatous lesions; thyroid, parathyroid, and thymic development round out the differential diagnosis; dermoid or epidermoid cysts are rare in the lateral neck.
E. Consider morphology: in addition to margins, edema, cystic nature (above), consider density, T1- or T2-weighted signal intensity, enhancement, vascularity, blood products, calcifications.

Clinical Points Of Importance And Supplemental Information

The occurrence of carcinoma in a branchial cleft cyst is *very rare.* Cystic masses containing squamous cell carcinoma should be considered metastases from an unknown (occult) primary tumor when a primary tumor is not found, even after direct panendoscopy and careful imaging. Patients with such an unknown primary tumor require treatment of the entire pharynx and neck or treatment of the neck and diligent follow-up to see if the primary "declares itself."

Answers To Questions

1. Lateral
2. Inflammatory
3. Antibiotics. Resolution of acute inflammatory component. Second branchial cleft cyst

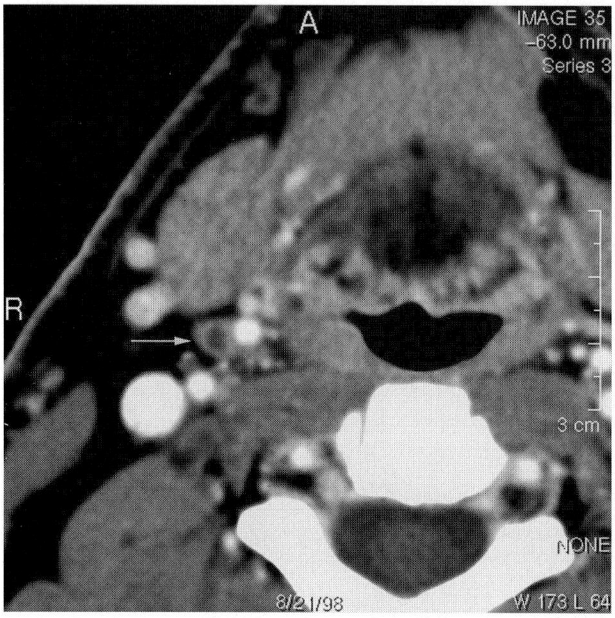

Figure 90G. Patient 1 with a fistula of the second branchial cleft anomaly, showing a tract (*arrow*) of the fistula between the internal and external carotid arteries, indicating second branchial cleft anomaly. Contrast-enhanced computed tomography image.

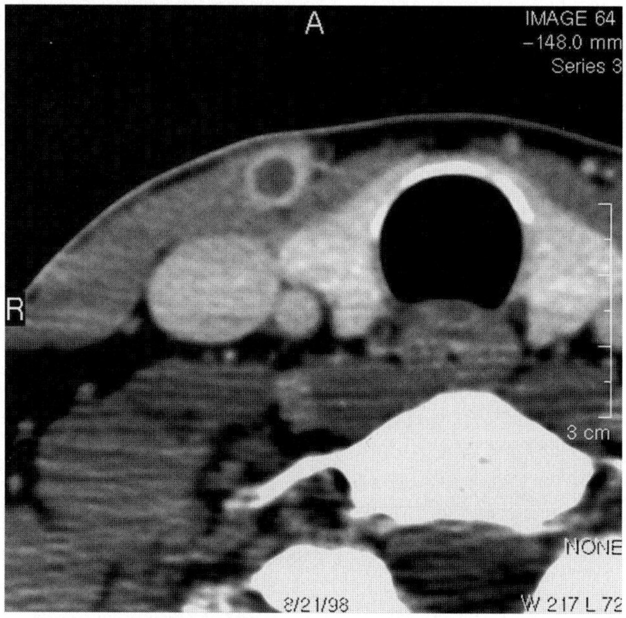

Figure 90H. Patient 1 with a fistula of the second branchial apparatus anomaly. Contrast-enhanced computed tomography image inferior to Fig. 90F showing the tract extending to the anterior edge of the sternocleidomastoid muscle.

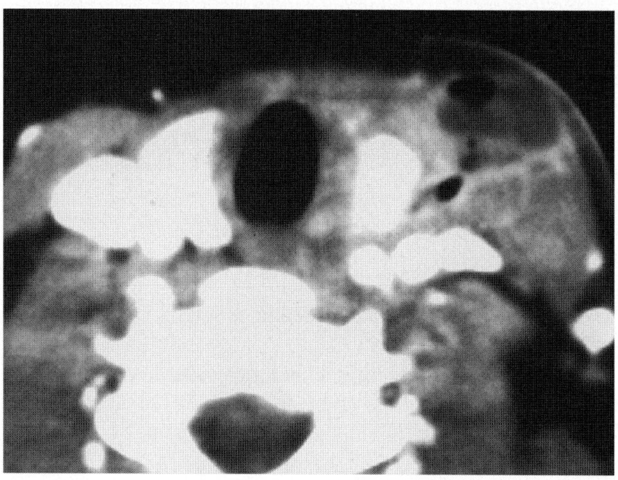

Figure 90I. Patient 2 with recurrent infection in the left lateral neck caused by a fourth branchial cleft anomaly, showing an abscess anterolateral to the left lobe of the thyroid gland. Contrast-enhanced computed tomography image.

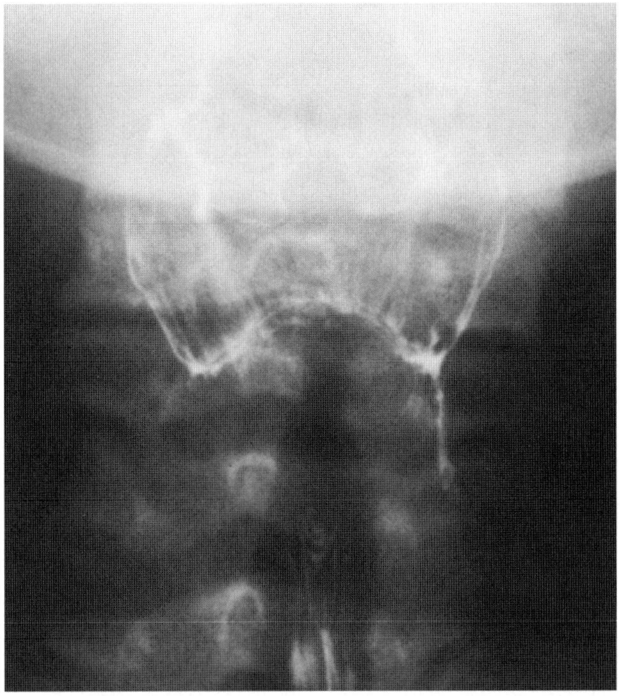

Figure 90J. Patient 2 with recurrent infection in the left lateral neck caused by a fourth branchial cleft anomaly. Pharyngography with Valsalva's maneuver showing the fistula extending from the apex of the left pyriform sinus, representing a presumed fourth branchial cleft anomaly.

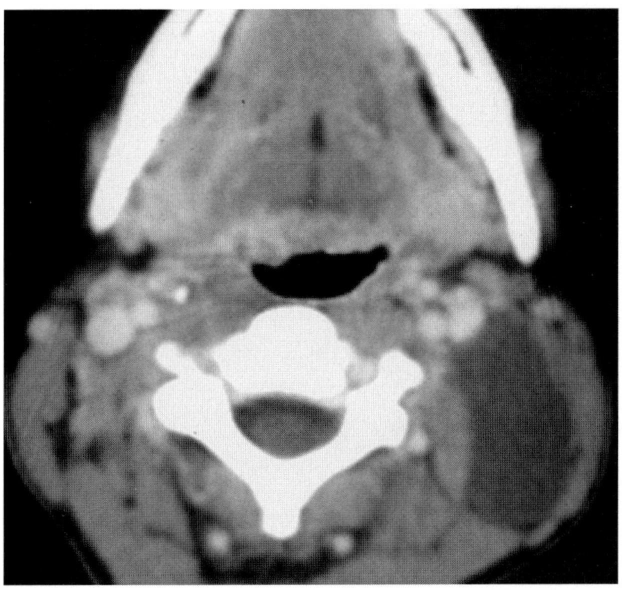

Figure 90K. Patient 3 with a third branchial cleft cyst, showing a unilocular cystic mass posterior to the carotid artery and internal jugular vein, involving the posterior triangle on the left.

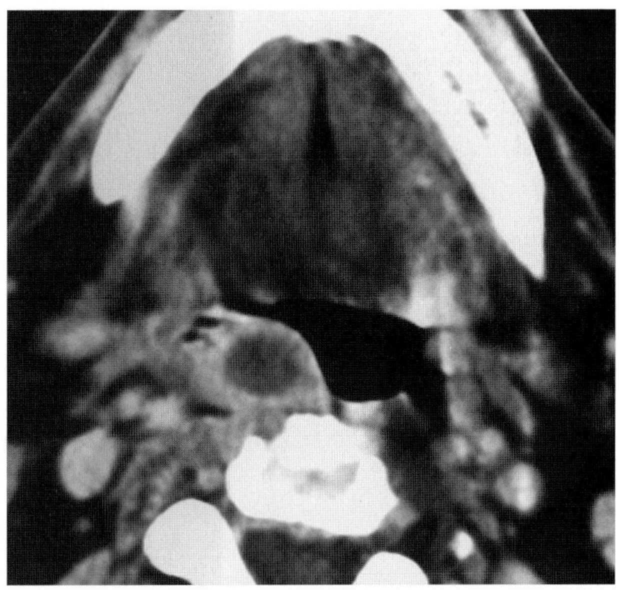

Figure 90L. Patient 4 with a Bailey type IV second branchial cleft cyst showing unilocular cystic mass within pharyngeal wall on the right. Contrast-enhanced computed tomography image.

CHAPTER 10

LARYNX AND HYPOPHARYNX

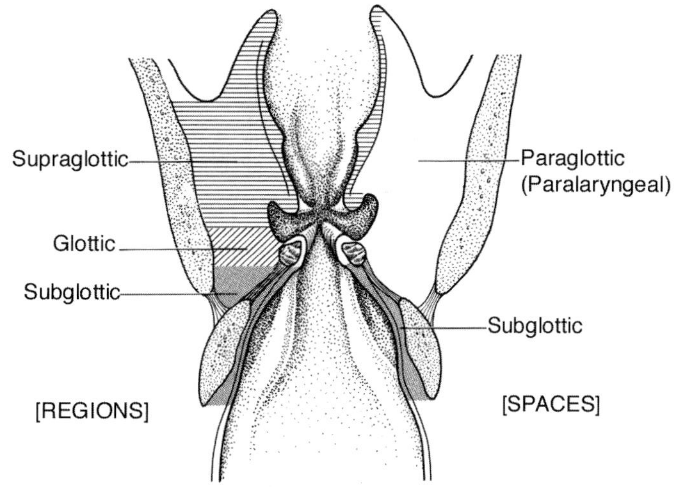

CASE 91

Clinical History: A 51-year-old man presents with left vocal cord paralysis.

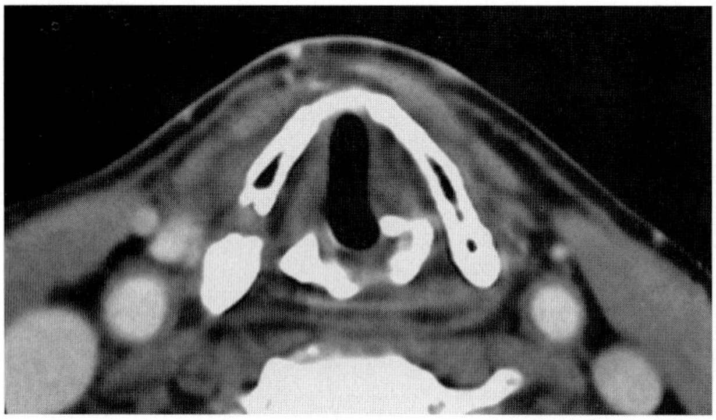

Figure 91A

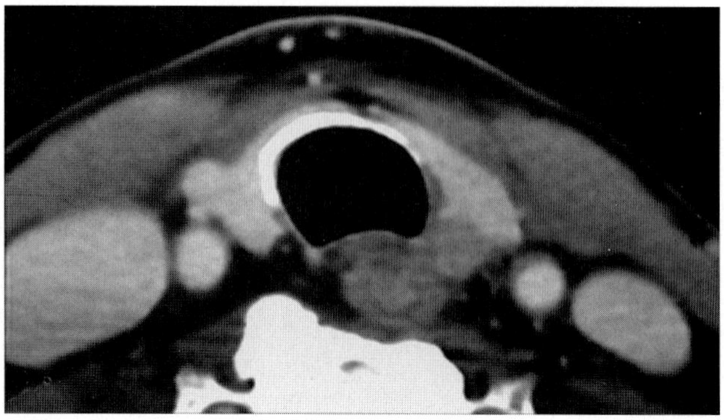

Figure 91B

1. What is the primary responsibility of the radiologist in evaluating a patient with vocal cord paralysis? (Hint: vagal nerve deficit.)
2. Where is the causative lesion?
3. Name four anatomic areas where causes for isolated vocal cord paralysis (on the left) are likely to be found.
4. What radiologic study should be done *before* a magnetic resonance imaging (MRI) or computed tomography (CT) study for this patient?

Findings

An abnormal soft tissue lesion arising from the posterior aspect of the left lobe of the thyroid gland. It directly involves the tracheoesophageal groove where the left recurrent nerve ascends. A CT image at the level of the true vocal cords shows an anteromedial position of the vocal process of the left arytenoid cartilage in association with a medial position of the true vocal cord and a possibly partially atrophic thyroarytenoid muscle.

Problem

A middle-aged man with left vocal cord paralysis and an infiltrating mass in the left tracheoesophageal groove

Anatomy

A. Course of the vagus and recurrent laryngeal nerve: brainstem (see Fig. 18F), medullary cistern, jugular fossa, poststyloid parapharyngeal space, carotid sheath to the thoracic inlet, recurrent laryngeal nerve (aortopulmonary window on left or subclavian artery on right), ascending in the tracheoesophageal groove on both sides to penetrate the cricothyroid membrane
B. Larynx: intrinsic musculature

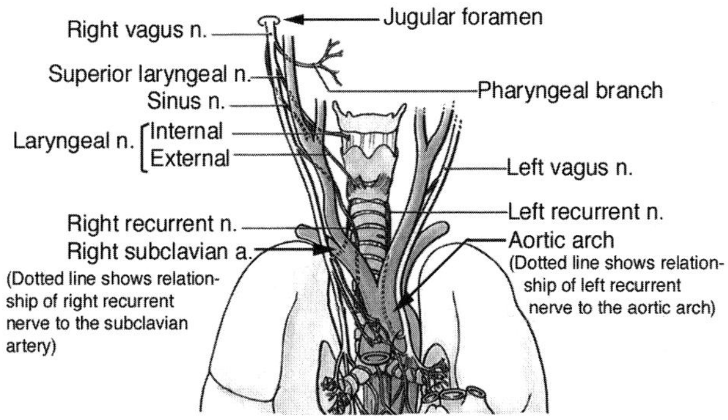

Figure 91C

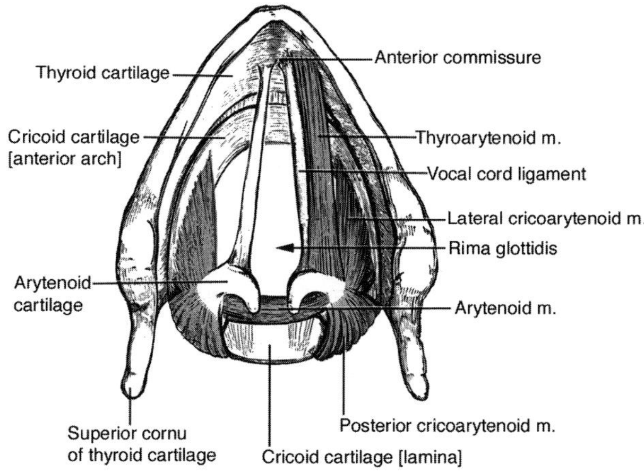

Figure 91D

Differential Diagnosis

Not appropriate for this specific case; by site, some causative lesions would include:

1. Brainstem: glioma
2. Medullary cistern: meningioma
3. Jugular fossa, poststyloid parapharyngeal space, carotid sheath: paraganglioma, schwannoma
4. Thoracic inlet: metastases, superior sulcus tumor
5. A-P window: lung cancer (nodal metastases or central primary tumor)
6. Tracheoesophageal groove: thyroid cancer
7. Larynx: submucosal malignancy, old trauma

Diagnosis

Thyroid carcinoma infiltrating the recurrent laryngeal nerve, with secondary vocal cord paralysis

Diagnostic Imaging Approach

A. Look for a mass or infiltrating process in all anatomic locations listed in the *Anatomy* section above.
B. Determine the site, structure, or organ of origin of the disease process.
C. Evaluate morphology: margins (for aggressiveness), associated edema, density, T1- or T2-weighted signal intensity, enhancement, vascularity, blood products, calcifications.

Clinical Points Of Importance And Supplemental Information

A. Imaging evaluation of cranial nerve deficits requires study of the entire course of the nerve at risk, from its brainstem nucleus(i) of origin to its end organ.
B. In many cases of vocal cord paralysis, the cause goes unproved. Careful imaging, however, is necessary to exclude a structural lesion along the nerve or within the larynx.

Answers To Questions

1. Study the vagus and recurrent laryngeal nerves from their nuclei of origin to end organs
2. Thyroid gland
3. Medullary cistern(s), jugular fossa, aortopulmonary window, larynx
4. Chest x-ray study

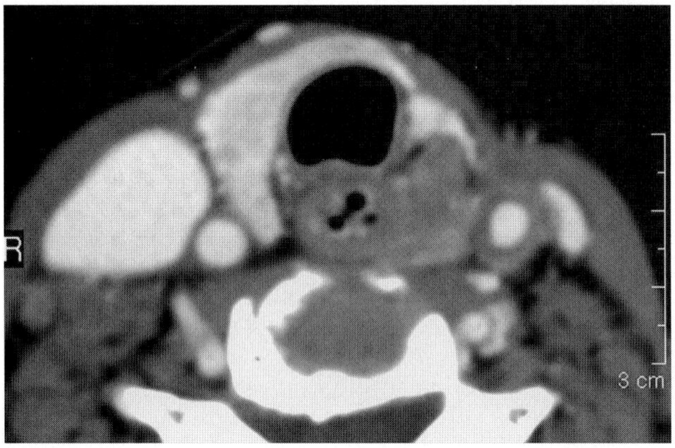

Figure 91E. Patient 1 with true vocal cord paralysis caused by recurrent nerve palsy from carcinoma of the cervical esophagus, showing an infiltrative mass involving the tracheoesophageal groove on the left. Contrast-enhanced computed tomography image.

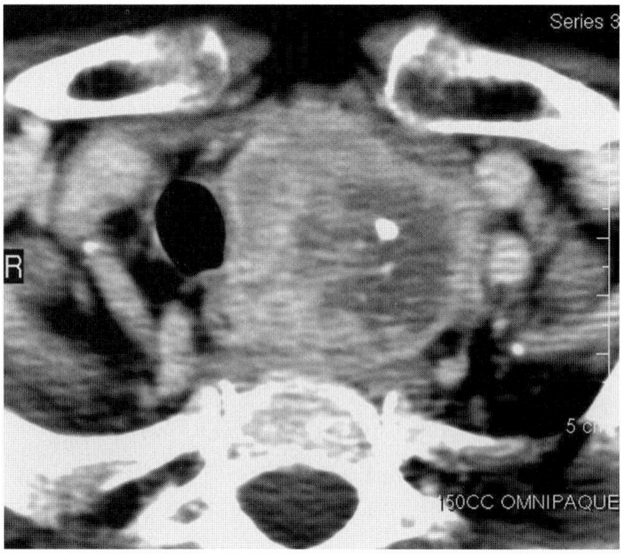

Figure 91F. Patient 2 with true vocal cord paralysis caused by recurrent nerve palsy from anaplastic carcinoma of the thyroid gland, showing an infiltrative mass arising from the left lobe of the thyroid gland with involvement of the left tracheoesophageal groove. Contrast-enhanced computed tomography image.

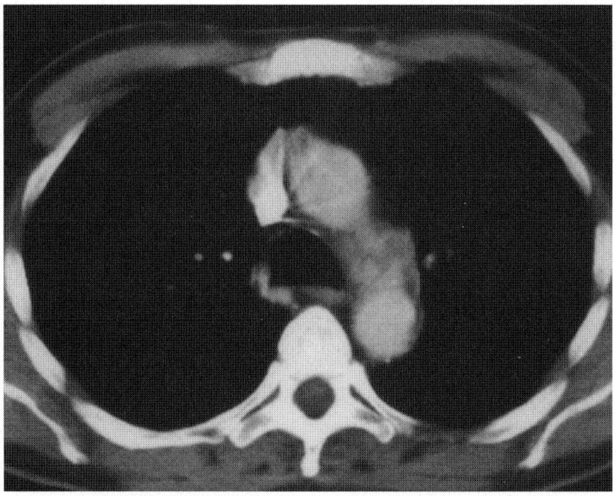

Figure 91G. Patient 3 with metastasis to the aortopulmonary window from lung carcinoma, showing the enlarged aortopulmonary window lymph nodes. (The first clinical presentation was the recurrent nerve palsy. Chest plain radiograph was negative at that time.) Contrast-enhanced computed tomography image.

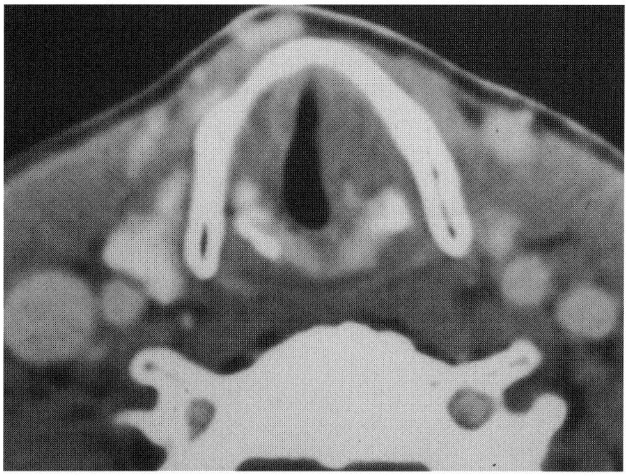

Figure 91H. Patient 4 in whom is seen clinical suspicion of the true vocal cord paralysis even after laryngoscopy until this study showed a submucosal infiltrative process involving the left true cord that was eventually proved to be non-Hodgkin lymphoma. Contrast-enhanced computed tomography image.

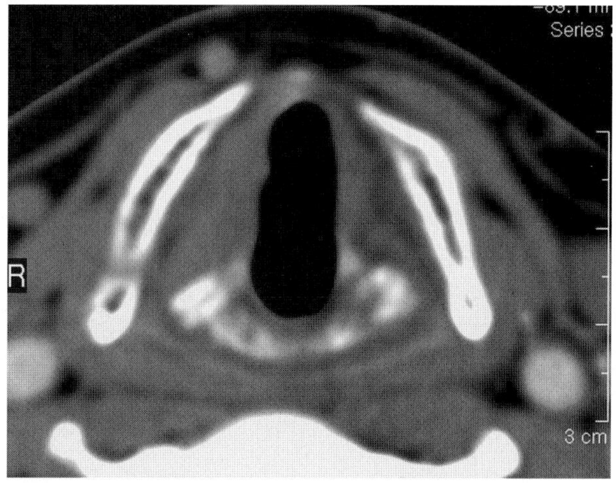

Figure 91I. Patient 5 with vocal cord paralysis of unknown cause, showing atrophic change (fatty infiltration) of the lateral and medial thyroarytenoid muscles on the left. Contrast-enhanced computed tomography image.

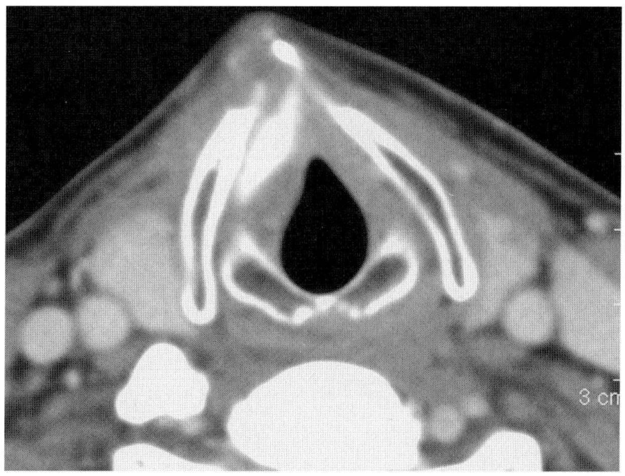

Figure 91J. Patient 6 with cranial nerve X palsy. Contrast-enhanced computed tomography image at the level of the undersurface of the true cord showing radioopaque material injected into the right paraglottic space to compensate atrophied true cord.

CASE 92

Clinical History: A 52-year-old woman presents with hoarseness, dysphagia, and a submucosal laryngeal mass.

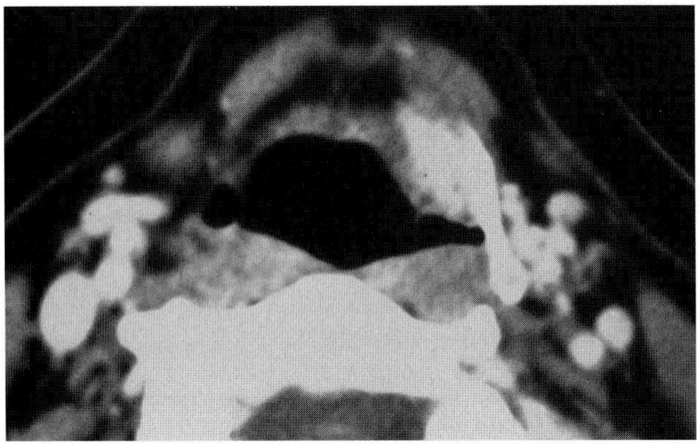

Figure 92A

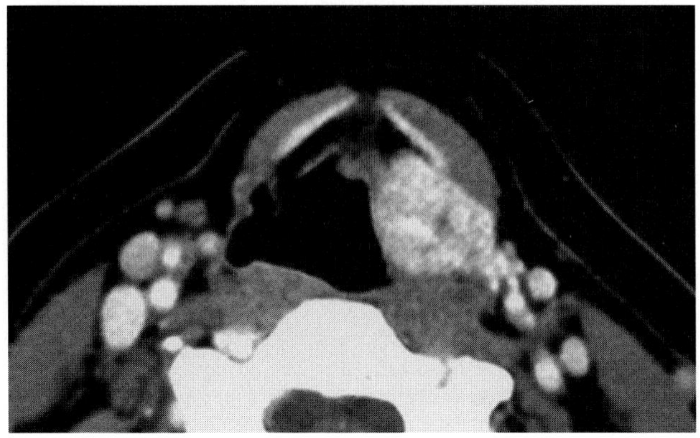

Figure 92B

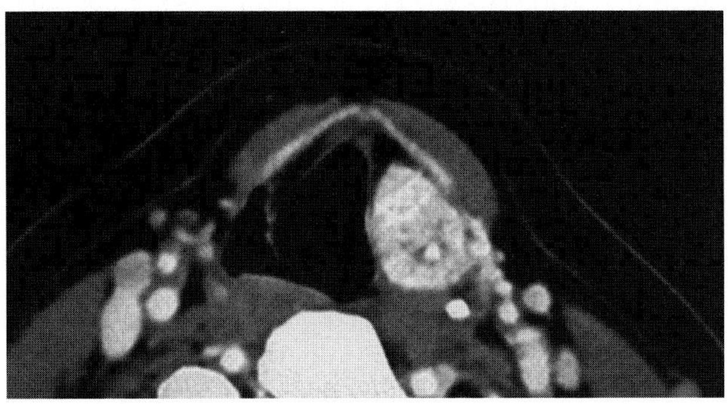

Figure 92C

1. What subdivision of the larynx is involved?
2. List the three main causes of a submucosal laryngeal mass.
3. List three reasons why a mass in the larynx might be submucosal.

Findings

An intensely enhancing mass in left aryepiglottic fold, false vocal cord, and adjacent paraglottic space of the supraglottic larynx. No extralaryngeal spread is noted. The superior laryngeal vessels are markedly enlarged and a prominent vascular pedicle is seen in the mass.

Problem

A middle-aged woman with an intensely enhancing, submucosal mass of the supraglottic larynx

Anatomy

A. Larynx: supraglottis, glottis, and subglottis, including all major mucosal landmarks, deep spaces, cartilages, and connecting membranes or ligaments
B. Superior laryngeal neurovascular bundle
C. Hypopharynx: pyriform sinus, posterior pharyngeal wall, postcricoid region

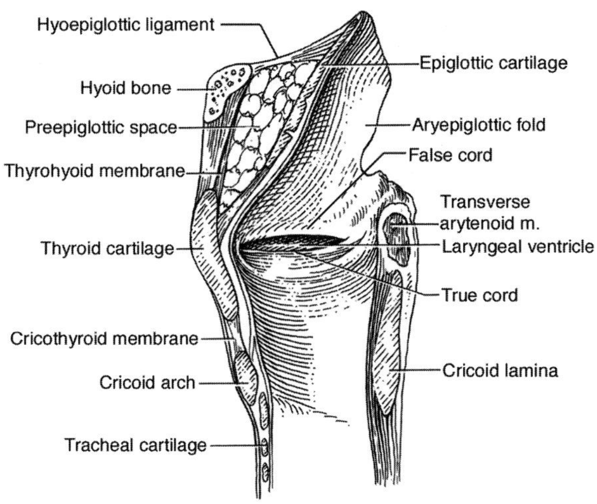

Figure 92D

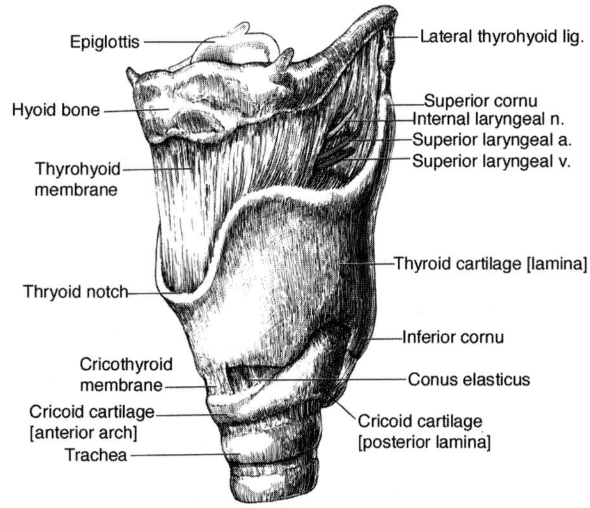

Figure 92E

Differential Diagnosis

Squamous cell carcinoma, arising in laryngeal ventricle or saccule; adenocarcinoma, adenoidcystic carcinoma, or mucoepidermoid carcinoma arising in minor salivary rests within the paraglottic or preepiglottic space (also benign salivary gland tumors); laryngocele or laryngopyocele caused by obstruction of the laryngeal saccule; chondrosarcoma from cartilages (cricoid being the most common origin); sarcoma from mesenchymal elements; old trauma or congenital deformities of the laryngeal skeleton causing a "pseudomass"

Diagnosis

Paraganglioma of the aryepiglottic fold (supraglottic larynx)

Diagnostic Imaging Approach

A. Identify the specific site of origin within the larynx.
B. Identify morphologic characteristics that might be atypical for squamous cell carcinoma, such as excessive enhancement, extensive edema, obviously cystic character, calcified matrix.

Clinical Points Of Importance And Supplemental Information

Entirely submucosal masses of the larynx are very uncommon; 50% will be squamous cell carcinomas, 25% will be laryngoceles, with the other 25% scattered among the causes listed under *Differential Diagnosis* (above).

Answers To Questions

1. Supraglottic
2. Carcinoma, laryngocele, and chondroid lesion of the cricoid or thyroid cartilage
3. Begins submucosally, or in the ventricle, or the source is the laryngeal skeleton

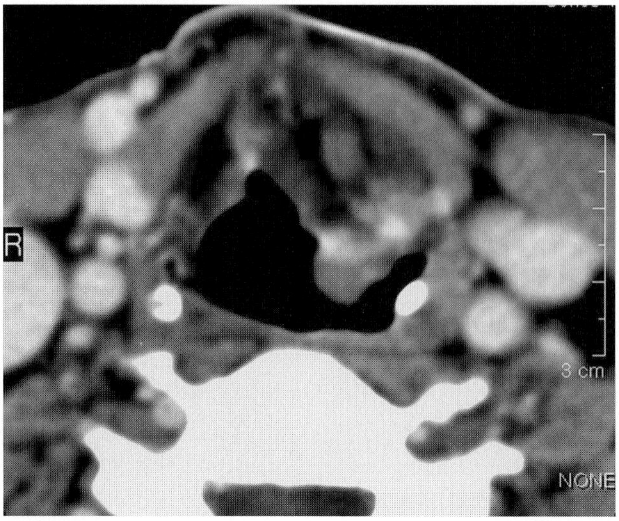

Figure 92F. Patient 1 with a cavernous vascular malformation of the larynx, showing an enhancing, submucosal lesion involving the aryepiglottic fold on the left. Contrast-enhanced computed tomography image.

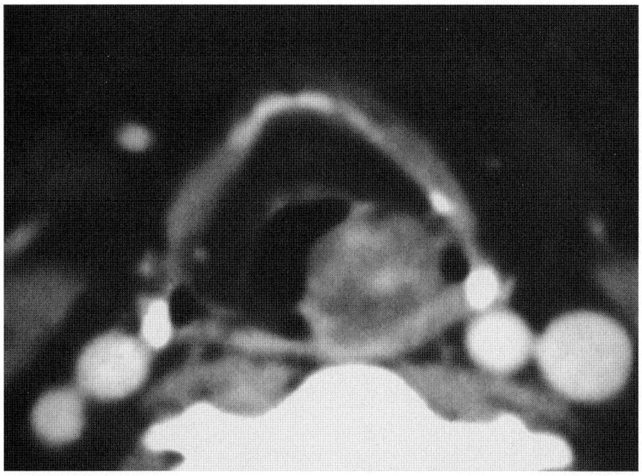

Figure 92G. Patient 2 with cavernous vascular malformation of the supraglottis, showing the enhancing mass involving the aryepiglottic fold on the left. Contrast-enhanced computed tomography image.

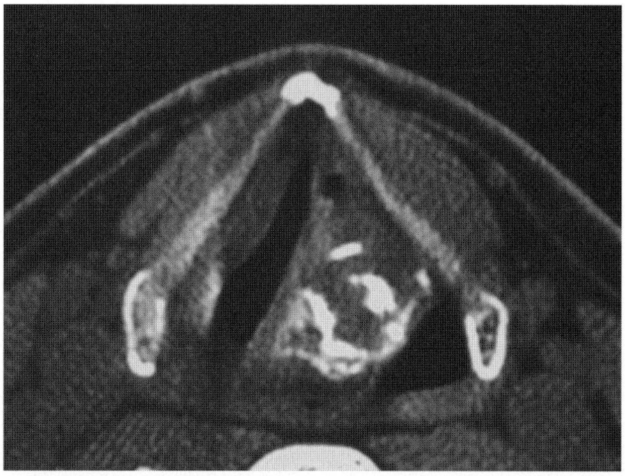

Figure 92H. Patient 3 with low-grade chondrosarcoma of the cricoid cartilage, showing a mass with mineralization in the paraglottic space, displacing the arytenoid cartilage posteromedially. Computed tomography image without contrast.

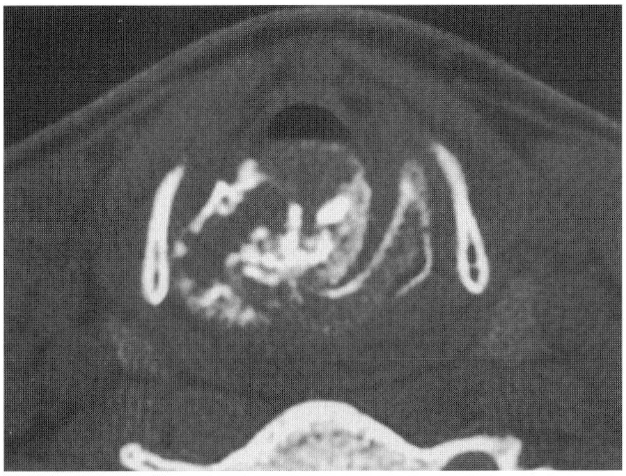

Figure 92I. Patient 3 with low-grade chondrosarcoma of the cricoid cartilage. Computed tomography image inferior to Fig. 92H showing the mass arising from the superolateral aspect of the lamina of cricoid cartilage on the right and protruding into the subglottic larynx.

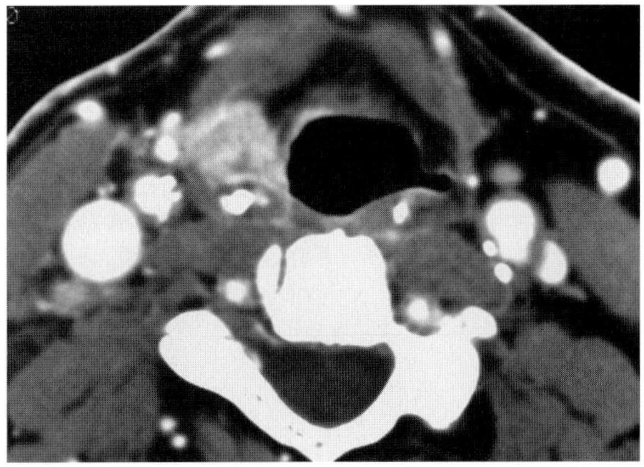

Figure 92J. Patient 4 with a largely submucosal laryngeal carcinoma, showing an infiltrative, enhancing mass involving the upper aryepiglottic fold and paraglottic space on the right, with early extralaryngeal spread via the superior laryngeal neurovascular bundle through the thyrohyoid membrane. Contrast-enhanced computed tomography image.

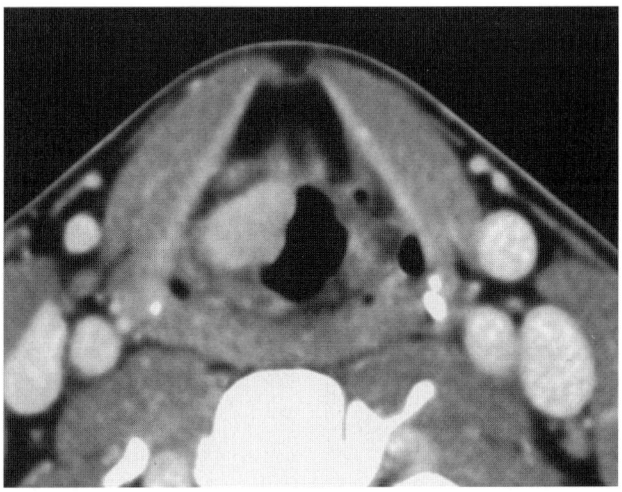

Figure 92K. Patient 5 with leiomyoma of the supraglottic larynx. Contrast-enhanced computed tomography image showing a partially exophytic, relatively well-defined mass involving the false cord on the right.

CASE 93

Clinical History: A 69-year-old man presents with hoarseness and a biopsy proved squamous cell carcinoma of the larynx.

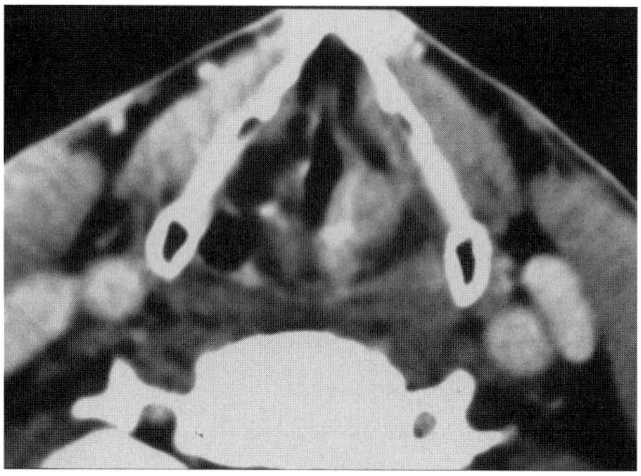

Figure 93A

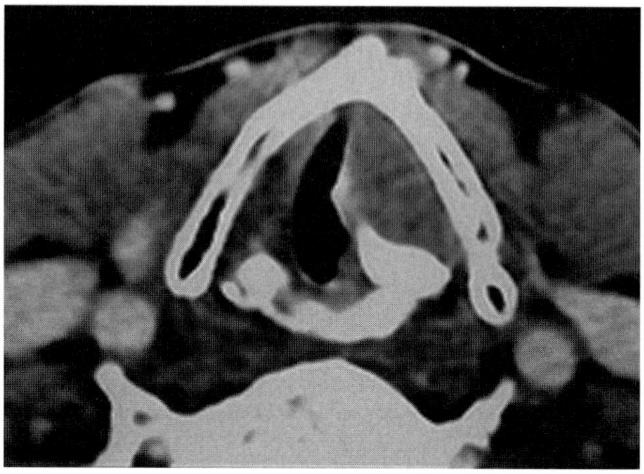

Figure 93B

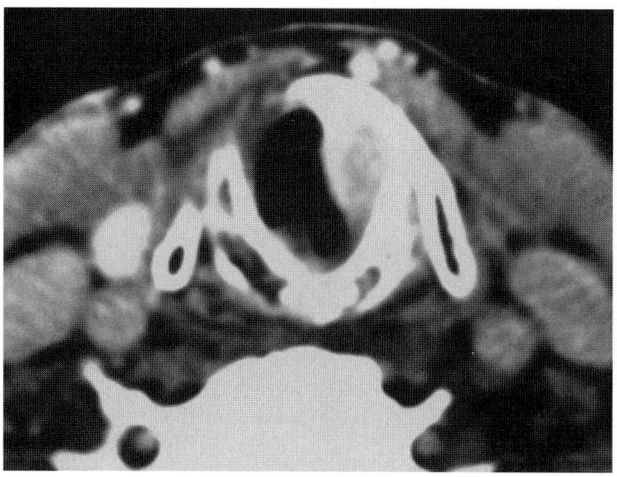

Figure 93C

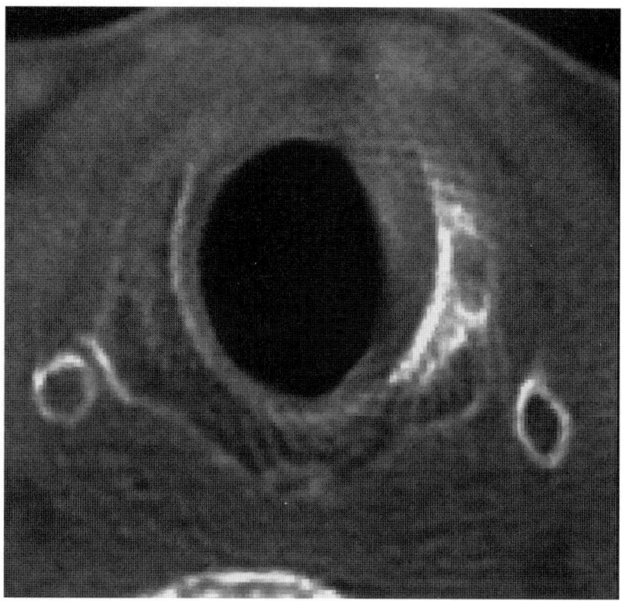

Figure 93D

1. What part (subdivision) of the larynx is involved?
2. Is the patient suitable for a vertical hemilaryngectomy? The decision *can* be made on the basis of these four images. Defend your answer with one or two good reasons.
3. The cricoid cartilage is sclerotic. What are the chances it is invaded based on that finding?

Findings

An abnormal soft tissue mass centered in left true vocal cord invading the paraglottic space and extending superiorly along the left aryepiglottic fold to the posterior aspect of the left false vocal cord. The lesion involves the left cricoarytenoid joint and extends into subglottic space. The left lateral aspect of the cricoid cartilage is sclerotic.

Problem

A patient with laryngeal squamous cell carcinoma and a need to determine if the lesion is suitable for voice conservation surgery

Anatomy

A. True vocal cord: anterior commissure, paraglottic space, arytenoid (all parts)
B. Subglottis: define its limits, cricothyroid membrane
C. Laryngeal ventricle
D. False vocal cord: paraglottic space
E. Cricoid cartilage: arches, lamina
F. Thyroid cartilage

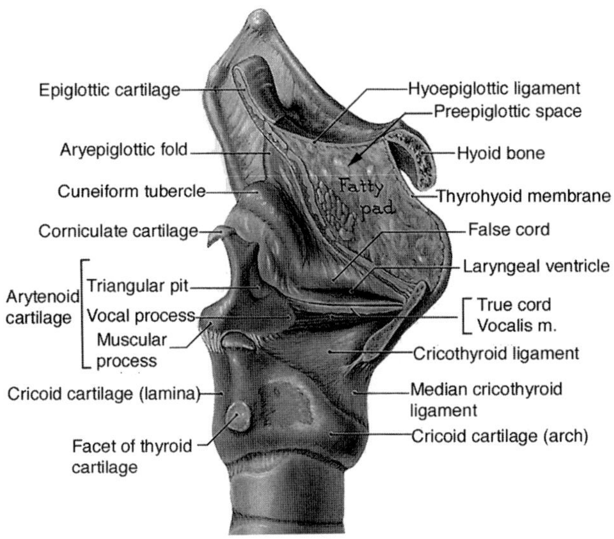

Figure 93E

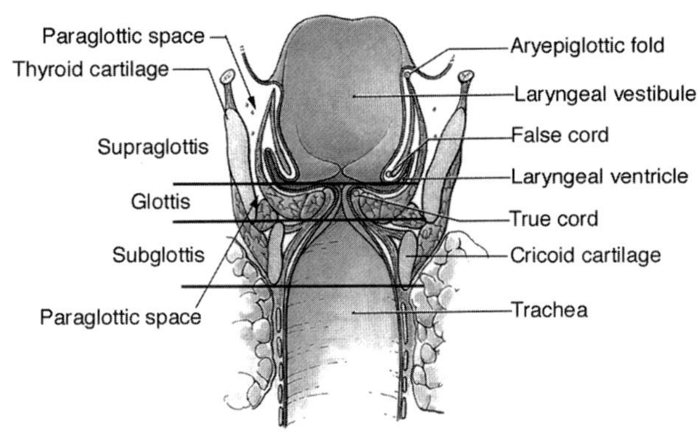

Figure 93F

Differential Diagnosis

Not applicable

Diagnosis

True vocal cord carcinoma, with subglottic spread; the cartilage sclerosis indicates an approximately 50% chance of cartilage invasion

Diagnostic Imaging Approach

A. Identify the specific site of origin.
B. Evaluate the local extent: anterior commissure, paraglottic space, ventricle, false cord, and amount of subglottic spread.
C. Is there cartilage involvement (thyroid, cricoid, arytenoid)?
D. Is there extralaryngeal spread?
E. Is there regional adenopathy?
F. Is there a second primary tumor?

Clinical Points Of Importance And Supplemental Information

A. A tumor adjacent to the cricoid cartilage (subglottic spread) makes the patient unsuitable for vertical hemilaryngectomy; surgical treatment would have to include a total laryngectomy, based on the imaging findings.
B. The relatively high risk of cartilage invasion would also suggest total laryngectomy as the best surgical option.

C. Treatment with radiotherapy would preserve the larynx, but a lesion with this imaging profile has only a 40% to 50% chance of local control, so that postradiotherapy surveillance would have to be very diligent and include periodic follow-up imaging.
D. Care surveillance helps detect recurrent tumor, whereas local control by total laryngectomy is still likely to be successful.

Answers To Questions

1. Glottic and subglottic
2. No. The tumor is next to the cricoid and interarytenoid cartilage.
3. 50%

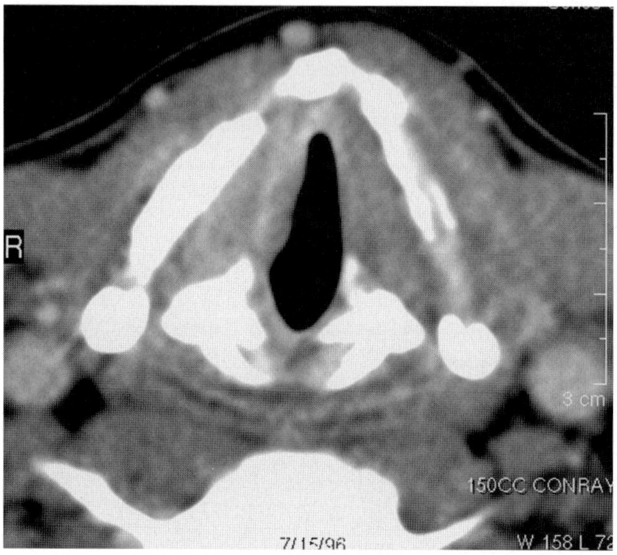

Figure 93G. Patient 1 with glottic carcinoma, showing irregular thickening of the right true cord and anterior commissure, with obliteration of a fat plane in the paraglottic space on the right. Contrast-enhanced computed tomography image at the level of the true vocal cord.

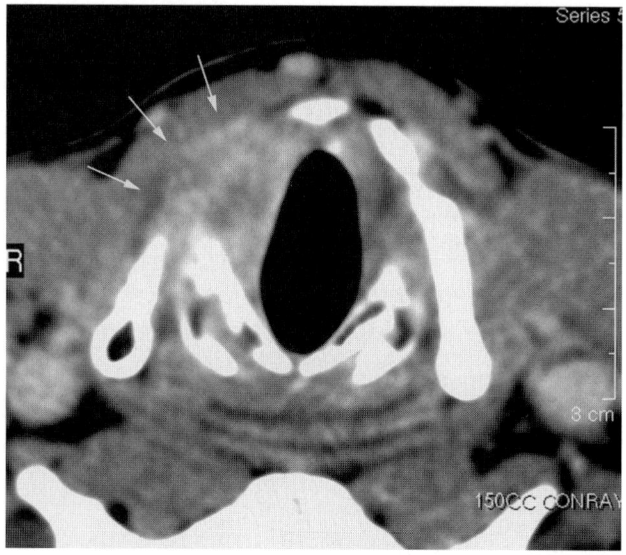

Figure 93H. Patient 1 with glottic carcinoma. Contrast-enhanced computed tomography at the level of the undersurface of the true vocal cord showing inferior spread of the tumor directly abutting on the inner surface of the cricoid cartilage, with extralaryngeal spread (*arrows*) through the cricothyroid membrane on the right.

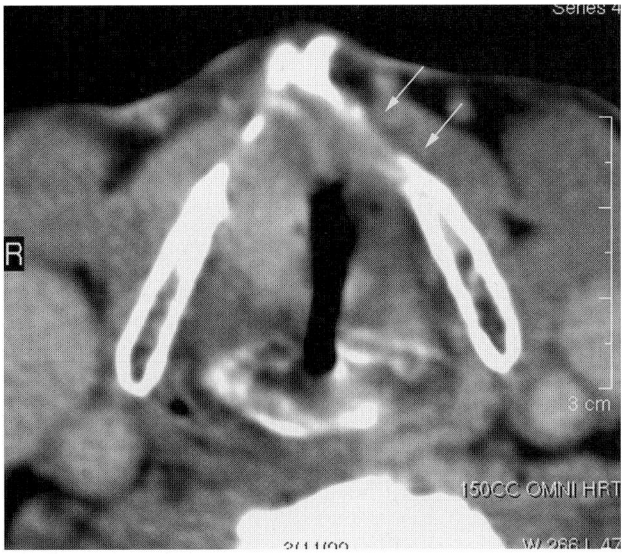

Figure 93I. Patient 2 with glottic carcinoma, showing an infiltrative process involving the anterior two thirds of the right true vocal cord, with obliteration of the fat plane in the paraglottic space. Also noted is obliteration of a fat plane external to the right lamina of thyroid cartilage anteriorly (see the normal one on the left side [*arrows*]), which is suggestive of early extralaryngeal spread. Contrast-enhanced computed tomography image.

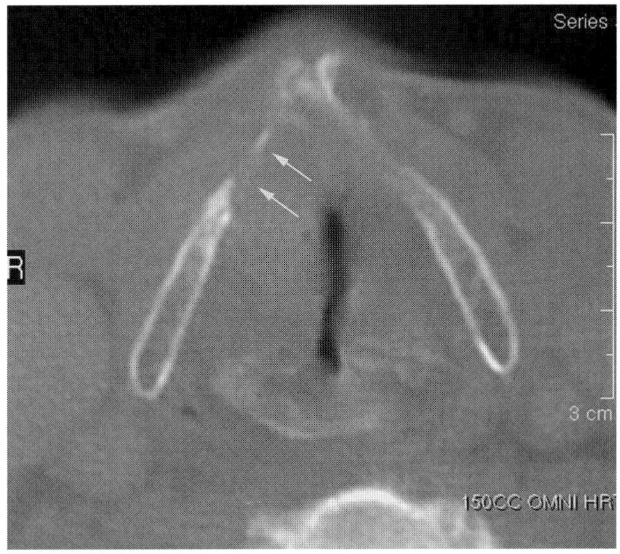

Figure 93J. Patient 2 with glottic carcinoma. Computed tomography image at the same level as Fig. 93I at bone window setting showing erosion at the inner surface of the thyroid lamina on the right.

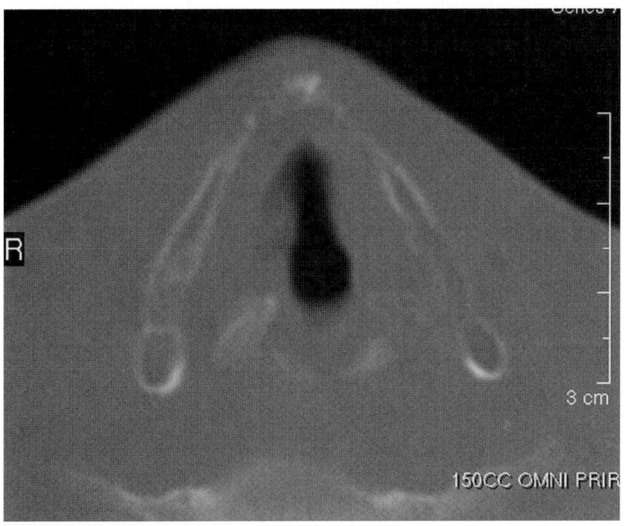

Figure 93K. Patient 3 with transglottic carcinoma. Computed tomography image at bone window setting showing sclerotic change of the arytenoid cartilage and, possibly, of the thyroid cartilage. Irregularity of the thyroid cartilage in the area of the anterior commissure is equivocal for cartilage invasion.

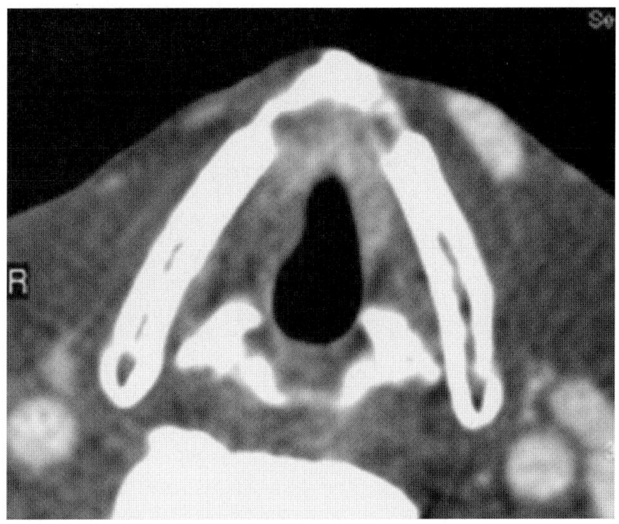

Figure 93L. Patient 4 with glottic carcinoma. Contrast-enhanced computed tomography image at the true vocal cord level showing an infiltrative process involving the left true vocal cord and extending into the anterior one third of the right true vocal cord across the anterior commissure. Early erosion of the thyroid cartilage is suspicious.

CASE 94

Clinical History: A 71-year-old man presents with dysphagia, hoarseness, and biopsy proved squamous cell carcinoma of the larynx.

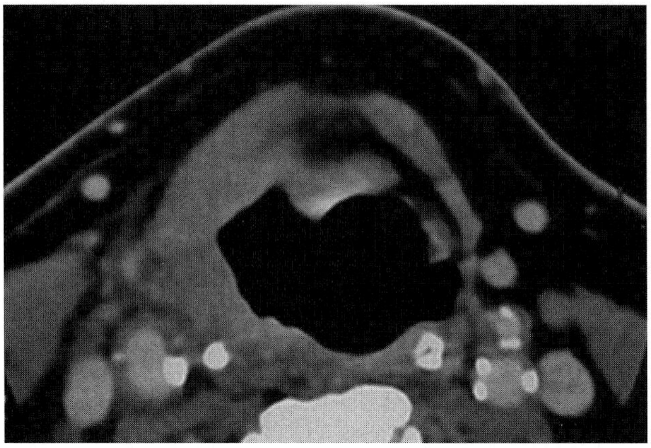

Figure 94A

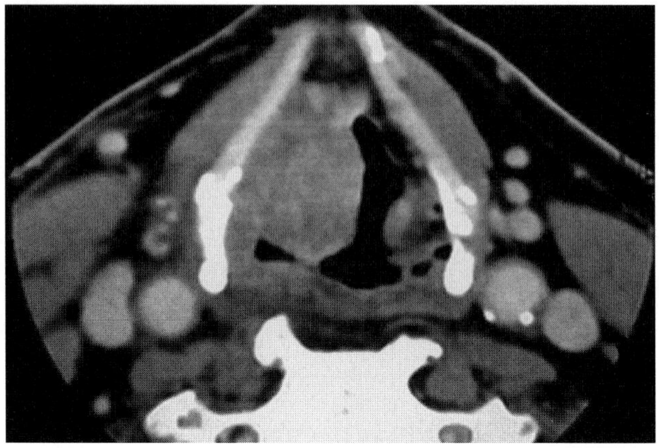

Figure 94B

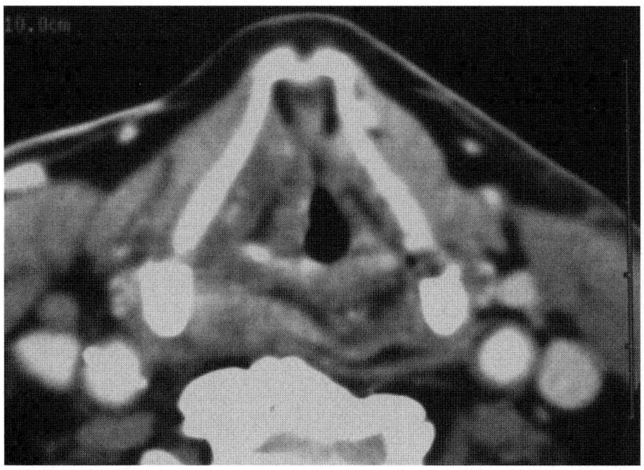

Figure 94C

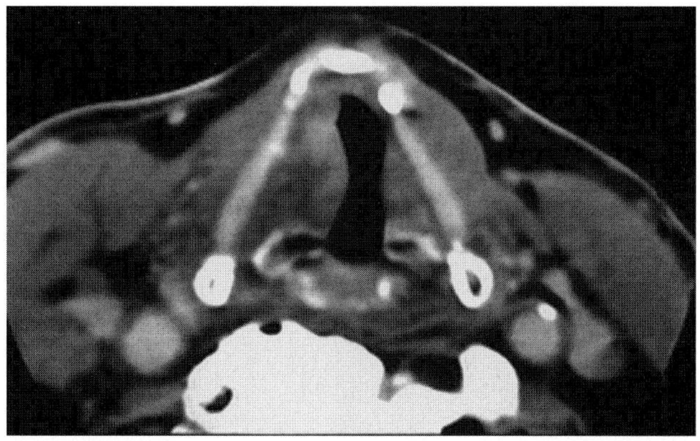

Figure 94D

1. What subdivision of the larynx is the site of origin?
2. Is the lesion suitable for partial (horizontal supraglottic) laryngectomy? The decision can be made on the basis of the images seen here. Defend your answer with two specific reasons (i.e., two critical areas are either involved or uninvolved).
3. What are the chances (in percentage) of nodal metastases from this primary tumor?
4. If nodal metastases are present with gross capsular penetration of the nodal disease, how is the prognosis affected? State this in terms of reduced survival for each finding.

Findings

An invasive soft tissue mass mainly in the right paraglottic space and the aryepiglottic fold with minimal preepiglottic space involvement. The lesion crosses the laryngeal ventricle to involve the anterior commissure anteroinferiorly and, within the right paraglottic space, has spread to the pharyngeal wall involving the right pyriform sinus posterolaterally at its apex and just above the apex.

Problem

A man with squamous cell carcinoma of the supraglottic larynx. Can the larynx be preserved with surgery (horizontal supraglottic laryngectomy)?

Anatomy

A. Supraglottic larynx: false vocal cords, epiglottis, aryepiglottic folds, paraglottic (paralaryngeal) space, preepiglottic space, thyroid cartilage, thyrohyoid membrane, hyoid bone, vallecula (see Fig. 92D)
B. Superior laryngeal neurovascular bundle (see Fig. 92E)
C. Hypopharynx: pyriform sinus, posterior pharyngeal wall, postcricoid region, esophageal verge (inlet)

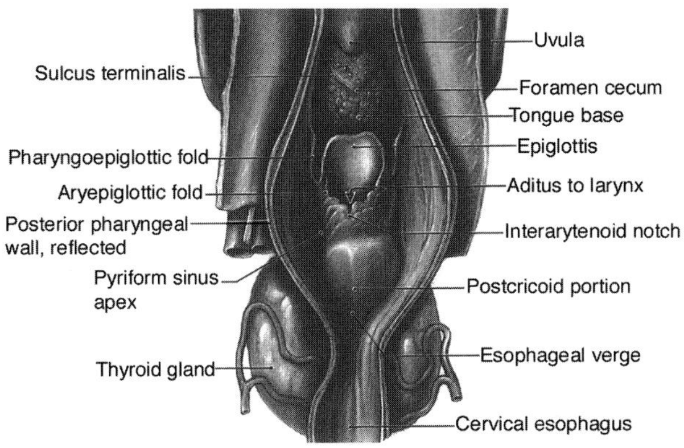

Figure 94E

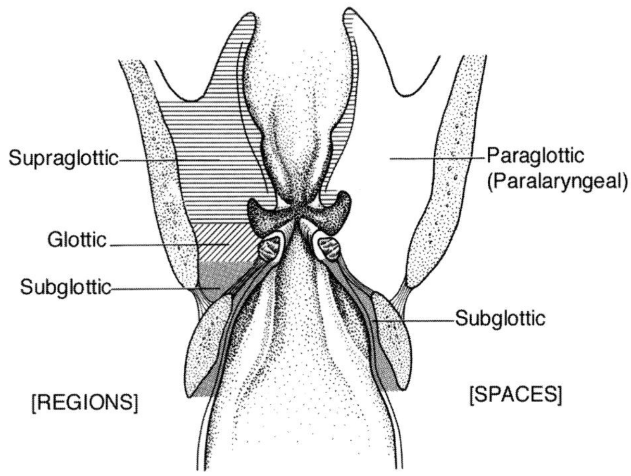

Figure 94F

Differential Diagnosis

Not applicable

Diagnosis

Squamous cell carcinoma of the supraglottic larynx (probably arising on the aryepiglottic fold—the so-called marginal supraglottic lesion), with early extralaryngeal spread and involvement of the anterior commissure and anterior third of the true vocal cord

Diagnostic Imaging Approach

A. Identify the laryngeal subdivision of origin.
B. Identify the specific site of origin (e.g., false vocal cord, aryepiglottic fold, epiglottis).
C. Determine the cephalocaudal extent of the lesion:
   1. True vocal cord involvement
   2. Proximity (in mm) from anterior commissure
   3. Proximity to arytenoid
   4. Vallecula or tongue base involvement
D. Is the pharynx involved?
E. Thyroid, cricoid, or arytenoid invasion?
F. Is there extralaryngeal spread (e.g., through thyrohyoid membrane, along the superior laryngeal neurovascular bundle)?
G. What are the first and second echelon nodes for supraglottic primary tumors? Are they involved?
H. If the nodes are involved, is there capsular penetration?
I. If capsular penetration is present, what is the extent of extranodal disease (e.g., perinodal fat, carotid fixation, fixation to the floor of the neck)?

Clinical Points Of Importance And Supplemental Information

Horizontal supraglottic laryngectomy requires at least a 3-mm tumor-free margin *above* the anterior commissure, with no thyroid cartilage invasion or extralaryngeal spread.

Answers To Questions

1. Supraglottic
2. No. The anterior commissure is involved and early extralaryngeal spread is likely.
3. At least 50%
4. Survival is cut in half in N+ vs. N− patients, and is cut in half again if gross nodal capsular penetration is also present

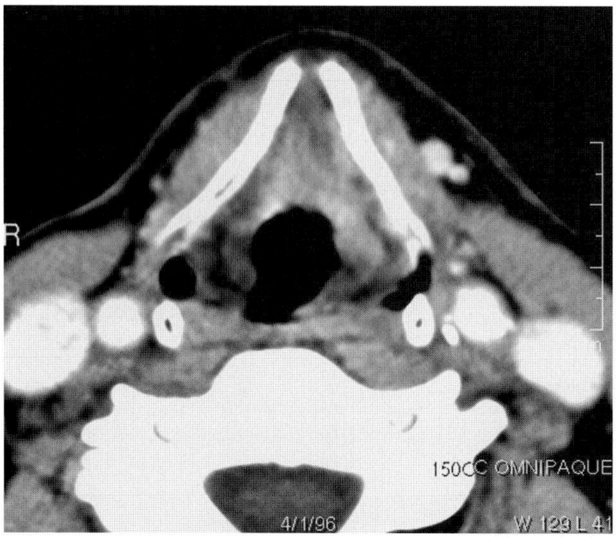

Figure 94G. Patient 1 with supraglottic carcinoma, showing an infiltrative process involving the low preepiglottic and left paraglottic spaces from the infrahyoid portion of epiglottis. Contrast-enhanced computed tomography image.

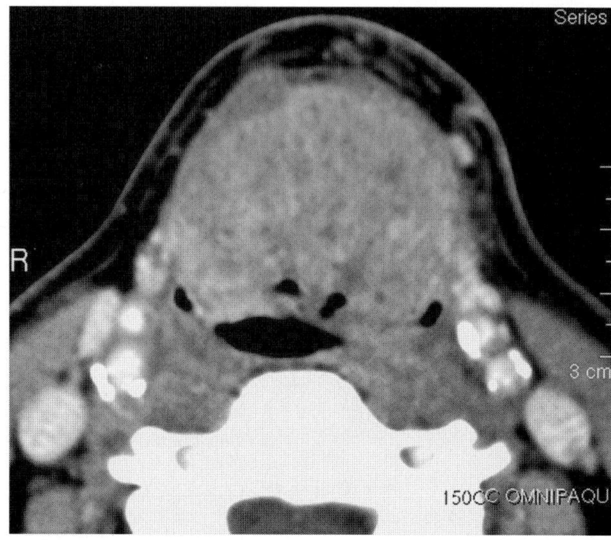

Figure 94H. Patient 1 with supraglottic carcinoma. Contrast-enhanced computed tomography image superior to Fig. 94E showing the tumor involving the entire preepiglottic space.

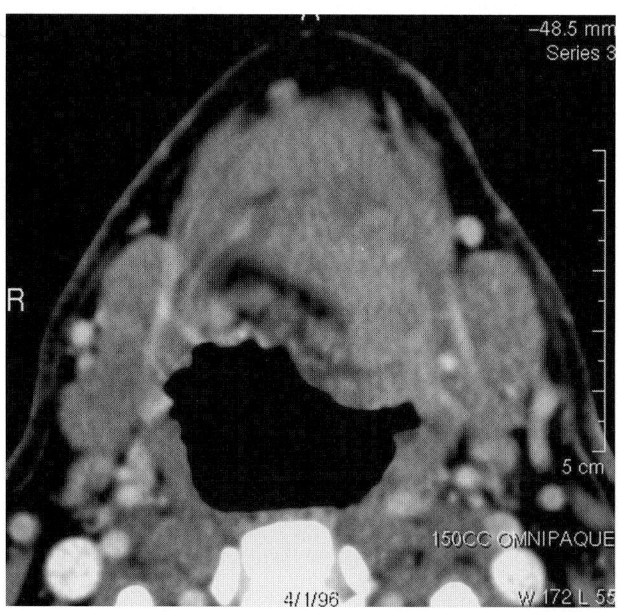

Figure 94I. Patient 1 with supraglottic carcinoma. Contrast-enhanced computed tomography image superior to Fig. 94F showing the tumor involving the tongue base on the left, with most of this extension being submucosal and clinically inapparent.

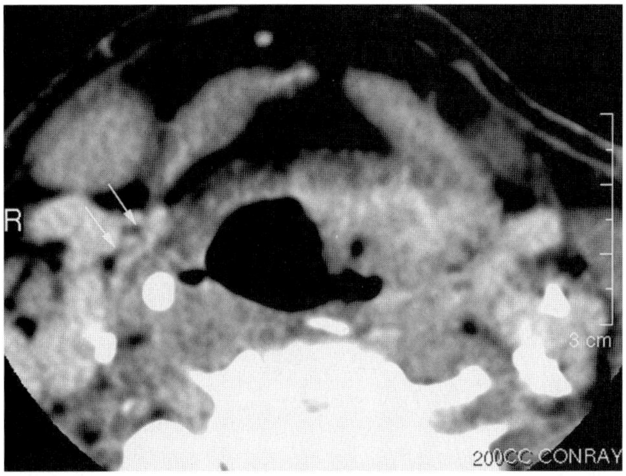

Figure 94J. Patient 2 with supraglottic carcinoma of the aryepiglottic fold, showing an infiltrative mass centered on the left aryepiglottic fold, with early extralaryngeal spread through the thyrohyoid membrane, probably along the superior laryngeal neurovascular bundle (see the normal superior laryngeal artery on the right [*arrows*]). Contrast-enhanced computed tomography image.

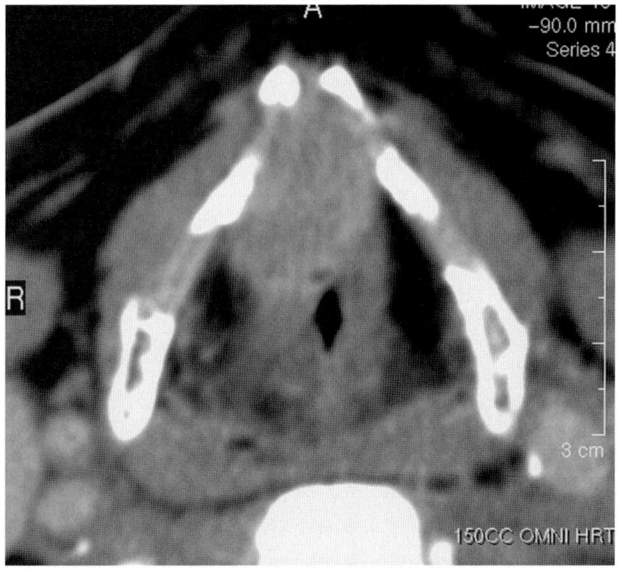

Figure 94K. Patient 3 with an anterior commissure-type transglottic carcinoma, showing an entirely submucosal mass involving the inferior portion of the preepiglottic space.

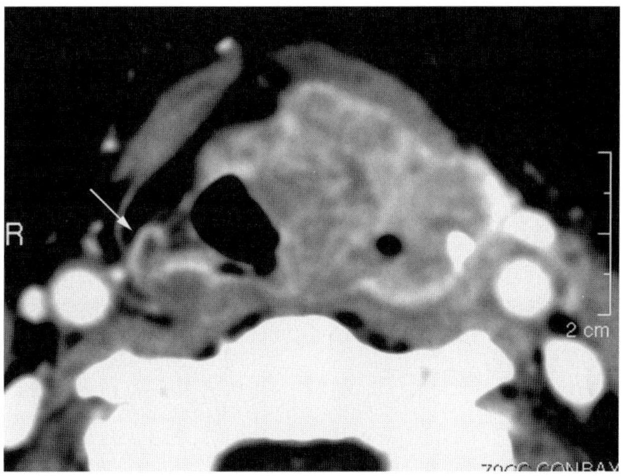

Figure 94L. Patient 4 with a hybrid type carcinoma of the supraglottic and pyriform sinus, showing an infiltrative mass involving the upper pyriform sinus and supraglottis, with extralaryngeal spread along the superior laryngeal neurovascular bundle (*arrows* on the opposite side) into the soft tissue of the neck.

CASE 95

Clinical History: A 65-year-old man with dysphagia presents. He had been told that he has an incurable cancer that is causing this symptom.

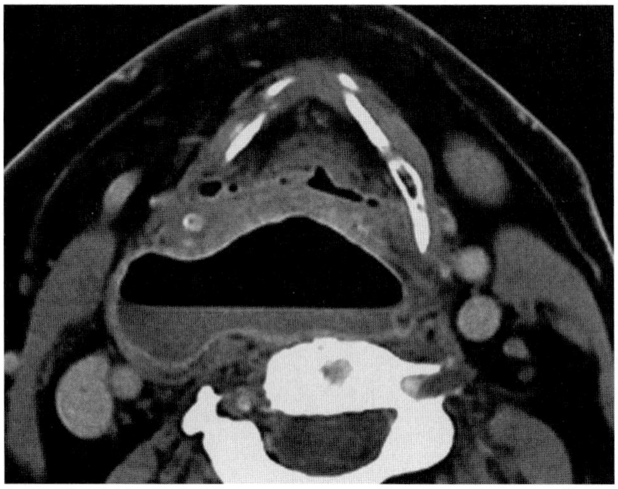

Figure 95A

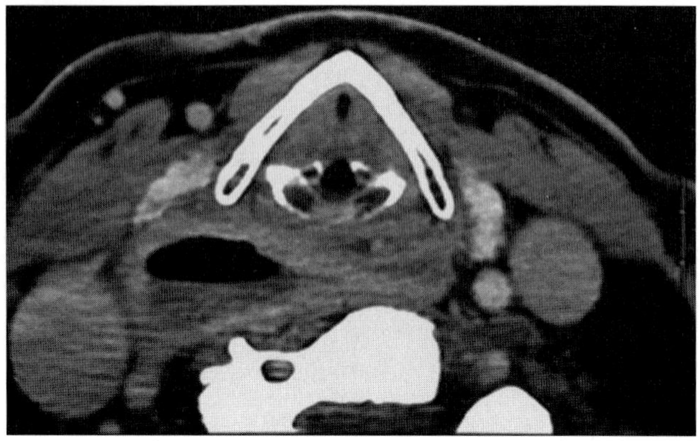

Figure 95B

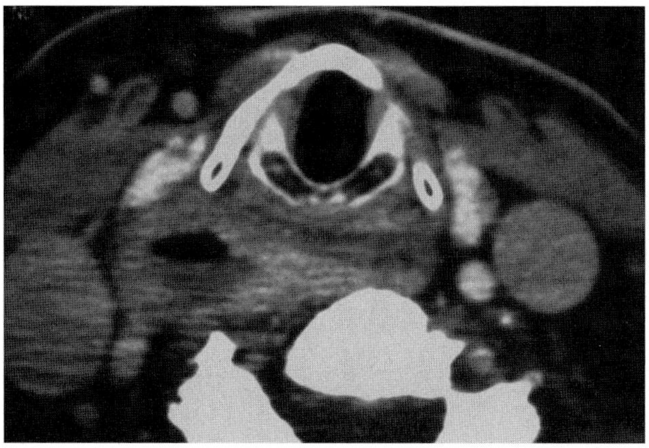

Figure 95C

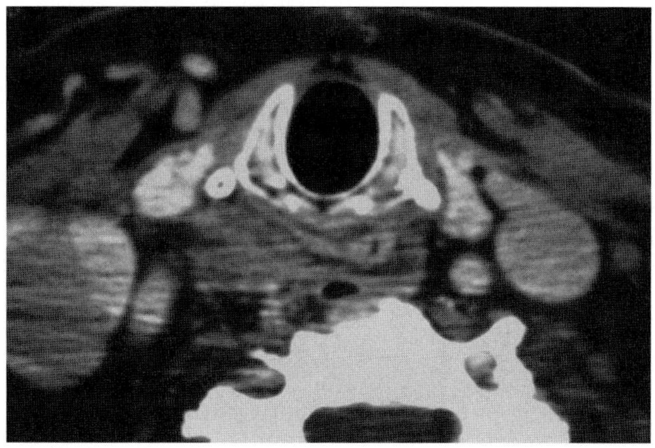

Figure 95D

1. What compartment(s) or space(s) is involved?
2. What is the specific diagnosis?
3. What is the better study—magnetic resonance imaging (MRI) or computed tomography (CT)—for identifying a mass in the wall of the postcricoid hypopharynx or cervical esophagus?

Findings

A unilocular cystic mass with an air–fluid level between the posterior pharyngeal wall and prevertebral muscles (in the retropharyngeal space) from at least the upper hypopharynx (it actually extended to the low oropharynx level) to the postcricoid level of the hypopharynx. The wall thickness of the mass is generally thin and smooth.

Problem

An older man with a fluid- and gas-filled, well-circumscribed mass, inseparable from the pharynx and apparently involving the retropharyngeal space

Anatomy

A. Retropharyngeal space: visceral fascia, prevertebral fascia, contents (see Fig. 89E)
B. Hypopharynx: limits, subdivisions (pyriform sinus, posterior pharyngeal wall, postcricoid region), middle and inferior constrictor muscles
C. Cervical esophagus: esophageal verge (inlet); esophageal mucosa and position (normal variants) of each
D. Tracheoesophageal groove: nodal groups, recurrent laryngeal nerve, inferior thyroid artery

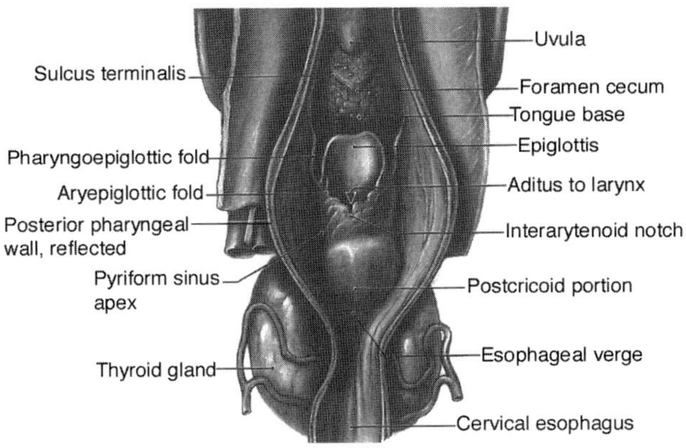

Figure 95E

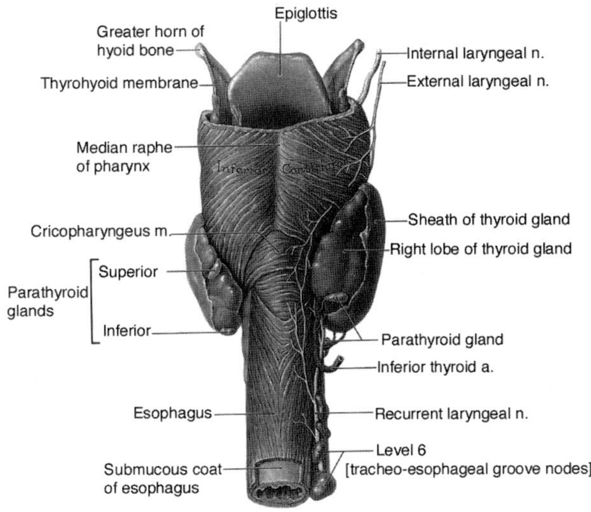

Figure 95F

Differential Diagnosis

Zenker's diverticulum; communicating esophageal duplication or neuroenteric cyst (doubtful); retropharyngeal abscess

Diagnosis

Large Zenker's diverticulum

Diagnostic Imaging Approach

A. Identify the space, structure (organ), or both of origin.
B. Does the morphology (i.e., aggressive margins) or associated findings (e.g., adenopathy) suggest a neoplastic origin?
C. Is there an inflammatory morphology?
D. Evaluate the full cephalocaudal extent of the lesion.
E. Consider other morphologic features: density, T1- or T2-weighted signal intensity, enhancement, vascularity, blood products, calcifications.

Clinical Points Of Importance And Supplemental Information

A. Submucosal pharyngeal wall masses should always be imaged before biopsy or definitive management.
B. The diagnosis of Zenker's diverticulum is usually easily confirmed on a barium swallow examination.
C. MRI is preferred over CT for evaluating lesions within the muscular wall of the postcricoid hypopharynx and esophagus; MRI is usually performed as an adjunct to CT in cases where the gross inferior extent of the cancer of the hypopharynx must be determined precisely and CT is not considered definitive in this regard.

Answers To Questions

1. Visceral and retropharyngeal
2. Zenker's diverticulum
3. MRI

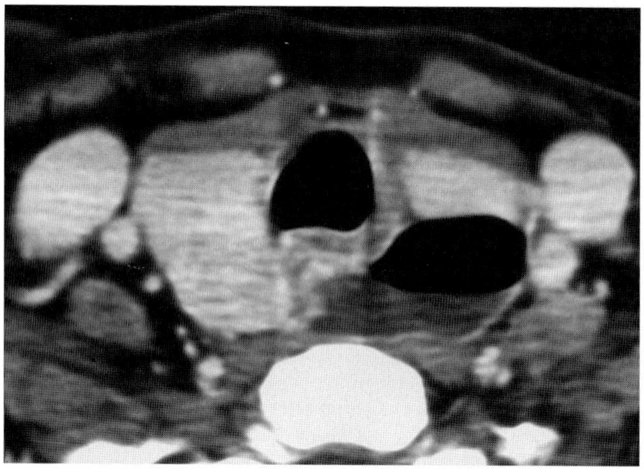

Figure 95G. Patient 1 with Zenker's diverticulum, showing a cystic mass with an air–fluid level centered in left posterolateral aspect of the cervical esophagus. Contrast-enhanced computed tomography image.

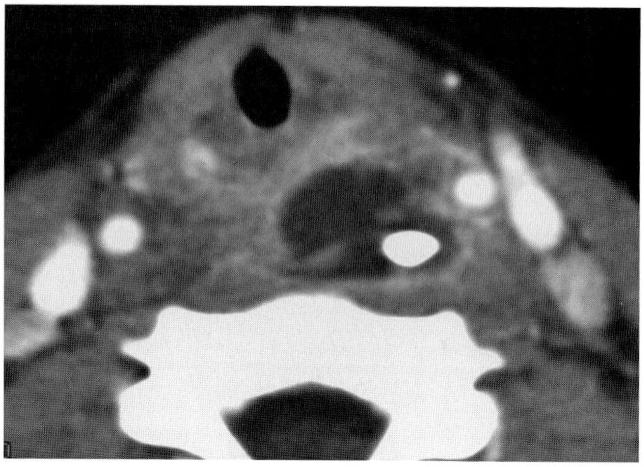

Figure 95H. Patient 2 with a retropharyngeal abscess caused by trauma, showing a loculated cystic mass involving the retropharyngeal space that contains a radiodense foreign body (chicken bone). An inflammatory change is noted in the surrounding soft tissue. Contrast-enhanced computed tomography image.

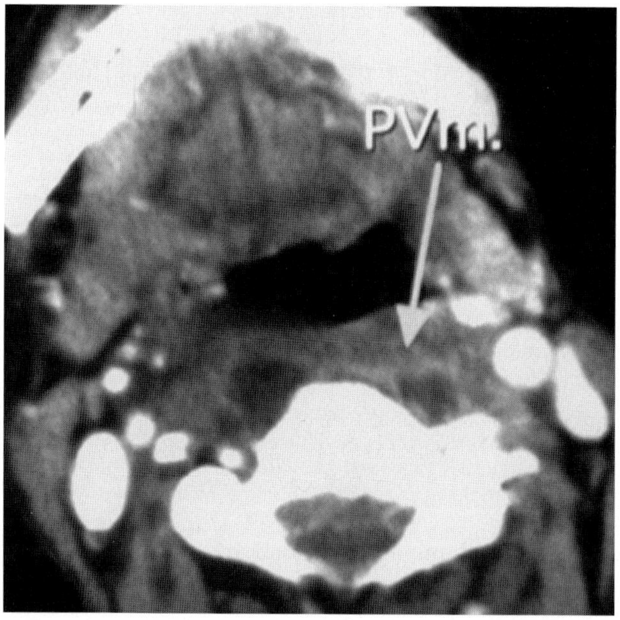

Figure 95I. Patient 3 with abscess in the prevertebral space, showing an abscess formation deep to the prevertebral muscle (PV m.) and epidural abscess within the spinal canal displacing the thecal sac posteriorly. Contrast-enhanced computed tomography image.

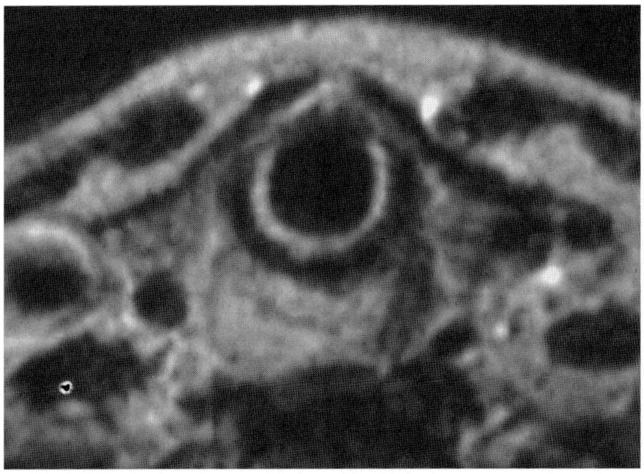

Figure 95J. Patient 4 with dysphagia caused by an entirely submucosal carcinoma of the cervical esophagus. Two endoscopic biopsies were negative for tumor, and a computed tomography-directed percutaneous biopsy was eventually needed for diagnosis. T2-weighted axial image at the level of the esophageal verge showing an infiltrative mass involving the cervical esophagus replacing all but a small rim of the muscular esophageal wall.

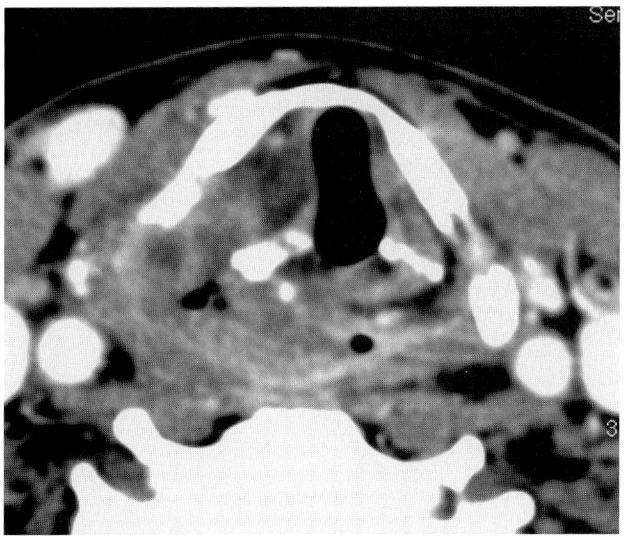

Figure 95K. Patient 5 with pyriform sinus carcinoma. Contrast-enhanced computed tomography image showing the tumor grossly involving the apex of pyriform sinus and posterior pharyngeal wall. The tumor extends into the paraglottic space through the thyroarytenoid gap (anteriorly) and extralaryngeal soft tissue of the neck along the attachment of inferior pharyngeal constrictor muscle (laterally), with destruction at the posterior edge of the lamina of thyroid cartilage.

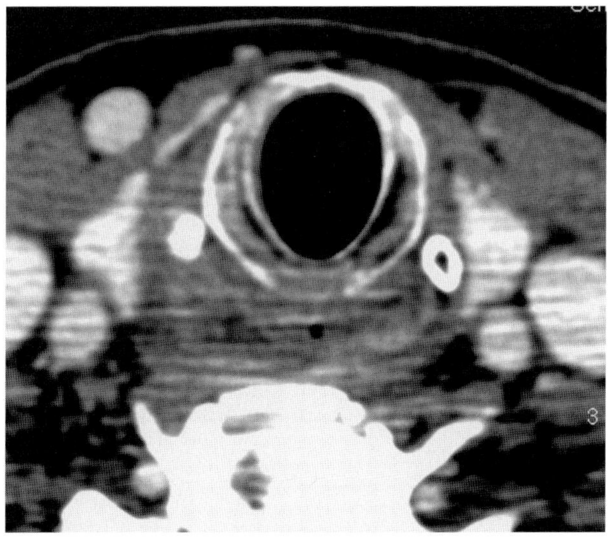

Figure 95L. Patient 5 with pyriform sinus carcinoma. Contrast-enhanced computed tomography image inferior to Fig. 95K showing the inferior extent of the tumor involving the postcricoid portion of hypopharynx to the esophageal verge.

CASE 96

Clinical History: A 57-year-old man presents with a slightly tender upper neck mass.

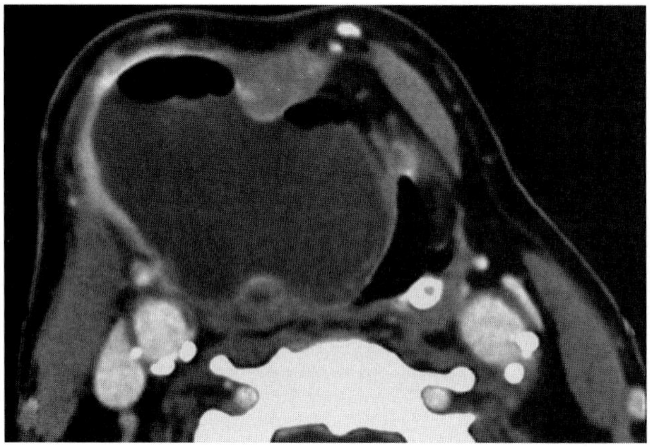

Figure 96A

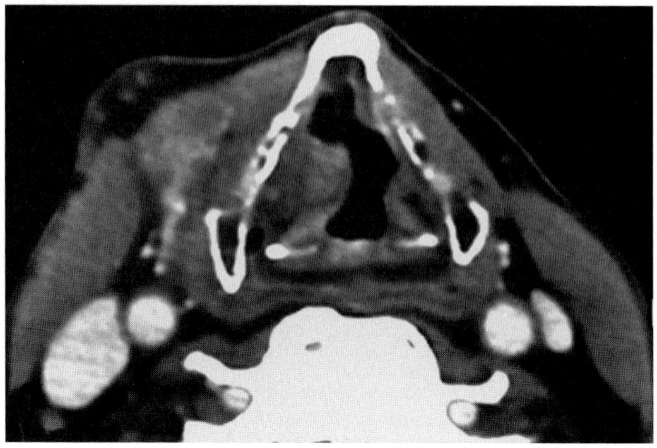

Figure 96B

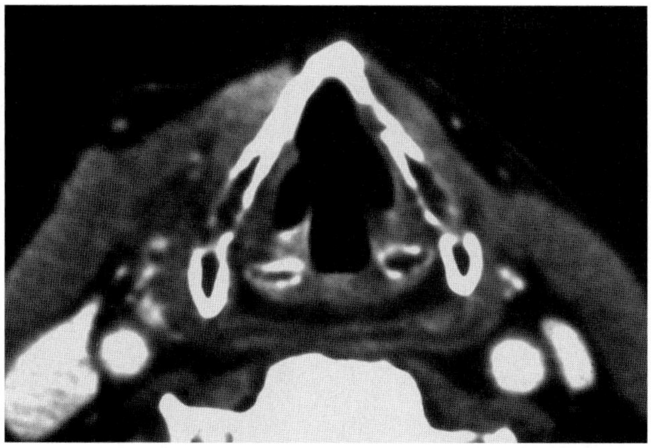

Figure 96C

1. What is the compartment of origin?
2. Give one specific diagnosis.
3. What is the prime responsibility of the radiologist after correctly diagnosing this condition?

Findings

A large cystic mass with an air–fluid level in the right paraglottic space, with extralaryngeal extension via the thyrohyoid membrane, and presenting in the anterior triangle region. Computed tomography (CT) image at level of the false vocal cord shows a possible small soft tissue lesion in the right paraglottic space just above the laryngeal ventricles; those ventricles are seen on the lowest section.

Problem

A middle-aged man with a cystic appearing, tender anterior triangle neck mass arising from the visceral compartment (larynx)

Anatomy

A. Compartments of the neck (see Fig. 89E)
   1. Visceral: within the middle (visceral) layer of deep cervical fascia—larynx, pharynx, thyroid, parathyroids, esophagus, infrahyoid strap muscles
   2. Lateral: paired within the investing (superficial) layer of deep cervical fascia
   3. Posterior: within the prevertebral (deep) layer of deep cervical fascia
B. Supraglottic larynx: laryngeal ventricle, false vocal cord, paraglottic space, thyrohyoid membrane
C. Laryngeal saccule: normal variants

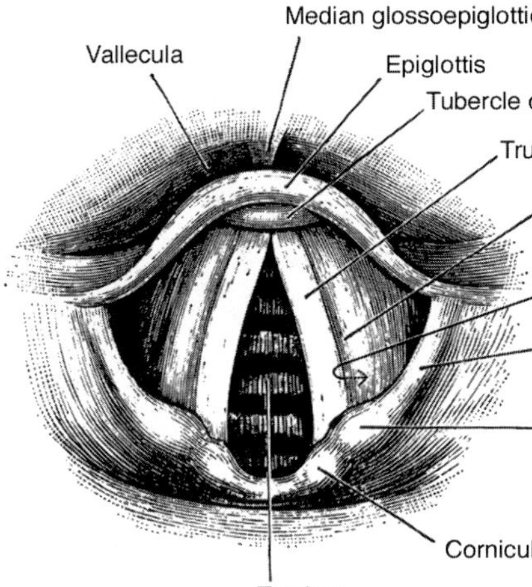

Figure 96D

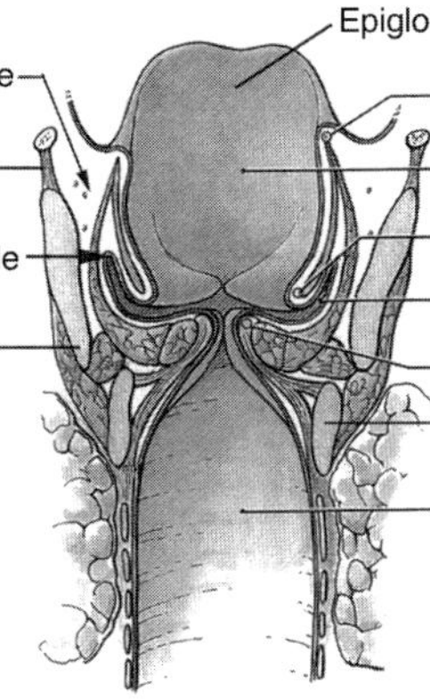

Figure 96E

Differential Diagnosis

None

Diagnosis

Laryngopyocele, possibly, with a small obstructing mass lesion at the false vocal cord or ventricle level

Diagnostic Imaging Approach

A. Establish the compartment of origin.
B. Determine the specific organ or structure of origin.
C. What is the precise cephalocaudal extent?
D. Is there aggressive morphology?
E. Is there inflammatory morphology?
F. This lesion is predominantly cystic and arises from within the laryngeal saccule; is an obstructing mass lesion the cause? If so, any morphologic features of this mass seen that aid in the diagnosis?
G. Are there associated abnormalities (e.g., nodal metastases) that help in the differential diagnosis?

Clinical Points Of Importance And Supplemental Information

A. About one half of all *entirely submucosal* laryngeal masses are caused by a laryngocele or laryngopyocele. Most will not have an obstructing mass as a cause; however, the radiologist must carefully scrutinize the image for such a lesion, which might also be submucosal.
B. The otolaryngologist will also look for an obstructing mass at the time of drainage and marsupialization of the laryngo(pyo)cele.

Answers To Questions

1. Visceral
2. Laryngopyocele with a possible obstructing mass
3. Exclude an obstructing mass at the laryngeal ventricle opening of the saccule

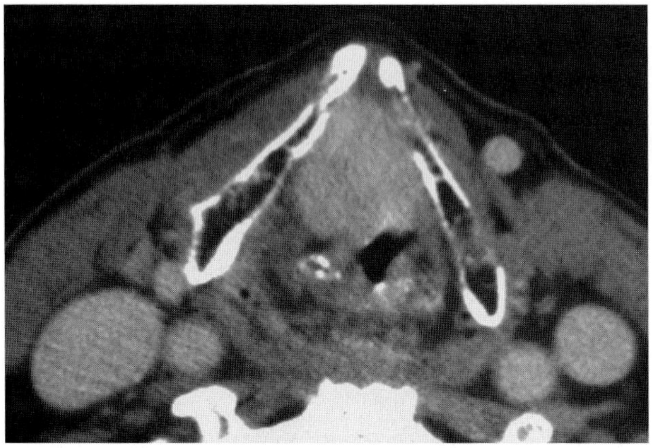

Figure 96F. Patient 1 with a laryngeal sarcoma, showing a mass involving the lower preepiglottic and paraglottic spaces, more on the right. Contrast-enhanced computed tomography image.

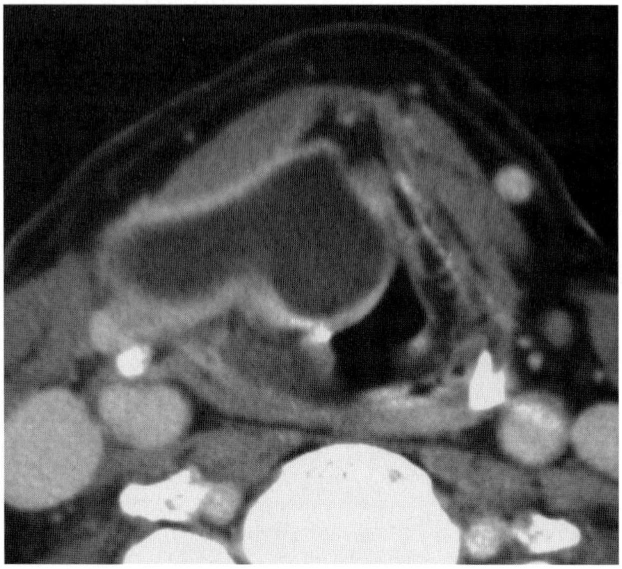

Figure 96G. Patient 1 with laryngeal sarcoma. Contrast-enhanced computed tomography image superior to Fig. 96F showing mixed type laryngocele on the right caused by obstruction of the laryngeal ventricle from sarcoma. Enhancement of the wall suggests superinfection (laryngopyocele).

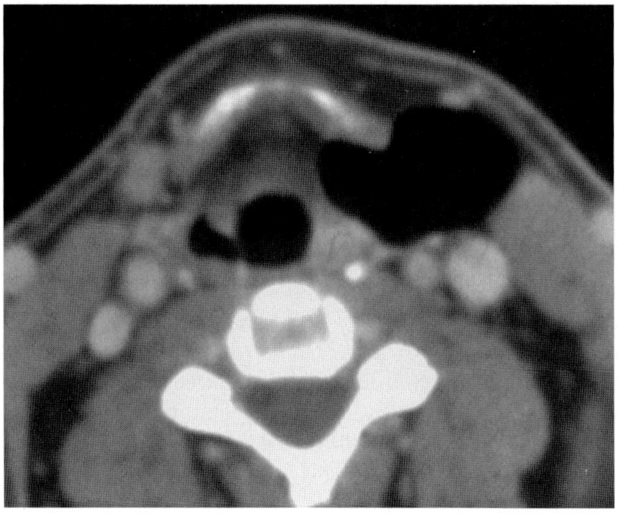

Figure 96H. Patient 2 with mixed type laryngocele, showing an air-filled cystic mass in the paralaryngeal space on the left, with extension into the lateral compartment of the neck via thyrohyoid membrane. Computed tomography image with contrast.

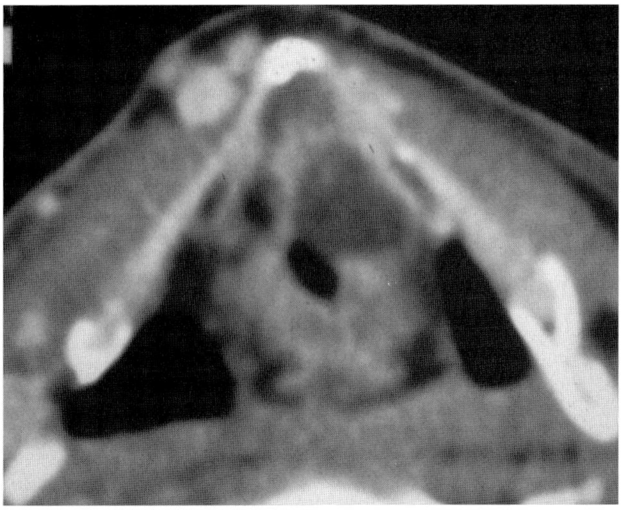

Figure 96I. Patient 3 with internal laryngocele, showing a cystic mass centered in the anterior portion of paraglottic space on the left. Contrast-enhanced computed tomography image.

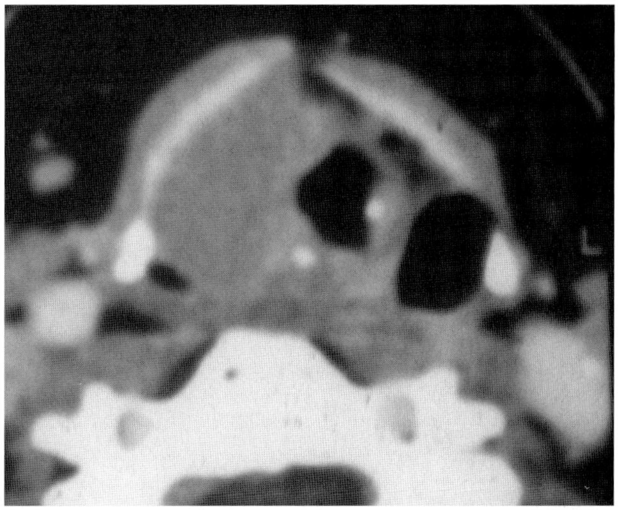

Figure 96J. Patient 4 with entirely submucosal, transglottic laryngeal carcinoma clinically mimicking laryngocele, showing an infiltrative mass involving the paraglottic space on the right. Contrast-enhanced computed tomography image.

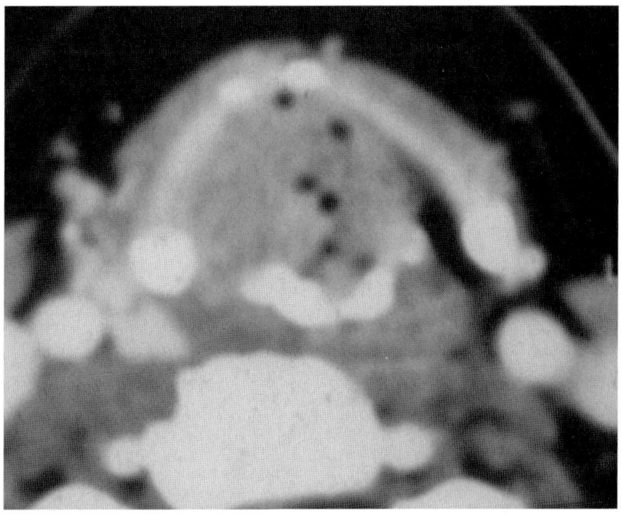

Figure 96K. Patient 4 with entirely submucosal, transglottic laryngeal carcinoma. Contrast-enhanced computed tomography image inferior to Fig. 96J showing an infiltrating mass involving the paraglottic space at the level of the true vocal cord.

CASE 97

Clinical History: A 42-year-old man who had suffered trauma to the neck in a car accident presents 3 months after the accident because he is still hoarse and is aspirating.

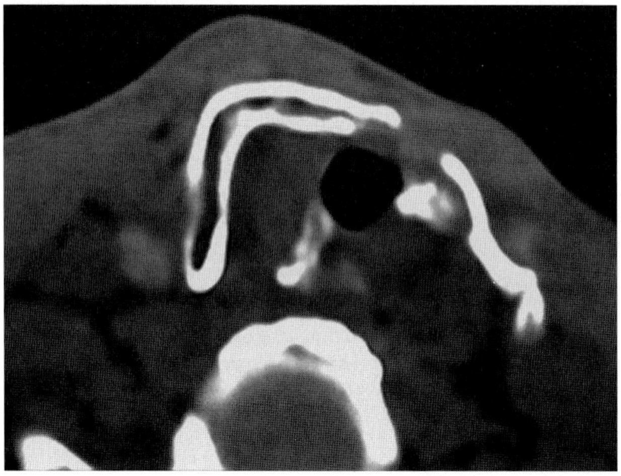

Figure 97A

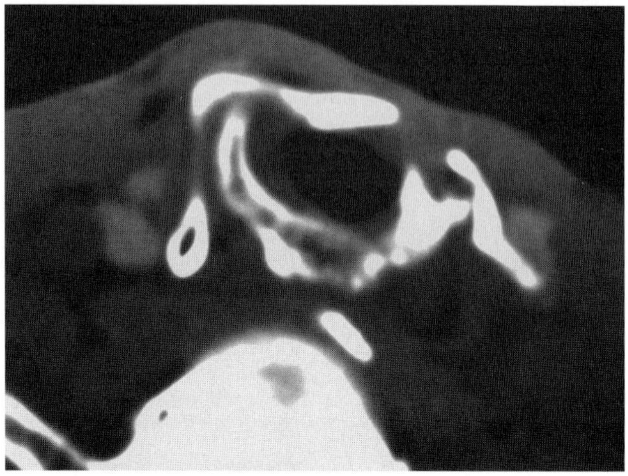

Figure 97B

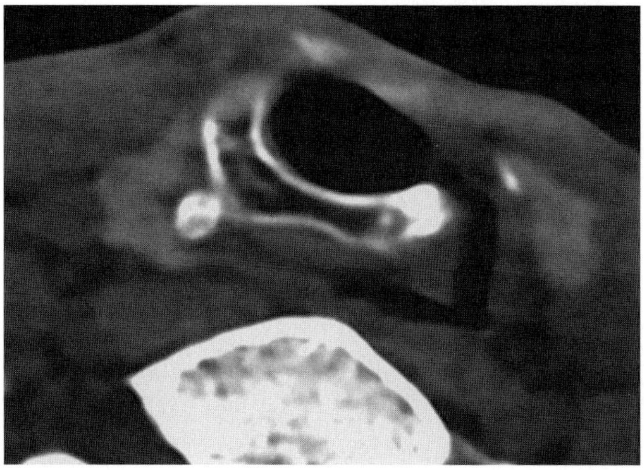

Figure 97C

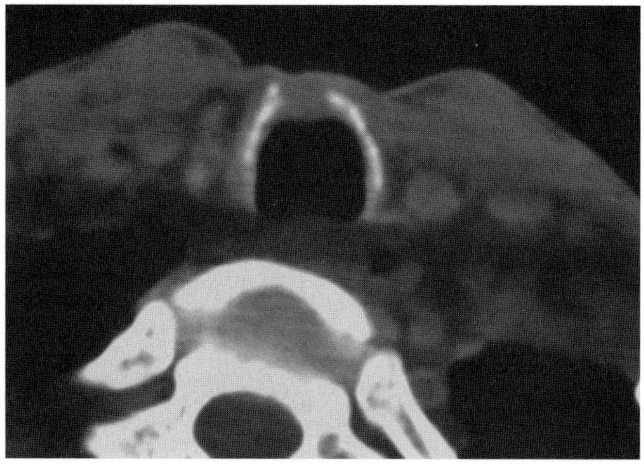

Figure 97D

1. What is the prime indicator of prognosis for return of normal laryngeal function following blunt trauma to the larynx?
2. Why is the patient hoarse?
3. Why is the patient aspirating?

Findings

A fracture-dislocation of the left ala of the thyroid cartilage and arch of the cricoid cartilage in association with an obvious distortion of laryngeal structures. An anterolateral dislocation is noted of the left cricoarytenoid joint, with scarring of the true vocal cords. A fistula is present between the subglottic larynx and the postcricoid region of the hypopharynx, with dislocation of left thyrocricoid joint where the left recurrent laryngeal nerve enters the larynx.

Problem

An adult who has sustained laryngeal trauma has a severely injured larynx based on his persistent symptoms and the computed tomography (CT) study.

Anatomy

A. Laryngeal skeleton: thyroid cartilage, cricoid cartilage, cricothyroid joint, thyrohyoid membrane, cricothyroid membrane, glottis, subglottis
B. Pharynx: postcricoid region and esophageal inlet, inferior constrictor and the "cricopharyngeus" muscle
C. Recurrent laryngeal nerve (see Fig. 95F)

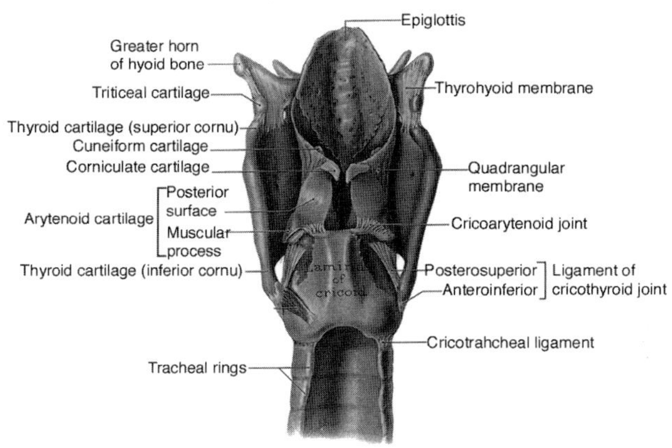

Figure 97E

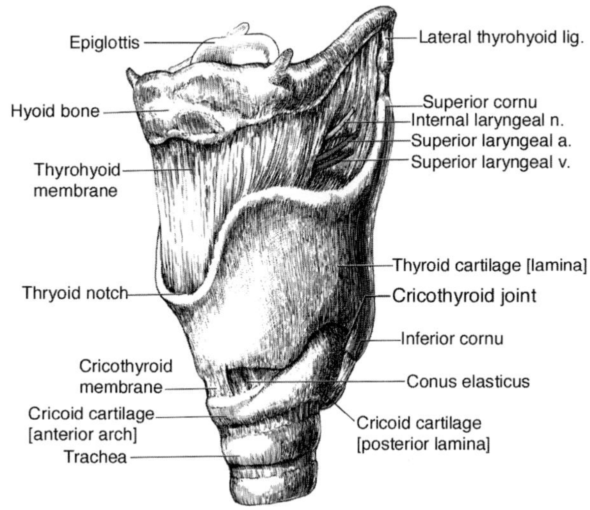

Figure 97F

Differential Diagnosis

Not applicable

Diagnosis

Markedly displaced fractures of the thyroid and cricoid cartilages; lateralization of the arytenoid, probably caused by fibrosis; and a fistula from the subglottis to the low postcricoid or esophageal verge region.

Diagnostic Imaging Approach

A. Evaluate soft tissues: extraluminal air, mucosal laceration, hematoma, secondary airway narrowing.
B. Try to identify false passages or fistula; however, this is usually not possible.
C. Are there displaced fractures of the thyroid or cricoid cartilages or hyoid bone?
D. Any evidence of cricoarytenoid dislocation or epiglottic avulsion?
E. Is there possible cricotracheal separation?

Clinical Points Of Importance And Supplemental Information

A. Laryngeal trauma should be evaluated and repaired within 7 to 10 days of injury. CT should be the primary imaging study.
B. The status of the cricoid cartilage is the most important determinant in predicting the likelihood of return to full laryngeal function (voice, airway maintenance, and swallowing without aspiration).

Answers To Questions

1. Status of the cricoid cartilage
2. Scarring and fixation of the true vocal cord
3. Scarring and fixation of the true vocal cord and fistula from pharynx to larynx

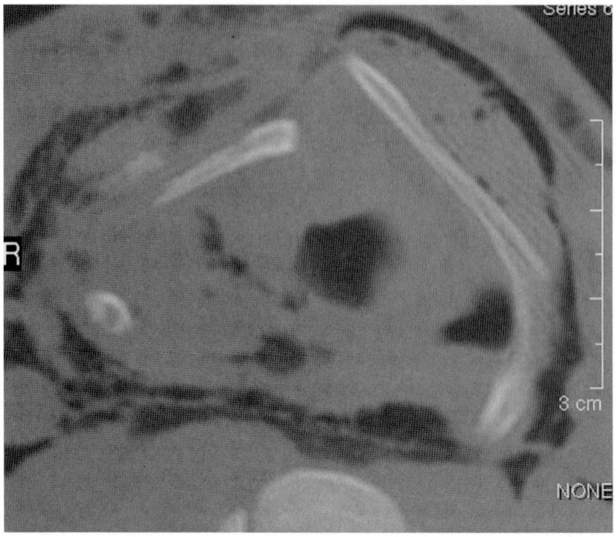

Figure 97G. Patient 1 with laryngeal trauma, showing a comminuted and depressed fracture of the thyroid cartilage and extensive soft tissue emphysema. Computed tomography image at bone window setting.

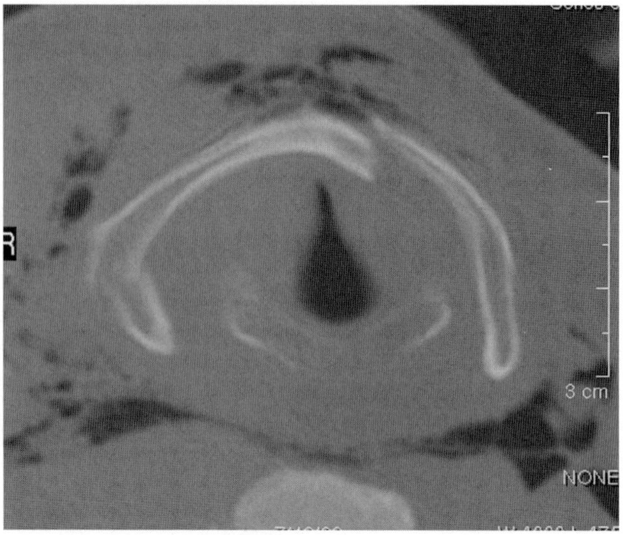

Figure 97H. Patient 1 with laryngeal trauma, showing dislocation of the cricothyroid joint on the right. Computed tomography image inferior to Fig. 97E.

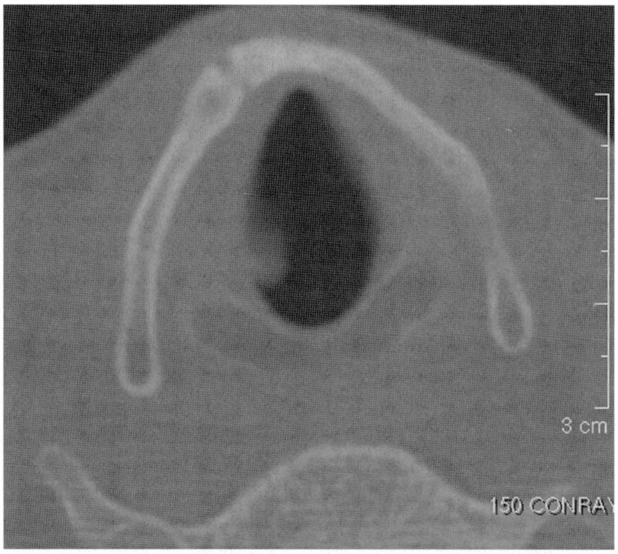

Figure 97I. Patient 2 with sudden onset of the true vocal cord paralysis. (The patient immediately "blew out his voice" when he was yelling loudly.) Image shows a nondisplaced fracture, with callus formation of the thyroid cartilage. Computed tomography image at bone window setting.

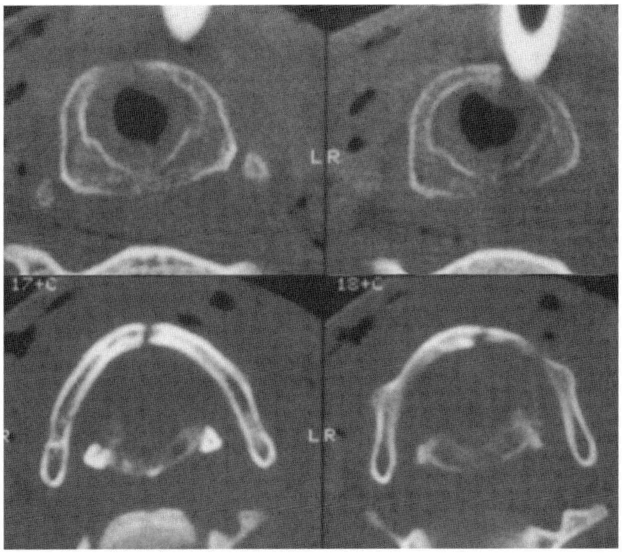

Figure 97J. Patient 3 with laryngeal trauma, showing a fracture involving the junction between the right and left laminae of thyroid cartilage without obvious displacement. Another nondisplaced fracture involves the posterior lamina of the cricoid cartilage and, possibly, left cricoarytenoid joint dislocation. Computed tomography images at bone window setting.

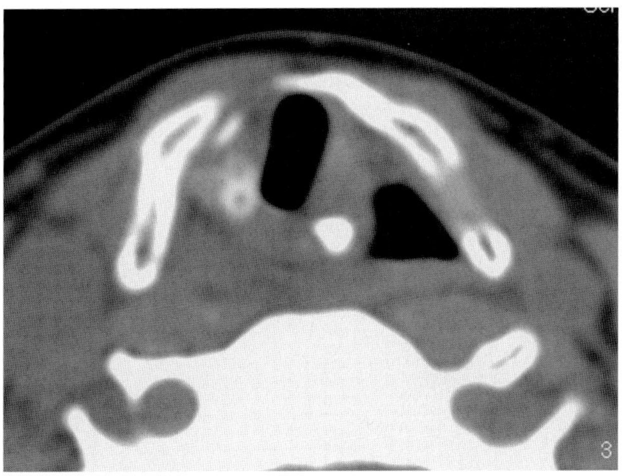

Figure 97K. Patient 4 with an old laryngeal injury, showing an old displaced fracture of the thyroid cartilage distorting the laryngeal skeleton. Computed tomography image without contrast.

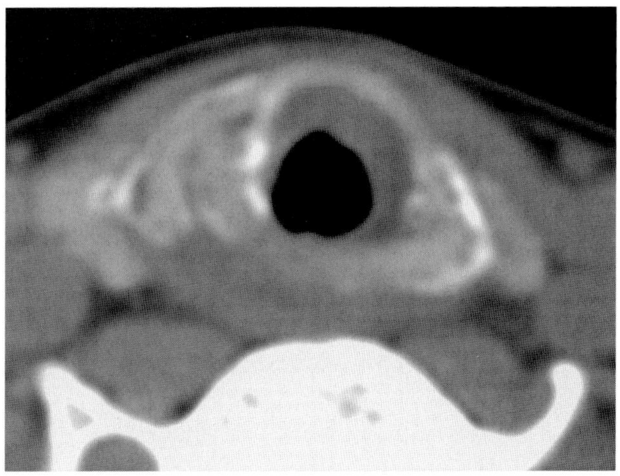

Figure 97L. Patient 4 with an old laryngeal injury, showing posttraumatic subglottic stenosis and a dislocated right cricothyroid joint. Computed tomography image inferior to Fig. 97K.

CHAPTER 11

THYROID

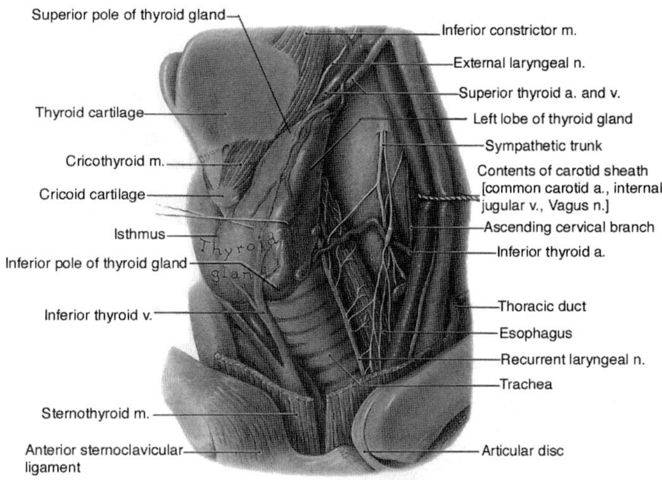

CASE 98

Clinical History: A 60-year-old man presents with an enlarged lower right neck node.

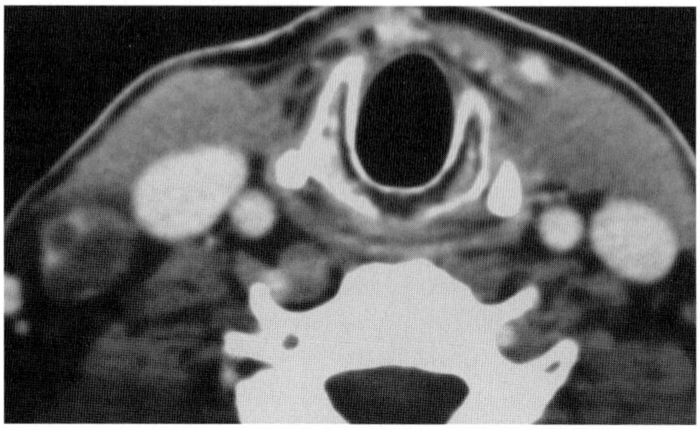

Figure 98A

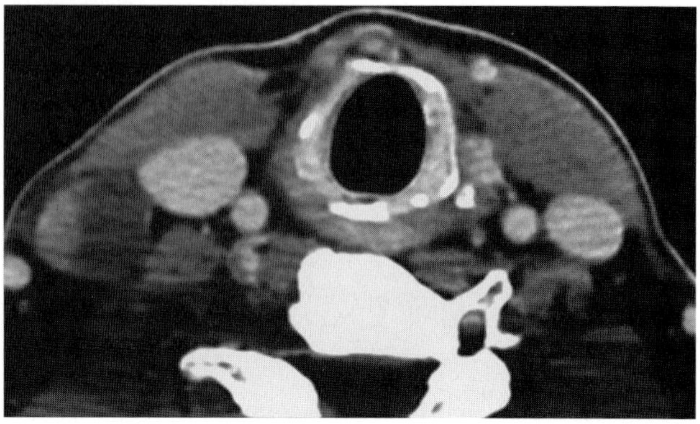

Figure 98B

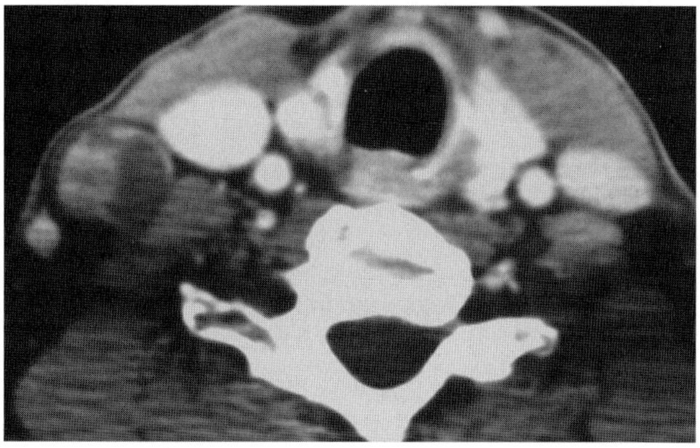

Figure 98C

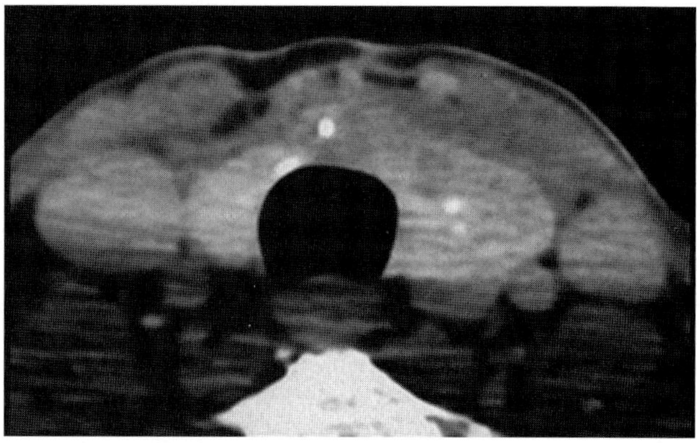

Figure 98D

1. To what nodal group (I-VI) does the enlarged node belong?
2. What head and neck primary sites commonly metastasize to this nodal group?
3. Does the node morphology (enhancing "mural nodule" with a large cyst) help in the differential diagnosis?

Findings

A cystic mass (node) with an enhancing mural nodule posterolateral to the right internal jugular vein at the level of the cricoid cartilage. A lobulated slightly low-attenuation mass involves the isthmus and left lobe of the thyroid gland. Several calcific densities lie scattered in the mass.

Problem

An older man with lower neck adenopathy that appears on computed tomography (CT) to be partially cystic, with an "enhancing nodule" and a thyroid mass

Anatomy

A. Thyroid gland: upper and lower poles, isthmus, pyramidal lobes, incidence of "incidental" nodules
B. Trachea: normal size, shape, muscular wall, how to count rings
C. Tracheoesophageal groove: nodes, recurrent laryngeal nerve, inferior thyroid artery or vein
D. Group IV nodes

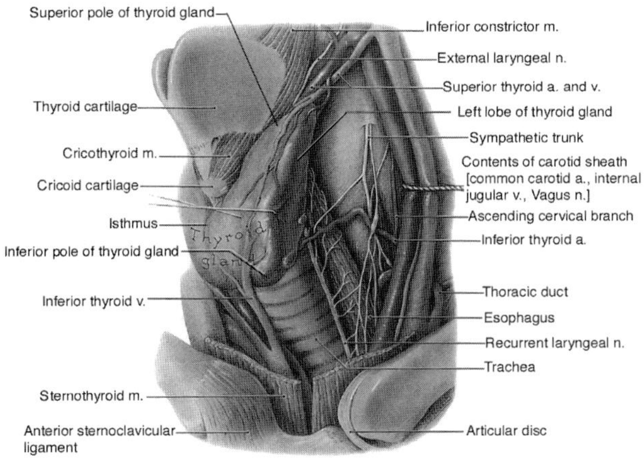

Figure 98E

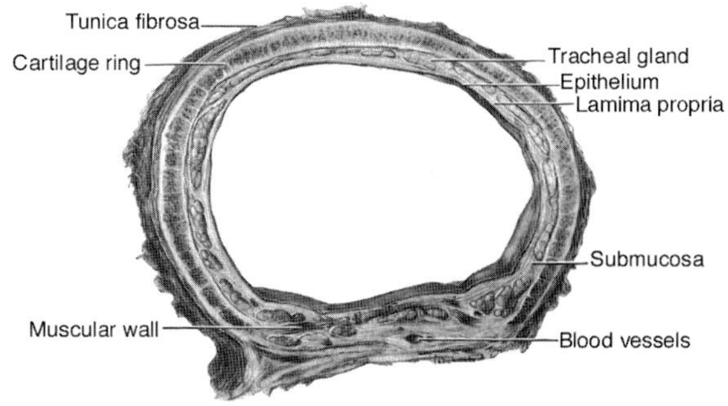

Figure 98F

Differential Diagnosis

Nodal metastasis (thyroid); nodal metastasis (other); lymphoma (doubtful); reactive adenopathy (extremely unlikely)

Diagnosis

Differentiated (probably mainly papillary) carcinoma of the thyroid gland, with a group IV metastasis

Diagnostic Imaging Approach

A. Is the mass nodal or nonnodal?
B. If nodal, does the morphology or location help determine a possible cause?
C. Are other nodes or nodal groups involved?
D. Are there associated findings (e.g., thyroid mass) that might suggest a cause or help with the differential diagnosis?

Clinical Points Of Importance And Supplemental Information

A. When lymph node morphology such as that seen on the CT in this case, suspect cancer in the thyroid gland as a possible primary site.
B. Isolated, neoplastic low neck and supraclavicular adenopathy is more likely to be caused by a thyroid malignancy, lymphoma, or an infraclavicular primary tumor than to a pharyngeal or laryngeal primary tumor.

Answers To Questions

1. IV or V
2. Thyroid, hypopharynx; advanced glottic-subglottic with other sites less common except with group II and III involvement
3. Yes; the thyroid gland is virtually a certain source

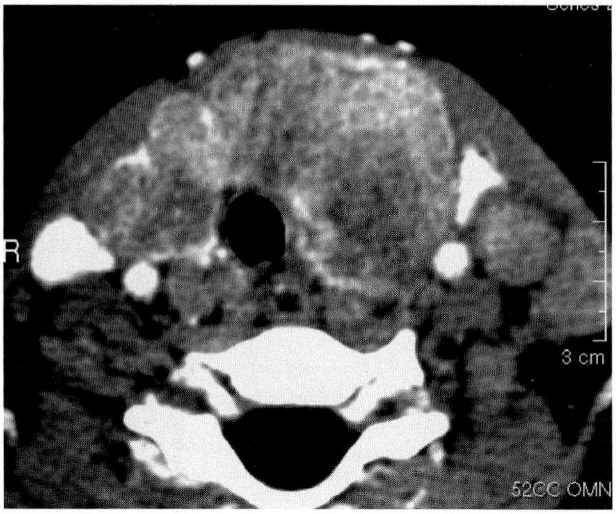

Figure 98G. Patient 1 with papillary carcinoma of the thyroid gland, showing an infiltrative mass diffusely involving the thyroid gland with, lymph node metastases to level IV, V, and VI. Contrast-enhanced computed tomography image.

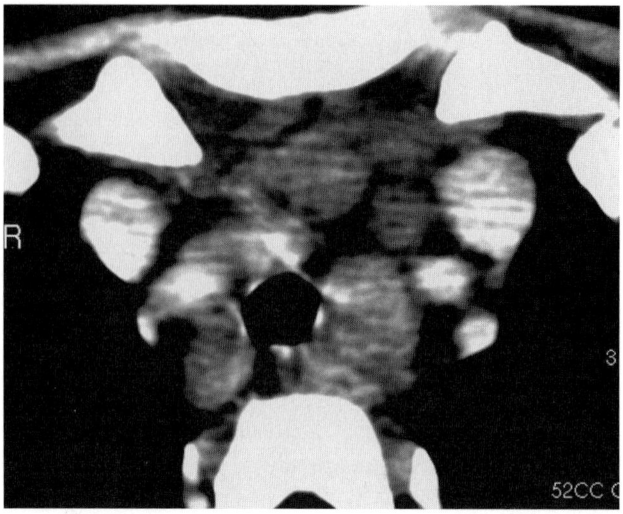

Figure 98H. Patient 1 with papillary carcinoma of the thyroid gland. Contrast-enhanced computed tomography image at the level of the superior mediastinum showing metastases to the paratracheal lymph nodes.

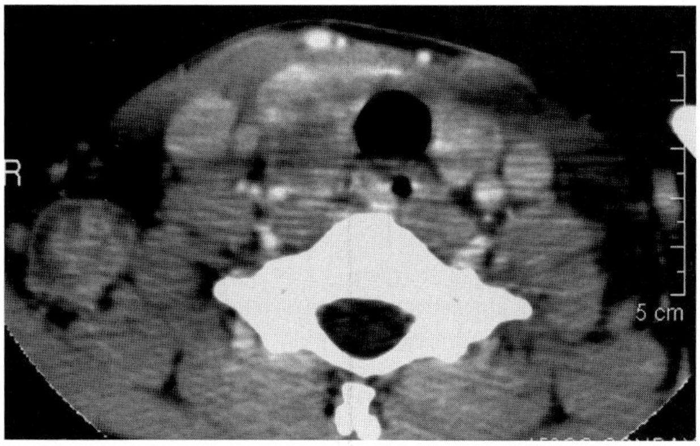

Figure 98I. Patient 2 with papillary carcinoma of the thyroid gland, showing an inhomogeneous mass involving the right lobe of the thyroid gland. An isolated enlarged level V lymph node is seen with enhancing nodules and admixed cystic zones on the right. Contrast-enhanced computed tomography image.

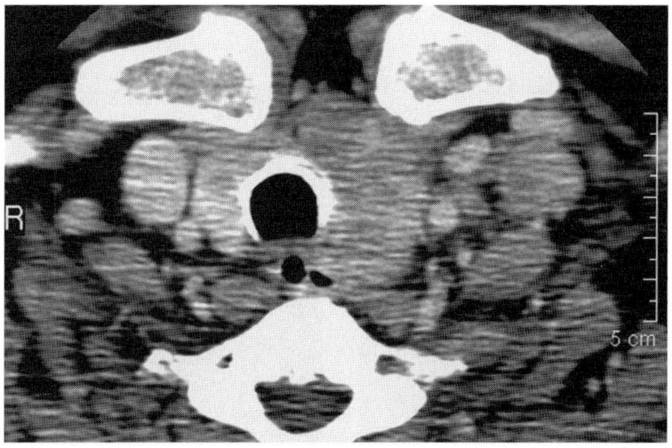

Figure 98J. Patient 3 with papillary carcinoma of the thyroid gland, showing an inhomogeneous mass arising from the left lobe of the thyroid gland, with metastasis to the supraclavicular lymph node on the left. Contrast-enhanced computed tomography image.

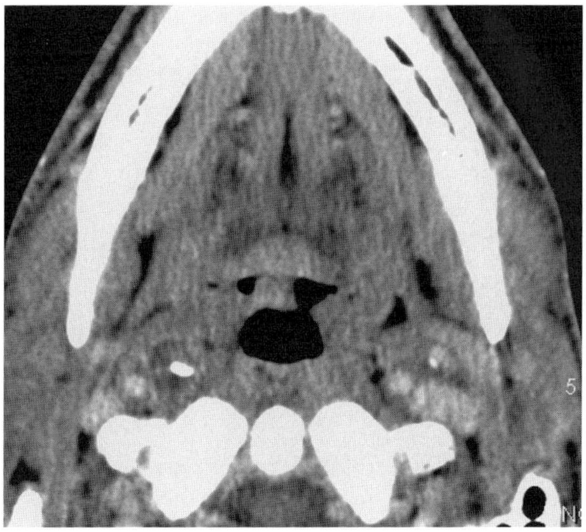

Figure 98K. Patient 4 with papillary carcinoma of the thyroid gland, showing cystic masses with calcification in the expected position of the lateral retropharyngeal lymph node on either side, representing metastases from the thyroid carcinoma. Contrast-enhanced computed tomography image.

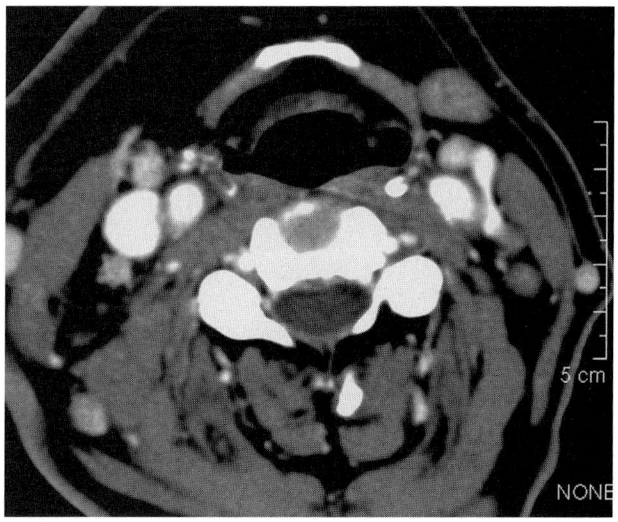

Figure 98L. Patient 5 with papillary carcinoma of the thyroid gland, showing several lymph nodes in the areas of level III and V that have a tendency to enhance more than is usually seen in squamous cell carcinoma. Some of the nodes have an irregular margin, which is suggestive of extracapsular spread. Contrast-enhanced computed tomography image.

CASE 99

Clinical History: A 47-year-old woman presents with a low neck mass.

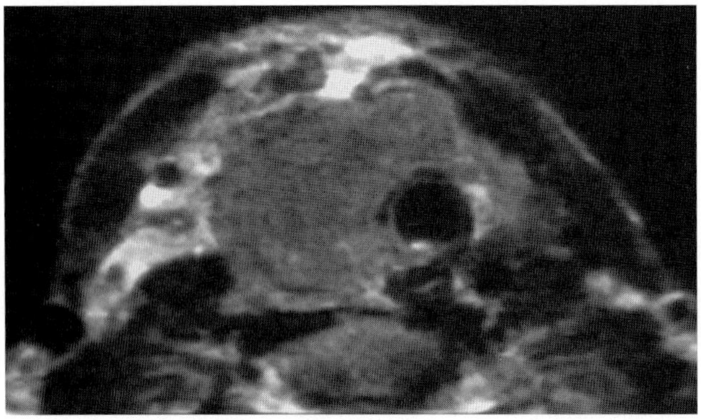

Figure 99A

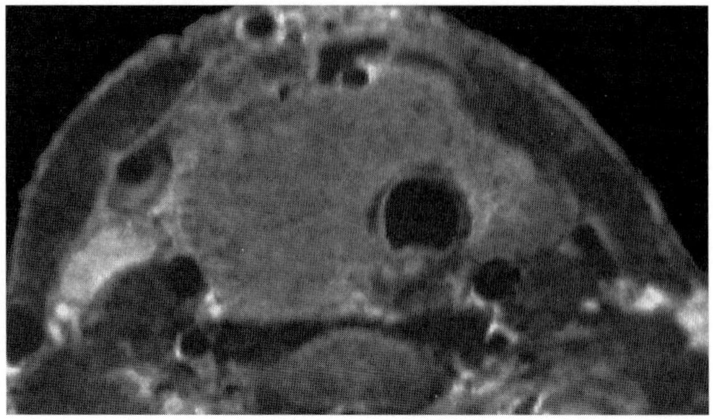

Figure 99B

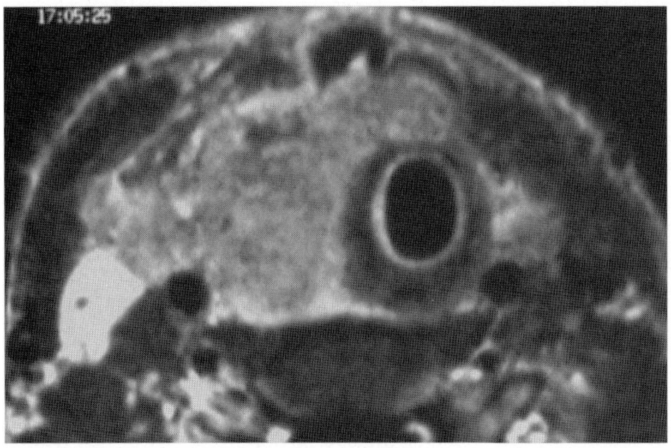

Figure 99C

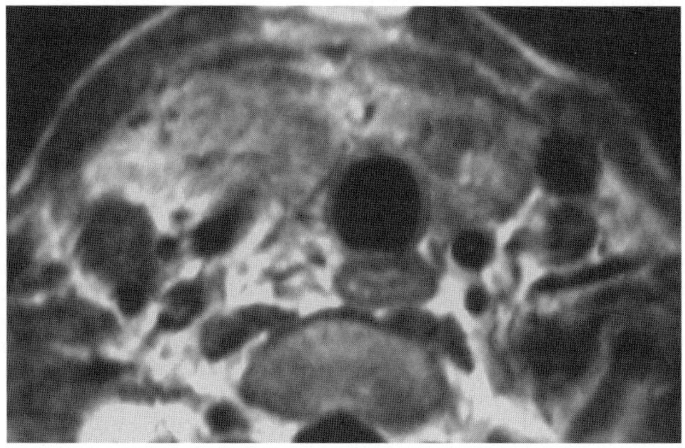

Figure 99D

1. What is the compartment and organ of origin?
2. Are there any signs of aggressive behavior present?
3. What is the diagnosis?

Findings

An intermediate signal intensity bulky mass involving the thyroid gland—mainly of the right lobe and the isthmus. The lesion directly invades both cartilaginous and membranous portions of the trachea and an outer surface of the cervical esophagus (posteriorly) and the infrahyoid strap muscles (anteriorly). Several separate nodular lesions are present around the right internal jugular vein.

Problem

A middle-aged woman with an aggressive thyroid mass

Anatomy

A. Thyroid gland: relationship to trachea, larynx, esophagus
B. Trachea: normal appearance on computed tomography (CT) and magnetic resonance imaging (MRI)
C. Esophagus: normal appearance on CT and MRI
D. Tracheoesophageal groove: nodes, recurrent laryngeal nerve, inferior thyroid artery and vein
E. Cervical nodes: groups IV and V and their relationship to supraclavicular nodes, scalene node; prethyroid, prelaryngeal, and pretracheal nodes

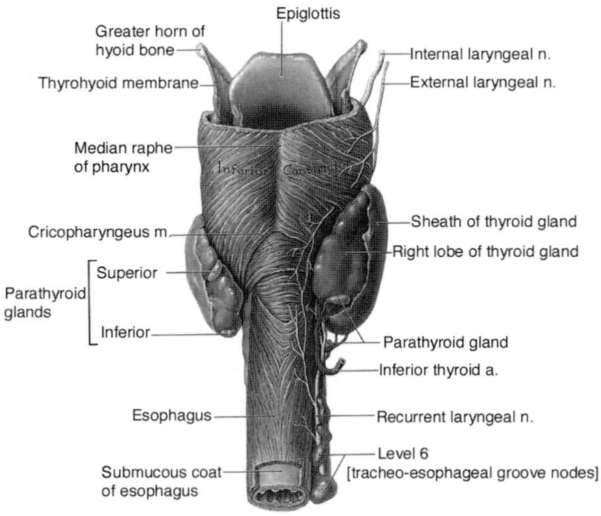

Figure 99E

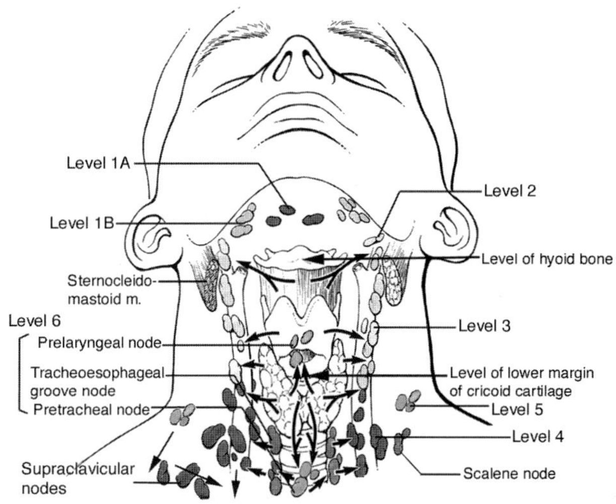

Figure 99F

Differential Diagnosis

Papillary and/or follicular carcinoma, poorly differentiated carcinoma, anaplastic carcinoma (usually in patients >50 years of age), lymphoma; inflammatory disease—unlikely

Diagnosis

Poorly differentiated carcinoma of the thyroid gland, with invasion of the trachea and, at least, adherence to the esophagus with metastatic adenopathy

Diagnostic Imaging Approach

A. Identify compartment and, if possible, specific organ or structure of origin.
B. If a thyroid mass is present:
   1. Diffuse enlargement or focal mass?
   2. Full cephalocaudal extent (upper neck to mediastinum)?
   3. Airway encroachment?
   4. Local signs of aggressive behavior: extension through gland capsule, nodal metastases?
C. If there is an aggressive thyroid mass:
   1. Extent of extraglandular spread: invasion of trachea, esophagus, larynx?
   2. Carotid encasement, jugular or other vascular invasion (rare)?
   3. Spread relative to course of recurrent laryngeal nerve?
   4. Precise accounting of all lymph node groups at risk.
D. Are there associated findings (i.e., if mass is of unknown cause) that might suggest a cause or help with the differential diagnosis?

Clinical Points Of Importance And Supplemental Information

A. MRI (assuming good quality images) is much better than CT for determining tracheal cartilage and esophageal wall invasion.
B. Ultrasound may be a good study to begin the evaluation of a low neck mass because thyroid-related pathology is a frequent cause.

Answers To Questions

1. Visceral
2. Yes; tracheal and esophageal invasion
3. Anaplastic carcinoma or lymphoma

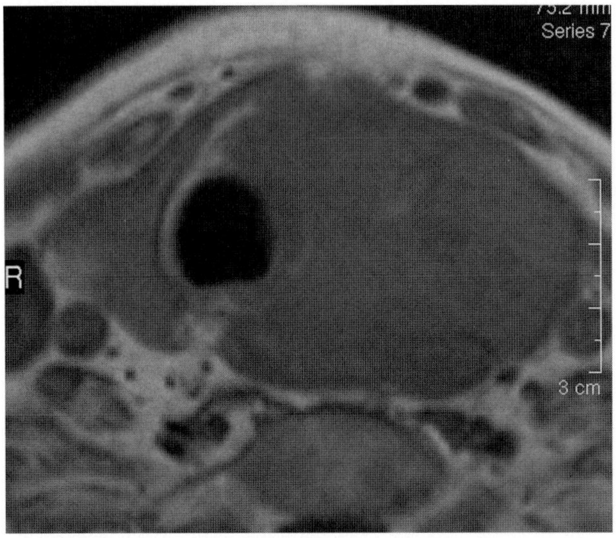

Figure 99G. Patient 1 with medullary carcinoma of the thyroid gland, showing an infiltrative mass centered in the left lobe of the thyroid gland, with extension beyond the capsule and direct invasion to the adjacent cervical esophagus and tracheal wall well manifested by loss of normal layered architecture of the trachea. T1-weighted axial image without contrast.

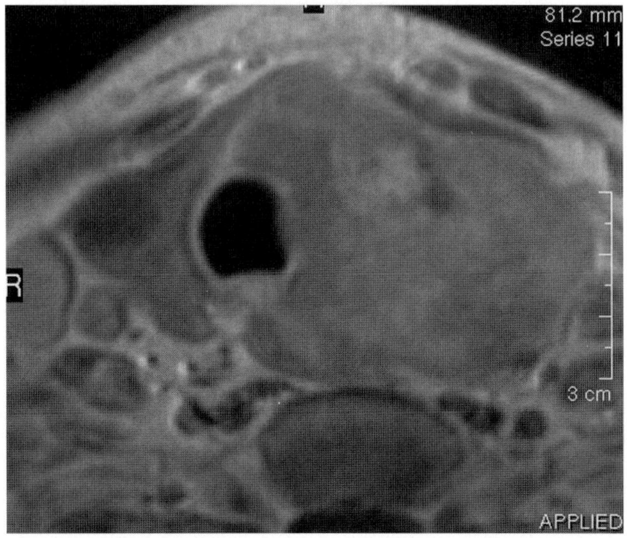

Figure 99H. Patient 1 with medullary carcinoma of the thyroid gland. T1-weighted axial image with contrast showing inhomogeneous enhancement of the mass.

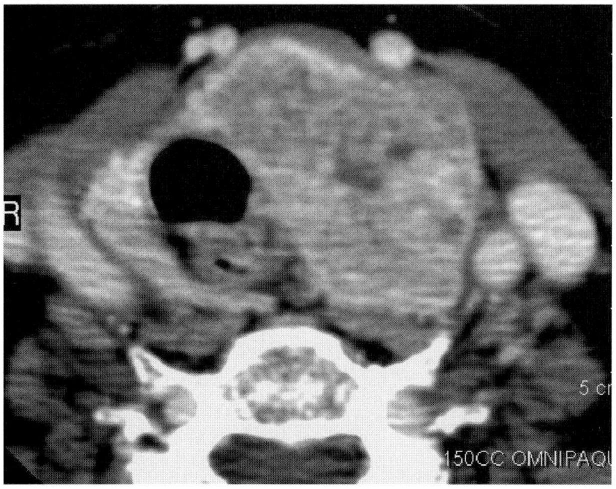

Figure 99I. Patient 2 with anaplastic carcinoma of the thyroid gland, showing an inhomogeneous mass involving the left lobe of the thyroid gland without obvious invasion to the trachea or cervical esophagus seen on this image. Contrast-enhanced computed image.

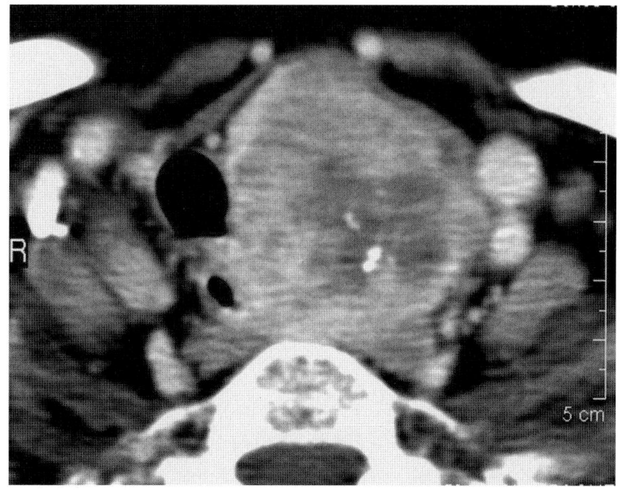

Figure 99J. Patient 2 with anaplastic carcinoma of the thyroid gland, showing possible invasion to the cervical esophagus, prevertebral muscle, and tracheal wall. Contrast computed tomography image inferior to Fig. 99I.

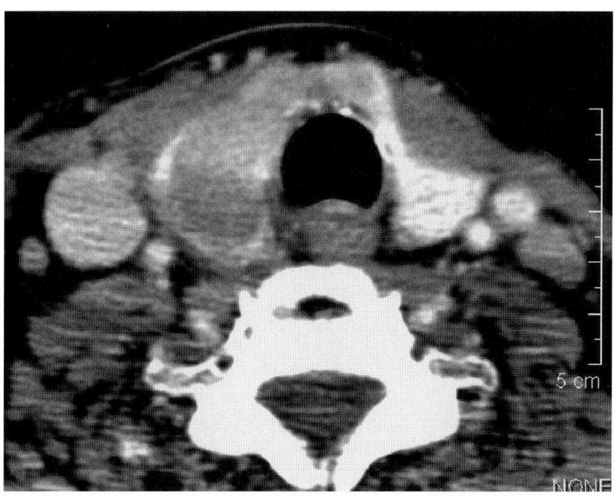

Figure 99K. Patient 3 with Hürthle cell carcinoma of the thyroid gland, showing a low-attenuation mass involving the right lobe and isthmus of the thyroid gland, that is still contained within the capsule of thyroid gland. An enlarged level IV node is seen on the left. Contrast-enhanced computed tomography image.

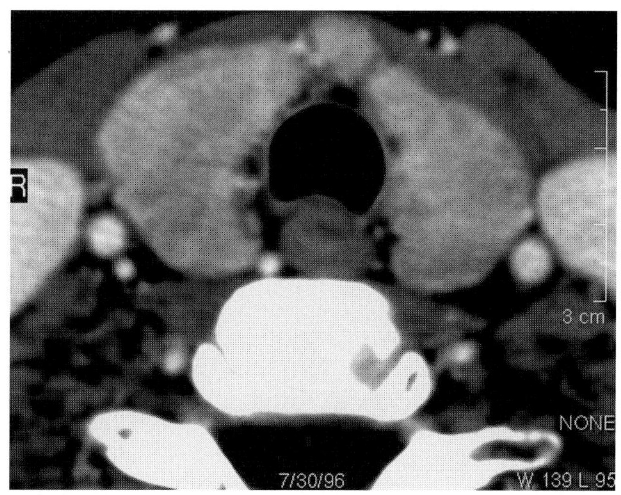

Figure 99L. Patient 4 with primary non-Hodgkin's lymphoma (large cell type) of the thyroid gland, showing a diffusely infiltrative process involving the entire thyroid gland. Such finding can be easily missed. Contrast-enhanced computed tomography image.

CHAPTER 12

PARATHYROID

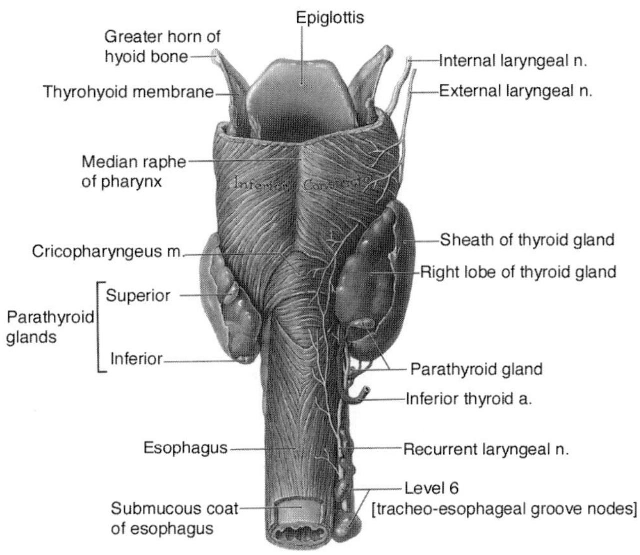

CASE 100

Clinical History: A 45-year-old woman presents with gastrointestinal complaints, depression, and an elevated serum calcium level.

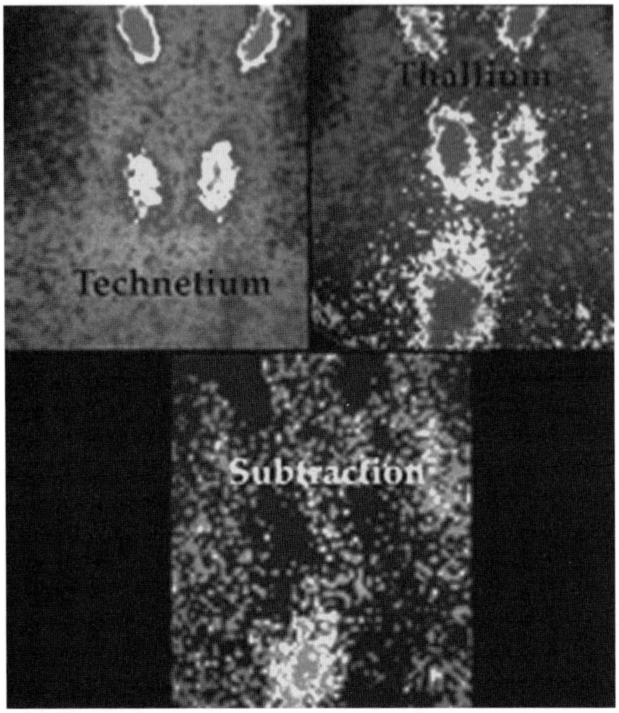

Figure 100A

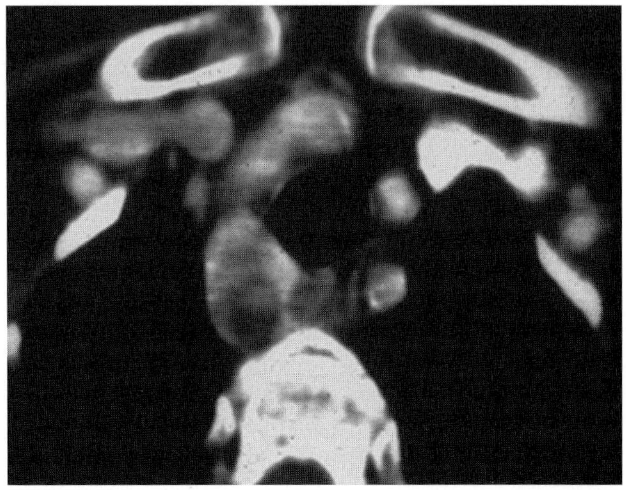

Figure 100B

1. What laboratory test *must* be done before the imaging studies shown here?
2. What is the complete diagnosis?
3. How might these findings limit the cost of patient management? Give two reasons, one general and one specifically related to this case.

Findings

An abnormal soft tissue nodule in the superior tracheoesophageal groove of the superior mediastinum is seen on computed tomography (CT) image. Dual scintigraphic scans were performed with ^{99m}Tc and ^{201}Tl. Subtraction image shows increased tracer activity in the expected area of the right superior mediastinum, which confirms ectopic parathyroid adenoma.

Problem

A middle-aged woman with hyperparathyroidism (parathyroid hormone level was also elevated, but this information was withheld)

Anatomy

A. Thyroid gland
B. Parathyroid glands: normal variation in position (e.g., from carotid bifurcation to mediastinum), the most common location of ectopic parathyroid tissue
C. Thoracic inlet: brachiocephalic vessels (arteries and veins) and their relationship to the scalene muscles and brachial plexus; tracheoesophageal groove (size of normal tracheoesophageal groove nodes)

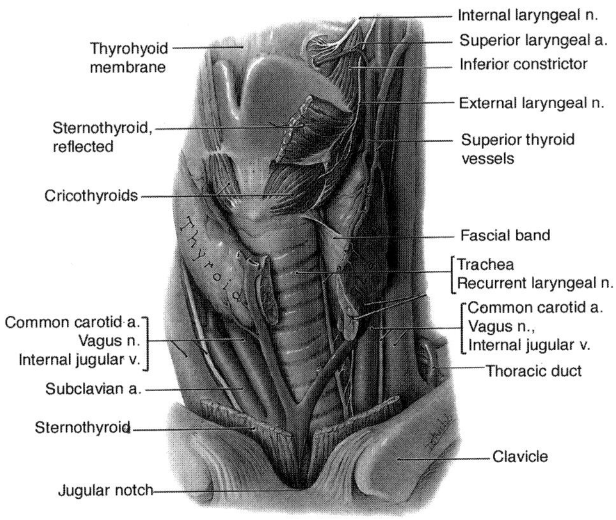

Figure 100C

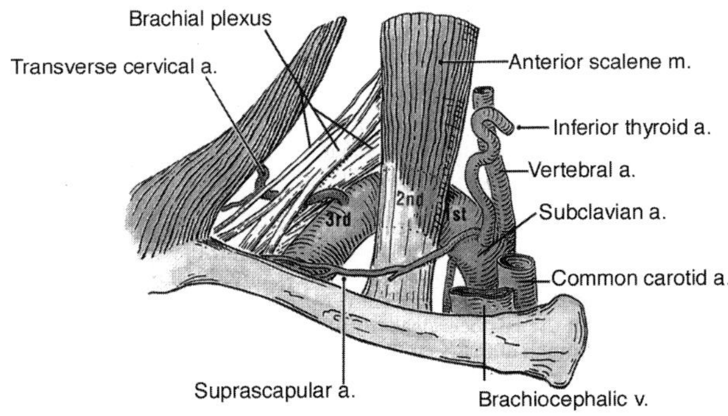

Figure 100D

Differential Diagnosis

Not applicable

Diagnosis

Ectopic parathyroid adenoma localized in the superior mediastinum

Diagnostic Imaging Approach

A. Elevated parathormone levels must be confirmed.
B. Determine if this is initial evaluation or being done for recurrent primary hyperparathyroidism following previous parathyroid surgery.
C. Be sure that the diagnostic study, usually ultrasound, radionuclide, or magnetic resonance imaging, covers all ectopic sites (within the study's capability)—from the carotid bifurcation to the tracheal bifurcation.
D. Identify potential adenomatous or hyperplastic glands and differentiate from other findings (e.g., tracheoesophageal groove nodes, thyroid nodules).
E. If this is recurrent disease, confirm the abnormality on two studies.

Clinical Points Of Importance And Supplemental Information

A. Many clinicians do not desire parathyroid localization in previously untreated patients. Virtually all will workup the patient with recurrent disease before a second surgical procedure.
B. Potential cost saving exists in finding ectopic lesions. Also, a surgeon who will limit exploration to one side of the neck, based on a localization study in a previously untreated patient, potentially saves some cost.

Answers To Questions

1. Parathormone level
2. Ectopic (mediastinal) parathyroid adenoma
3. Limit operative time if only one side is explored. Finding the ectopic adenoma saves prescription failure.

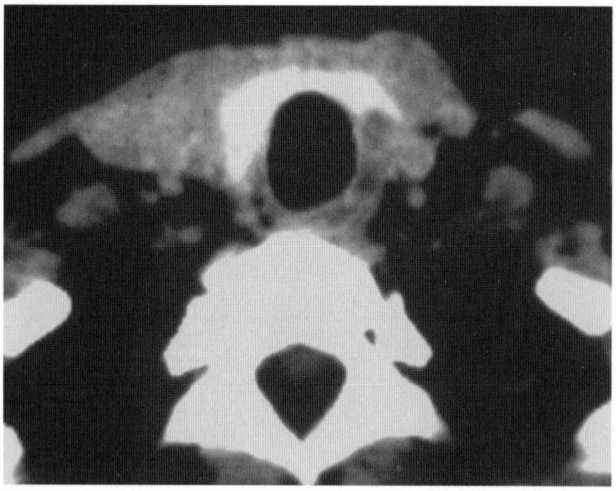

Figure 100E. Patient 1 with a surgically proved intrathyroid parathyroid adenoma, showing a low-attenuation nodule in the inferior pole of the left lobe of the thyroid gland. Computed tomography image without contrast.

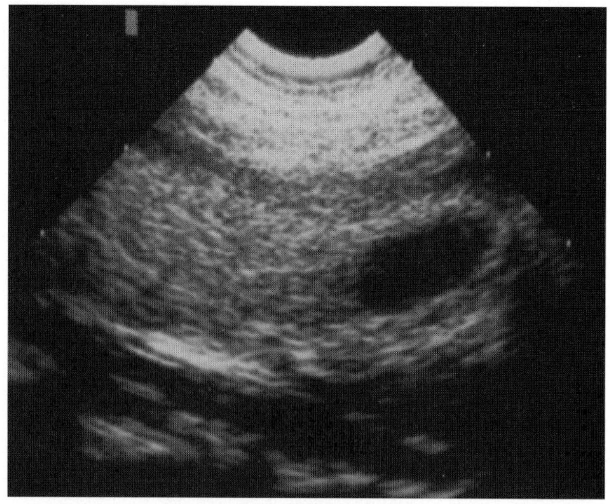

Figure 100F. Patient 1 with a surgically proved intrathyroid parathyroid adenoma. Ultrasonographic image along the long axis of the left lobe of thyroid gland showing a hypoechoic nodule in the inferior pole.

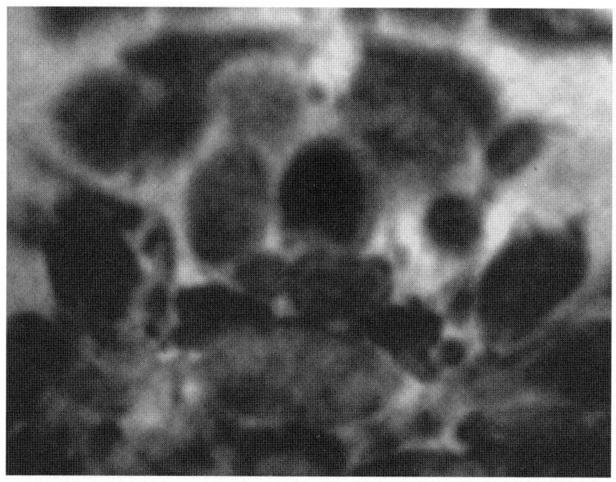

Figure 100G. Patient 2 with parathyroid hyperplasia, showing two well-circumscribed nodular lesions lateral to the trachea and in the tracheoesophageal groove on the right. T1-weighted axial image without contrast.

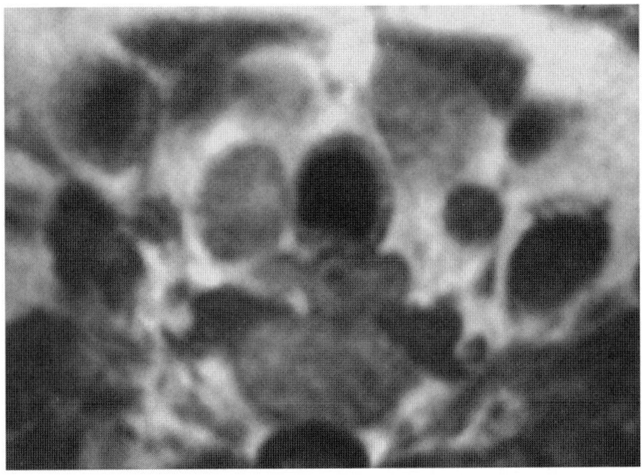

Figure 100H. Patient 2 with parathyroid hyperplasia. T1-weighted axial image with contrast showing enhancement of the nodular lesions.

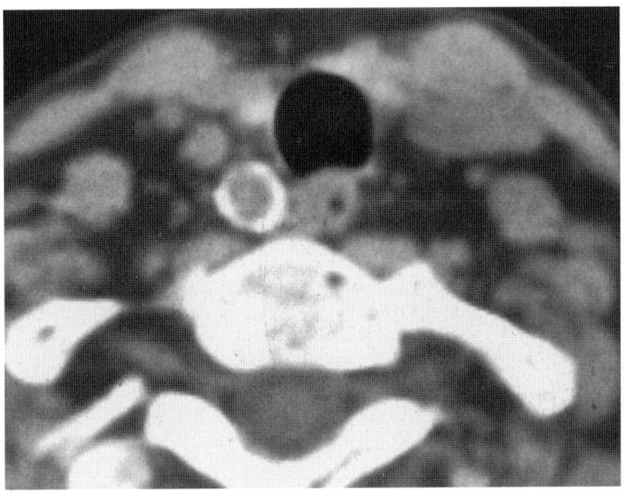

Figure 100I. Patient 3 with "calcified" parathyroid adenoma, showing a nodule with rim-calcification inferoposterior to the inferior pole of right lobe of the thyroid gland. Computed tomography image without contrast.

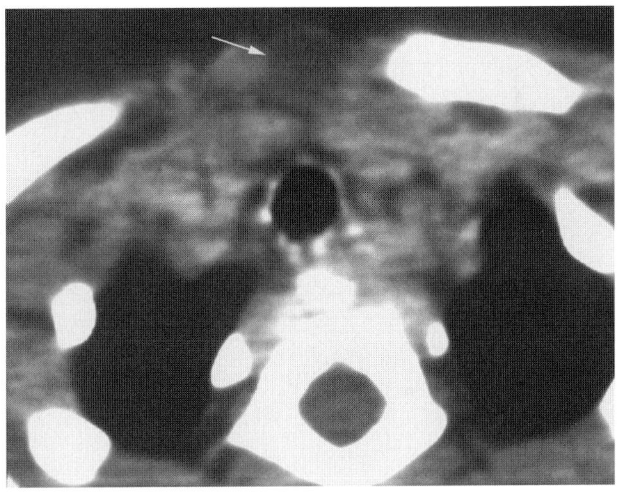

Figure 100J. Patient 4 with epidermoid in the anterior low neck, showing a unilocular cystic mass in the suprasternal notch. Differential diagnosis includes epidermoid vs. thymobranchial cyst. Computed tomography image without contrast.

SUBJECT INDEX

G

H

I

J

R

S

T

V

W

Z